CLINICAL COMPANION TO

Lewis's Medical-Surgical Nursing

12TH EDITION

ASSESSMENT AND MANAGEMENT OF CLINICAL PROBLEMS

Prepared by

Debra Hagler, PhD, RN, ACNS-BC, CNE, CHSE, ANEF, FAAN
Clinical Professor
Edson College of Nursing and Health Innovation
Arizona State University
Phoenix, Arizona

Mariann M. Harding, PhD, RN, CNE, FAADN
Professor of Nursing, Kent State University Tuscarawas,
New Philadelphia, Ohio

Jeffrey Kwong, DNP, MPH, RN, ANP-BC, FAANP, FAAN
Professor, Division of Advanced Nursing Practice, School of Nursing,
Rutgers University, Newark, New Jersey

Courtney Reinisch, DNP, RN, FNP-BC
Associate Professor, School of Nursing, Montclair State University, Montclair,
New Jersey

ELSEVIER

T0195354

Elsevier
3251 Riverport Lane
St. Louis, Missouri 63043

Notice

Practitioners and researchers must always rely on their own experience and knowledge in evaluating and using any information, methods, compounds or experiments described herein. Because of rapid advances in the medical sciences, in particular, independent verification of diagnoses and drug dosages should be made. To the fullest extent of the law, no responsibility is assumed by Elsevier, authors, editors or contributors for any injury and/or damage to persons or property as a matter of products liability, negligence or otherwise, or from any use or operation of any methods, products, instructions, or ideas contained in the material herein.

Previous editions copyrighted 2020, 2017, 2014, 2011, 2007, 2004, 2000, 1996.

Executive Content Strategist: Lee Henderson
Director, Content Development: Laurie Gower
Senior Content Development Specialist: Rebecca M. Leenhouts
Senior Book Production Executive: Manchu Mohan
Book Designer: Brian Salisbury

Printed in Canada
Last digit is the print number: 9 8 7 6 5 4 3 2 1

PREFACE

The *Clinical Companion* to Harding, Kwong, Hagler, and Reinisch's *Lewis's Medical-Surgical Nursing: Assessment and Management of Clinical Problems*, 12th edition, is an updated and condensed reference to essential information on almost 200 medical-surgical patient problems and clinical care topics. The 12th edition of this pocket-sized book provides nurses and nursing students with quick access to current, concise, and important information for patient care.

The book is divided into three sections. Part One contains common medical-surgical patient problems arranged alphabetically and organized in an easy-to-use format. Part Two contains brief explanations of common medical-surgical treatments and procedures (e.g., pacemakers, oxygen therapy) in which the role of the nurse is emphasized. Part Three contains reference material frequently used in clinical nursing practice (e.g., heart and breath sounds, medication administration, blood and urine laboratory values). An extensive index provides for easy location of information.

The *Clinical Companion* can be used separately as a reference or in conjunction with *Lewis's Medical-Surgical Nursing*, 12th edition. We strongly believe the *Clinical Companion* will serve as an important resource to help nurses meet the challenges and opportunities in caring for patients and their caregivers.

Debra Hagler

Our greatest weakness lies in giving up. The most certain way to succeed is to try just one more time.
Thomas Edison

CONTENTS

Part Two: Treatments and Procedures

Part Three: Reference Appendix

PART ONE

Disorders

ABDOMINAL PAIN, ACUTE

Description

Acute abdominal pain is pain of recent onset. It may signal a life-threatening problem requiring immediate attention. Causes include damage to organs in the abdomen and pelvis, which may lead to inflammation, infection, obstruction, bleeding, or perforation. Common causes of acute abdominal pain are listed in Table 1.

Clinical Manifestations

Pain is the most common symptom of an acute abdominal problem. Patients may have nausea, vomiting, diarrhea, constipation, flatulence, fatigue, fever, rebound tenderness, and bloating.

Diagnostic Studies

Diagnosis begins with a complete history and physical examination. Description of the pain (frequency, timing, duration, location), accompanying symptoms, and sequence of symptoms (e.g., pain before or after vomiting) provide vital clues about the problem. Physical examination should include both rectal and pelvic examinations in addition to an abdominal examination.

- Complete blood count, urinalysis, abdominal X-ray, and an electrocardiogram are done initially, along with an ultrasound or CT scan.

TABLE 1 Causes of Acute Abdominal Pain	
Gynecologic Problems • Pelvic inflammatory disease • Ruptured ectopic pregnancy • Ruptured ovarian cyst Infectious disease • *Escherichia coli* O157:H7 • *Giardia* • *Salmonella* Inflammation • Appendicitis • Cholecystitis • Diverticulitis • Gastritis • Inflammatory bowel disease • Pancreatitis • Pyelonephritis	Vascular Problems • Mesenteric vascular occlusion • Ruptured aortic aneurysm Other • Obstruction or perforation of abdominal organ • Gastrointestinal bleeding or ischemia • Myocardial infarction • Trauma

- A pregnancy test is done to rule out ectopic pregnancy in women of childbearing age.

Interprofessional Management

The goal of management is to identify and treat the cause and monitor and treat complications, especially shock. See Shock.

- A diagnostic laparoscopy may be performed to inspect the surface of abdominal organs, obtain biopsy specimens, perform laparoscopic ultrasounds, and remove organs.
- A laparotomy is used when laparoscopic techniques are inadequate. If the cause of the acute abdomen can be surgically removed (e.g., inflamed appendix) or surgically repaired (e.g., ruptured abdominal aneurysm), surgery is considered definitive therapy.

Nursing Management

Goals

The patient will have relief of abdominal pain, resolution of inflammation, freedom from complications (especially hypovolemic shock), and normal nutritional status.

Nursing Interventions

Conduct ongoing assessments of vital signs, intake and output, and level of consciousness, which are key indicators of hypovolemic shock. General care involves management of fluid and electrolyte imbalances, pain, and anxiety. Assess the quality and intensity of pain at regular intervals, and provide medication and other comfort measures. Maintain a calm environment and provide information to help allay anxiety.

General care of the preoperative patient is described in Chapter 18 of Harding et al., *Lewis' Medical-Surgical Nursing*, ed 12.

Postoperative care depends on the type of surgical procedure performed. Laparoscopic procedures result in lower rates of postoperative complications (e.g., poor wound healing, paralytic ileus), earlier diet advancement, and shorter hospital stays compared with open surgical procedures.

A nasogastric (NG) tube with low suction may be used to empty the stomach and prevent gastric distention. If the upper gastrointestinal tract was entered, drainage from the NG tube may be dark brown to dark red for the first 12 hr. Later, it should be light yellowish brown or greenish. If a dark red color continues or if bright red blood is observed, notify the surgeon of the possibility of hemorrhage. "Coffee ground" granules in the drainage indicate blood that has been changed by acidic gastric secretions.

- Nausea and vomiting are common after a laparotomy and may result from the surgery, decreased peristalsis, or pain medication. Antiemetics such as ondansetron (Zofran) may be given (see Nausea and Vomiting).
- Monitor fluid and electrolyte status along with vital signs.
- Swallowed air and decreased peristalsis from decreased mobility, manipulation of abdominal organs during surgery, and anesthesia can lead to abdominal distention and gas pains. Early ambulation helps restore peristalsis, expel flatus, and reduce gas pain.

▼ **Patient and Caregiver Teaching**

Preparation for discharge begins soon after surgery. Teach the patient and caregiver about modifications in activity, care of the incision, diet, and drug therapy.

- Clear liquids are progressed to a regular diet.
- Normal activities should be resumed gradually, with planned rest periods and restrictions on lifting.
- Both patient and caregiver should be aware of possible complications. Teach them to notify the surgeon immediately if fever is higher than 101°F (38.3°C) or if pain, weight loss, incisional drainage, or changes in bowel function occur.

ACUTE CORONARY SYNDROME

Description

Acute coronary syndrome (ACS) develops when myocardial ischemia is prolonged and not immediately reversible. ACS includes the spectrum of non-ST elevation acute coronary syndrome (unstable angina [UA], non-ST segment elevation myocardial infarction [NSTEMI]), and ST segment elevation myocardial infarction (STEMI) (Fig. 1).

Pathophysiology

ACS occurs when a previously stable atherosclerotic plaque ruptures, releasing the lipid core into the vessel. This causes platelet aggregation and thrombus formation. The vessel may be partially blocked by a thrombus (manifesting as UA or NSTEMI) or totally blocked by a thrombus (manifesting as STEMI). It is unclear what causes the plaque to suddenly become unstable. Systemic inflammation (described earlier) may play a role. Patients with suspected ACS need immediate hospitalization.

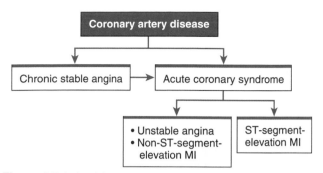

Figure 1 Relationships among coronary artery disease, chronic stable angina, and acute coronary syndrome. *MI*, myocardial infarction.

Unstable Angina

UA is chest pain that is new in onset, occurs at rest, or occurs with increasing frequency, duration, or less effort than the patient's chronic stable angina pattern. The pain usually lasts 10 min or more. The patient with chronic stable angina may develop UA, or UA may be the first clinical sign of coronary artery disease (CAD). Unlike chronic stable angina, UA is unpredictable and must be treated immediately.

- The patient with previously diagnosed chronic stable angina describes a significant change in the pattern of angina. It occurs with increasing frequency and is easily provoked by minimal exertion, during sleep, or even at rest.
- The patient without previously diagnosed angina describes chest pain that has progressed rapidly in the past few hours, days, or weeks, often ending in pain at rest.

Ischemic electrocardiogram (ECG) changes that may be seen with UA include ST depression and/or T wave inversion.

Myocardial Infarction: ST-Elevation and Non-ST-Elevation

A *myocardial infarction* (MI) occurs because of an abrupt stoppage of blood flow through a coronary artery with a thrombus caused by platelet aggregation. This causes irreversible myocardial cell death (necrosis). Serum cardiac biomarkers are released into the blood. Most MIs occur in the setting of preexisting CAD. The location of an MI correlates with the involved coronary circulation. For example, inferior wall infarctions result from occlusions in the right coronary artery. The majority of MIs affect the left ventricle.

Damage can occur in more than one location (e.g., anterolateral MI, anteroseptal MI).

- A STEMI, caused by an occlusive thrombus, creates ST elevation in the ECG leads facing the area of infarction. A STEMI is an emergency. To limit the infarct size, the artery must be opened within 90 min of presentation to restore blood and O_2 to the heart muscle and limit the infarct size. This can be done either by percutaneous coronary intervention (PCI) or with thrombolytic (fibrinolytic) therapy. PCI is the first-line treatment, if available. Cardiac catheterization confirms which artery has the occlusive thrombus so it can be opened with a balloon and stent. Thrombolytic therapy is done in hospitals that do not have a catheterization laboratory for PCI. If the patient does not seek treatment quickly, the STEMI will evolve.

- NSTEMI, caused by a nonocclusive thrombus, does not cause ST segment elevation on the 12-lead ECG. The ECG may or may not show ST depression and/or T wave inversion in the leads facing the area of infarction. NSTEMI patients do not need an emergent catheterization but usually undergo the procedure within 12–72 hr. Thrombolytic therapy is not a treatment option.

- Cardiac cells can withstand ischemic conditions for approximately 10 min before cellular death (necrosis) begins. The acute MI process evolves over hours to days. The earliest tissue to become ischemic is the subendocardium (the innermost layer of tissue in the heart muscle). If ischemia persists, it takes around 4–6 hr for the entire thickness of the heart muscle to necrose. If the thrombus is not completely blocking the artery, the time to complete necrosis may be as long as 12 hr.

- The degree of collateral circulation influences the severity of the MI. A person with a long history of CAD may have developed good collateral circulation to the tissue surrounding the infarction site.

The body's response to cell death is the inflammatory process. Within 24 hr, leukocytes infiltrate the area. Enzymes are released from the dead cardiac cells and are important diagnostic indicators (markers) of MI. Proteolytic enzymes from neutrophils and macrophages remove necrotic tissue by the fourth day.

- The necrotic zone is identifiable by ECG changes (e.g., ST segment elevation, pathologic Q wave) and by nuclear scanning after the onset of symptoms. The necrotic zone of a STEMI is identified by ECG changes (e.g., lowering of the initially elevated ST segments, T wave inversion, and/or a pathologic Q wave) within a day or two.

- At 10–14 days after MI, the new scar tissue is still weak. The heart muscle is vulnerable to increased stress during this time. At the same time, the patient's activity level may be increasing, so special caution and assessment are necessary.
- By 6 weeks after MI, scar tissue has replaced necrotic tissue, and the injured area is considered healed.

Changes in the infarcted heart muscle also cause changes in the unaffected areas. To try to compensate for the damaged muscle, the normal myocardium hypertrophies and dilates. This process is called *ventricular remodeling*. Remodeling of normal myocardium can lead to the development of late heart failure (HF), especially in the person with atherosclerosis of other coronary arteries and/or an anterior MI. Angiotensin-converting enzyme (ACE) inhibitor drugs are given to limit ventricular remodeling.

Clinical Manifestations

Unstable Angina

The chest pain associated with UA is new in onset, occurs at rest, or has a worsening pattern.

Myocardial Infarction

Severe and persistent chest pain not relieved by rest or nitrate administration may mean the patient is having an MI.

- Unlike any other pain, it is usually described as a heavy, pressure, tight, burning, constricted, or crushing feeling. Common locations are the substernal or epigastric area. The pain may radiate to the neck, lower jaw, and arms or to the back. When epigastric pain is present, the patient may relate it to indigestion, take antacids without relief, and therefore delay seeking treatment.
- It may occur while the patient is active or at rest, asleep, or awake. Pain often occurs in the early morning hours. It usually lasts for 20 min or longer.
- Some patients may not have pain but may have "discomfort," weakness, nausea, indigestion, or shortness of breath. Some women may have atypical discomfort, shortness of breath, or fatigue.
- Patients with diabetes may have silent (asymptomatic) MIs because of cardiac neuropathy or have atypical symptoms (e.g., shortness of breath).
- An older patient may have a change in mental status (e.g., confusion), shortness of breath, pulmonary edema, dizziness, or a dysrhythmia. The patient's skin may be ashen, clammy, and cool (cold sweat). The patient may have nausea and vomiting. Fever occurs within the first 24 hr (up to 100.4°F [38°C]) and

may continue for 4–5 days. BP and pulse rate are elevated initially. The BP may then drop, with decreased urine output, lung crackles, hepatic engorgement, and peripheral edema. Jugular veins may be distended, with obvious pulsations.

Complications

Dysrhythmias are the most common complication after an MI and are the most common cause of death in patients in the prehospital period. Dysrhythmias are caused by conditions that affect the myocardial cell's sensitivity to nerve impulses, such as ischemia, electrolyte imbalances, and sympathetic nervous system stimulation. Life-threatening dysrhythmias occur most often with anterior wall infarction, heart failure, and shock. Complete heart block is seen in a massive infarction (see Dysrhythmias).

- *Ventricular tachycardia and ventricular fibrillation* are lethal dysrhythmias that most often occur within the first 4 hr after the onset of pain. Premature ventricular contractions may precede ventricular tachycardia and fibrillation. Life-threatening ventricular dysrhythmias must be treated immediately.
- *HF* occurs when the heart's pumping action is reduced. Left-sided HF occurs initially with subtle signs, such as mild dyspnea, restlessness, agitation, or slight tachycardia. Other signs indicating the onset of left-sided HF include pulmonary congestion on chest X-ray, S3 or S4 heart sounds on auscultation of the heart, crackles on auscultation of the lungs, paroxysmal nocturnal dyspnea (PND), and orthopnea. Signs of right-sided HF include jugular venous distention, hepatic congestion, and lower extremity edema. (See Heart Failure, XXX).
- *Cardiogenic shock* occurs when inadequate oxygen and nutrients are supplied to the tissues because of severe left ventricular (LV) failure, papillary muscle rupture, ventricular septal rupture, LV free wall rupture, or right ventricular infarction. Cardiogenic shock requires aggressive management including control of dysrhythmias, intraaortic balloon pump therapy, and support of contractility with vasoactive drugs.

Other complications include papillary muscle rupture, ventricular rupture, ventricular aneurysm, and pericarditis. (See Pericarditis, Acute).

Diagnostic Studies

In addition to the patient's history of pain, risk factors, and health history, the primary diagnostic studies used to determine whether a person has UA or an MI include an ECG and serum cardiac markers. Other diagnostic measures can include coronary angiography, exercise stress testing, and echocardiogram.

Electrocardiogram

- When patients first present with chest pain, ST elevations on the 12-lead ECG most likely indicate a STEMI. Compare the new ECG to a previous ECG whenever possible. ST elevation represents myocardial injury that is potentially reversible but, if not treated, will likely evolve to permanent necrosis (tissue death) of the myocardium.
- A patient with STEMI tends to have a more extensive MI that is associated with prolonged and complete coronary occlusion. A pathologic Q wave develops on the ECG.
- Patients with UA or NSTEMI may or may not have ST segment depression and/or T wave inversion on the ECG. For patients with chest pain who do not have ST segment elevation or ST–T wave changes on the ECG, it is difficult to distinguish between UA and NSTEMI until we evaluate serum cardiac biomarkers.
- A patient with UA or NSTEMI usually has transient thrombosis or incomplete coronary occlusion, and the ECG typically does not develop pathologic Q waves.
- Serial ECGs often reveal the evolution and time sequence of ischemia, injury, infarction, and resolution of the infarction.

Cardiac Biomarkers

Serum cardiac biomarkers are proteins released into the blood from necrotic heart muscle after an MI.

- A high-sensitivity cardiac troponin test (hs-cTn) provides more rapid detection of MI compared with the conventional cardiac-specific troponin assays, allowing for a quicker diagnosis. Serum levels of hs-cTn rise within 1 hr of cardiac injury and stay high for 7–14 days. A second hs-cTn is drawn 2–3 hr after the first one if STEMI is ruled out. These markers are highly specific indicators of MI and have greater sensitivity and specificity for myocardial injury than creatine kinase (CK)-MB or myoglobin.

Interprofessional Management

A patient with ACS needs rapid diagnosis and treatment to preserve cardiac muscle. Initial management of the patient with chest pain most often occurs in the emergency department (ED).

- Obtain a 12-lead ECG and start continuous ECG monitoring.
- Position the patient in an upright position unless contraindicated and start O_2 by nasal cannula to keep O_2 saturation above 93%.
- Obtain intravenous (IV) access for drug administration.

A

- Give sublingual nitroglycerin (NTG) and 162–325 mg of chewable aspirin if not given before arrival at the ED. Morphine is given for pain unrelieved by NTG.
- A high-dose statin (e.g., atorvastatin [Lipitor]) is given.
- The patient usually receives ongoing care in a critical care or telemetry unit where continuous ECG monitoring is available and dysrhythmias can be treated.
- Monitor vital signs, including pulse oximetry, frequently during the first few hours after admission and closely thereafter. Maintain bed rest and limit activity for 12–24 hr, with a gradual increase in activity unless contraindicated.
- If the ECG shows ST elevation, the patient with STEMI is taken directly to the cardiac catheterization laboratory in PCI-capable hospitals. Glycoprotein IIb/IIIa inhibitors may be used during PCI for STEMI patients. Thrombolytic therapy is started if the patient is unable to be quickly transported to a PCI capable hospital.
- If the ECG shows ST depression and/or T wave inversion, the patient is usually transferred to a critical care unit or telemetry unit for ongoing care. Dysrhythmias are treated according to agency protocols.
- UA and NSTEMI patients are started on heparin. Some patients with UA or NSTEMI start on glycoprotein IIb/IIIa inhibitors (e.g., eptifibatide [Integrilin]) either before catheterization or at the time of PCI.
- For a patient with UA or NSTEMI, aspirin and heparin (unfractionated heparin [UH] or low-molecular-weight heparin [LMWH]) are recommended. Dual antiplatelet therapy (e.g., with aspirin and clopidogrel) and heparin are recommended for NSTEMI. Cardiac catheterization with possible PCI is considered as treatment for both UA and NSTEMI once the patient is stabilized, or if angina returns or increases in severity.

Traditional *coronary artery bypass graft* (CABG) surgery places conduits to transport blood between the aorta, or other major arteries, and the myocardium distal to the obstructed coronary artery (or arteries). It requires a sternotomy (opening of the chest cavity) and the use of cardiopulmonary bypass (CPB). It is a palliative treatment for CAD and not a cure. Newer techniques include minimally invasive direct coronary artery bypass, off-pump coronary artery bypass, totally endoscopic coronary artery bypass (TECAB), and transmyocardial laser revascularization. These surgical procedures and related nursing care are further discussed in Chapter 37 of Harding et al., *Lewis' Medical-Surgical Nursing*, ed 12.

Drug therapy includes IV nitroglycerin, aspirin, β-adrenergic blockers, and anticoagulation. Systemic anticoagulation may be achieved with LMWH given subcutaneously or IV UH. If PCI is anticipated, glycoprotein IIb/IIIa inhibitors may be used. ACE inhibitors are added for some patients after an MI. Calcium channel blockers may be used if the patient is already taking adequate doses of β-blockers or does not tolerate these blockers.

Nursing Management

Goals

The patient with an ACS will experience pain relief, quick and appropriate treatment, and preservation of heart muscle. During the hospitalization, the overall goals include effective coping with illness-associated anxiety, participation in a rehabilitation plan, and reducing risk factors. See eNursing Care Plan 37-1 for the patient with ACS on the website.

Interventions

Proper management decreases the O_2 needs of the patient's compromised myocardium. Institute measures to avoid the hazards of immobility while encouraging rest.

- Provide nitroglycerin, morphine, and supplemental O_2 as needed to eliminate or reduce chest pain.
- Maintain continuous ECG monitoring while the patient is in the ED and intensive care unit (ICU) and after transfer to a step-down or general care unit. Dysrhythmias need to be identified and treated quickly.
- If the patient is receiving thrombolytic therapy, monitor for reperfusion dysrhythmias. If signs and symptoms of major bleeding occur (e.g., drop in BP, increase in HR, sudden change in the patient's mental status, blood in the urine or stool), stop the drug and notify the HCP.
- In addition to frequent vital signs, evaluate intake and output. Assess lung and heart sounds and inspect for evidence of early heart failure (e.g., dyspnea, tachycardia, pulmonary congestion, distended neck veins).
- Assess oxygenation status frequently. If the patient is receiving O_2, check the nares for irritation or dryness (see Oxygen Therapy).
- Plan to ensure adequate rest periods free from interruption. There is no evidence for prolonged bed rest for the patient with an uncomplicated MI, but bed rest may be ordered for a few days after a large STEMI.
- Anxiety is usually present in patients with ACS. Identify the source of anxiety and assist the patient in reducing it. If the patient is afraid of being alone, allow a caregiver to sit quietly by the bedside or check in frequently with the patient.

▼Patient and Caregiver Teaching

The patient will need teaching at every stage of hospitalization and recovery (e.g., ED, telemetry unit, home care). The purpose of teaching is to give the patient and caregiver the tools to make informed health decisions (Table 2).

- Prepare the patient and caregiver for the usual course of recovery and rehabilitation to promote their sense of control.
- Teach patients to count their HR or use technology (e.g., cell phone applications, fitness trackers) to check their HR. Tell the patient that the HR should return to the resting HR within a few minutes of stopping exercise. Tell the patient to stop exercising and rest if chest pain or shortness of breath occurs.
- Encourage participation in an outpatient or home-based cardiac rehabilitation program.
- Include sexual counseling for cardiac patients and their partners. Tell the patient that resumption of sex depends on the emotional readiness of both the patient and partner and on the health care provider (HCP)'s assessment of recovery. It is generally safe to resume sexual activity 7–10 days after an uncomplicated MI. Sexual activity for most middle-aged men and women with their usual partners is a moderate-energy activity equivalent to climbing two flights of steps or walking briskly.

TABLE 2   Patient and Caregiver Teaching: Acute Coronary Syndrome

Include the following information in the teaching plan for the patient with acute coronary syndrome and the caregiver.

- Signs and symptoms of angina and MI and what to do should they occur (e.g., take nitroglycerin)
- When and how to seek help (e.g., contact ERS)
- Anatomy and physiology of the heart and coronary arteries
- Cause and effect of CAD
- Definition of terms (e.g., CAD, angina, MI, sudden cardiac death, heart failure)
- Identification of and plan to decrease risk
- Reasons for tests and treatments (e.g., ECG monitoring, blood tests, cardiac catheterization), activity limitations and rest, diet, and drugs
- Appropriate expectations about recovery (anticipatory guidance)
- Resumption of work, physical activity, sexual activity
- Measures to promote recovery and health (e.g., cardiac rehabilitation)
- Importance of the gradual, progressive resumption of activity

---

CAD, coronary artery disease; *ECG,* electrocardiogram; *ERS,* emergency response system; *MI,* myocardial infarction.

ACUTE RESPIRATORY DISTRESS SYNDROME

Description

Acute respiratory distress syndrome (ARDS) is a sudden and progressive form of respiratory failure in which the alveolar-capillary membrane becomes damaged and more permeable to intravascular fluid. ARDS accounts for about 10% of all adult ICU admissions. Despite supportive therapy, the mortality rate from ARDS is around 35%.

Etiology and Pathophysiology

Direct lung injury may cause ARDS, or ARDS may develop as a result of indirect injury, such as from multiple organ dysfunction syndrome (MODS) (see Systemic Inflammatory Response Syndrome and Multiple Organ Dysfunction Syndrome). The most common cause is sepsis. Table 3 lists conditions that predispose patients to developing ARDS. The pathophysiologic changes in ARDS are divided into three phases: (1) injury (exudative) phase; (2) reparative (proliferative) phase; and (3) fibrotic (chronic or late) phase.

TABLE 3   Conditions Predisposing to Acute Respiratory Distress Syndrome

Direct Lung Injury	Indirect Lung Injury
Common Causes	
• Aspiration (gastric contents or other substances) • Bacterial or viral pneumonia • Sepsis	• Massive trauma • Sepsis and septic shock (especially gram-negative infection) • Severe TBI • Shock states (hypovolemic, cardiogenic)
Less Common Causes	
• Chest trauma (blunt or penetrating) • Embolism: fat, air, amniotic fluid, thrombus • Inhalation of toxic substances • Near-drowning • O_2 toxicity • Radiation pneumonitis	• Acute pancreatitis • Cardiopulmonary bypass • Disseminated intravascular coagulation • Opioid drug overdose • Transfusion-related acute lung injury (e.g., multiple blood transfusions) • Urosepsis

The *injury (exudative) phase* usually occurs 24–72 hr after the initial injury and lasts up to 7 days.

- Engorgement of the peribronchial and perivascular interstitial space causes interstitial edema. Fluid in the parenchyma of the lung surrounding the alveoli crosses the alveolar membrane and enters the alveolar space. V/Q mismatch and intrapulmonary shunt develop because the alveoli fill with fluid. Blood in the capillary network cannot be oxygenated.
- Alveolar cells that produce surfactant are damaged by the changes caused by ARDS. This damage, in addition to further fluid and protein accumulation, results in surfactant dysfunction. When surfactant synthesis is decreased or surfactant is inactivated, alveoli become unstable and collapse. This causes atelectasis, further decreases lung compliance, compromises gas exchange, and worsens hypoxemia.
- Necrotic cells, protein, and fibrin form hyaline membranes that line the inside of each alveolus. In ARDS, the hyaline membrane thickens. This causes more atelectasis, further impairing gas exchange and reducing lung compliance.

Severe V/Q mismatch and shunting result in hypoxemia that is not responsive to increasing fraction of inspired oxygen (FiO_2). This is the classic sign of ARDS, called *refractory hypoxemia*. Despite receiving higher O_2 concentrations, the patient's condition continues to get worse. The *reparative (proliferative) phase* of ARDS begins 1–2 weeks after the initial lung injury.

- During this phase, there is a continued influx of granulocytes, monocytes, lymphocytes, and fibroblasts as part of the inflammatory response.
- Increased pulmonary vascular resistance and pulmonary hypertension may occur because fibroblasts and inflammatory cells destroy the pulmonary vasculature.
- Lung compliance continues to decrease because of interstitial fibrosis. Hypoxemia worsens because of the thickened alveolar membrane.
- If this phase persists, widespread fibrosis results. If this phase is stopped, the lesions resolve.

The *fibrotic* (chronic or late) *phase* may start as early as 24 hr after the initial lung injury. Not all patients who develop ARDS enter the fibrotic stage.

- For those that never fully recover from ARDS, the lung is completely remodeled by collagenous and fibrous tissues. Diffuse scarring of the lungs, interstitial fibrosis, and alveolar duct fibrosis result in decreased lung compliance and reduced surface area for gas exchange. Hypoxemia continues.

- Pulmonary vascular destruction and fibrosis cause varying degrees of pulmonary hypertension.

The progression of ARDS varies. Some survive the acute phase of lung injury. Pulmonary edema resolves, and complete recovery occurs within a week or so. The chance for survival is lower for those who enter the fibrotic stage. Patients may need several weeks of long-term mechanical ventilation.

Clinical Manifestations and Diagnostic Studies

At the time of the initial injury, and for 24–72 hr, the patient may not have respiratory symptoms or only exhibit mild dyspnea, tachypnea, cough, and restlessness. Lung auscultation may be normal or reveal fine, scattered crackles. Arterial blood gases (ABGs) may show mild hypoxemia and respiratory alkalosis caused by hyperventilation. The chest X-ray may be normal or show diffusely scattered but minimal interstitial infiltrates.

As ARDS progresses, symptoms worsen. Respiratory distress becomes evident as work of breathing (WOB) increases. Tachypnea and intercostal and suprasternal retractions may be present. Tachycardia, diaphoresis, changes in mental status, cyanosis, and pallor may be seen. Lung auscultation usually reveals scattered to diffuse crackles and coarse crackles on expiration.

- After 72 hr, the chest X-ray often shows diffuse and extensive bilateral interstitial and alveolar infiltrates.
- Refractory hypoxemia is the hallmark characteristic of ARDS. The partial pressure of oxygen in arterial blood (PaO_2) remains lower than expected despite increasing FiO_2.
- Hypercapnia often signifies respiratory muscle fatigue and hypoventilation with imminent respiratory failure.
- Severe hypoxemia, hypercapnia, metabolic acidosis, and manifestations of organ dysfunction often accompany ARDS.
- Complications may develop as a result of ARDS or its treatment. Besides the lungs, the vital organs most often involved are the kidneys, liver, and heart. The main cause of death in ARDS is MODS, often accompanied by sepsis.

Nursing and Interprofessional Management
Goals

The overall goals for the patient with ARDS include PaO_2 within normal limits for age or at baseline on room air, O_2 saturation in arterial blood (SaO_2) > 90%, resolution of the precipitating factor(s), and clear lungs on auscultation.

The care for acute respiratory failure is applicable to ARDS (see Respiratory Failure, Acute). Patients with ARDS are commonly cared for in critical care units. Best practices for care of the patient with ARDS include (1) O_2 administration; (2) mechanical ventilation; (3) low tidal volume ventilation; (4) permissive hypercapnia; (5) positive end-expiratory pressure (PEEP); (6) prone positioning; and (7) extracorporeal membrane oxygenation (ECMO).

O_2 Administration

The primary goal of O_2 therapy is to correct hypoxemia (see Oxygen Therapy). At first, the use of a high-flow system that delivers higher O_2 concentrations to maximize O_2 delivery may be all that is needed. Continuously monitor O_2 saturation (SpO_2) to assess the effectiveness of O_2 therapy.

For most patients diagnosed with ARDS, high-flow O_2 delivery, including bilevel positive airway pressure (Bi-PAP), is only a temporary measure. Patients with moderate to severe ARDS and refractory hypoxemia need mechanical ventilation (see Artificial Airways: Endotracheal Tubes) to keep the PaO_2 at or close to near normal levels. Even with mechanical ventilation, the patient may need a FiO_2 of 70%, 80%, or higher, to keep the PaO_2 at least 60 mmHg. Most health care professionals (HCPs) agree that in the injury and reparative phases, they may have to accept a lower than normal PaO_2 (e.g., PaO_2 55–80 mmHg) and SpO_2 (88%–95%).

Mechanical Ventilation

Mechanical ventilation is often delivered via a pressure control type of ventilation. Pressure control ventilation helps keep the inspiratory and plateau pressures from becoming too high. This prevents alveolar overdistention and rupture.

- Patients with ARDS are ventilated with a low tidal volume (VT) of 4–8 mL/kg to minimize additional injury to the stiff lungs. As a result, the $PaCO_2$ level will slowly rise above normal limits, known as permissive hypercapnia.
- During mechanical ventilation, it is common to apply PEEP at 5 cm H_2O to compensate for loss of glottic function caused by the endotracheal tube. PEEP increases functional residual capacity, or the volume of air left in the lungs at the end of a normal expiration. PEEP also helps open up ("recruit") collapsed alveoli. PEEP set at higher levels can improve ventilation in respiratory units that collapse at low airway pressures. This may allow the FiO_2 to be lowered.

ECMO is used most often in specialized ICUs. A large blood vessel is cannulated (most often the internal jugular, femoral artery, or femoral vein), and a catheter is inserted. ECMO and extracorporeal CO_2 removal pass blood across a gas-exchanging membrane outside the body and return oxygenated blood back to the body.

Positioning

Prone positioning is an option for patients with refractory hypoxemia who do not respond to other strategies. Special attention must be given to securing and maintaining the airway before, during, and after proning. By turning the patient prone, perfusion may be better matched to ventilation. Air-filled alveoli in the anterior part of the lung become dependent. Alveoli in the posterior part of the lungs are "recruited" (given the opportunity to reexpand), improving oxygenation. Another positioning strategy to consider for management of ARDS is continuous lateral rotation therapy, which provides continuous, slow, side-to-side turning of the patient by rotating the actual bed frame <40 degrees.

Promoting Tissue Perfusion

Maintaining fluid balance and hemodynamic stability is challenging in the patient with ARDS. Increasing pulmonary capillary permeability results in pulmonary edema. At the same time, the patient may be intravascularly volume depleted and at risk for hypotension and decreased CO from mechanical ventilation and PEEP.

Hemodynamic monitoring allows you to see trends, detect changes, and adjust therapy as needed. BP and mean arterial pressure (MAP) are important indicators of the adequacy of CO. Newer technologies permit monitoring stroke volume variation, CO, and mixed venous oxygen saturation ($ScvO_2$ or SvO_2) noninvasively. Closely monitor BP and indicators of CO and tissue perfusion (SaO_2, $ScvO_2$, or SvO_2) with changes in mechanical ventilation. Decreased CO is treated with IV fluids, drugs, or both.

Analgesia and Sedation

Assess for treatable causes of anxiety or restlessness (e.g., hypoxemia, pain, delirium). Often, restlessness and mental status changes are the first signs of hypoxemia or patient-ventilator dyssynchrony. You should address the causes and not depend solely on the use of analgesics and sedatives.

- Provide reassurance, spend time at the bedside, and ensure that the patient can obtain assistance immediately (e.g., call light and tools for alternate communication strategy while intubated). Anxiety also may be reduced through instruction in and use of progressive relaxation, guided imagery, and music therapy.
- Explain to the patient any expected sensations that may be encountered with each new experience (e.g., suctioning, drawing ABGs) so that coping strategies can be purposefully selected.
- Analgesia and sedation decrease the discomfort associated with the presence of an endotracheal tube, help reduce WOB, and prevent ventilator dyssynchrony. IV benzodiazepines (e.g.,

lorazepam, midazolam) and opioids (e.g., morphine, fentanyl) may decrease anxiety, restlessness, and pain. Start these drugs at the lowest dose possible.

Patients with ventilator dyssynchrony may need an adjustment of inspiratory flow rates or other settings. Patients with dyssynchrony despite aggressive analgesia and sedation may need a neuromuscular blocking agent (NMBA), such as vecuronium, pancuronium (Pavulon), or cisatracurium (Nimbex), to relax skeletal muscles and promote breathing with the ventilator. Remember that a patient receiving neuromuscular blockade can appear to be asleep, but still be awake and in pain. For this reason, simultaneous administration of analgesia and sedation with NMBAs is essential.

ADDISON DISEASE

Description

Addison disease is a primary adrenocortical insufficiency. All three classes of adrenal steroids—glucocorticoids, mineralocorticoids, and androgens—are reduced because of adrenal cortex hypofunction.

- Secondary adrenocortical insufficiency is due to lack of pituitary adrenocorticotropic hormone (ACTH) secretion. In this case, corticosteroids and androgens are deficient, but mineralocorticoids are usually sufficient.

Up to 80% of Addison disease cases in the United States are caused by an autoimmune response in which antibodies destroy the adrenal cortex. This results in loss of glucocorticoid, mineralocorticoid, and adrenal androgen hormones.

- Addison disease presenting along with other endocrine disorders is known as *autoimmune polyglandular syndrome.*

Other causes of Addison disease include amyloidosis, fungal infections (e.g., histoplasmosis), acquired immunodeficiency syndrome (AIDS), and metastatic cancer. Iatrogenic Addison disease may be due to adrenal hemorrhage, often related to anticoagulant therapy, chemotherapy, or bilateral adrenalectomy.

Clinical Manifestations

Manifestations include a slow onset of anorexia, nausea, progressive weakness, fatigue, and weight loss. Skin hyperpigmentation is seen primarily in sun-exposed areas of the body; at pressure points; over joints; and in the creases, especially palmar creases. Other manifestations include severe vomiting, abdominal pain, diarrhea, headache, orthostatic hypotension, salt craving, and pain in the lower back and legs.

Patients with adrenocortical insufficiency are at risk for *addisonian crisis* (acute adrenal insufficiency), a life-threatening emergency caused by critically low levels of adrenocortical hormones.

- Addisonian crisis may be triggered by stress (e.g., from infection, surgery), sudden withdrawal of corticosteroid hormone therapy, adrenal surgery, or sudden pituitary gland destruction.
- Hypotension may cause shock, especially during stress. Circulatory collapse is often unresponsive to the usual treatment (vasopressors and fluid replacement).

Diagnostic Studies

- Plasma cortisol levels are low or fail to rise with an ACTH stimulation test. A positive response to ACTH stimulation indicates a functioning adrenal gland and points to pituitary disease rather than adrenal disease.
- Urine levels of free cortisol and aldosterone are low.
- Laboratory findings include hyperkalemia, hypochloremia, hyponatremia, hypoglycemia, anemia, and increased BUN levels.
- CT and MRI are used to localize other causes including tumors, fungal infections, tuberculosis, or adrenal calcification.

Interprofessional and Nursing Management

Treatment of adrenocortical insufficiency focuses on managing the underlying cause when possible. The mainstay is often lifelong hormone therapy with glucocorticoids and mineralocorticoids.

- Hydrocortisone, the most commonly used form of hormone therapy, has both glucocorticoid and mineralocorticoid properties. Glucocorticoids are usually given in divided doses, two-thirds in the morning and one-third in the afternoon to reflect normal circadian rhythm and decrease side effects. The dosage is increased in stressful situations to prevent addisonian crisis.
- Mineralocorticoids are replaced with fludrocortisone and increased dietary salt intake. Mineralocorticoids are given once daily, preferably in the morning.
- Women need androgen replacement with dehydroepiandrosterone (DHEA), as their only source of androgen production is the adrenal glands.

- Teach patients using mineralocorticoid therapy (fludrocortisone) how to take their BP, increase salt intake, and report any significant changes to their health care provider (HCP).

The patient in addisonian crisis requires immediate aggressive shock management and high-dose hydrocortisone replacement. Large volumes of 0.9% saline solution and 5% dextrose are administered to reverse hypotension and electrolyte imbalances.

- Assess vital signs and signs of fluid volume deficit. Monitor trends in serum glucose, sodium, and potassium.
- The patient cannot cope with stress because corticosteroids cannot be produced. Protect the patient from noise, bright light, and environmental temperature extremes.
- If hospitalization was caused by an adrenal crisis, patients usually respond to IV high-dose hydrocortisone replacement by the second day and can start oral corticosteroid replacement.

▼ Patient and Caregiver Teaching

The serious nature of Addison disease and the need for lifelong hormone therapy require a comprehensive teaching plan.

- Teach patients the signs and symptoms of corticosteroid deficiency and excess and to contact their HCP for dosage adjustment.
- Teach about conditions requiring increased medication. Examples of situations requiring corticosteroid adjustment are fever, influenza, tooth extraction, and rigorous physical activity, such as playing sports on a hot day or distance running. If vomiting or diarrhea occurs, as may happen with gastroenteritis, the patient should notify the HCP at once. They may need electrolyte replacement and IV cortisol administration.
- Teach prevention of infection and need for prompt and vigorous treatment of existing infections.
- It is critical that the patient wear a medical identification (Medic Alert) bracelet and carry a wallet card stating the patient has Addison disease, so that appropriate therapy can be initiated in an emergency.
- Patients should carry an emergency kit with 100 mg of IM methylprednisolone (Solu-Medrol), syringes, and instructions for use when hormone therapy cannot be taken orally. Have the patient practice IM injections.
- Provide management instructions for patients who have diabetes and those who have elevated blood glucose levels when taking corticosteroids.

ALZHEIMER DISEASE

Description

Alzheimer disease (AD) is a chronic, progressive, irreversible neurodegenerative brain disease. It most often affects persons aged 65 and older. More than 6.2 million people are currently living with AD in the United States (US).

AD progresses slowly. It has a long preclinical phase, which may last up to 20 years. The average clinical duration is 4–8 years. There are some patients who have lived for 20 years after diagnosis.

Etiology and Pathophysiology

The exact cause of AD is unknown. Although age is the greatest risk factor, AD is not a normal part of aging, and age alone is not sufficient to cause the disease. When AD develops in someone younger than 60 years, it is referred to as *early-onset AD*. AD that becomes evident after the age of 60 years is called *late-onset AD*.

- Family history of AD is an important risk factor. Other risk factors include cardiovascular disease and head trauma.

Characteristic findings of AD related to changes in the brain's structure and function include amyloid plaques, neurofibrillary tangles, loss of connections between neurons, and neuron death.

Amyloid plaques consist of insoluble deposits of a protein called β-*amyloid*, other proteins, remnants of neurons, nonnerve cells, such as microglia, and other cells. In AD, the plaques develop first in brain areas used for memory and cognitive function. Eventually the cerebral cortex, especially the areas responsible for language and reasoning, is affected. Genetic factors may play a critical role in the way that the brain processes the β-amyloid protein, an important risk factor for AD. Abnormally high levels of β-amyloid cause cell damage directly or through an inflammatory response and neuron death.

Neurofibrillary tangles are abnormal collections of twisted protein threads inside nerve cells. The main component of these structures is a protein called *tau*. Normally, tau proteins maintain cellular structure by holding intracellular microtubules together. In AD, the tau protein is altered, and the microtubules twist together, forming neurofibrillary tangles.

- Plaques and neurofibrillary tangles are also found in the brains of people without cognitive impairment. However, they are more abundant in the brains of those with AD.

The other feature of AD is the loss of connections between neurons and neuron death. These processes result in structural damage. Affected parts of the brain begin to shrink in a process called *brain atrophy*. By the final stage of AD, brain tissue has shrunk significantly.

Diabetes, hypertension, current smoking, hypercholesterolemia, obesity, and trauma are associated with an increased risk for dementia including AD.

Clinical Manifestations

Pathologic changes often precede signs of dementia by at least 15 years. Early warning signs of AD are listed in Table 4. The rate of progression from mild to severe is highly variable, ranging from 3 to 20 years.

Initial changes are usually related to changes in cognitive functioning. Patients may have memory loss, mild disorientation, and/or trouble with words and numbers. Often a family member reports the patient's declining memory to the health care provider (HCP).

- Memory loss initially relates to recent events, with remote memories still intact. With progression of AD, memory loss includes both recent and remote memory and affects the ability to perform self-care.
- Behavioral manifestations (e.g., agitation, aggression) are from changes within the brain. The behaviors are not intentional or controllable by the person with AD. Some people develop delusions and hallucinations.
- As AD progresses, the person may develop more cognitive impairments, such as *dysphasia* (difficulty comprehending language and oral communication), *apraxia* (inability to manipulate objects or perform purposeful acts), *visual agnosia* (inability to recognize objects by sight), and *dysgraphia* (difficulty communicating by writing).
- Later in the disease, long-term memories cannot be recalled. The person does not recognize family members and may lose the abilities to communicate and perform activities of daily living (ADLs). Some tend to wander.
- In the late or final stages, the patient is unresponsive and incontinent and needs total care.

TABLE 4 Patient and Caregiver Teaching: Early Warning Signs of Alzheimer Disease (AD)

Include the following information in the teaching plan for the patient with AD and the caregiver.

1. Memory loss that affects job skills
   - Frequent forgetfulness or unexplainable confusion at home or in the workplace may signal that something is wrong.
   - This type of memory loss goes beyond forgetting an assignment, colleague's name, deadline, or phone number.
2. Problems with abstract thinking
   - For the patient with AD, this goes beyond challenges, such as balancing a checkbook.
   - The patient with AD may not be able to recognize numbers or do basic calculations.
3. Difficulty doing familiar tasks
   - It is normal for most people to become distracted and to forget something (e.g., leave something on the stove too long).
   - People with AD may cook a meal and then forget not only to serve it but also that they made it.
4. Poor or decreased judgment
   - Many people from time to time may choose not to dress appropriately for the weather (e.g., not bringing a coat or sweater on a cold evening).
   - The patient with AD may dress inappropriately in more noticeable ways, such as wearing a bathrobe to the store or a sweater on a hot day.
5. Problems with language
   - Most people have trouble finding the "right" word from time to time.
   - People with AD may forget simple words or substitute inappropriate words, making their speech difficult to understand.
6. Misplacing things
   - For many people, temporarily misplacing keys, purses, or wallets is a normal, albeit frustrating, event.
   - The patient with AD may put items in inappropriate places (e.g., eating utensils in clothing drawers), but have no memory of how they got there.
7. Changes in mood
   - Most people have mood changes.
   - The patient with AD tends to have more rapid mood swings for no apparent reason.
8. Changes in personality
   - As most people age, they may have some change in personality (e.g., become less tolerant).
   - The patient with AD can change dramatically, either suddenly or over time. For example, someone who is easygoing may become angry, suspicious, or fearful.
9. Loss of initiative
   - The patient with AD may become and remain uninterested and uninvolved in many or all their usual pursuits.

Adapted from Alzheimer's Association: *Early warning signs*, Chicago, The Association. www.alz.org/alzheimers_disease_know_the_10_signs.asp.

Diagnostic Studies

The diagnosis of AD is primarily a diagnosis of exclusion. When all other possible conditions that can cause mental impairment have been excluded, the diagnosis of AD can be made.

- Comprehensive health history, physical examination, neurologic and mental status assessments, and laboratory tests are done. Neuropsychologic testing is important for diagnostic purposes and to establish a baseline for evaluating changes over time.
- Brain imaging tests include CT or MRI scan, which may show brain atrophy in the later stages. However, this finding occurs in other diseases and in people without cognitive impairment.
- Positron emission tomography (PET) scanning can be used to differentiate AD from other forms of dementia.
- Cerebrospinal fluid neurochemical markers for β-amyloid and tau proteins show the level of β-amyloid accumulation in the brain.
- Definitive diagnosis of AD usually requires finding neurofibrillary tangles and neuritic plaques at autopsy.

Genetic testing for family members of patients with early-onset AD may be appropriate. Testing should be done only with formal genetic counseling, especially when asymptomatic family members are involved. If a person tests positive for apolipoprotein E-4 (ApoE-4) allele on chromosome 19, it does not mean they will develop AD.

Interprofessional Management

At this time, there is no cure for AD. Treatment does not stop the deterioration of brain cells. Management of AD is aimed at controlling undesirable behaviors that the patient may exhibit and providing support for the family caregivers. Current drugs have no effect on overall disease progression.

- Cholinesterase inhibitors block cholinesterase, the enzyme responsible for the breakdown of acetylcholine in the synaptic cleft. Cholinesterase inhibitors include donepezil (Aricept), rivastigmine (Exelon), and galantamine (Razadyne). Rivastigmine is available as a patch.
- Memantine (Namenda) protects brain nerve cells by blocking the damaging effects of glutamate, which is released in large amounts by cells damaged by AD.
- Treating depression associated with AD may improve the patient's cognitive ability. Drugs include selective serotonin

reuptake inhibitors (SSRIs), such as fluoxetine (Prozac), sertraline (Zoloft), and citalopram (Celexa). The antidepressant trazodone may help with sleep problems.

- Antipsychotic drugs have been shown to increase the risk of death and cognitive decline in older patients with AD.

Nursing Management

Goals

The patient with AD will maintain functional ability for as long as possible, be in a safe environment with a minimum of injuries, have personal care needs met, and have dignity maintained. The overall goals for the caregiver of a patient with AD are to reduce caregiver stress, maintain personal, emotional, and physical health, and cope with the long-term effects of caregiving.

Interventions

The diagnosis of AD is traumatic for both the patient and family.

- Assess family caregivers and their ability to accept and cope with the diagnosis. You are in an important position to assess for depression.
- Collaborate with caregivers and patients to manage manifestations, which change over time.
- Teach the caregiver to perform the tasks required to manage the patient's care.
- Adult day care is an option to provide respite for the family and a safe environment for the patient.
- As the disease progresses, the demands on the caregivers eventually exceed their resources. The person with AD may need to be in a special dementia unit of a long-term care facility.
- Support groups for caregivers and family members can provide an atmosphere of understanding and give current information about the disease itself and related topics, such as safety, legal, ethical, and financial issues. The Alzheimer's Association has educational and support systems available (www.alz.org).

Hospitalization of the patient with AD can be traumatic. Patients with AD who are hospitalized in the acute care setting need to be observed more closely, frequently oriented to place and time, and given reassurance. Anxiety or disruptive behavior may be reduced by consistent nursing staff.

A family and caregiver teaching guide based on the disease stages is provided in Table 5.

TABLE 5   Family and Caregiver Teaching: Alzheimer Disease

A

Include the following instructions when teaching families and caregivers the management of the patient with Alzheimer disease.

Mild Stage

- Many treatable (and potentially reversible) conditions can mimic dementia. Try to establish a diagnosis.
- Get the patient to stop driving. Confusion and poor judgment can impair driving skills and potentially put others at risk.
- Encourage activities such as visiting with friends and family, listening to music, enjoying hobbies, and exercising.
- Provide cues in the home, establish a routine, and determine a specific location where essential items (e.g., eyeglasses) need to be kept.
- Do not correct misstatements or faulty memory.
- Register with MedicAlert + Alzheimer's Association Safe Return, a program established by the MedicAlert Foundation and the Alzheimer's Association to locate those who wander from their homes.
- Make plans in terms of advance directives, care options, financial concerns, and personal preferences for care.

Moderate Stage

- Install door locks for patient safety.
- Provide protective wear for urinary and fecal incontinence.
- Ensure that the home has good lighting, install handrails in stairways and bathroom, and remove area rugs.
- Label drawers and faucets (hot and cold) to ensure safety.
- Develop ways, such as distraction and diversion, to cope with behavioral problems. Identify and reduce potential triggers (e.g., reduce stress, extremes in temperature) for disruptive behavior.
- Provide memory triggers, such as pictures of family and friends.

Severe Stage

- Provide a regular schedule for toileting to reduce incontinence.
- Provide care to meet needs, including oral care and skin care.
- Monitor diet and fluid intake to ensure their adequacy.
- Continue communication through talking and touching.
- Consider placement in a long-term care facility when providing total care becomes too difficult.

AMYOTROPHIC LATERAL SCLEROSIS

Amyotrophic lateral sclerosis (ALS) is a rare, progressive neuromuscular disease marked by loss of motor neurons. ALS usually leads to death 3–5 years after diagnosis, but a few patients survive more than 10 years. The median age of onset is 55 years.

- This disease became known as *Lou Gehrig disease* after the famous baseball player was stricken with it in 1939. Perhaps the best-known patient with ALS is physicist Stephen Hawking, who lived with ALS for over 50 years.

In ALS, motor neurons in the brainstem and spinal cord gradually degenerate for unknown reasons. Early in the disease, mitochondrial changes occur, and excess glutamate (an excitatory neurotransmitter) damages the neurons. Destroyed motor neurons cannot produce or transport signals to muscles. Progressive muscle weakness and atrophy are the classic signs of ALS.

- Factors that we suspect affect ALS include smoking, athleticism, metals, solvents, radiation, electromagnetic fields, pesticides, and viruses.
- Some have "limb-onset ALS," initially affecting the arms or legs. The person may have trouble with tasks requiring fine motor skills (e.g., writing, typing) or notice they are tripping, dropping things, or stumbling more often.
- Those who first have problems with slurred speech or swallowing have "bulbar-onset" ALS.
- Muscle wasting and involuntary contractions and twitching result from the denervation of the muscles and lack of stimulation and use. Eventually the patient may not be able to communicate. As the ability to move decreases, swallowing is impaired, leading to aspiration.
- Other symptoms include pain, sleep disorders, spasticity and hyperreflexia, drooling, emotional lability, constipation, and esophageal reflux.
- ALS does not affect a patient's intelligence, but affected people may have depression and problems with decision-making and memory.
- Death often results from compromised respiratory function caused by muscle weakness and paralysis.

The course of ALS is devastating because the patient is cognitively intact while wasting away. No cure exists for ALS. Two drugs may slow the decline.

- Riluzole (Rilutek) reduces damage to motor neurons by decreasing the release of glutamate.

- Edaravone (Radicava) is a free radical scavenger that we think
  relieves effects of oxidative stress, a likely factor in progression
  of ALS. It is given IV in 14-day cycles.

  Nursing interventions include facilitating communication, reducing
  risk of aspiration, facilitating early identification of respiratory insufficiency, decreasing pain from muscle weakness, decreasing risk of
  injury related to falls, providing diversional activities, such as reading
  and companionship, and providing compassionate end-of-life care.
- Help the patient and family manage the disease process, including grieving related to the loss of motor function and impending death. Discuss artificial methods of ventilation and advance
  directives with the patient and caregivers.
- Provide the patient and caregiver with support and resources to
  combat the stressors they experience.

ANAL CANCER

Anal cancer is uncommon in the general population, but the incidence is increasing. In the United States, around 8700 people are
diagnosed with anal cancer each year. It is more common in people over 50 years. Human papillomavirus is associated with about
90% of the cases. Those at high risk include smokers, HIV-positive
homosexual men, people who are immunocompromised (e.g., post-
transplant immunosuppression), and women with cervical, vaginal,
or vulvar cancer.
- Rectal bleeding is the most common presenting sign. Other
  symptoms include rectal pain, itching, pressure, or a full feeling. Symptoms may be constant and worsen with sex or bowel
  movements. There may be a change in bowel frequency or size
  with increased straining.

It is especially important to screen high-risk persons using digital rectal examination and anal Pap tests. In an anal Pap test, the
anal lining is swabbed, and the cells examined to identify any cell
changes (e.g., dysplasia, neoplasia). High-resolution anoscopy
allows for visualization of the mucosa and biopsy. An endoanal
(endorectal) ultrasound may be done.

Treatment of anal cancer depends on the size and depth of the
lesions. It is primarily treated with a combination of low-dose
radiation and chemotherapy. Chemotherapy regimens include combinations of mitomycin, cisplatin, and fluorouracil. Options for
precancerous lesions are surgical removal or treatment with topical
imiquimod (Aldara) and fluorouracil. If the tumor involves the rectum and is large enough to require removing the anal sphincters, the
anus will be sutured shut and a permanent ostomy created.

ANEMIA

Description

Anemia is a deficiency in the number of red blood cells (RBCs), or erythrocytes, quantity of hemoglobin (Hgb), and/or volume of packed RBCs (hematocrit). It is a common condition with diverse causes, such as blood loss, impaired production of erythrocytes, or increased destruction of erythrocytes.

- Because RBCs transport O_2, erythrocyte disorders can lead to tissue hypoxia. Hypoxia accounts for many of the signs and symptoms of anemia.
- Anemia is not a specific disease; it is a manifestation of a pathologic process.
- Anemia can result from primary hematologic problems or can develop secondary to disorders in other body systems.
  The various types of anemias are classified according to morphology (cell characteristics) or etiology.
- *Morphologic classification* is based on RBC size and color (Table 6).
- *Etiologic classification* is based on clinical conditions causing the anemia (Table 7).

Diagnostic Studies

- Anemia is diagnosed using a complete blood count, reticulocyte count, and peripheral blood smear. Further investigation may determine its specific cause.

TABLE 6   Morphologic Classification of Anemia

RBC Morphology	Etiology
Normocytic, normochromic (normal size and color) MCV 80–95 fL, MCH 27–31 pg	Acute blood loss, hemolysis, chronic kidney disease, chronic disease, cancers, endocrine disorders, starvation, aplastic anemia, sickle cell anemia, pregnancy
Microcytic, hypochromic (small size, pale color) MCV <80 fL, MCH <27 pg	Iron deficiency anemia, vitamin B_6 deficiency, copper deficiency, thalassemia, lead poisoning
Macrocytic (megaloblastic), normochromic (large size, normal color) MCV >95 fL, MCH >31 pg	Cobalamin (vitamin B_{12}) deficiency, folic acid deficiency, liver disease (including effects of alcohol abuse)

MCH, mean corpuscular hemoglobin; *MCV*, mean corpuscular volume; *RBC*, red blood cell.

- The Hgb level is decreased in all types of anemias. Other laboratory results are characteristic of specific types of anemias (Table 8).

Clinical Manifestations

Signs and symptoms of anemia result from the body's response to tissue hypoxia (Table 9). Specific manifestations vary depending

TABLE 7	Etiologic Classification of Anemia
Decreased RBC Production	*Chronic*
Decreased Hemoglobin Synthesis	• Gastritis
• Iron deficiency	• Hemorrhoids
• Sideroblastic anemia (decreased porphyrin)	• Menstrual flow
• Thalassemias (decreased globin synthesis)	**Increased RBC Destruction (Hemolytic Anemias)**
Decreased Number of RBC Precursors	*Acquired (Extrinsic)*
• Aplastic anemia and inherited disorders (e.g., Fanconi syndrome)	• Antibodies against RBCs
• Anemia of myeloproliferative diseases (e.g., leukemia) and myelodysplasia	• Infectious agents (e.g., malaria) and toxins
• Chronic diseases or disorders	• Physical destruction
• Medications and chemicals (e.g., chemotherapy, lead)	• Disseminated intravascular coagulopathy
• Radiation	• Extracorporeal circulation
	• Prosthetic heart valves
Defective DNA Synthesis	• Thrombotic thrombocytopenic purpura
• Cobalamin (vitamin B_{12}) deficiency	*Hereditary (Intrinsic)*
• Folic acid deficiency	• Abnormal hemoglobin (sickle cell disease)
Blood Loss	• Enzyme deficiency (G6PD)
Acute	• Membrane abnormalities (paroxysmal nocturnal hemoglobinuria, hereditary spherocytosis)
• Blood vessel rupture	
• Splenic sequestration crisis	
• Trauma	

G6PD, glucose-6-phosphate dehydrogenase; *RBC*, red blood cell.

TABLE 8 Laboratory Results in Anemias

Etiology of Anemia	Hgb/Hct	MCV	Reticulocytes	Serum Iron	TIBC	Transferrin	Ferritin	Bilirubin	Serum B$_{12}$	Folate
Acute blood loss	↓	N or ↓	N or ↑	N	N	N	N	N	N	N
Aplastic anemia	↓	N or slight ↑	↓	N or ↑	N or ↑	N	N	N	N	N
Chronic blood loss	↓	↓	N or ↑	↓	↑	N	N	N or ↓	N	N
Chronic disease	↓	N or ↓	N or ↓	N or ↑	↓	N or ↓	N or ↑	N	N	N
Cobalamin deficiency	↓	↑	N or ↓	N or ↑	N	Slight ↑	↑	N or slight ↑	↓	N
Folic acid deficiency	↓	↑	N or ↓	N or ↑	N	Slight ↑	↑	N or slight ↑	N	↓
Hemolytic anemia	↓	N or ↑	↑	N or ↑	N or ↓	N	N or ↑	↑	N	N
Iron deficiency	↓	↓	N or slight ↓ or ↑	↓	↑	N or ↓	↓	N or ↓	N	N
Sickle cell anemia	↓	N	↑	N or ↑	N or ↓	N	N	↑	N	↓
Thalassemia major	↓	N or ↓	↑	↑	↓	↓	N or ↑	↑	N	↓

Hgb/Hct, hemoglobin/hematocrit; *MCV,* mean corpuscular volume; *N,* normal; *TIBC,* total iron-binding capacity.

TABLE 9	Manifestations of Anemia		
	SEVERITY OF ANEMIA		
Body System	**Mild (Hgb 10–12 g/dL [100–120 g/L])**	**Moderate (Hgb 6–10 g/dL [60–100 g/L])**	**Severe (Hgb <6 g/dL [<60 g/L])**
Cardiovascular	Palpitations	↑ Palpitations, bounding pulse	↑ HR, ↑ pulse pressure, systolic murmurs, intermittent claudication, angina, HF, MI
Eyes	None	None	Icteric conjunctiva and sclera, retinal hemorrhage, blurred vision
GI	None	None	Anorexia, hepatomegaly, splenomegaly, problems swallowing, sore mouth
General	None or mild fatigue	Fatigue	Sensitivity to cold, weight loss, lethargy
Mouth	None	None	Glossitis, smooth tongue
Musculoskeletal	None	None	Bone pain
Pulmonary	Exertional dyspnea	Dyspnea	Tachypnea, orthopnea, dyspnea at rest
Neurologic	None	"Roaring in the ears"	Headache, vertigo, irritability, depression, impaired thought processes
Skin	None	None	Pallor, jaundice, itching

GI, gastrointestinal; *HF*, heart failure; *Hgb*, hemoglobin; *HR*, heart rate; *MI*, myocardial infarction.

on how fast the anemia has evolved, its severity, and any coexisting disease. Hgb levels may determine the severity of anemia.

- *Mild anemia* (Hgb 10–12 g/dL [100–120 g/L]) may not cause symptoms. Signs and symptoms are usually caused by an underlying disease or a compensatory response to heavy exercise. Symptoms may include palpitations, dyspnea, and mild fatigue.

- In *moderate anemia* (Hgb 6–10 g/dL [60–100 g/L]), cardiopulmonary signs and symptoms (e.g., increased heart rate) may be present with rest as well as activity.
- In *severe anemia* (Hgb <6 g/dL [60 g/L]), patients display many clinical manifestations involving multiple body systems.

Nursing and Interprofessional Management

The goals of care for the patient with anemia include assuming normal activities of daily living, maintaining adequate nutrition, and developing no complications related to anemia. See eNursing Care Plan 34.1 for the patient with anemia (available on the website).

Implement nursing interventions specific to the patient's needs and type of anemia.

- Acute interventions may include blood transfusions, drug therapy (e.g., iron supplements), and O_2 therapy to stabilize the patient.
- For the patient with fatigue, encourage alternate rest and activity periods. Help the patient prioritize activities according to energy levels. Arrange activities (e.g., avoid activity right after meals) to reduce competition for O_2 supply to vital functions.
- Aid with regular activities (e.g., ambulation, transfers, personal care) to minimize fatigue and risk for injury from falls. Monitor the patient's cardiorespiratory response to activity (e.g., tachycardia, dysrhythmias, dyspnea, diaphoresis, pallor, tachypnea).
- Diet and lifestyle changes can reverse some anemias.

ANEMIA, APLASTIC

Description

Aplastic anemia is a disease in which the patient has peripheral blood *pancytopenia* (decrease in number of all blood cell types—red blood cells [RBCs], white blood cells [WBCs], and platelets) and hypocellular bone marrow. The spectrum of the anemia can range from a moderate condition managed with erythropoietin or blood transfusions to severe with potentially fatal bleeding and sepsis.

Pathophysiology

About 70% of aplastic anemias are caused by autoimmune activity by autoreactive T lymphocytes. The cytotoxic T cells destroy the patient's own hematopoietic stem cells. Other anemias may be acquired from toxic injury to bone marrow stem cells or a result of an inherited stem cell defect. Causes of aplastic anemia include chemical agents and toxins; drugs; radiation; and viral or bacterial infections.

Clinical Manifestations

Aplastic anemia can manifest abruptly over days or develop insidiously over weeks and months. The patient may have symptoms caused by suppression of any or all bone marrow elements.

- General manifestations of anemia, such as fatigue and dyspnea, as well as cardiovascular and cerebral signs, may be seen (see Table 9).
- The patient with neutropenia (low neutrophil count) is susceptible to infection and at risk for development of septic shock and death.
- Thrombocytopenia may lead to bleeding (e.g., petechiae, ecchymoses, epistaxis).

Diagnostic Studies

Diagnosis is confirmed by laboratory studies.

- Hgb, WBC, and platelet values are often decreased (see Table 8). Reticulocyte count is low.
- Serum iron and total iron-binding capacity may be high as initial signs of decreased RBC production.
- Bone marrow examination findings include a hypocellular marrow with increased yellow marrow (fat content).

Nursing and Interprofessional Management

Management of aplastic anemia is based on identifying and removing the causative agent (when possible) and providing supportive care until pancytopenia reverses.

Nursing interventions for the patient with pancytopenia from aplastic anemia are presented in the nursing care plans (on the website) for patients with anemia (see eNursing Care Plan 34.1), thrombocytopenia (eNursing Care Plan 34.2), and neutropenia (eNursing Care Plan 34.3). Nursing actions are directed at preventing complications from infection and hemorrhage.

- The prognosis for severe untreated aplastic anemia is poor. Early consideration of a hematopoietic stem cell transplant (HSCT) is critical. The best treatment outcomes for those who receive an HSCT occur in younger patients who have had limited blood transfusions. Prior transfusions increase the risk for HSCT graft rejection.
- Patients ineligible for HSCT may receive immunosuppressive therapy with antithymocyte globulin and cyclosporine. Eltrombopag (Promacta), an oral thrombopoietin receptor agonist, can increase platelet counts. High-dose cyclophosphamide, alemtuzumab, or androgens may be helpful in select patients who do not respond to other treatments.

ANEMIA, COBALAMIN (VITAMIN B$_{12}$) DEFICIENCY

Description

Cobalamin (vitamin B$_{12}$) deficiency causes a type of megaloblastic anemia, which results in defective red blood cell (RBC) maturation. The most common cause of cobalamin deficiency is *pernicious anemia,* which results from an absence of *intrinsic factor* (IF). Pernicious anemia is a disease of insidious onset that begins in middle age or later.

Pathophysiology

Normally, the parietal cells of the gastric mucosa secrete IF, which promotes cobalamin (extrinsic factor) absorption in the distal ileum. In pernicious anemia, the gastric mucosa does not secrete IF because of either gastric mucosal atrophy or autoimmune destruction of parietal cells. Without the hydrochloric acid (HCl) secretion by parietal cells, IF is not secreted and cobalamin is not absorbed.

Cobalamin deficiency can occur in patients who had gastrointestinal (GI) surgery (e.g., gastrectomy, gastric bypass) or a small bowel resection involving the ileum. Others at risk include those with Crohn disease, ileitis, celiac disease, diverticula of the small intestine, or chronic atrophic gastritis. In these cases, cobalamin deficiency results from the loss of IF-secreting gastric mucosal cells or impaired absorption of cobalamin in the distal ileum. Cobalamin deficiency also occurs with excess alcohol or hot tea ingestion, smoking, long-term use of H$_2$-histamine receptor blockers and proton pump inhibitors, and in those who are strict vegetarians.

Clinical Manifestations

Manifestations of anemia related to cobalamin deficiency develop as a result of tissue hypoxia (see Table 9).
- GI manifestations include a sore, red, beefy, and shiny red tongue, anorexia, nausea, vomiting, and abdominal pain.
- Neuromuscular manifestations include weakness, paresthesias of feet and hands, reduced vibratory and position senses, ataxia, muscle weakness, and impaired cognition.

Diagnostic Studies

Laboratory data reflective of cobalamin deficiency anemia are presented in Table 8.
- RBCs appear large (macrocytic) with abnormal shapes. This structure contributes to RBC destruction because the cell membrane is fragile.

- Serum cobalamin levels are reduced.
- Normal serum folate levels with low cobalamin levels suggest that megaloblastic anemia is caused by a cobalamin deficiency.
- A serum test for anti-IF antibodies may be done that is specific for pernicious anemia.
- An upper GI endoscopy and biopsy of the gastric mucosa may also be done.

Interprofessional and Nursing Care

Lifelong administration of cobalamin is needed. Most patients need parenteral vitamin B_{12} (cyanocobalamin, hydroxocobalamin) or intranasal cyanocobalamin (Nascobal).

- A typical treatment schedule consists of 1000 mcg/day of cobalamin IM for 2 weeks, and then weekly until the hemoglobin is normal, and then monthly for life.
- Follow-up evaluation is essential to assess for neurologic deficits that were not corrected by cobalamin replacement therapy. Physical therapy may be useful.
- A diminished sensation to heat and pain as a result of neurologic impairment increases the risk for injury. Teach the patient to protect extremities from burns and trauma.
- Nursing interventions for the patient with anemia are also appropriate for the patient with cobalamin deficiency (see Anemia).

ANEMIA, FOLIC ACID DEFICIENCY

Folic acid (folate) deficiency can cause megaloblastic anemia. Folic acid is needed for DNA synthesis leading to red blood cell formation and maturation. Common causes of folic acid deficiency are dietary deficiency, especially a lack of leafy green vegetables and citrus fruits; malabsorption syndromes; drugs that interfere with absorption/or use of folic acid (e.g., methotrexate, phenobarbital, phenytoin); chronic alcohol use; and chronic hemodialysis.

Clinical Manifestations

The manifestations of folic acid deficiency are similar to cobalamin deficiency. Symptoms may be attributed to other coexisting problems (e.g., cirrhosis, esophageal varices). Gastrointestinal problems may include stomatitis, cheilosis, dysphagia, flatulence, and diarrhea. Thiamine deficiency, which is often present with folate deficiency, can cause neurologic symptoms.

In folic acid deficiency, the serum folate level is low (normal is 5–25 ng/mL [11–57 nmol/L]), with a normal serum cobalamin level.

Interprofessional and Nursing Management

Folic acid deficiency is treated by replacement therapy. The usual dosage is 1–5 mg/day by mouth. Teach the patient to eat foods high in folic acid (e.g., leafy green vegetables, breakfast cereals, breads, pasta).

Nursing interventions for the patient with anemia are also appropriate for the patient with folic acid deficiency (see Anemia).

ANEMIA, IRON DEFICIENCY

Description

Iron deficiency anemia is the most common nutritional disorder in the world. Those most susceptible to iron deficiency anemia are the very young, those on poor diets, and women in their reproductive years.

Pathophysiology

Iron deficiency may develop from inadequate dietary intake, malabsorption, blood loss, or hemolysis. Dietary iron is enough to meet the needs of men and older women. It may be inadequate for those with higher iron needs (e.g., menstruating or pregnant women).

Iron absorption occurs in the duodenum. Absorption can be altered by disease or by surgical procedures that remove or bypass the duodenum.

Blood loss is a major cause of iron deficiency in adults. Major sources of chronic blood loss are from the gastrointestinal (GI) and genitourinary (GU) systems.

- GI bleeding is often not obvious. It may exist for a long time before the problem is found. A loss of 50–75 mL of blood from the upper GI tract is enough for stools to appear black *(melena)*. The black color results from the iron in the red blood cells (RBCs).
- Common causes of GI blood loss are peptic ulcer, esophagitis, diverticula, hemorrhoids, and cancer. GU blood loss occurs primarily from menstrual bleeding.
- In addition to anemia of chronic kidney disease, dialysis treatment for chronic kidney disease may induce iron deficiency anemia because of the blood lost in the dialysis equipment and frequent blood sampling.

Clinical Manifestations

In the early course of iron deficiency anemia, the patient may not have any symptoms. As the disease becomes chronic, general manifestations of anemia may develop (see Table 9). In addition, specific signs and symptoms may occur with iron deficiency anemia.

- Pallor is the most common finding, and glossitis (inflammation of the tongue) is the second most common. Another finding is cheilitis (inflammation of the lips).
- The patient may report headache, paresthesia, and a burning sensation of the tongue.

Diagnostic Studies

Laboratory abnormalities characteristic of iron deficiency anemia are presented in Table 8. Other diagnostic studies are done to determine the cause of iron deficiency. Endoscopy and colonoscopy may be used to detect GI bleeding.

Interprofessional and Nursing Management

Consider groups who are at increased risk for development of iron deficiency anemia, including premenopausal and pregnant women, people from lower socioeconomic backgrounds, older adults, and those who have had blood loss. Diet teaching, with an emphasis on foods high in iron and ways to maximize absorption, is important for these groups.

The main goal is to treat the underlying problem causing iron loss, reduced iron intake (e.g., malnutrition, alcohol use), or poor absorption of iron. Efforts are directed toward replacing iron. Oral or occasionally parenteral iron supplements are used. If iron deficiency is from acute blood loss, transfusion of packed RBCs may be required. Nursing measures are presented in eNursing Care Plan 34.1 on the website.

- Parenteral iron supplements require special considerations. We give a test dose of IV iron dextran and then observe the patient for 1 hr before giving the rest of dose so we can monitor for anaphylaxis. Because IM iron solutions may stain the skin, use separate needles for withdrawing the solution and injecting the medication. Use a Z-track injection technique.
- Monitor patients who require lifelong iron supplementation for potential liver problems related to iron storage.

▼ **Patient and Caregiver Teaching**
- Discuss the need for diagnostic studies to identify the cause of anemia and to evaluate response to therapy.
- Teach the patient about good food sources of iron (lean beef, turkey, pork, chicken, fish, legumes, dark green leafy vegetables, whole-grain and enriched bread and cereals, beans).
- Stress adherence with dietary and drug therapy. To replenish the body's iron stores, the patient needs to take iron therapy for 2–3 months after the hemoglobin (Hgb) level returns to normal.

- Oral iron supplements should be taken about an hour before meals. Taking iron with vitamin C (ascorbic acid) or orange juice enhances iron absorption. Iron may be taken with meals if absolutely needed to decrease GI side effects.
- Dilute liquid iron and have the patient drink it through a straw to avoid staining the teeth.
- GI side effects of oral iron supplements include heartburn, constipation, and diarrhea. Have the patient stay upright for 30 minutes after taking oral forms. Constipation is common. The patient should start on stool softeners and laxatives, if needed.
- Tell patients that iron supplements will cause their stools to become black because the GI tract excretes excess iron.

ANEURYSM, AORTIC

Description

One of the most common problems affecting the aorta is an *aneurysm*, which is a permanent, localized outpouching or dilation of the vessel wall. Aneurysms occur in men more often than in women and in whites more often than in blacks. The incidence increases with age.

Aneurysms may occur in more than one location. Aortic aneurysms may involve the aortic arch, thoracic aorta, and/or abdominal aorta. Three-fourths of aortic aneurysms occur in the abdominal aorta. Most *abdominal aortic aneurysms* (AAAs) occur below the renal arteries.

Pathophysiology

A variety of disorders are associated with aortic aneurysms. The main causes are classified as degenerative, congenital, infectious, mechanical (e.g., penetrating or blunt trauma), or inflammatory (e.g., aortitis). The larger the aneurysm, the greater the risk of rupture.

- Risk factors for aortic aneurysms include age, male gender, hypertension, coronary artery disease, family history, tobacco use, high cholesterol, lower extremity peripheral artery disease, carotid artery disease, previous stroke, and excess weight or obesity. Tobacco use is the most important modifiable risk factor.
- Aortic aneurysm and dissection have a strong genetic component. The familial tendency is related to congenital anomalies, such as bicuspid aortic valve, coarctation of the aorta, Turner syndrome, and autosomal dominant polycystic kidney disease. Aneurysms are classified as true and false aneurysms.
- A *true aneurysm* is one in which the wall of the artery forms the aneurysm, with at least one vessel layer still intact. A *fusiform*

aneurysm is circumferential and relatively uniform in shape. A *saccular aneurysm* is pouch-like, with a narrow neck connecting the bulge to one side of the arterial wall.

- A *false aneurysm*, or *pseudoaneurysm*, is not an aneurysm, but a disruption of all wall layers with bleeding that is contained by surrounding structures. False aneurysms may result from trauma, infection, after peripheral artery bypass graft surgery at the site of the graft-to-artery anastomosis, or arterial leakage after removal of cannulae (e.g., femoral artery catheters, intraaortic balloon pump devices).

Clinical Manifestations

Thoracic aortic aneurysms are usually asymptomatic. When symptoms present, the most common is deep, diffuse chest pain that may extend to the interscapular area.

Aneurysms in the ascending aorta and aortic arch can cause (1) angina from decreased blood flow to the coronary arteries; (2) transient ischemic attacks from decreased blood flow to the carotid arteries; and (3) coughing, shortness of breath, hoarseness, and/or dysphagia (difficulty swallowing) from pressure on the laryngeal nerve. Compression of the superior vena cava by the aneurysm can cause distended neck veins and face and arm edema.

AAAs are often asymptomatic, found during routine physical examination or on evaluation for an unrelated problem (e.g., abdominal X-ray). A pulsatile mass in the periumbilical area slightly to the left of midline may be present. Bruits may be auscultated over the aneurysm. Physical findings may be harder to detect in obese persons.

- AAA symptoms may mimic pain associated with abdominal or back disorders. Compression of nearby structures and nerves may cause symptoms, such as back pain, epigastric discomfort, altered bowel elimination, and intermittent claudication.
- Sometimes, aneurysms spontaneously embolize plaque, causing "*blue toe syndrome*," (patchy mottling of the feet and toes in the presence of peripheral pulses).

Complications

Smokers with an aortic aneurysm are more likely to experience aortic rupture.

- If rupture occurs into the retroperitoneal space, bleeding may be controlled by surrounding structures, preventing exsanguination and death. The patient has severe back pain and may have back and/or flank ecchymosis *(Grey Turner sign)*.
- If rupture occurs into the thoracic or abdominal cavity, the patient can die from massive hemorrhage. For patients admitted with a ruptured AAA, in-hospital mortality is high at 53%.

- The patient who reaches the hospital will be in hypovolemic shock with tachycardia; hypotension; pale, clammy skin; decreased urine output; altered sensorium; and abdominal tenderness. Simultaneous resuscitation and immediate surgical repair are needed.

Diagnostic Studies

- Chest X-rays reveal abnormal widening of the thoracic aorta. Abdominal X-rays may show calcification in the aortic wall.
- Echocardiography assesses the function of the aortic valve.
- Ultrasound is useful for aneurysm screening and to monitor aneurysm size.
- CT or MRI may help assess the location and severity of aneurysms.

Interprofessional Management

The goal of management is to prevent aneurysm rupture. Conservative therapy of small, asymptomatic AAAs (<5.5 cm) is the best practice.

- Risk factor modification is recommended (ceasing tobacco use, decreasing BP, optimizing lipid profile, gradually increasing physical activity).
- Aneurysm size is monitored using ultrasound or CT every 6–12 months. Monitoring by ultrasound every 2–3 years is recommended for patients with AAAs smaller than 4.0 cm in diameter.
- Patients should receive medical management for hypertension, hyperlipidemia, diabetes, and other cardiovascular risk factors.

Aneurysms 5.5 cm in diameter or larger are surgically repaired. Surgical intervention may occur sooner if the patient has a genetic disorder (e.g., Marfan), if the aneurysm expands rapidly or becomes symptomatic, or if the risk of rupture is high.

- Open aneurysm repair (OAR) involves a large abdominal incision through which the surgeon: (1) cuts into the diseased aortic segment; (2) removes any thrombus or plaque; (3) sutures a synthetic graft to the aorta proximal and distal to the aneurysm; and (4) sutures the native aortic wall around the graft to act as a protective cover.
- An alternative to OAR is the minimally invasive endovascular aneurysm repair. This procedure involves placement of a sutureless aortic graft into the abdominal aorta inside the aneurysm via a femoral artery cutdown.

The most common complication of aneurysm repair is *endoleak*, the seepage of blood back into the old aneurysm. This may result from an inadequate seal at either graft end, a tear through the graft fabric, or leakage between overlapping graft segments. Repair may require coil embolization (insertion of beads) for hemostasis.

Nursing Management

Goals

The patient undergoing aortic surgery will have normal tissue perfusion, intact motor and sensory function, and no complications related to surgical repair, such as infection, rupture, or thrombosis.

Interventions

Encourage the patient to reduce cardiovascular risk factors, including controlling BP, smoking cessation, and maintaining normal body weight and serum lipid levels. Counsel the patient about taking part in moderate physical activity.

- Before surgery, provide emotional support and teaching to the patient and caregivers. Briefly explain the disease process, the planned surgical procedure(s), preoperative routines, what to expect immediately after surgery (e.g., recovery room, tubes/drains), and usual postoperative timelines.
- After surgery, in addition to the usual goals of care for a postoperative patient (e.g., maintaining adequate respiratory function, fluid and electrolyte balance, pain control), check for graft patency and renal perfusion. Watch for and intervene to limit or treat dysrhythmias, ischemia, venous thromboembolism, infections, and neurologic complications.
- A potentially lethal complication in an emergency repair of a ruptured AAA is the development of intraabdominal hypertension (IAH) with associated abdominal compartment syndrome. Persistent IAH reduces blood flow to the viscera. IAH is confirmed by measuring the patient's intraabdominal pressure indirectly through a catheter and transducer system.

▼ Patient and Caregiver Teaching

Teach the patient and caregiver to gradually increase activities at home. Fatigue, poor appetite, and irregular bowel habits are common.

- Teach the patient to avoid heavy lifting for 6 weeks after surgery. Any redness, swelling, increased pain, drainage from incisions, or fever >100°F (37.8°C) should be reported to a health care provider.
- Teach the patient and the caregiver to observe for changes in color or warmth of the extremities and changes in peripheral pulses.
- Sexual problems in male patients are common after aortic surgery. Referral to a urologist, and counseling may be useful if erectile dysfunction occurs.

ANGINA, CHRONIC STABLE

Description

Chronic stable angina refers to chest pain that occurs intermittently over a long period with a similar pattern of onset, duration, and intensity of symptoms. Chronic stable angina is a clinical manifestation of coronary artery disease (CAD).

Pathophysiology

Angina, or chest pain, is a result of myocardial ischemia when the demand for myocardial oxygen exceeds the ability of the coronary arteries to supply the heart muscle with oxygen. The primary cause of myocardial ischemia is insufficient blood flow to the myocardium through coronary arteries narrowed by atherosclerosis (see Coronary Artery Disease).

Variants of chronic stable angina include the following:

- *Silent ischemia,* in which ischemia occurs in the absence of any subjective symptoms.
- *Prinzmetal angina* (variant angina), which often occurs at rest, usually in response to spasm of a major coronary artery. Risk factors include a history of migraine headaches, Raynaud phenomenon, or heavy smoking. It is usually caused by spasm of a major coronary artery, with or without CAD.
- *Microvascular angina* occurs in the absence of significant coronary atherosclerosis or coronary spasm, especially in women. In these patients, chest pain is related to myocardial ischemia from atherosclerosis or spasm of the small distal branch vessels of the coronary microcirculation. This is known as *coronary microvascular disease (MVD).* Often the angina is prolonged and brought on by physical exertion. Prevention and treatment of MVD follow the same recommendations as for CAD.

Clinical Manifestations

The pain or discomfort of chronic angina is often provoked by physical exertion, stress, or emotional upset. Patients may describe a pain, pressure, or ache in the chest often described as a constrictive, squeezing, heavy, tight, or suffocating sensation (Table 10). Many people report severe indigestion or epigastric burning. Although most angina pain is substernal, the sensation may occur in the neck or radiate to the jaw, neck, shoulders, and arms. Chronic angina pain usually does not change with position or breathing and is rarely described as sharp or stabbing.

TABLE 10	PORST Assessment of Angina	A

Use the following memory aid to obtain information from the patient who has chest pain.

Factor	Questions to Ask Patient
P Precipitating events	What events or activities precipitated the pain or discomfort (e.g., argument, exercise, resting)?
Q Quality of pain	What does the pain or discomfort feel like (e.g., pressure, dull, aching, tight, squeezing, heaviness)?
R Region (location) and radiation of pain	Can you point to where the pain or discomfort is located? Does the pain or discomfort radiate to other areas (e.g., back, neck, arms, jaw, shoulder, elbow)?
S Severity of pain	On a scale of 0–10, with 0 indicating no pain and 10 being the most severe pain you could imagine, what number would you give the pain or discomfort?
T Timing	When did the pain or discomfort begin? Has it changed since this time? Have you had pain/discomfort like this before?

- Some patients, especially women and older adults, report atypical symptoms including dyspnea, nausea, and/or fatigue. This presentation is referred to as "angina equivalent."
- Often people will report pain between the shoulder blades and dismiss it as not being related to the heart.
- The pain usually lasts for only a few minutes (5–15 minutes) and often subsides with rest, calming down, and/or using sublingual nitroglycerin (NTG) (e.g., Nitrostat).
- An electrocardiogram (ECG) usually reveals ST segment depression and/or T wave inversion, indicating ischemia. The ECG pattern returns to baseline when blood flow is restored and the pain is relieved.

Diagnostic Studies

Diagnostic studies used to evaluate angina are the same as those used to diagnose CAD (see Coronary Artery Disease). For patients with known CAD and chronic stable angina, common diagnostic studies include 12-lead ECG, echocardiography, exercise stress testing, and pharmacologic nuclear imaging.

Interprofessional Management

The goal of treatment for a patient admitted with angina is to decrease O_2 demand and/or increase O_2 supply. Reducing modifiable CAD risk factors is a priority. In addition to antiplatelet and cholesterol-lowering drug therapy, the most common interventions for chronic stable angina are nitrates, angiotensin-converting enzyme (ACE) inhibitors, β-blockers, and calcium channel blockers.

Drug Therapy

- Aspirin is given in the absence of contraindications (such as an aspirin allergy).
- Short-acting nitrates are first-line therapy for the treatment of angina. Nitrates produce their principal effects by dilating peripheral blood vessels, coronary arteries, and collateral vessels. Sublingual NTG tablets or spray will usually relieve pain in approximately 3 minutes and lasts approximately 30–60 minutes. If symptoms are unchanged or worse after 5 minutes, the patient should activate the emergency response system. Sublingual NTG also can be used before undertaking an activity that the patient knows may precipitate angina.
- Long-acting nitrates, such as isosorbide dinitrate and isosorbide mononitrate, can reduce the frequency of anginal attacks. Long-acting nitrates are available in oral preparations, ointments, and transdermal controlled-release patches. Tolerance to long-acting NTG can develop. To limit this, schedule your patients for a 10- to 14-hr nitrate-free period every day.
- ACE inhibitors (e.g., lisinopril) are prescribed for patients with chronic stable angina who are at high risk for a cardiac event (e.g., ejection fraction 40% or less, diabetes, hypertension, or chronic kidney disease). These drugs result in vasodilation and reduced blood volume. Most important, they can prevent or reverse ventricular remodeling. For patients who are intolerant of ACE inhibitors (e.g., cough, angioedema), angiotensin receptor blockers (e.g., losartan) are used.
- Patients with left ventricular dysfunction or elevated BP or those who have had a myocardial infarction (MI) take β-blockers, such as carvedilol (Coreg), metoprolol (Toprol XL), and bisoprolol (Zebeta). These medications reduce myocardial oxygen demand by decreasing myocardial contractility, heart rate (HR), systemic vascular resistance, and BP.
- Calcium channel blockers, such as nifedipine, verapamil, diltiazem, and nicardipine, are used if β-adrenergic blocking agents

are contraindicated, are poorly tolerated, or do not control symptoms. The dihydropyridines (e.g., amlodipine) have more vasodilatory effects, and the nondihydropyridines (e.g., verapamil, diltiazem) have more rate and contractility effects.

A

- Ranolazine (Ranexa), a sodium current inhibitor, is used to treat chronic angina in patients who have not had an adequate response with other medications. Ranolazine does not affect the BP or HR. It can prolong the QT interval.
- Other medications, such as lipid-lowering drugs, are used to manage the underlying CAD.

Cardiac Catheterization

If a coronary blockage is amenable to treatment, coronary revascularization with percutaneous coronary intervention (PCI) may be recommended. PCI may be done at the same time as the cardiac catheterization.

- During PCI, a catheter with a deflated balloon tip is inserted into the blocked coronary artery. The deflated balloon is positioned inside the blockage and inflated. This compresses the plaque against the artery wall, resulting in vessel dilation and a larger vessel diameter. This procedure is called *balloon angioplasty.*
- *Intracoronary stents* are usually inserted to prevent abrupt closure and restenosis after balloon angioplasty. A stent is an expandable, mesh-like structure designed to keep the vessel open by supporting the arterial walls. Because stents are thrombogenic, drugs are used to prevent platelet aggregation within the stent and acute stent thrombosis. Many stents are coated with a drug (e.g., everolimus, zotarolimus) that helps to prevent stent restenosis.
- Drugs commonly used during PCI are unfractionated heparin or low-molecular-weight heparin, a direct thrombin inhibitor (e.g., bivalirudin [Angiomax]), and/or a glycoprotein IIb/IIIa inhibitor (e.g., eptifibatide [Integrilin]). After PCI, the patient receives dual antiplatelet therapy (e.g., aspirin [indefinitely] and ticagrelor or clopidogrel [Plavix]) until the intimal lining grows over the stent and provides a smooth vascular surface.

The most serious complications from stent placement are abrupt closure and vascular injury. Less common complications include acute MI, stent embolization, coronary spasm, contrast medium allergy, renal compromise, bleeding (e.g., retroperitoneal), infection, stroke, and emergent coronary artery bypass graft surgery. The risk for dysrhythmias during and after PCI is high.

Nursing Management

Goals

Goals for the patient with chronic stable angina are the same as those for acute coronary syndrome (see Acute Coronary Syndrome).

Interventions

If your patient has chest pain but you are unsure if the pain is from chronic stable angina, UA, or an MI, plan to perform the following measures: (1) position the patient upright unless contraindicated and apply supplemental O_2; (2) assess vital signs; (3) apply a continuous ECG monitor; (4) obtain a 12-lead ECG; (5) provide prompt pain relief, first with SL or IV NTG, followed by an IV opioid analgesic, if needed; (6) obtain cardiac biomarkers; (7) assess heart and breath sounds; and (8) obtain a chest X-ray.

- Ask the patient to describe the pain and rate it on a scale of 0–10 before and after treatment to evaluate the effectiveness of the interventions. Use the same words that the patient uses to describe the symptoms (e.g., tightness, pressure).
- The patient may be anxious and may have pale, cool, clammy skin. The BP and HR may be high. Assess for other signs of pain, such as restlessness; ECG changes; high HR, respiratory rate, or BP; clutching of the bed linens; or other nonverbal cues.
- Support and reassure the patient. Use a calm approach to help reduce the patient's anxiety.

▼ Patient and Caregiver Teaching

Reassure the patient with a history of chronic stable angina that a long, productive life is possible. Heart models, video recordings, and written information are important tools for teaching.

- Assist the patient to identify factors that precipitate angina and how to avoid or control these factors.
- Help the patient identify and plan to modify personal risk factors for CAD.
- Teach the patient and caregivers about diets low in sodium and saturated fats. Maintaining ideal body weight is important in controlling angina, because excess weight increases myocardial workload.
- Advise about a regular, individualized exercise program that conditions rather than stresses the heart. For example, many patients can walk briskly on a flat surface at least 30 minutes a day on most days of the week.
- Teach the patient and caregivers about the proper storage and use of NTG. It should be always easily accessible to the patient. Store the tablets away from light and heat sources, including body heat, to protect them from degradation. Keep tablets in

their original bottles. Once opened, the tablets lose potency. They should be replaced every 6 months.

- Patients may feel a threat to their roles, identity, and self-esteem. If needed, arrange for counseling to support adjustment of the patient and caregiver to the diagnosis of CAD and resulting angina.

ANKYLOSING SPONDYLITIS

Description and Pathophysiology

Ankylosing spondylitis (AS), also known as *axial spondyloarthritis*, is a chronic inflammatory disease that primarily affects the axial skeleton, including the sacroiliac joints, intervertebral spaces, and costovertebral articulations. Inflammation in joints and adjacent tissue causes the formation of granulation tissue (pannus) and the development of dense fibrous scars that lead to joint fusion. Inflammation can affect the eyes, lungs, heart, kidneys, and peripheral nervous system.

- The human leukocyte antigen HLA-B27 antigen is found in about 90% of whites with AS, but only 8% of those without the disease. This suggests genes play an important role in AS. Along with whites, Asians, and Hispanics are more likely to have AS than other ethnic groups.

Clinical Manifestations and Complications

The patient typically reports lower back pain, stiffness, and limitation of motion that are worse during the night and in the morning but decrease with mild activity. In women, early symptoms may include pain and stiffness in the neck rather than the lower back. Patients with AS may have chest pain and sternal/costal cartilage tenderness.

- Uveitis is the most common nonskeletal symptom. It can appear years before arthritic symptoms develop.

Postural abnormalities and deformity can cause significant disability. Aortic insufficiency and pulmonary fibrosis are frequent complications. Cauda equina syndrome can also result, contributing to lower extremity weakness and bladder dysfunction. The patient is at risk for spinal fracture from osteoporosis.

Diagnostic Studies

- X-rays are limited in ability to detect early sacroiliitis or subtle changes in posterior vertebrae.
- MRI can be useful in assessing early cartilage abnormalities.

- Increased erythrocyte sedimentation rate and mild anemia may be seen.
- When the suspicion for AS is high, the presence of the HLA-B27 antigen improves the likelihood of the diagnosis.

Interprofessional Management

Prevention of AS is not possible. However, families with other diagnosed HLA-B27-positive rheumatic diseases (e.g., acute anterior uveitis, juvenile spondyloarthritis) should be alert to signs of lower back pain and arthritis symptoms for early identification and treatment of AS.

Care of the patient is aimed at maintaining maximal mobility while decreasing pain and inflammation. Heat applications, nonsteroidal antiinflammatory drugs and salicylates, and disease-modifying antirheumatic drugs, such as sulfasalazine or methotrexate, can help in relieving symptoms. Etanercept, a biologic response modifier, inhibits the action of tumor necrosis factor (TNF) and has been shown to reduce active inflammation and improve spinal mobility. Additional anti-TNF agents (infliximab, adalimumab, or golimumab) may also be effective.

Good posture and stretching exercises of the back, neck, and chest help minimize spinal deformity. Hydrotherapy may decrease pain and facilitate spinal extension. Surgery may be needed for severe deformity and mobility impairment. Spinal osteotomy and total joint replacement are the most common procedures.

Nursing Management

A key responsibility is to teach the patient about the nature of the disease and principles of therapy. The home management program consists of local moist heat, regular exercise, and knowledgeable use of drugs.

- Discourage excessive exertion during periods of active inflammation.
- Evaluate chest expansion as part of baseline range-of-motion (ROM) assessment. Encourage smoking cessation to decrease the risk for lung complications.
- Physical therapy should include gentle, graded stretching and strengthening exercises to preserve and improve ROM.
- Encourage the patient to use a firm mattress and sleep on the back with a flat pillow to avoid flexion deformity.
- Stress the need to avoid spinal flexion (e.g., leaning over a desk), heavy lifting, and prolonged walking, standing, or sitting. Encourage sports that involve stretching, such as swimming and racquet games.
- Family counseling and vocational rehabilitation are important.

AORTIC DISSECTION

Description

Aortic dissection, often misnamed "dissecting aneurysm," is not a type of aneurysm. Rather, aortic dissection results from the creation of a false lumen between the intima (inner layer) and media (middle layer) of the arterial wall.

Aortic dissection is classified according to the location of the dissection and duration of symptoms. Type A dissection affects the ascending aorta and arch, requiring emergency surgery. Type B dissection begins in the descending aorta, allowing for potential conservative management. Dissections are also classified as acute (first 14 days), subacute (14–90 days), or chronic (>90 days) based on symptom onset.

- Hypertension is the most important risk factor for aortic dissection.
- Men are at a higher risk of developing aortic dissection than women.
- Other predisposing factors include age, aortic diseases (e.g., aortitis, coarctation, arch hypoplasia), atherosclerosis, blunt trauma, tobacco use, cocaine or methamphetamine use, congenital heart disease (e.g., bicuspid aortic valve), connective tissue disorders (e.g., Marfan syndrome), family history, history of heart surgery, and pregnancy.

Pathophysiology

Most nontraumatic aortic dissections are attributed to weakened elastic fibers in the medial layer. Chronic hypertension accelerates the degradation process. In aortic dissection, the inner wall of the aorta tears. Blood surges through this tear, causing the inner and middle layers to separate (dissect). If the blood-filled channel ruptures through the outside aortic wall, aortic dissection is often fatal.

As the heart contracts, each pulsation increases the pressure on the damaged area, which worsens the dissection. Extension of the dissection may cut off blood supply to the brain, kidneys, spinal cord, and extremities. The false lumen may remain patent, become thrombosed (clotted), rejoin the true lumen by way of a distal tear, or rupture.

Clinical Manifestations and Complications

About 80% of patients with an acute type A aortic dissection report an abrupt onset of severe anterior chest pain or back pain. Patients with acute type B aortic dissection are more likely to report pain in the back, abdomen, or legs. Pain location may overlap between type A and B dissections. The pain may be described as "sharp" and "worst ever," or as "tearing," "ripping," or "stabbing." Dissection pain can be distinguished from myocardial infarction (MI) pain, which is more gradual in onset and intensity.

- Older patients are more likely to have hypotension and vague symptoms. In some cases, aortic dissection may be painless.
- If the aortic arch is involved, the patient may have neurologic deficits, including altered level of consciousness and dizziness, with weakened or absent carotid and temporal pulses.
- Type A aortic dissection usually disrupts coronary artery blood flow and causes aortic valvular insufficiency.
- When either subclavian artery is involved, the pulse quality and BP readings may differ between the left and right arms.
- As dissection progresses down the aorta, the abdominal organs and lower extremities show evidence of altered tissue perfusion.

A life-threatening complication of an acute ascending aortic dissection is *cardiac tamponade*, which occurs when blood from the dissection leaks into the pericardial sac. Manifestations include hypotension, narrowed pulse pressure, distended neck veins, muffled heart sounds, and pulsus paradoxus.

- An aorta weakened by dissection may rupture into the mediastinal, pleural, or abdominal cavity.
- Dissection can lead to occlusion of the blood supply to the spinal cord, kidneys, and abdominal structures. Spinal cord ischemia leads to weakness and decreased sensation. Renal ischemia can lead to renal failure. Signs of abdominal (mesenteric) ischemia include abdominal pain, decreased bowel sounds, and altered bowel elimination.

Diagnostic Studies

Studies to detect aortic dissection are similar to those performed for suspected aneurysms.

- Chest X-ray indicates widening of the mediastinum and pleural effusion.
- Three-dimensional (3-D) CT scanning, transesophageal echocardiography, or MRI may be used to diagnose acute aortic dissection.

Interprofessional Management

Reducing the heart rate (HR), BP, and myocardial contractility limits extension of the acute dissection.

- An IV β-blocker (e.g., esmolol) or calcium channel blocker (e.g., diltiazem) is often titrated to a target HR under 60 beats/minute, or to a systolic BP between 100 and 110 mm Hg.
- Morphine decreases sympathetic nervous system stimulation and relieves pain.

Patients with acute aortic dissection are managed in the intensive care unit. An acute ascending aortic dissection is considered a surgical emergency. Otherwise, surgery is indicated when conservative therapy is ineffective or when complications (e.g., heart failure) occur. Because the aorta is fragile after dissection, surgical intervention is delayed when possible to allow time for edema to decrease and to permit clotting of the blood in the false lumen.

- Surgery involves resection of the aortic segment containing the intimal tear and replacement with a synthetic graft.

Even with prompt surgical intervention, the in-hospital mortality rate for acute aortic dissection is high. Causes of death include aortic rupture, mesenteric ischemia, MI, sepsis, and multiorgan failure.

The patient with an acute or chronic type B descending aortic dissection without complications can be managed nonsurgically. Such conservative treatment includes pain relief, HR and BP control, and cardiovascular disease risk factor modification along with close surveillance imaging with CT or MRI.

- Endovascular repair is a treatment option for an acute descending aortic dissection with complications (e.g., hemodynamic instability) or a chronic descending aortic dissection with complications (e.g., peripheral ischemia).

Nursing Management

Before surgery, nursing care includes keeping the patient in bed in a semi-Fowler position and maintaining a quiet environment. These measures help keep the HR and systolic BP at the lowest possible level that maintains vital organ perfusion (typically HR < 60 beats/minute and systolic BP of 100–120 mm Hg). Manage pain and anxiety, which can cause elevations in the HR and systolic BP. Give opioids and sedatives as prescribed.

- Titrating IV administration of antihypertensive agents requires continuous electroencephalogram and intraarterial BP monitoring. Monitor vital signs frequently, sometimes as often as every 2–3 minutes, until target HR and BP are reached. Look for changes in peripheral pulses and signs of increasing pain, restlessness, and anxiety.

Postoperative care is similar to that after open aneurysm repair (see Aneurysm, Aortic, p. XX).

▼ **Patient and Caregiver Teaching**

- Teach patients and caregivers about taking antihypertensive drugs daily for lifelong control of HR and BP.
- Tell the patient to discuss any side effects (e.g., dizziness, depression, fatigue, erectile dysfunction) with the heath care provider (HCP) before discontinuing prescribed drugs.
- Follow-up with regularly scheduled MRI or CT scans is essential.
- Tell patients that if the pain or other symptoms return, they should contact the emergency response system for immediate care.

APPENDICITIS

Description

Appendicitis is an inflammation of the appendix, a narrow blind tube that extends from the inferior part of the cecum. It is most common in those 10–30 years of age. It is the most common reason for emergency abdominal surgery.

Pathophysiology

Appendicitis is thought to be caused by luminal obstruction. Obstruction results in distention, venous engorgement, and the accumulation of mucus and bacteria. This can lead to gangrene, perforation, and peritonitis.

Clinical Manifestations and Complications

Appendicitis typically begins with dull periumbilical pain, followed by anorexia, nausea, and vomiting. The pain is persistent and continuous, eventually shifting to the right lower quadrant and localizing at McBurney's point (halfway between the umbilicus and right iliac crest).

- Further assessment reveals rigidity, rebound tenderness, and muscle guarding. Coughing, sneezing, and deep inhalation magnify the pain.
- Positive psoas (pain with extension of right thigh), obturator (pain with passive internal rotation of the flexed thigh), and Rovsing signs (increased right lower quadrant pain occurring with left lower quadrant palpation) lend to the diagnosis.
- The patient usually prefers to lie still, often with the right leg flexed.
- A low-grade fever may develop.

If diagnosis and treatment are delayed, the appendix can rupture. The resulting peritonitis can be fatal.

Diagnostic Studies

- White blood cell count is usually high.
- Urinalysis is done to rule out genitourinary conditions that mimic appendicitis.
- CT scan and ultrasound may be used.

Interprofessional Management

Treatment is immediate surgical removal of the appendix (appendectomy) if the inflammation is localized. If the appendix has ruptured and there is evidence of peritonitis or an abscess, giving antibiotics and IV fluids for 6–8 h before the appendectomy helps prevent sepsis and dehydration.

Nursing Management

- Nothing should be taken by mouth to ensure that the stomach will be empty if surgery is needed.
- Postoperative nursing management is similar to postoperative care of a patient after laparotomy (see Abdominal Pain, Acute).
- Patients are usually discharged within 24 h after an uncomplicated laparoscopic appendectomy. Those who had a perforation have a longer length of stay and need IV antibiotics. Ambulation begins a few hours after surgery, and the diet is advanced as tolerated. Most patients resume normal activities in 2–3 weeks.

ASTHMA

Description

Asthma is a disease characterized by bronchial hyperreactivity with reversible expiratory airflow limitation, either spontaneously or with treatment. Signs and symptoms can be variable. For example, there may be mild shortness of breath and chest tightness with a minor asthma attack. A major asthma attack may include severe shortness of breath, accessory muscle use, stridor, and severe hypoxemia. If left untreated, respiratory and/or cardiac arrest can occur.

- Asthma affects an estimated 25 million adult Americans. More than 4000 people die each year from asthma. In adulthood, asthma affects more women.

Risk factors for asthma and triggers of asthma attacks are listed in Table 11.

Pathophysiology

Asthma involves persistent but variable airway inflammation. Exposure to allergens or irritants initiates the inflammatory cascade. Airflow is limited because inflammation results in bronchoconstriction, airway hyperresponsiveness (hyperactivity), and airway edema.

- As the inflammatory process begins, mast cells in the bronchial wall release multiple inflammatory mediators, including leukotrienes, histamine, cytokines, prostaglandins, and nitric oxide.
- Inflammatory mediators have effects on the (1) blood vessels, causing vasodilation, and increasing capillary permeability (runny nose); (2) nerve cells, causing itching; (3) smooth

TABLE 11   Triggers of Asthma Attacks

Air Pollutants
- Aerosol sprays
- Cigarette smoke
- Exhaust fumes
- Oxidants
- Perfumes
- Sulfur dioxides

Allergen Inhalation
- Animal dander (e.g., cats, mice, guinea pigs)
- Cockroaches
- House dust mites
- Molds
- Pollens

Drugs
- Aspirin
- Nonsteroidal antiinflammatory drugs
- β-Adrenergic blockers

Food Additives
- Sulfites (bisulfites and metabisulfites)
- Beer, wine, dried fruit, shrimp, processed potatoes
- Monosodium glutamate
- Tartrazine

Occupational Exposure
- Agriculture, farming
- Paints, solvents
- Laundry detergents
- Metal salts
- Wood and vegetable dusts
- Industrial chemicals and plastics
- Pharmaceutical agents

Other Factors
- Exercise and cold, dry air
- Stress
- Hormones, menses
- Gastroesophageal reflux disease

Viral or Bacterial Infection
- Sinusitis, allergic rhinitis
- Viral upper respiratory tract infection

muscle cells, causing bronchial spasms and airway narrowing; and (4) goblet cells, causing mucus production.

- The *early-phase response* in asthma occurs within minutes after exposure to a trigger or irritant.
- A *late-phase response* occurs in about 50% of people with asthma. Symptoms can recur 4–6 hr after the early response because of the influx of inflammatory cells and the further release of inflammatory mediators.
- Bronchoconstriction with symptoms lasts for 24 hr or more. Corticosteroids are often effective in treating inflammation in this phase.

Chronic inflammation may cause structural changes in the bronchial wall known as "remodeling." A progressive loss of lung function is not fully reversed by therapy.

Clinical Manifestations

Asthma signs and symptoms can differ for each patient. The most common manifestations include cough, shortness of breath (dyspnea), wheezing, chest tightness, and variable airflow obstruction. The presence of any of these (usually in combination) can indicate that an asthma episode or attack is occurring. Attacks may last for a few minutes to several hours.

- Characteristic manifestations are wheezing, cough, dyspnea, and chest tightness. Expiration may be prolonged, with an inspiratory/expiratory (I/E) ratio of 1:3 or 1:4.
- Wheezing is an unreliable sign to gauge the severity of an attack because many patients with minor attacks wheeze loudly, whereas others with severe attacks do not wheeze.
- Diminished breath sounds may indicate a significant decrease in air movement. Severely diminished breath sounds or a "silent chest" when the patient is struggling after a period of wheezing is an ominous sign, indicating severe obstruction and impending respiratory failure.
- In some patients with asthma, cough is the only symptom. The cough may be nonproductive with secretions so thick, tenacious, and gelatinous that their removal is difficult.
- During an acute attack, the patient usually sits upright or slightly bent forward, using accessory muscles of respiration. The more difficult the breathing becomes, the more anxious the patient feels.
- The patient is hypoxemic early on, with decreased partial pressure of CO_2 in arterial blood ($PaCO_2$) and increased pH (respiratory alkalosis) caused by hyperventilation.
- Signs of hypoxemia include restlessness, increased anxiety, confusion, increased pulse, and BP.
- As the airflow limitation worsens with air trapping, the patient works much harder to breathe. The $PaCO_2$ normalizes as the patient tires and then increases to produce respiratory acidosis, which is an ominous sign of respiratory failure.

Classification of Asthma

Asthma can be classified as intermittent, mild persistent, moderate persistent, or severe persistent (Table 12). Asthma severity is used to guide treatment decisions. Patients may have different levels of severity over the course of the disease.

TABLE 12 Classification of Asthma Severity

Components of Severity	Intermittent	ASTHMA SEVERITY			
		Mild	Moderate	Severe	
			PERSISTENT		
Impairment					
Symptoms	≤2 days/week	>2 days/week, not daily	Daily	Continuous	
Nighttime awakenings	≤2/mo	3–4/mo	>1/week, not nightly	Often 7/week	
SABA use for symptoms	≤2 days/week	>2 days/week, not daily	Daily	Several times per day	
Interference with normal activity	None	Minor limitation	Some limitation	Extremely limited	
Lung function[a]	Normal FEV$_1$ between attacks FEV$_1$ > 80% FEV$_1$/FVC normal	FEV$_1$ >80% predicted FEV$_1$/FVC normal	FEV$_1$ 60%–80% predicted FEV$_1$/FVC reduced by 5%	FEV$_1$ < 60% predicted FEV$_1$/FVC reduced by 5%	
Risk					
Attacks requiring oral corticosteroids	0–1/year	≥2/year even in the absence of impairment			
		Consider severity and interval since last attack			
		Frequency and severity may fluctuate over time			
		Relative annual risk of exacerbation may be related to FEV$_1$			

A

Recommended Step for Initiating Treatment	Step 1	Step 2	Step 3[b]	Step 4 or 5[b]
		Reevaluate asthma control in 2–6 weeks and adjust therapy accordingly		

Guidelines for Using Table

- Patients should be assigned to the most severe step in which any feature occurs. Clinical features for may overlap across steps. Determine level of severity by assessment of both impairment and risk. Assess impairment by previous 2–4 week spirometry results.
- A person's classification should change over time with treatment. After treatment, the focus switches to the level of control, not the classification of severity.
- Patients at any level of severity of chronic asthma can have mild, moderate, or severe asthma attacks. Some patients with intermittent asthma have severe and life-threatening attacks separated by long periods of normal lung function and no symptoms.

FEV$_1$, forced expiratory volume in 1 s; FVC, forced vital capacity; SABA, short-acting β_2-adrenergic agonist.
[a]Percent predicted values for FEV$_1$, or ratio of FEV$_1$/FVC. Normal FEV$_1$/FVC: 8–19 year, 85%; 20–39 year, 80%; 40–59 year, 75%; 60–80 year, 70%.
[b]Consider short-term corticosteroid therapy.
Adapted from National Asthma Education and Prevention Program, National Heart, Lung, and Blood Institute: *Expert Panel Report 3: guidelines for the diagnosis and management of asthma*, NIH pub no 08-4051, Bethesda, MD, 2007, National Institutes of Health.

Complications

In severe asthma exacerbations, the patient is dyspneic at rest and speaks in single words because of the difficulty breathing.

- The patient is often agitated, sitting forward to maximize the diaphragmatic movement and using accessory muscles in the neck to lift the chest wall. Respiratory rate may be > 30 breaths/minute and pulse >120 beats/minute. The peak flow (PEFR [peak expiratory flow rate]) is <50% of the patient's personal best.
- A life-threatening medical emergency, *status asthmaticus* is the most extreme form of an acute asthma attack. It is characterized by hypoxia, hypercarbia, and acute respiratory failure unresponsive to treatment with bronchodilators and corticosteroids. The patient may have chest tightness, a severely marked increase in shortness of breath, or suddenly be unable to speak. Hypotension, bradycardia, respiratory, and/or cardiac arrest may occur. The patient needs immediate intubation and mechanical ventilation.

Diagnostic Studies

Underdiagnosis of asthma is common. The history is important to determine if a person has had similar attacks, which are often precipitated by a known trigger.

- The PEFR measured by the peak flow meter (at home or in a health care setting) is a test of current lung function.
- Spirometry determines the reversibility of bronchoconstriction. Spirometry, oximetry, and arterial blood gases provide information about the severity of the attack and response to treatment.
- Chest X-ray during an attack shows hyperinflation.
- Sputum specimen can be used to rule out bacterial infection.
- High serum immunoglobulin E levels and eosinophil counts suggest allergy.
- Allergy skin testing can be used to determine sensitivity to specific allergens.

Interprofessional Management

The goal of asthma treatment is to achieve and maintain control of the disease. The health care provider (HCP) steps down the medication, as the patient achieves control of the symptoms or steps it up as the symptoms worsen.

Drug Therapy

The classification of asthma severity (see Table 12) helps determine which types of medications are best suited to control the symptoms.

- Guidelines recommend using inhaled corticosteroids (ICSs) as first-line agents in an acute asthma attack and as the first step in acute asthma management. They are the most effective short-term controller drugs for asthma.
- Patients in all classifications of asthma require a rescue medication for *short-term*, immediate control of symptoms. Short-acting β_2-adrenergic agonists (SABAs) (e.g., albuterol [ProAir HFA, Proventil HFA, Ventolin HFA]) are the most effective class of drugs used as rescue medications. Patients with persistent asthma must also be on a long-term or controller medication.
- For *long-term* control of moderate to severe persistent asthma, long-acting β_2-adrenergic agonists (LABAs) are added to daily ICSs (e.g., fluticasone [Flovent]). Like SABAs, LABAs should not be used alone as primary treatment. They should only be used only if the patient does not respond to medium-dose ICS. Examples of LABAs used in the treatment of asthma attacks include salmeterol and formoterol.

Acute Asthma Exacerbations

Asthma exacerbations may be mild to life-threatening. Patients with mild or moderate asthma attacks are often seen in the community at an outpatient clinic. A severe acute asthma attack is usually frightening enough for patients to go to the emergency department. In many cases, a severe asthma attack will warrant hospital admission.

- Management of the patient with a severe asthma attack focuses on correcting hypoxemia and continually observing and/or improving ventilation. Supplemental O_2 is given by nasal cannula or mask to achieve a PaO_2 of at least 60 mm Hg or O_2 saturation >93%. O_2 monitoring should be continuous with pulse oximetry.

Nursing Management

Goals

The patient with asthma will have minimal symptoms during the day and night, acceptable activity levels (including exercise), greater than 80% of personal best PEFR, few or no adverse effects of drug therapy, no acute asthma attacks, and adequate knowledge to carry out the treatment plan.

Nursing Interventions

A goal in asthma care is to maximize the patient's ability to safely manage acute asthma attacks via an action plan developed with the HCP.

- If a patient's PEFR is in the green zone (usually 80%–100% of the patient's personal best), the patient should take their usual medications. A PEFR within the yellow zone (usually

50%–80% of personal best) indicates caution. A PEFR in the red zone (50% or less of personal best) indicates a serious problem. In other words, something is triggering the patient's asthma (e.g., viral infection). The patient should seek out their HCP as soon as possible.

- During an acute attack requiring care, monitor the respiratory and cardiovascular systems. This includes auscultating lung sounds and monitoring heart rate and respiratory rate, BP, pulse oximetry, and peak flow.
- The patient may feel anxious or have a sense of panic. Stay with the patient. A calm, quiet, reassuring attitude may help the patient relax. Position the patient comfortably (usually sitting) to maximize chest expansion.
- Maintain eye contact and use a firm, calm voice to coach the patient in pursed-lip breathing, which keeps the airways open by maintaining positive pressure.
- See eNursing Care Plan 31.1 on the website.

▼ **Patient and Caregiver Teaching**

A patient and caregiver teaching guide for the patient with asthma is presented in Table 13 (Fig. 2).

TABLE 13   Patient and Caregiver Teaching: Asthma

Include the following information in a teaching plan for the patient with asthma and the caregiver. It will help improve the patient's quality of life and promote lifestyle changes that support successful living with asthma.

What is Asthma?
- Basic anatomy and physiology of lung
- Pathophysiology of asthma
- Relationship of pathophysiology to signs and symptoms
- Measurement and correlation of spirometry and peak expiratory flow rate

What is Good Asthma Control?
- Personal ideas of good control
- Use Asthma Control Test available at *www.asthmacontroltest.com.*

Obstacles to Asthma Treatment and Control
- Discuss possible obstacles (e.g., denial, poor perception of asthma severity, cost of medications) with patient and caregiver

TABLE 13   Patient and Caregiver Teaching: Asthma—cont'd

Environmental and Trigger Control

- Identify possible triggers and possible preventive measures (use triggor diary)
- Avoid allergens and other triggers
- Maintain good hydration

Medications

- Classes (include mechanism of action)
- Terms: Controller, reliever, and alternate reliever
- Correct use of inhalers, spacer, and nebulizer
- Write out a medication list, identify schedule

Asthma Action Plan (Fig. 31.11 in Harding et al., *Lewis' Medical-Surgical Nursing,* ed 12)

- Peak flow zones
- Patient-centered care asthma action plan with HCP and patient
- Early recognition of infection
- Building a partnership with the health care provider

Pursed-lip Breathing

- See Chapter 28 in Harding et al., *Lewis' Medical-Surgical Nursing,* ed 12)

Correct Use of Peak Flow Meter

- See Table 31.14 in Harding et al., *Lewis' Medical-Surgical Nursing,* ed 12

For more information, visit the American Lung Association website at http://www.lung.org/lung-disease/asthma.

Using an inhaler seems simple, but most patients do not use it the right way. When you use your inhaler the wrong way, less medicine gets to your lungs. (Your physician may give you other types of inhalers.)

For the next 2 weeks, read these steps aloud as you do them or ask someone to read them to you. Ask your physician or nurse to check how well you are using your inhaler.

Use your inhaler in one of the three ways pictured below (**A** or **B** is best, but **C** can be used if you have trouble with **A** or **B**).

Steps for Using Your Inhaler

Getting ready   1. Take off the cap and shake the inhaler.
2. Breathe out all the way.
3. Hold your inhaler the way your doctor said (**A**, **B**, or **C** below).

Breathe in slowly   4. As you start breathing in **slowly** through your mouth, press down on the inhaler **one** time. (If you use a holding chamber, first press down on the inhaler. Within 5 seconds, begin to breathe in slowly.)
5. Keep breathing in **slowly**, as deeply as you can.

Hold your breath   6. Hold your breath as you count to 10 slowly, if you can.
7. For inhaled quick-relief medicine (β_2-agonists), wait about 1 minute between puffs. There is no need to wait between puffs for other medicines.

A. Hold inhaler 1 to 2 inches in front of your mouth (about the width of two fingers).

B. Use a spacer/holding chamber. These come in many shapes and can be useful to any patient.

C. Put the inhaler in your mouth.

Clean Your Inhaler as Needed

Look at the hole where the medicine sprays out from your inhaler. If you see "powder" in or around the hole, clean the inhaler. Remove the metal canister from the L-shaped plastic mouthpiece. Rinse only the mouthpiece and cap in warm water. Let them dry overnight. In the morning, put the canister back inside. Put the cap on.

Know When to Replace Your Inhaler

For medicines you take each day (an example): Say your new canister has 200 puffs (number of puffs is listed on canister) and you are told to take 8 puffs per day.

$$8 \text{ puffs per day} \overline{) \begin{array}{c} 25 \text{ days} \\ 200 \text{ puffs} \\ \text{in canister} \end{array}}$$

So this canister will last 25 days. If you started using this inhaler on May 1, replace it on or before May 25. You can write the date on your canister.

For quick-relief medicine take as needed and count each puff.

Do not put your canister in water to see if it is empty, as water may enter MDI and impair inhaler.

Figure 2 How to use your metered-dose inhaler.

BELL PALSY

Description

Bell palsy is an acute, usually temporary, facial paresis (or palsy) resulting from damage or trauma of the facial nerve (CN VII). CN VII is a mixed cranial nerve with motor, sensory, and autonomic function.

Bell palsy can affect one or both sides of the face. It is the most common facial nerve disorder.

- Most patients recover within 2 weeks–6 months.
- In some cases, there may be residual effects, including facial asymmetry or abnormal facial movements.

B

Pathophysiology

It is believed that reactivation of a dormant viral infection, such as herpes simplex virus 1 or herpes zoster virus, may trigger Bell palsy. The viral infection causes inflammation, leading to nerve compression and clinical features such as facial paralysis. Another cause may be acute demyelination similar to what happens in Guillain-Barré syndrome.

- There is a high incidence of Bell palsy during pregnancy and in persons with upper respiratory tract conditions (e.g., flu, colds). Risk factors include obesity, diabetes, and hypertension.

Clinical Manifestations

The key feature is the acute onset of unilateral lower motor facial weakness. Pain around and behind the ear and neck is present in 50%–60% of patients. Other manifestations include drooping of the eyelid and corner of the mouth, drooling, facial twitching, dryness of the eye or mouth, facial numbness, altered taste, hearing loss, and excessive tearing in one eye. Most often, these symptoms begin suddenly and reach their peak within 48–72 hr.

- The diagnosis is based on clinical examination and history.
- Quality of life is often decreased due to problems with eating, swallowing, speech, and taste. Patients may have psychologic withdrawal because of changes in appearance, muscle stretching, and facial spasms and contractures. They may have malnutrition, dehydration, mucous membrane trauma, or corneal abrasions.

Interprofessional and Nursing Management

Care is primarily focused on relief of symptoms, protection of the eye on the affected side, and prevention of complications.

- Oral corticosteroid therapy to reduce inflammation and swelling should be started within 72 hr of onset. Some patients receive an antiviral agent, such as acyclovir (Zovirax), in addition to the steroid therapy.
- A facial sling may be fitted by an occupational or physical therapist to support affected muscles, improve lip alignment, and facilitate eating.
- Surgical decompression of the facial nerve is controversial.

Methods of treatment include moist heat, gentle massage, electrical stimulation of the nerve, and prescribed exercises. Mild analgesics can relieve pain. When function begins to return, active facial exercises are performed several times per day.

- Tell the patient to protect the face from cold and drafts because *trigeminal hyperesthesia* (extreme sensitivity to pain or touch) may occur.

- Maintenance of good nutrition is important. Teach the patient to chew on the unaffected side of the mouth to avoid trapping food and improve taste. Thorough oral hygiene after each meal helps to prevent development of parotitis, caries, and periodontal disease from residual food.

- Dark glasses may be worn for protective and cosmetic reasons. Artificial tears (methylcellulose) can be instilled frequently during the day to prevent corneal drying. Ointment and an impermeable eye shield or taping the eyelid shut at night helps protect from corneal injury.

The change in physical appearance as a result of Bell palsy can be devastating. Support from family and friends is important. Reassure the patient that chances for a full recovery are good.

BENIGN PAROXYSMAL POSITIONAL VERTIGO

Benign paroxysmal positional vertigo (BPPV) is a condition in which free-floating debris "ear rocks" in the semicircular canal causes vertigo with specific head movements, such as getting out of bed, rolling over in bed, and sitting up from lying down. The debris is composed of small calcium carbonate crystals that may develop in the inner ear due to head trauma, infection, the aging process, or from an unknown cause.

Symptoms are intermittent and include dizziness, vertigo, lightheadedness, loss of balance, and nausea. There is no hearing loss. Symptoms of BPPV may be confused with those of Ménière disease. Diagnosis is based on auditory and vestibular testing results.

A person experiencing BPPV is at risk for falls. A trained health care provider can teach the patient how to perform a repositioning maneuver that may provide symptom relief (See Chapter 23 in Harding et al., *Lewis's Medical-Surgical Nursing*, ed 12 for a description of the procedure.)

BENIGN PROSTATIC HYPERPLASIA

Description

Benign prostatic hyperplasia (BPH) is a condition in which the prostate gland increases in size, disrupting the flow of urine from the bladder through the urethra. Half of men will develop some signs of BPH by the age of 50 years. That number increases to more than 70% for men 60–69 years old.

Pathophysiology

As men age, decreased testosterone levels result in a higher proportion of estrogen within the prostate gland. This increases the activity of substances, including dihydroxytestosterone (DHT), which promote prostate cell growth. BPH usually develops in the inner part of the prostate. As the prostate enlarges, it gradually compresses the urethra, leading to partial or complete obstruction.

- The location of the enlargement is significant. Even mild prostate enlargement can cause severe symptoms.
- Risk factors for BPH include aging, obesity (especially increased waist circumference), lack of physical activity, a high amount of red meat and animal fat, alcohol use, erectile dysfunction (ED), smoking, and diabetes. A family history of BPH in a first-degree relative may also be a risk factor.

Clinical Manifestations

Symptoms of BPH can include lower urinary tract symptoms. As the severity of urethral obstruction increases, the symptoms gradually worsen. Symptoms can be divided into two groups: obstructive and irritative.

- *Obstructive symptoms* of BPH caused by urinary retention include a decrease in the caliber and force of the urinary stream, difficulty in initiating voiding, intermittency (stopping and starting stream several times while voiding), and dribbling at the end of urination.
- *Irritative symptoms,* including nocturia, urinary frequency, urgency, dysuria, bladder pain, and incontinence, are related to inflammation and infection.

Complications

- Acute urinary retention is a sudden and painful inability to urinate. Treatment involves the insertion of a bladder catheter. Surgery may also be indicated.

- Urinary tract infection and pyelonephritis can result from incomplete bladder emptying, which provides an environment for bacterial growth.
- Calculi may develop in the bladder because of alkalinization of the residual urine.
- Hydronephrosis from back pressure of urine in an obstructed system may lead to renal failure.

Diagnostic Studies

- Physical examination including a digital rectal examination (DRE) to determine prostate size, symmetry, and consistency
- Urinalysis with culture to determine the presence of infection
- Postvoid residual urine volume to assess the degree of urine flow obstruction
- Prostate-specific antigen (PSA) blood test to rule out prostate cancer
- Uroflowmetry studies
- Transrectal ultrasound scan of prostate, possibly with biopsy, or renal ultrasound
- Cystoscopy to visualize the urethra and bladder

Interprofessional Management

The goals of collaborative care are to restore bladder drainage, relieve the patient's symptoms, and prevent or treat the complications of BPH. Treatment is generally based on the degree of symptoms or complications, rather than on the size of the prostate.

- Dietary changes (decreasing intake of bladder irritants such as caffeine, alcohol, carbonated drinks, artificial sweeteners, and spicy or acidic foods), avoiding medications such as decongestants and anticholinergics, and restricting evening fluid intake may reduce symptoms.
- A timed voiding schedule (also referred to as "bladder retraining") may reduce symptoms.

If the patient has signs or symptoms that indicate an increase in obstruction, further treatment is indicated. See Table 14 for descriptions of minimally invasive and surgical treatment options.

Drug Therapy

Drugs are used to treat BPH with variable results.

- 5α-Reductase inhibitors reduce the size of the prostate gland. Finasteride (Proscar) blocks the enzyme needed to convert testosterone to DHT, the principal intraprostatic androgen. This results in a regression of hyperplastic tissue. Serum PSA levels may decrease by almost 50% in patients taking finasteride.

TABLE 14 Treatment for Benign Prostatic Hyperplasia

Description	Advantages	Disadvantages
Minimally Invasive		
Laser Enucleation of the Prostate		
Laser beams used to rapidly vaporize and coagulate prostate tissue. Laser does not penetrate deep tissue. Two types of lasers in this class: Holmium laser enucleation of the prostate and thulium laser enucleation of the prostate.	• Outpatient procedure • Better coagulative properties in tissue compared with TURP • Comparable results to TURP and PVP • Minimal bleeding • Fast recovery time	• Catheter needed after for 24–48 h • Irritative voiding symptoms, urinary incontinence • Hematuria • Retrograde ejaculation • May be more difficult to perform compared with PVP
Photoselective Vaporization of the Prostate (PVP)		
Uses a laser beam to cut or destroy part of the prostate. May be more effective for small- to moderate-sized prostates.	• Short procedure • Comparable results to TURP • Minimal bleeding • Fast recovery time • Rapid symptom improvement • Very effective	• Catheter needed up to 7 days after due to edema and urinary retention • Delayed sloughing of tissue • Takes several weeks to reach optimal effect • Retrograde ejaculation
Prostatic Urethral Lift (PUL)		
Permanent transprostatic implants/tension sutures placed transurethrally via cystoscope. Mechanically opens the prostatic urethra by compressing the prostate tissue/parenchyma.	• Outpatient procedure • Erectile dysfunction (ED), urinary incontinence, and retrograde ejaculation are minimal • No change in PSA since no prostate tissue ablated	• Lack of long-term durability/results • Treatment response rates slightly lower when compared with TURP • If unsuccessful, may need repeat PUL or TURP in the future

Continued

TABLE 14   Treatment for Benign Prostatic Hyperplasia—cont'd

Description	Advantages	Disadvantages
Transurethral Microwave Thermotherapy		
Use of microwave radiating heat to produce coagulative necrosis of the prostate.	• Outpatient procedure • ED, urinary incontinence, and retrograde ejaculation are rare • Mild effects: bladder spasm, hematuria, dysuria	• Potential for damage to surrounding tissue • Urinary catheter needed after for 2–7 days • Not appropriate for men with rectal problems
Transurethral Needle Ablation		
Low-wave radiofrequency used to heat the prostate, causing necrosis.	• Outpatient procedure • ED, urinary incontinence, and retrograde ejaculation are rare • Precise delivery of heat to desired area • Very little pain • Early return to activities	• Urinary retention common • Irritative voiding symptoms • Hematuria for up to a week • May need a catheter for a short time after
Transurethral Vaporization of Prostate		
Electrosurgical modification of the standard TURP. Vaporization and desiccation are used together to destroy prostatic tissue. Can use a variety of energy delivery mediums (e.g., button, rollerball, VaporTrode).	• Minimal risks • Minimal bleeding and sloughing	• Retrograde ejaculation • Intermittent hematuria

TABLE 14   Treatment for Benign Prostatic Hyperplasia—cont'd

Description	Advantages	Disadvantages
Water Vapor Thermal Therapy		
Heated water vapor/steam used to destroy obstructive prostate tissue. Delivered transurethrally via handheld device with a retractable needle that releases the water vapor in 9-second doses.	• Outpatient procedure • Can be done in an outpatient office setting • ED, urinary incontinence, and retrograde ejaculation are rare • Precise delivery of steam to desired area • Very little pain	• Relatively new, so lack of long-term durability/results • Irritative voiding symptoms and urinary tract infection • Hematuria
Surgical Therapy		
Transurethral Incision of Prostate		
Involves transurethral incisions into prostatic tissue to relieve obstruction. Effective for small to moderate prostates.	• Outpatient procedure • Minimal complications • Low occurrence of ED or retrograde ejaculation • Outcomes similar to TURP	• Urinary catheter needed after
Transurethral Resection of Prostate (TURP)		
Use of excision and cauterization to remove prostate tissue via cystoscope. Standard for treatment of benign prostatic hyperplasia.	• ED unlikely	• Bleeding, clot retention • Retrograde ejaculation • Catheter needed after

Continued

TABLE 14 Treatment for Benign Prostatic Hyperplasia—cont'd

Description	Advantages	Disadvantages
Simple Prostatectomy (Open, Laparoscopic, or Robotic-Assisted)		
Surgery of choice for men with large prostates (often >100 g), bladder damage, or other complicating factors. If open, involves an external incision with two possible approaches (either retropubic or perineal). If laparoscopic and/or robotic-assisted, involves several small abdominal incisions and one slightly larger incision near the umbilicus.	• Complete visualization of the prostate and surrounding tissue	• ED • Bleeding • Pain • Risk for infection

■ Dutasteride (Avodart) is a dual inhibitor of 5α-reductase type 1 and 2 isoenzymes.

■ α-Adrenergic receptor blockers are used, including alfuzosin (Uroxatral), doxazosin (Cardura), prazosin (Minipress), tamsulosin (Flomax), and silodosin (Rapaflo). These drugs offer symptom relief by relaxing the smooth muscle of the prostate that surrounds the urethra, but do not decrease the overall size of the prostate.

■ Tadalafil (Cialis) has been shown to be effective in reducing symptoms for both BPH and ED.

■ Saw palmetto has been shown to have no benefit over a placebo in reducing BPH symptoms. Advise patients to discuss all herbal therapies being used with their health care provider (HCP).

Nursing Management

The focus of nursing management is on health promotion for early detection and treatment, preoperative care, and postoperative care.

Goals

Overall preoperative goals for the patient having prostatic surgery are to restore urinary drainage, resolve urinary tract infection, and understand the upcoming surgery. Overall postoperative goals are that the patient will have no complications, restoration of urinary control, complete bladder emptying, and satisfying sexual expression.

Nursing Interventions

When symptoms of prostatic hyperplasia become evident, further diagnostic screening may be necessary.

- Consuming alcohol and caffeine may increase prostatic symptoms because of the diuretic effect that increases bladder distention.
- Compounds found in common cough and cold remedies, such as pseudoephedrine (e.g., Sudafed) and phenylephrine, often worsen the symptoms of BPH.
- Advise patients with obstructive symptoms to urinate every 2–3 hr or when they first feel the urge, to minimize urinary stasis and acute urinary retention.

Preoperative Care. Urinary drainage must be restored before surgery. A urethral catheter, such as a coudé (curved-tip) catheter, may be needed.

- Any infection of the urinary tract must be treated before surgery. Restoring drainage and encouraging a high fluid intake (2–3 L/day) are helpful.
- Patients are often concerned about the impact of surgery on sexual function. Provide an opportunity for the patient and his partner to express concerns.

Postoperative Care. Adjust the plan of care to the type of surgery, reasons for surgery, and patient response to surgery.

- After surgery, bladder irrigation is often done to remove clotted blood from the bladder and ensure drainage of urine. The bladder is irrigated either manually, on an intermittent basis, or as continuous bladder irrigation with sterile normal saline solution or another prescribed solution. Monitor the inflow and outflow of the irrigant. The infusion of the continuous bladder irrigation fluid should be at a rate to keep the urine drainage light pink without clots.
- The catheter should be connected to a closed drainage system and not disconnected unless it is being removed, changed, or irrigated. Blood clots are expected for the first 24–36 hr.

However, large amounts of bright red blood in the urine can indicate hemorrhage.

- Painful bladder spasms occur as a result of irritation of the bladder mucosa. Tell the patient not to urinate around the catheter because this increases the chance of spasm. If bladder spasms develop, check the catheter for clots. If present, remove the clots by manual irrigation so urine flows freely. Belladonna and opium suppositories, along with relaxation techniques, are used to relieve pain and spasms.

- Sphincter tone may be poor after catheter removal, resulting in urinary incontinence or dribbling. Have the patient practice Kegel exercises (pelvic floor muscle technique) 10 to 20 times per hour while awake. Continence can improve for up to 12 months.

- Observe for signs of postoperative infection. If an external wound is present, observe the area for redness, heat, swelling, and purulent drainage. Rectal procedures, such as rectal temperatures and enemas (except insertion of well-lubricated belladonna and opium suppositories), should be avoided.

- A diet high in fiber and stool softeners is important to prevent straining with bowel movements.

- Activities that increase abdominal pressure, such as sitting or walking for prolonged periods and straining to have a bowel movement (Valsalva maneuver), should be avoided.

▼ Patient and Caregiver Teaching

Discharge planning and home care issues are important aspects of care after prostate surgery.

- Instructions include (1) caring for an indwelling catheter, if one is in place; (2) managing urinary incontinence; (3) maintaining oral fluid intake; (4) observing for signs and symptoms of urinary tract and wound infection; (5) preventing constipation; (6) avoiding heavy lifting (more than 10 lb [more than 4.5 kg]); and (7) refraining from driving or sexual intercourse as directed by the HCP.

- Retrograde ejaculation may occur due to trauma to the internal sphincter. Semen is discharged into the bladder at orgasm and may produce cloudy urine when the patient urinates after orgasm. Discuss these changes with the patient and partner and allow them to ask questions and express their concerns.

- Sexual counseling and treatment options may be needed if ED becomes a chronic issue.

- The bladder may take up to 2 months to return to its normal capacity. Teach the patient to drink at least 2–3 L of fluid per day and to urinate every 2–3 hr to flush the urinary tract.

- Teach the patient to avoid or limit bladder irritants such as caffeine products, citrus juices, and alcohol.

■ Advise the patient to discuss the need for a yearly DRE with the HCP if prostate tissue was not completely removed. Hyperplasia or cancer can occur in the remaining prostatic tissue.

BLADDER CANCER

Description

Bladder cancer is the most common cancer of the urinary system. Most bladder tumors are papillomatous growths. The most frequent cancerous tumor of the urinary tract is transitional cell cancer of the bladder.

■ About half of bladder cancers are related to cigarette smoking. Other risk factors include workplace exposure to certain chemicals. Others at risk include those treated with pelvic radiation for cancer; patients who received cyclophosphamide or aristolochic acid; and those who have indwelling catheters for long periods. People with chronic, recurrent urinary tract stones, often in the bladder, and chronic lower UTIs have an increased risk for nonurethral bladder cancer such as squamous cell carcinoma.

Ninety percent of cases occur in those over the age of 55 years. Bladder cancer is more common in men and in whites.

Clinical Manifestations and Diagnostic Studies

Microscopic or gross, painless hematuria (chronic or intermittent) is the most common clinical finding. Dysuria, frequency, and urgency may occur because of bladder irritability.

■ Urine specimens may contain cancer or atypical cells.
■ Ultrasound, CT, or MRI may be used to detect bladder cancer.
■ Cystoscopy and biopsy are used to confirm a diagnosis of bladder cancer.

Pathologic grading systems are used to classify the cancer potential of tumor cells on a scale ranging from well-differentiated to undifferentiated.

Interprofessional and Nursing Management

The majority of bladder cancers are diagnosed at an early stage when the cancer is treatable. Low-stage, low-grade, superficial bladder cancers are most common and most responsive to treatment.

Surgical therapies include a variety of procedures:

■ *Transurethral resection of the bladder tumor* (TURBT) is used for superficial lesions of the bladder's inner lining. This procedure is also used to control bleeding in the patient who is at post

operative risk or who has advanced tumors. The primary disadvantages of TURBT include the chance of incomplete tumor
removal, bleeding, and bladder perforation.

- A segmental cystectomy *(partial cystectomy)* is used to treat
larger tumors or those that involve only one area of the bladder.
The part of the bladder wall containing the tumor is removed
along with a margin of normal tissue.
- A *radical cystectomy* involves removal of the bladder, prostate,
and seminal vesicles in men and the bladder, uterus, cervix,
anterior vagina, and ovaries in women. After a radical cystectomy, a new way for urine to leave the body, or *urinary diversion*, must be created.

Postoperative management for any of these procedures includes
instructions to drink large amounts of fluid, use opioid analgesics
and stool softeners if necessary, and take sitz baths to promote muscle relaxation and reduce urinary retention.

Radiation therapy can be used in combination with cystectomy or
as the primary therapy when the cancer is inoperable or the patient
declines surgery. Chemotherapy is often used in combination with
radiation. Targeted therapy includes FGFR inhibitors (e.g., erdafi-
tinib) that affect proteins that help the cancer cells grow. Immunotherapy can be used to treat bladder cancer. Options include
immune checkpoint inhibitors, PD-1 and PD-L1 inhibitors, and
intravesical Bacillus Calmette-Guérin (BCG).Other intravesical
chemotherapy agents include mitomycin, epirubicin, gemcitabine,
and valrubicin.

After intravesical therapy, most patients have irritative voiding
symptoms and hemorrhagic cystitis.

- Encourage patients to increase daily fluid intake and to quit smoking. Assess the patient for a secondary UTI and stress the need
for routine urologic follow-up care. Address fears or concerns the
patient may have about sexual activity or bladder function.

BONE TUMORS

Description

Primary *bone tumors*, both benign and malignant, are rare in adults.
They account for only about 3% of all tumors. Metastatic bone
cancer, in which the cancer has spread from another site, is more
common.

- Benign bone tumors, such as osteochondroma, osteoclastoma,
and enchondroma, are often removed by surgery.

- Primary bone cancer is called *sarcoma*. The more common types of primary bone cancer are osteosarcoma, chondrosarcoma, and Ewing sarcoma. Primary malignant tumors occur most often during childhood and young adulthood. They cause bone destruction and have rapid metastasis.

Osteochondroma

Osteochondroma is the most common primary benign bone tumor. It is characterized by an overgrowth of cartilage and bone near the end of the bone at the growth plate. It is more often found in the pelvis, scapula, or long bones of the leg.

- Clinical manifestations of osteochondroma include a painless, hard, and immobile mass; lower-than-normal-height for age; sore muscles near the tumor; one leg or arm longer than the other; and pressure or irritation with exercise. Patients may be asymptomatic.
- Diagnosis is confirmed using X-ray, CT scan, and MRI.
- No treatment is necessary. If the tumor is causing pain or neurologic manifestations because of compression, surgical removal is usually done. Patients should have regular screenings to detect progression to cancer.

Osteosarcoma

- Osteosarcoma is an extremely aggressive bone cancer that rapidly metastasizes. It usually occurs in the pelvis or metaphyseal region of long bones of the extremities, especially in the distal femur, proximal tibia, and proximal humerus. It is the most common malignant bone tumor affecting children and young adults. It is often associated with Paget disease and radiation.
- The gradual onset of pain and swelling in the affected bone are the most common manifestations. The pain may be worse at night and increase with activity. A minor injury does not cause the cancer but may bring the condition to medical attention.
- Diagnosis is confirmed from tissue biopsy, increased serum alkaline phosphatase and calcium levels, and X-ray, CT or positron emission tomography scans, and MRI findings.
- Metastasis is present in 10%–20% of people when they are diagnosed with osteosarcoma.

Preoperative chemotherapy may decrease tumor size before surgery. Limb-salvage surgical procedures are usually considered if there is a clear (no cancer present) 6- to 7-cm margin surrounding the lesion. Chemotherapy after surgery has increased the 5-year survival rate to 70% in patients without metastasis. Chemotherapy includes combinations of methotrexate, doxorubicin, cisplatin, ifosfamide, cyclophosphamide, and etoposide.

Metastatic Bone Cancer

Metastatic bone cancer is the most common type of malignant bone tumor. It occurs as a result of metastasis from a primary tumor. Common sites for the primary tumor include the breast, colon, prostate, lungs, kidney, and thyroid. Metastatic bone lesions are often found in the spine, ribs, or pelvis.

■ Pathologic fractures at the site of metastasis are common because the bone is weak. High serum calcium occurs as damaged bones release calcium.

■ Radionuclide bone scans may detect metastatic lesions before they are visible on X-ray. The lesions may occur at any time (even years later) after treatment of the primary tumor.

■ Bone metastasis should be suspected in any patient who has local bone pain and a history of cancer.

■ Palliative treatment consists of radiation and pain management. Surgical stabilization may be indicated for a fracture or high risk of fracture. Prognosis depends on the primary type of cancer and other sites of metastasis.

Nursing Management: Bone Cancer

Nursing care of the patient with bone cancer does not differ significantly from the general care of the patient with cancer. Anemia and decreased mobility may cause weakness. Prevent fractures by careful handling and support of the affected extremity and logrolling the patient.

■ Monitor the tumor site for swelling, changes in circulation, and decreased movement, sensation, or joint function.

■ Pain caused by the tumor pressing against nerves and other organs near the bone can be very severe. Carefully monitor the patient's pain and ensure adequate pain medication. Sometimes, radiation therapy is used to shrink the tumor and decrease the pain.

■ The patient may be reluctant to take part in activities because of weakness and fear of pain. Provide rest periods between activities.

■ Special attention is needed for problems of pain and disability, side effects of chemotherapy, and postoperative care (e.g., after spinal cord decompression or amputation).

BRAIN TUMORS

Description

Brain tumors may be primary, arising from tissues within the brain, or secondary, as a metastasis from cancer elsewhere in the body. Secondary tumors are more common. The cancers that most often metastasize to the brain are lung and breast cancers.

Meningiomas are the most common primary brain tumor. Other common brain tumors are gliomas (e.g., astrocytoma, glioblastoma [most common form of glioma]).

- More than half of brain tumors are malignant. They infiltrate the brain tissue and are not amenable to complete surgical removal. Other tumors may be histologically benign but are located where complete removal is not possible.
- Brain tumors rarely metastasize outside the central nervous system (CNS) because they are contained by structural (meninges) and physiologic (blood-brain) barriers.

Clinical Manifestations

A wide range of manifestations are possible with brain tumors, depending on the location and size.

- Headache is common. Tumor-related headaches tend to be worse at night and may awaken the patient. The headaches are usually dull and constant but may be throbbing.
- Seizures are common with gliomas and brain metastases.
- Brain tumors can cause nausea and vomiting from increased intracranial pressure (ICP). See Increased Intracranial Pressure.
- Cognitive problems, including memory loss and mood or personality changes, are common with brain metastases. Expanding tumors may produce signs of increased ICP, cerebral edema, or obstruction of cerebrospinal fluid (CSF) pathways.

Diagnostic Studies

- Extensive history and a comprehensive neurologic examination are essential.
- CT (with contrast) and MRI assist in tumor location.
- MRI and positron emission tomography (PET) scans allow for detection of very small tumors.
- Other tests include angiography, magnetic resonance spectroscopy, and single-photon emission computed tomography (SPECT).

Correct diagnosis of a brain tumor is made by obtaining tissue for histologic study. In most patients, tissue is obtained at time of surgery.

Interprofessional Management

Surgical removal is the preferred treatment for brain tumors. Outcome depends on the type, size, and location of the tumor. Meningiomas and oligodendrogliomas can usually be completely removed. The more invasive gliomas and medulloblastomas can be only partially removed.

- Even if complete tumor removal is not possible, surgery can reduce the tumor mass to decrease ICP, provide symptom relief, and extend survival time.

Hydrocephalus due to a tumor obstructing the CSF flow can be treated by placing a ventricular shunt. A catheter with one-way valves is placed in the lateral ventricle and then tunneled under the skin to drain CSF into the peritoneal cavity.

- Rapid decompression of ICP can cause total body collapse and weakness. Headache may be prevented by gradually introducing the patient to the upright position.
- Manifestations of shunt malfunction, which are related to increased ICP, include decreasing LOC, restlessness, headache, blurred vision, or vomiting. This may require shunt revision or replacement. Infection may occur, as exhibited by high fever, persistent headache, and stiff neck. Antibiotics are used to treat the infection. In some situations, the shunt must be replaced. CSF drainage is managed with an extraventricular drainage system while the infection is treated.

Radiation therapy is used as a follow-up measure after surgery. Radiation seeds can also be implanted into the brain. Cerebral edema and rapidly increasing ICP may be complications of radiation therapy, but they can be managed with high doses of corticosteroids (dexamethasone or methylprednisolone [Solu-Medrol]).

- Stereotactic radiosurgery delivers a highly concentrated dose of radiation precisely to a location within the brain. It may be used when conventional surgery has failed or is not an option because of the tumor location.

Normally the blood-brain barrier prohibits the entry of most drugs into brain tissue. Cancerous tumors can cause a breakdown of the blood-brain barrier in the area, thus allowing chemotherapy drugs to reach the tumor.

- Temozolomide (Temodar) is an oral chemotherapy agent that can cross the blood-brain barrier. Chemotherapy drug-laden biodegradable wafers implanted during surgery can deliver chemotherapy directly to the tumor site. Intrathecal administration also allows direct delivery of chemotherapeutic drugs to the CNS.
- Bevacizumab (Avastin) is used to treat patients with glioblastoma when this type of brain cancer continues to progress after

standard therapy. Bevacizumab is a targeted therapy agent that inhibits the action of vascular endothelial growth factor (substance that helps form new blood vessels).

Nursing Management
Goals
The patient with a brain tumor will maintain normal ICP, maximize neurologic functioning, achieve control of pain and discomfort, and be aware of the long-term implications with respect to prognosis and cognitive and physical functioning.
Interventions
Behavioral changes associated with a frontal lobe lesion, such as loss of emotional control, confusion, memory loss, and depression, are often not perceived by the patient but can be disturbing and frightening to the family. Assist the caregiver and family in understanding what is happening.
- Use a calm and reassuring approach, closely supervise activity, and provide padded side rails.
- Minimize environmental stimuli. Create a routine and use reality orientation for the confused patient.
- Seizures often occur with brain tumors. Institute seizure precautions for the protection of the patient (see Seizure Disorders).
- Motor and sensory dysfunctions interfere with the activities of daily living. Encourage the patient to provide as much self-care as physically possible. Self-image often depends on the patient's ability to take part in care within the limitations of the physical deficits.
- Motor (expressive) or sensory (receptive) dysphasia may occur. Disturbances in communication can be frustrating for the patient and may interfere with your ability to meet patient needs. Establish a communication system that can be used by both the patient and staff.
- Tumors in the temporal lobe can cause hallucinations, which may be confused with dementia or delirium.
- Nutritional intake may be decreased because of the patient's inability to eat, loss of appetite, or loss of desire to eat. Assess the nutritional status of the patient. The patient may need encouragement to eat or may need enteral or parenteral nutrition (see Enteral Nutrition and Parenteral Nutrition).

Social workers and home health nurses may be needed to aid the caregiver with discharge planning.
- Help the family adjust to role changes and psychosocial and socioeconomic factors and discuss palliative and end-of-life care.

BREAST CANCER

Description

Breast cancer is the most common cancer in women in the United States except for skin cancer and is second only to lung cancer as the leading cause of death from cancer in women. In the United States, 276,480 new cases of invasive breast cancer and more than 48,530 cases of in situ breast cancer are diagnosed annually. Another 2620 cases of breast cancer happen in men.

Etiology and Risk Factors

Risk factors for breast cancer appear to be cumulative and interacting (Table 15). The presence of multiple risk factors may greatly increase the overall risk. A breast cancer risk assessment tool for health care providers (HCPs) is available through the National Cancer Institute (www.cancer.gov/bcrisktool).

TABLE 15 Risk Factors for Breast Cancer	
Risk factor	**Comments**
Age ≥55 yr	Majority found in postmenopausal women
	After age 60, ↑ in incidence
Alcohol use	Drinking ≥1 alcoholic beverage per day may have an ↑ risk
Benign breast disease with atypical epithelial hyperplasia, lobular carcinoma in situ	Atypical changes in breast biopsy ↑ risk
Chemicals in environment, cosmetics (parabens, phthalates), food	Emerging risk: may be hormone disruptors
Early menarche (before age 12), late menopause (after age 55)	A long menstrual history ↑ risk
Exposure to ionizing radiation	Radiation damages DNA (e.g., prior treatment for Hodgkin's lymphoma)
Family history	Breast cancer, ovarian, pancreatic and high grade prostate cancer in a first-degree relative, particularly when premenopausal or bilateral

TABLE 15 Risk Factors for Breast Cancer—cont'd

Risk factor	Comments
Female	Women account for 99% of breast cancer cases
First full-term pregnancy after age 30, nulliparity, no breastfeeding	Prolonged exposure to unopposed estrogen ↑ risk
Genetic factors *(BRCA1, BRCA2, P53, PTEN, PALB2, ATM, CHEK2, NBM)*	Gene mutations play a role in up to 10% of breast cancer cases
Hair chemicals in permanent dyes and hair -straightening products	Emerging risk: especially in black women
Height, being taller	May be due to factors related to early growth
Hormone use	Use of estrogen and/or progesterone as hormone therapy, especially in postmenopausal women
Light exposure at night	Emerging risk: seen in night shift workers
Long-term heavy smoking	May ↑ risk, especially in women who begin smoking before first pregnancy
Obesity, weight gain after menopause	Fat cells store estrogen, which ↑ the risk for developing breast cancer
Personal history of breast, colon, endometrial, or ovarian cancer	Personal history significantly ↑ risk for breast cancer, risk for cancer in other breast, and recurrence
Physical inactivity	Risk ↑s most after menopause
Race and ethnicity	White and black women have the highest incidence of breast cancer. Black women have lower survival rates from breast cancer than white women, even when diagnosed at an early stage. Hispanic and black women are more likely to be diagnosed at a later stage of breast cancer than white women.

B

- Combined hormone therapy (estrogen plus progesterone) increases the risk of breast cancer after as little as 2-years use and increases the risk of having a larger, more advanced breast cancer at diagnosis. However, this risk decreases within 5 years of stopping hormone therapy. Using estrogen therapy alone for longer than 15 years (for women with a prior hysterectomy) increases a woman's long-term risk.
- A link also exists between oral contraceptive use and increased risk of breast cancer. This risk decreases when use is stopped and is gone after 10 years.
- Up to 10% of all breast cancers are hereditary, related to mutations in *BRCA1* and *BRCA2* genes.
- Modifiable risk factors include excess weight gain during adulthood, sedentary lifestyle, smoking, dietary fat intake, obesity, night-shift work, and alcohol intake. Environmental factors, such as radiation exposure and using hair dyes and straighteners, may play a role.
- Risk factors for breast cancer in men include estrogen use, hyperestrogenism, a family history of breast cancer, and radiation exposure.

In general, breast cancer arises from the epithelial lining of the ducts *(ductal carcinoma)* or from the epithelium of the lobules *(lobular carcinoma)*. Breast cancers may be in situ (within the duct) or invasive (invading through the wall of the duct). Breast cancer can be classified as noninvasive or invasive and as ductal or lobular (Table 16).

- Factors that affect cancer prognosis are tumor size, axillary node involvement (the more nodes involved, the worse the prognosis), tumor differentiation (morphology of malignant cells), estrogen and progesterone receptor status, and human epidermal growth factor receptor 2 (HER-2; a protein that helps regulate cell growth).

Breast cancer is usually detected as a lump in the breast or mammographic abnormality. It occurs most often in the upper outer quadrant of the breast because that is the location of most of the glandular tissue.

- If palpable, breast cancer is characteristically hard and may be irregularly shaped, poorly delineated, nonmobile, and nontender.
- A small number of breast cancers cause clear or bloody nipple discharge, usually unilateral. Nipple retraction may occur.
- Plugging of the dermal lymphatics can give the skin the appearance of an orange peel (peau d'orange).

In large cancers, infiltration, induration, and dimpling of the overlying skin may occur.

Recurrence may be local or regional (skin or soft tissue near mastectomy site, axillary lymph nodes) or distant metastases (most commonly bone, brain, lung, and liver).

TABLE 16   Classification of Breast Cancer

Based on tissue type

- Ductal carcinoma (affects milk ducts)
  - Medullary
  - Tubular
  - Colloid (mucinous)
- Lobular carcinoma (affects milk-producing glands)
- Other
  - Inflammatory
  - Paget disease
  - Phyllodes tumor

Based on invasiveness
Noninvasive (in situ)

- Ductal carcinoma in situ (DCIS)
- Pure Paget disease

Invasive (spreading to other locations)

- Invasive ductal carcinoma
- Invasive lobular carcinoma

Based on hormone receptor and genetic status
Estrogen and progesterone receptor status

- Estrogen receptor-positive
- Estrogen receptor-negative
- Progesterone receptor-positive
- Progesterone receptor-negative

HER-2 genetic status

- HER-2-positive
- HER-2-negative

HER-2, Human epidermal growth factor receptor 2.

Diagnostic Studies
Screening

- Physical examination of breast and lymphatics
- Mammography and ultrasound
- Breast MRI
- Biopsy including fine-needle aspiration and stereotactic core biopsy

Postdiagnosis

Axillary lymph node analysis is often performed to determine if cancer has spread. The more nodes involved, the greater the risk of recurrence.

Sentinel lymph node (SLN) biopsy helps identify the lymph nodes that drain from the tumor site (sentinel node) and determine the extent of tumor spread. If the SLNs are positive, a complete *axillary lymph node dissection* (ALND) may be done.

- The larger the tumor, the poorer the prognosis. In general, poorly differentiated tumors are more aggressive.
- Estrogen and progesterone receptor status helps determine treatment decisions and prognosis. Receptor-positive tumors (1) often show histologic evidence of being well differentiated, (2) have a lower chance for recurrence, (3) often have a diploid (more normal) DNA content and low proliferative indices, and (4) are often hormone-dependent and responsive to hormone therapy. Receptor-negative tumors (1) are often poorly differentiated histologically, (2) often recur, (3) have a high incidence of aneuploidy (abnormally high or low DNA content) and higher proliferative indices, and (4) are usually unresponsive to hormone therapy.
- Ploidy status (number of chromosomes in a cell) correlates with tumor aggressiveness. Diploid tumors have a much lower risk for recurrence than aneuploid tumors.
- Overexpression of the HER-2 receptor has been associated with unusually aggressive tumor growth, a greater risk for recurrence, and a poorer prognosis. About 10%–20% of patients with breast cancer produce excessive HER-2. The presence of HER-2 helps in the selection and sequence of drug therapy and predicts the patient's response to treatment.
- Genomic assays (MammaPrint, Oncotype DX, PAM50 [Prosigna], EndoPredict, and the Breast Cancer Index) are used to analyze the activity of a group of genes.

A person whose breast cancer tests negative for all three receptors (estrogen, progesterone, and HER-2) has *triple-negative breast cancer*, an aggressive tumor with a poorer prognosis. The incidence of triple-negative breast cancer is higher in blacks, Hispanics, premenopausal women, and those with a *BRCA1* mutation.

Interprofessional Management

Prognostic factors are considered in treatment decisions. Tumor size (T), nodal involvement (N), and presence of metastasis (M) are used to stage breast cancer with the TNM system (see TNM Classification System). The stages range from 0 to IV, with stage 0 being in situ cancer with no lymph node involvement and no metastasis. Stage IV indicates metastatic spread, regardless of tumor size or lymph node involvement.

Surgical Therapy

The most common options for operable breast cancer are: (1) breast-conserving surgery (lumpectomy, segmental mastectomy), and (2) mastectomy with or without reconstruction. Most women with early-stage breast cancer (tumors smaller than 5 cm) are candidates for either surgery.

Breast-conserving surgery (lumpectomy) usually involves removal of the entire tumor along with a margin of normal tissue. After surgery, radiation therapy is delivered to the entire breast, ending with a boost to the tumor bed. If the risk for recurrence is high, chemotherapy may be given before radiation therapy.

A *total* or *simple mastectomy* removes the entire breast. *Modified radical mastectomy* includes removing the breast and axillary lymph nodes while preserving the pectoralis major muscle.

Radiation Therapy

Radiation therapy may be used to prevent local tumor recurrences after breast-conserving surgery, prevent local and nodal recurrences after mastectomy, or palliate pain caused by local, regional, and distant recurrence.

- A minimally invasive method of delivering internal radiation therapy uses small catheters or a balloon catheter to insert radioactive seeds into the breast after the tumor is removed.

Drug Therapy

Chemotherapy, hormone therapy, and targeted therapies are used.

- Chemotherapy. A combination of cytotoxic drugs is usually better than using a single drug. The incidence and severity of the side effects are influenced by the drug combinations, schedule, and doses (see Chemotherapy).
- Hormone Therapy. Estrogen can promote growth of breast cancer cells if cells are estrogen-receptor (ER) positive. Hormone receptor assays can identify women who are likely to respond to hormone therapy. Hormonal therapy can block ERs or suppress estrogen synthesis through inhibiting aromatase, an enzyme needed for estrogen synthesis (Table 17).
- Targeted Therapy. HER-2 inhibitors attach to the HER-2 receptors on the surface of the breast cancer cells and block them from receiving signals to proliferate. Kinase inhibitors prevent cells from dividing, thus slowing cancer growth. Other drugs work by blocking a protein that normally promotes cell growth and division (Table 17).

TABLE 17 Drug Therapy: Breast Cancer		
Drug class	**Mechanism of action**	**Indications**
Hormone therapy		
Aromatase inhibitors		
Anastrozole (Arimidex)	Prevents estrogen production by inhibiting aromatase	ER-positive breast cancer in postmenopausal women only
Exemestane (Aromasin)		
Letrozole (Femara)		
Estrogen receptor blockers		
Fulvestrant (Faslodex)	Blocks estrogen receptors (ERs) and increases their degradation	ER-positive breast cancer in postmenopausal women only
Tamoxifen	Selectively blocks ERs	ER-positive breast cancer in premenopausal and postmenopausal women
		Used as a preventive measure in high-risk premenopausal and postmenopausal women
Toremifene (Fareston)	Blocks ERs	ER-positive breast cancer in postmenopausal women only
Estrogen receptor modulator		
Raloxifene (Evista)	In breast, blocks the effect of estrogen. In bone, promotes effect of estrogen and prevents bone loss.	Postmenopausal women
Targeted therapy		
HER-2 inhibitors		
Lapatinib (Tykerb)	Blocks the function of HER-2 related kinases inside the cell	HER-2-positive breast cancer

TABLE 17 Drug Therapy: Breast Cancer—cont'd		
Drug class	**Mechanism of action**	**Indications**
Margetuximab-cmkb (Margenza)	Blocks HER-2 receptor	HER-2-positive breast cancer
Pertuzumab (Perjeta)		
Trastuzumab (Herceptin)		
Trastuzumab-pkrb (Herzuma)		
Trastuzumab-qyyp (Trazimera)		
Ado-trastuzumab emtansine (Kadcyla)	Trastuzumab with a chemotherapy drug called DM1	HER-2-positive breast cancer
Fam-traztuzumab-deruxtecan nxki (Enhertu)	HER-2 directed antibody and a topoisomerase inhibitor	Advance or metastatic HER-2 positive breast cancer after 2 other HER-2 therapies
Kinase inhibitors		
Abemaciclib (Verzenio)	CDK4/6 kinase inhibitors	ER-positive, HER-2-negative breast cancer in postmenopausal women
Palbociclib (Ibrance)		
Ribociclib (Kisqali)		
Neratinib (Nerlynx)	Tyrosine kinase inhibitor	Advanced or metastatic HER-2 positive breast cancer after 1 other HER-2 therapy, includes patients with brain metastasis
Tucatinib (Tukysa)		
Alpelisib (Piqray)	P13 kinase inhibitor	PIK3CA mutated, HER-2 negative advanced breast cancer
Everolimus (Afinitor)	mTOR inhibitor suppressing T cell activation and proliferation	ER-positive, HER-2-negative breast cancer in postmenopausal women
Olaparib (Lynparza)	PARP inhibitors	Patients with metastatic breast cancer positive for BRCA mutations
Talazoparib (Talzenna)		

B

Continued

TABLE 17 Drug Therapy: Breast Cancer—cont'd		
Drug class	**Mechanism of action**	**Indications**
Entrectinib (Rozlytrek) Larotrectinib (Vitrakvi)	NTRK inhibitors	In NTRK + breast cancers (very rare) when no other options exist
Immunomodulators		
Atezolizumab (Tecentriq)	PD-1 inhibitor	PD-L1 positive triple negative advanced or metastatic breast cancer
Pembrolizumab (Keytruda)	PD-1 inhibitor	Any MSI-H breast cancer when no other options exist
Sacituzumab govitecan-hziy (Trodelvy)	Monoclonal antibody that targets Trop-2 protein and a topoisomerase 1 inhibitor	Metastatic triple negative disease after 2 other therapies

EGFR, Epidermal growth factor receptor; *HER-2,* human epidermal growth factor receptor 2.

Follow-Up and Survivorship Care

After treatment for breast cancer, the patient will have ongoing survivorship care.

- A history and physical examination is recommended 1–4 times per year as clinically appropriate for 5 years, then annually thereafter.
- Teach breast cancer survivors to perform monthly breast self-examination (BSE) and chest wall self-examination and report any changes to their HCP. Local recurrence of breast cancer is usually at the surgical site.
- Breast cancer survivors should have an annual mammogram. Other breast imaging studies, such as a breast ultrasound or breast MRI, should only be done as an adjunct to mammography and not for annual routine surveillance.

Nursing Management

Goals

The patient with breast cancer will take part in the decision-making process related to treatment, adhere to the therapeutic plan, communicate about and manage the side effects of therapy, be supported by significant others and the health care team, and adhere to recommended follow-up and surveillance after treatment.

Interventions

The times of waiting for the initial biopsy results and waiting for treatment recommendations are difficult for patients and their families. Even after the HCP has discussed treatment options, the patient often relies on you to clarify and expand on these options.

- Explore the patient's usual decision-making processes. Help them evaluate the options and provide relevant information. Clarify any unresolved issues with the HCP. Provide support to the patient and family after they make decisions.
- Provide the patient with enough information to ensure informed consent. Preoperative teaching includes turning and deep breathing, a review of postoperative exercises, and an explanation of the recovery period.

The woman who has breast-conserving surgery usually has an uncomplicated postoperative course with variable pain intensity. After ALND or a mastectomy, patients are generally discharged home with drains in place.

- Teach the patient and family (including a return demonstration) how to manage the drains.

Restoring arm function on the affected side after mastectomy and axillary lymph node dissection is a key nursing goal.

- Place the patient in a semi-Fowler's position with the arm on the affected side elevated on a pillow. Flexing and extending the fingers should begin in the recovery room, with progressive increases in activity.
- Postoperative arm and shoulder exercises are instituted gradually. Discomfort can be minimized by administering analgesics about 30 min before initiating exercises. When able to shower, the warm water on the affected shoulder often has a muscle-relaxing effect and reduces joint stiffness.

Lymphedema (accumulation of lymph in soft tissue) can occur at any point after breast cancer treatment. The patient may have heaviness, pain, impaired motor function in the arm, and numbness and paresthesia of the fingers. Teach measures to prevent or reduce lymphedema including:

- No BP readings, venipunctures, or injections on the affected arm.
- The affected arm should not be dependent for long periods.
- Prevent infection, burns, or compromised circulation on the affected side.

- If trauma to the arm occurs, wash it thoroughly with soap and water. A topical antibiotic ointment and a bandage or other sterile dressing may be applied.
- Frequent elevation of the arm, regular use of a custom-fitted pressure sleeve, and treatment with an inflatable sleeve (pneumomassage) may be helpful.

Remain sensitive to the complex psychologic impact that a diagnosis of cancer and subsequent breast surgery can have.

- Help identify sources of support such as partner, family, and spiritual practices.
- Provide a safe environment for the expression of feelings.
- Encourage the patient to identify and learn individual coping strengths.
- Provide accurate and complete answers to questions about the disease, treatment options, reproductive or lactation issues, and breast reconstruction.
- Make resources available for mental health counseling.
- Offer information about community resources, such as local or national breast cancer organizations.

▼ **Patient and Caregiver Teaching**
- Emphasize the importance of ongoing monitoring and self-care.
- Immediately after surgery, advise the patient of symptoms to report to the HCP, including fever, inflammation at the surgical site, erythema, postoperative constipation, and unusual swelling.
- For women who have had a mastectomy without breast reconstruction, a variety of garment choice products are available, including camisoles with soft breast prosthetic inserts as well as a fitted prosthesis with bra.
- If you are comfortable, begin a discussion of sexuality by inviting questions about relationships or intimacy concerns.
- The partner or family members may need assistance in dealing with their emotional reactions to the diagnosis and surgery so that they can support the patient.
- Depression and anxiety may occur with the continued stress and uncertainty of a cancer diagnosis. The support of family and friends and participation in a cancer support group are important aspects of care that are often helpful in improving quality of life and have a significant impact on survival.
- Additional information on expected outcomes for the patient after breast cancer surgery is presented in eNursing Care Plan 56-1 (available on the website).

BRONCHIECTASIS

Description

Bronchiectasis is characterized by permanent, abnormal dilation of medium-sized bronchi. It results from inflammatory changes that destroy elastic and muscular structures supporting the bronchial wall. Airways can become colonized with microorganisms (e.g., *Pseudomonas*), which cause the bronchial walls to weaken and pockets of infection to form. Bacteria attract neutrophils, which enhance inflammation and cause edema. Impaired clearance of mucus by the cilia leads to stasis of thick mucus. This results in a reduced ability to clear mucus from the lungs and decreased expiratory airflow.

- Around 40% of cases have no known cause. Cystic fibrosis is the main cause of bronchiectasis in children. Bacterial infection of the lungs is the main cause in adults. It can follow a single episode of severe pneumonia or infection that was either not treated or received inadequate or delayed treatment.
- Other risk factors include airway obstruction with mucous plugs, impaired pulmonary defenses, and repeated aspiration. Several systemic problems, such as diabetes, inflammatory bowel disease, rheumatoid arthritis, immune disorders (e.g., acquired immunodeficiency syndrome), and alpha-1 antitrypsin deficiency, are risk factors.

Clinical Manifestations

The primary characteristic is a persistent cough with consistent production of thick, tenacious, purulent sputum. Other manifestations include pleuritic chest pain, dyspnea, wheezing, clubbing, weight loss, and anemia. Adventitious sounds are heard (e.g., crackles, wheezes) over the lung fields.

- Recurrent infections injure blood vessels. Large connections (anastomoses) may develop between blood vessels in the lungs, and hemoptysis may occur. In severe cases, bleeding can be life-threatening, weight loss, and anemia.
- Complications include pulmonary hypertension and repeated exacerbations of the condition, often accompanied by chronic inflammation and hypoxemia.

Diagnostic Studies

A person with a chronic productive cough and copious purulent sputum (which may be blood streaked) should be suspected of having bronchiectasis.

- A CT scan is considered the gold standard for diagnosing bronchiectasis.

- Chest X-ray shows nonspecific abnormalities.
- Spirometry usually shows an obstructive pattern, including a decrease in forced expiratory volume in 1 s (FEV1) and in the ratio of FEV1 to forced vital capacity.
- Sputum culture may provide additional information regarding active infection. Sputum samples are frequently found to contain *Haemophilus influenzae*, *Staphylococcus aureus*, or *Pseudomonas aeruginosa*.

Nursing and Interprofessional Management

Therapy is aimed at treating acute flare-ups and preventing a decline in lung function.

- Antibiotics are the mainstay of treatment and are often given for at least 14 days. Long-term antibiotic therapy is given to patients who have symptoms that recur a few days after stopping antibiotics.
- Bronchodilator therapy with short-acting beta-2 agonists, long-acting beta-2 agonists, or anticholinergics can prevent bronchospasm and stimulate mucus clearance.
- Patients may receive oral or inhaled corticosteroids depending on the severity of the condition.
- Maintaining hydration is important to liquefy secretions. Unless contraindicated, the patient should drink at least 2–3 L of fluid daily.
- Direct hydration of the respiratory system may help in expectorating secretions. Nebulized hypertonic saline may be prescribed. At home, a steamy shower can prove effective.
- Chest physiotherapy and other airway clearance techniques facilitate expectoration of sputum. Active bleeding is a contraindication to CPT.
- Rest is important to prevent overexertion.
- Teach the patient to reduce exposure to excessive air pollutants and irritants, avoid cigarette smoking, and obtain pneumococcal and influenza vaccinations.
- Teach the patient and caregiver manifestations to report to the health care provider (HCP). These include increased sputum production, increasing dyspnea, fever, chills, and chest pain. If the patient expectorates a moderate to large amount of blood, they should contact the HCP at once.
- If hemoptysis occurs in the acute care setting, contact the HCP immediately. Elevate the head of the bed and place the patient in a side-lying position with the suspected bleeding side down.
- Good nutrition may be difficult to maintain because the patient is often anorexic. Oral hygiene to cleanse the mouth and remove dried sputum crusts may improve the patient's appetite.

For select patients who are disabled despite maximal therapy, a lung transplant may be an option.

BURNS

Description

Burns are tissue injuries caused by heat, chemicals, electric current, or radiation. An estimated 486,000 Americans seek medical care each year for burns.

Types of Burn Injury

Various types of burns may be seen alone or in combination.

- *Thermal burns* are caused by flame, flash, scald, or contact with hot objects. Severity depends on the temperature of the burning agent and duration of contact.
- *Chemical burns* are the result of tissue injury and destruction from acids, alkalis (e.g., cement, oven cleaner), and organic compounds, such as petroleum products.
- *Smoke and inhalation injury* results from inhalation of hot air or noxious chemicals that damage the respiratory tract. These injuries include metabolic asphyxiation (carbon monoxide poisoning), upper airway injury, and lower airway injury.
- *Electrical burns* result from the intense heat of an electric current. An electric shock can cause immediate cardiac standstill or ventricular fibrillation. Other injuries may include falls when the electrical current causes sudden muscle contraction and spinal or extremity fractures.

Pathophysiology

Immediately after the burn injury occurs, there is increased blood flow to the area surrounding the wound. This is followed by the release of various vasoactive substances from burned tissue, which results in increased capillary permeability. Fluid then shifts from the intravascular compartment to the interstitial space, producing edema, hypovolemia, and (potentially) shock. After several days, diuresis from fluid mobilization occurs and tissue healing begins. Burn effects occur in three phases: emergent (resuscitative), acute (wound healing), and rehabilitative (restorative).

Emergent Phase

The greatest initial threat to a patient with a major burn is hypovolemic shock. Shivering (a result of heat loss or anxiety) and a paralytic ileus (if the burn area is large) may also be present. Full-thickness and deep partial-thickness burns are initially painless because nerve endings have been destroyed. Superficial to moderate partial-thickness burns are very painful. Blisters are common in partial-thickness burns. Unconsciousness or altered mental status is the result of inhalation injury or head trauma. Complications may include respiratory distress, dysrhythmias, venous thromboembolism, and acute tubular necrosis. The emergent phase ends when fluid mobilization and diuresis begin.

Acute Phase

Partial-thickness wounds form eschar. After eschar is removed, reepithelialization begins at wound margins and appears as red or pink scar tissue. Wound closure and healing usually occur within 10–21 days. Separation of eschar from full-thickness wounds takes longer, and these wounds require surgical debridement and skin grafting. Wound infection is a serious complication. Other possible complications include extreme disorientation and delirium, contractures, Curling ulcer, hyperglycemia, and pneumonia.

Rehabilitative Phase

Mature healing of burns occurs in about 12 months when suppleness has returned, and the color has faded to a slightly lighter hue than the surrounding unburned tissue. New scar tissue shrinks, causing a contracture if not prevented with range-of-motion (ROM) exercises. The healing site, which is extremely sensitive to trauma, may itch. Complications are skin and joint contractures and hypertrophic scarring.

Clinical Manifestations and Classification of Burn Injury

The treatment of burns is related to the severity of injury. A variety of methods exist for determining burn severity.

1. Depth of burn is described according to the depth of skin destruction (epidermis, dermis, or subcutaneous tissue). Table 18 compares the various burn classifications according to the depth of injury.

2. Extent of the burn wound is calculated as percent of total body surface area (TBSA) affected. Two common methods for determining the extent of a burn include:

   ■ *Lund-Browder chart,* which is considered the most accurate because it takes into account patient age in proportion to relative body area size (Fig. 3A).

   ■ *Rule of Nines chart,* which is often used for initial assessment because it is easy to remember (see Fig. 3B).

3. The location of the burn injury influences the severity. Face, neck, and chest burns may inhibit respiratory function. Hands, feet, joint, and eye burns may limit self-care and mobility.

4. Patients with chronic diseases have a poorer prognosis for recovery. Diabetes and peripheral vascular disease increase the risk of delayed healing.

TABLE 18 Classification of Burn Injury Depth

Classifi-cation	Appearance	Possible cause	Structures involved
Partial-thickness skin destruction			
Superficial (first-degree) burn	Erythema, blanching on pressure, pain and mild swelling, no vesicles or blisters (although after 24 h skin may blister and peel).	Quick heat flash Superficial sunburn	Superficial epidermal damage with hyperemia. Tactile and pain sensation intact.
Deep (second-degree) burn	Fluid-filled vesicles that are red, shiny, wet (if vesicles have ruptured). Severe pain caused by nerve injury. Mild to moderate edema.	Chemicals Contact burns Electric current Flame Flash Scald Tar, cement	Epidermis and dermis are involved in varying depths. Skin elements, from which epithelial regeneration occurs, remain viable.
Full-thickness skin destruction			
Third- and fourth-degree burns	Dry, waxy white, brown or charred, leathery, or hard skin. Visible thrombosed vessels. Insensitivity to pain because of nerve destruction. Possible muscle, tendon, and bone involvement.	Chemical Electric current Flame Scald Tar, cement	All skin elements and local nerve endings destroyed. Coagulation necrosis present. Surgical intervention required for healing.

B

The American Burn Association (ABA) has established referral criteria to determine which burn injuries should be treated in burn centers with specialized facilities (Table 19).

Diagnostic Studies

- Serum electrolytes, especially sodium (Na^+) and potassium (K^+), to monitor fluid and electrolyte shifts

Figure 3 (A) Lund-Browder chart. (B) Rule of Nines chart.

TABLE 19 Burn Center Referral Criteria

Burn injuries that should be referred to a burn center include the following:

1. Partial-thickness burns >10% of total body surface area (TBSA)
2. Burns that involve the face, hands, feet, genitalia, perineum, or major joints
3. Third-degree burns in any age group
4. Electrical burns, including lightning injury
5. Chemical burns
6. Inhalation injury
7. Burn injury in patients with preexisting medical disorders that could complicate management, prolong recovery, or affect mortality risk (e.g., heart or kidney disease)
8. Any patient with burns and concomitant trauma (e.g., fractures) in which the burn injury poses the greatest risk for morbidity or mortality. If trauma poses a greater immediate risk, the patient may be stabilized in a trauma center before being transferred to a burn center. HCP judgment will be necessary in such situations and should be in concert with the regional medical control plan and triage protocols.
9. Burned children in hospitals without qualified personnel or equipment for care of children
10. Burn injury in patients who will require special social, emotional, or long-term rehabilitative intervention

Source: American Burn Association: Guidelines for the operation of burn centers. Retrieved from http://ameriburn.org/wp-content/uploads/2017/05/burncenterreferralcriteria.pdf

- Chest X-ray, arterial blood gases (ABGs), and sputum for inhalation injury
- Urine output and serum creatinine to evaluate fluid replacement and detect acute tubular necrosis and/or renal ischemia
- Complete blood count (CBC) to detect anemia and immunologic response to injury
- White blood cell (WBC) count and wound cultures if infection is suspected

Nursing and Interprofessional Management

Burn management progresses through three phases: emergent, acute, and rehabilitative (Table 20).

Emergent Phase

Patient survival depends on rapid and thorough assessment and intervention.

- Assess adequacy of airway management. Provide IV fluids based on burn injury assessment and ongoing monitoring for cardiovascular

TABLE 20 Interprofessional Care: Burn Injury

Emergent phase	Acute phase	Rehabilitation phase
Fluid therapy • Assess fluid needs. • Begin IV fluid replacement. • Insert an indwelling urinary catheter. • Monitor urine output.	**Fluid therapy** • Continue to replace fluids, depending on the patient's clinical response.	• Continue to teach patients and caregivers about wound care. • Continue to encourage and aid the patient in resuming self-care. • Continue to prevent or minimize contractures. • Assess risk for scarring (surgery, physical and occupational therapy, splinting, pressure garments). • Discuss possible reconstructive surgery. • Prepare for discharge home or transfer to a rehabilitation hospital. • Discuss the possible need for home care nursing.
Wound care • Start daily shower and wound care. • Debride as needed. • Assess the extent and depth of burns. • Give tetanus toxoid or tetanus antitoxin.	**Wound care** • Continue daily shower and wound care. • Continue debridement (if needed). • Assess wound daily and adjust dressing protocols as needed. • Observe for complications (e.g., infection).	
Pain and anxiety • Assess and manage pain and anxiety.	**Early excision and grafting** • Provide temporary allografts. • Provide permanent autografts. • Care for donor sites.	
Physical and occupational therapy • Place the patient in a position that prevents contracture formation and reduces edema. • Assess the need for splints.	**Pain and anxiety** • Continue to assess for and treat pain and anxiety.	
Nutrition therapy • Assess nutrition needs and begin feeding patients by the most appropriate route as soon as possible.	**Physical and occupational therapy** • Begin a daily therapy program for maintenance of a range of motion. • Assess the need for splints and anticontracture positioning. • Encourage and aid patients with self-care as possible.	
Respiratory therapy • Assess oxygenation needs. • Provide supplemental oxygen as needed. • Intubate if needed. • Monitor respiratory status.	**Nutrition therapy** • Continue to assess diet to support wound healing.	
Psychosocial care • Provide support to patients and caregivers during the initial crisis phase.	**Respiratory therapy** • Continue to assess oxygenation needs. • Continue to monitor respiratory status. • Monitor for signs of complications (e.g., pneumonia).	
	Psychosocial care • Provide ongoing support, counseling, and teaching to patients and caregiver about physical and emotional aspects of care and recovery. • Begin discharge planning.	
	Drug therapy • Assess the need for drugs (e.g., antibiotics). • Continue to monitor effectiveness and adjust dosage as needed.	

response (www.mdcalc.com/parkland-formula-for-burns). Provide pain medication and wound care, and offer support to patient and family. Begin feeding patient by most appropriate route as soon as possible.

- Standard pulse oximetry (SpO2) does not distinguish oxyhemoglobin from carboxyhemoglobin. For patients with suspected or confirmed carbon monoxide exposure, use a carbon monoxide pulse oximetry (SpCO) device.

Acute Phase

Major interventions are wound care, excision and grafting, pain management, physical and occupational therapy, nutritional therapy, and psychosocial care.

- Wound care consists of ongoing observation, assessment, cleansing, debridement, and dressing reapplication.
- Pain assessment and management are critical.

Rehabilitative Phase

Care of the person with burns can be intense over a long period. Nurses should seek support from coworkers, a manager, or the employee assistance program as needed.

Encourage the patient and caregiver to actively participate in care.

- Encourage patient to perform physical and occupational therapy routines.
- Apply water-based moisturizers that penetrate the dermis on healed areas to keep skin supple.
- Assist patients in adapting to a realistic, yet positive appraisal focusing on what they can do instead of what they cannot do.

▼ Patient and Caregiver Teaching

- Describe the burn injury healing process and phases of burn management.
- Explain treatments, precautions, infection control measures, and visiting policy to elicit cooperation and decrease anxiety.
- Teach the patient to watch for injuries or signs and symptoms of infection in new skin.
- Teach caregivers how to perform dressing changes.
- Stress exercise and physical therapy. Plan a daily program with the patient and offer resources for a continuing activity program.
- Help the patient and caregiver know what to expect during recovery and set realistic future expectations.
- Assist the patient and caregivers to establish contact with family and patient support groups, such as the Phoenix Society (www.phoenix-society.org).

CARDIOMYOPATHY

Description

Cardiomyopathy (CMP) is a group of diseases that directly affect myocardial structure or function. CMP is classified as primary or secondary. *Primary CMP* refers to idiopathic conditions involving only the heart muscle. In *secondary CMP*, another disease process causes the myocardial disease. Common causes of secondary CMP are coronary artery disease (CAD), myocarditis, hypertension, cardiotoxic agents (alcohol, cocaine), valve disease, and metabolic and autoimmune disorders.

Three major types of CMP are *dilated, hypertrophic,* and *restrictive.* Each type has its own pathogenesis, clinical presentation, and treatment (Table 21). CMP that leads to cardiomegaly and heart failure (HF) is the main reason for heart transplants.

Dilated Cardiomyopathy

Pathophysiology

Dilated CMP is the most common type. It appears with diffuse inflammation and rapid degeneration of heart fibers. It results in ventricular dilation, impairment of systolic function, atrial enlargement, and blood stasis in the left ventricle. The ventricular walls do not hypertrophy.

- Dilated CMP often follows infectious myocarditis. Some evidence links dilated CMP with an autoimmune process or genetic causes. Other common causes include alcohol, cocaine, hypertension, and CAD.
- Sudden cardiac death (SCD) from dysrhythmias is a leading cause of death in idiopathic dilated CMP.

Clinical Manifestations

Signs and symptoms of dilated CMP may develop acutely after an infection or slowly over time. Most affected people eventually develop HF.

- Symptoms can include fatigue, dyspnea at rest, paroxysmal nocturnal dyspnea, and orthopnea. Dry cough, abdominal bloating, and anorexia may occur as the disease progresses.
- Signs can include an irregular heart rate with an abnormal S3 and/or S4, pulmonary crackles, edema, pallor, hepatomegaly, heart murmurs, dysrhythmias, and jugular venous distention.

Diagnostic Studies

A diagnosis is made on the basis of patient history and exclusion of other causes of HF.

- Doppler echocardiography is usually the basis for the diagnosis of dilated CMP.

TABLE 21	Types of Cardiomyopathy	
Dilated	**Hypertrophic**	**Restrictive**
Cardiac output		
Decreased	Normal or decreased	Normal or decreased
Cardiomegaly		
Moderate to severe	Mild to moderate	Mild
Contractility		
Decreased	Increased or decreased	Normal or decreased
Dysrhythmias		
Sinus tachycardia, atrial and ventricular dysrhythmias	Atrial and ventricular dysrhythmias	Atrial and ventricular dysrhythmias
Major manifestations		
Fatigue, weakness, palpitations, dyspnea	Exertional dyspnea, fatigue, angina, syncope, palpitations	Dyspnea, fatigue
Outflow tract obstruction		
None	Increased	None
Valvular incompetence		
Atrioventricular (AV) valves, especially mitral	Mitral valve	AV valves

C

- Chest X-ray may show cardiomegaly with pulmonary venous hypertension and pleural effusion.
- The electrocardiogram (ECG) may reveal tachycardia, bradycardia, and dysrhythmias with conduction disturbances.
- Serum levels of b-type natriuretic peptide (BNP) are increased in the presence of HF.
- Heart catheterization confirms or excludes CAD, and multiple gated acquisition (MUGA) nuclear scan determines ejection fraction (EF).

Interprofessional and Nursing Management

The goals of therapy are to keep the patient at an optimal level of functioning and out of the hospital. Interventions focus on controlling HF by enhancing myocardial contractility and decreasing preload and afterload. Observe for signs and symptoms of worsening HF, dysrhythmias, and embolus formation. A patient with secondary dilated CMP must be treated for the underlying disease process. For example, the patient with alcohol-induced dilated CMP must abstain from alcohol. All patients with CMP are at risk for infective endocarditis from any procedure that may cause bacteremia. Teach the patient about the need for prophylactic antibiotics.

Drug and nutritional therapy and cardiac rehabilitation may help alleviate symptoms of HF and improve cardiac output (CO) and quality of life. Monitor for drug effectiveness.

- Nitrates and loop diuretics decrease preload.
- Angiotensin-converting enzyme (ACE) inhibitors reduce afterload.
- β-Adrenergic blockers (e.g., metoprolol [Lopressor]) and aldosterone antagonists (e.g., spironolactone [Aldactone]) control the neurohormonal stimulation that occurs in HF.
- Antidysrhythmics (e.g., amiodarone) and anticoagulants are used as indicated.
- Anticoagulation therapy reduces the risk of systemic embolization from clots that form in the heart chambers.

Patients may also benefit from nondrug therapies. Cardiac resynchronization therapy and an implantable cardioverter defibrillator may be used. A ventricular assist device (VAD) allows the heart to rest and recover from acute HF. It may also serve as a bridge to heart transplantation.

- Currently, approximately 50% of heart transplantations performed are for treatment of CMP. Heart transplant recipients have a good prognosis.
- Encourage caregivers to learn cardiopulmonary resuscitation (CPR). Teach them when and how to activate emergency care.

Hypertrophic Cardiomyopathy

Pathophysiology

Hypertrophic cardiomyopathy (HCM) is asymmetric left ventricular hypertrophy without ventricular dilation. HCM is more common in men than in women. It is usually diagnosed in young adulthood and is often seen in active, athletic persons. HCM is the most common cause of sudden cardiac death (SCD) in otherwise healthy young people.

- The main characteristics of HCM result from massive ventricular hypertrophy: rapid, forceful contraction of the left ventricle; impaired relaxation (diastole); and obstruction to aortic outflow (not present in all patients). The end result is poor filling of the stiff ventricle. Decreased ventricular filling and obstruction to outflow result in decreased CO, especially during exertion.

Clinical Manifestations

Patients may be asymptomatic. The most common symptom is dyspnea, caused by an elevated left ventricular diastolic pressure. Other manifestations include exertional fatigue, angina, syncope, and dysrhythmias.

- Common dysrhythmias include atrial fibrillation, ventricular tachycardia, and ventricular fibrillation.
- Clinical findings on examination may be unremarkable. On chest palpation, the apical impulse can be exaggerated and displaced to the left. Auscultation may reveal an S4 and a systolic murmur between the apex and sternal border at the fourth intercostal space.

Diagnostic Studies

- Echocardiogram is the primary diagnostic tool to confirm HCM, showing left ventricular hypertrophy, wall motion abnormalities, and diastolic dysfunction.
- Heart catheterization and nuclear stress testing may help in diagnosing and guiding treatment.

Interprofessional and Nursing Management

Goals of care are to improve ventricular filling by reducing ventricular contractility and relieving left ventricular outflow obstruction. This can be achieved with β-blockers (e.g., metoprolol) or calcium-channel blockers (e.g., verapamil).

- Amiodarone and sotalol (Betapace) are effective antidysrhythmic drugs. However, their use does not prevent SCD. Patients at risk for SCD need an implantable cardioverter defibrillator.
- Atrioventricular pacing can reduce the degree of outflow obstruction by causing the septum to move away from the left ventricular wall.
- Patients with severe symptoms unresponsive to therapy may be candidates for ventriculomyotomy and myectomy of the hypertrophied septum. Most patients have an improvement in symptoms and exercise tolerance after surgery.
- An alternative nonsurgical procedure is percutaneous transluminal septal myocardial ablation (PTSMA). Ablation of the septal wall decreases the obstruction to flow, and the patient's symptoms decrease.

- Vasodilators, such as nitroglycerin, may worsen the chest pain by decreasing venous return and further increasing obstruction of blood flow from the heart.

Nursing interventions focus on relieving symptoms, observing for and preventing complications, and providing emotional support.

- Focus teaching on helping the patient plan to avoid strenuous activity and dehydration. Any activity that causes an increase in systemic vascular resistance (thus increasing obstruction to forward blood flow) is dangerous.
- Rest and elevation of the feet to improve venous return to the heart can help manage chest pain.

Restrictive Cardiomyopathy

Pathophysiology

Restrictive cardiomyopathy is a disease of the heart muscle that impairs diastolic filling and stretch. Several pathologic processes may be involved, including myocardial fibrosis, hypertrophy, and infiltration, which produce stiffness of the ventricular wall. The ventricles resist filling and require high diastolic filling pressures to maintain CO.

Clinical Manifestations

Classic manifestations of restrictive CMP are fatigue, exercise intolerance, and dyspnea. Other manifestations may include angina, orthopnea, syncope, palpations, and signs of HF. The most common dysrhythmias are atrial fibrillation and atrioventricular block.

Diagnostic Studies

Chest X-ray may appear normal or show cardiomegaly with pleural effusions and pulmonary congestion.

- Echocardiography may show a left ventricle of normal size with a thickened wall, a slightly dilated right ventricle, and dilated atria.
- Endomyocardial biopsy, CT scan, and nuclear imaging may help determine a diagnosis.

Interventions for restrictive CMP are aimed at improving diastolic filling and the underlying disease process. Treatment includes conventional therapy for HF and dysrhythmias. Heart transplantation may be an option.

Nursing care is similar to the care of a patient with HF. As with HCM, teach patients to avoid situations, such as strenuous activity and dehydration that impair ventricular filling and increase systemic vascular resistance.

CARPAL TUNNEL SYNDROME

Description

Carpal tunnel syndrome (CTS) is caused by compression of the median nerve, which enters the hand through the narrow carpal tunnel. The carpal tunnel is formed by ligaments and bones. CTS is often caused by pressure from trauma or edema due to inflammation of a tendon (tenosynovitis), cancer, rheumatoid arthritis, or soft tissue masses, such as ganglia.

- CTS is associated with hobbies or occupations that require continuous wrist movement (e.g., musicians, carpenters, computer users).
- Women are affected more often than men, possibly due to a smaller carpal tunnel. Hormones may be involved because CTS often occurs during the premenstrual period, pregnancy, and menopause.

Clinical Manifestations

Manifestations are impaired sensation, pain, numbness, or weakness in the distribution of the median nerve and clumsiness in performing fine hand movements. Numbness and tingling may awaken the patient at night. Shaking the hands often relieves the symptoms. Physical signs of CTS include Tinel's sign and Phalen's sign.

- *Tinel's sign* is elicited by tapping over the median nerve as it passes through the carpal tunnel in the wrist. A positive response is a sensation of tingling in the distribution of the median nerve over the hand.
- *Phalen's sign* is elicited by allowing the wrists to fall freely into maximum flexion for more than 60 s. A positive response is a sensation of tingling in the distribution of the median nerve over the hand.

In late stages, there is atrophy of the thenar muscles around the base of the thumb, resulting in recurrent pain and eventual dysfunction of the hand.

Interprofessional and Nursing Management

Teach employees and employers about risk factors for CTS.

- Adaptive devices, such as wrist splints, may relieve pressure on the median nerve.
- Special keyboard pads and mice are available for computer users. Other ergonomic changes include workstation modifications, change in body position, and frequent breaks from work-related activities.

Early symptoms of CTS can usually be relieved by stopping the aggravating movement and immobilizing the hand and wrist in a splint.

- Splints worn at night help keep the wrist in a neutral position and may reduce night pain and numbness.
- Physical therapy with hand and wrist exercises may lessen symptom severity.
- Injection of a corticosteroid drug directly into the carpal tunnel may give short-term relief.

If symptoms persist for more than 6 months, carpal tunnel release surgery may be recommended. Open release or endoscopic surgery is done in an outpatient setting under local anesthesia.

- After surgery, assess the neurovascular status of the hand regularly.
- Teach the patient about wound care and the assessments to perform at home.

Although symptoms may be relieved after surgery, full recovery may take months.

CATARACT

Description

A cataract is an opacity in the lens of one or both eyes, causing a gradual decline in vision. Cataract removal is the most common surgical procedure in the United States.

Pathophysiology

Most cataracts are age related (senile cataracts). Other factors include blunt or penetrating trauma, smoking, alcohol use, radiation or ultraviolet light exposure, certain drugs (e.g., steroids), and ocular inflammation. Patients with diabetes tend to develop cataracts at a younger age.

- In senile cataract formation, altered metabolic processes within the lens cause water accumulation and changes in the lens fiber structure. These changes affect lens transparency and vision.

Clinical Manifestations

- Patients may have decreased vision and abnormal color perception. Glare is worse at night.
- Visual decline is gradual.

Diagnostic Studies

- Lens opacity is observed by ophthalmoscopic or slit lamp microscopic examination
- Visual acuity measurement
- Glare testing
- Keratometry and A-scan ultrasound if surgery is planned

Interprofessional Management

Currently, no treatment "cures" cataracts other than surgical removal.

- Helpful measures include changing the eyeglass prescription, using strong reading glasses or magnifiers, increasing the amount of reading light, and avoiding nighttime driving if glare is worse at night.
- When these measures no longer provide an acceptable level of visual function, the patient is a candidate for surgery. Removal of the lens may also be medically necessary in patients with increased intraocular pressure and diabetic retinopathy.

Most patients have an intraocular lens (IOL) implanted at the time of cataract extraction surgery. The patient's eye may be covered with a patch or protective shield, which is removed during the first postoperative visit. IOL implants provide immediate visual improvement for most patients.

Nursing Management

Goals

- Before surgery, the patient will (1) make informed decisions about treatment options and (2) have minimal anxiety.
- After surgery, the overall goals are that the patient with a cataract will (1) understand and follow discharge instructions; (2) maintain an acceptable level of physical and emotional comfort; and (3) remain free of infection and other complications.

Interventions

For the patient who chooses not to have surgery, suggest vision enhancement techniques and a modification of activities and lifestyle to accommodate the visual deficit.

For the patient who elects surgery, provide information, support, and reassurance about the surgical experience to reduce or alleviate anxiety. After surgery, offer mild analgesics for slight scratchiness or mild eye pain.

▼ **Patient and Caregiver Teaching**

- Suggest ways to modify activities and the environment for safety. Suggestions may include getting assistance with stairs,

TABLE 22 Patient and Caregiver Teaching: After Eye Surgery

Include the following information in the teaching plan for the patient and caregiver after eye surgery.

- If a patch is used, the patient will not have depth perception until the patch is removed. Ask for assistance to walk on uneven ground or on stairs.
- Measures to cope with visual loss and promote safety, such as large screens, audiobooks, and additional lighting.
- Use proper hygiene to ensure that dressings and/or surgical wounds are not contaminated during eye care.
- Report signs and symptoms of infection (such as redness, increased or purulent drainage) to allow for early treatment.
- Follow postoperative restrictions on head positioning, bending, coughing, and Valsalva maneuver to prevent increased intraocular pressure.
- Instill eye medications using aseptic technique and adhere to prescribed eye medication routine to prevent infection.
- Monitor pain, take pain medication, and report pain not relieved by medication.
- Schedule recommended postoperative appointments to maximize visual outcomes.

removing area rugs and other obstacles, preparing meals for freezing before surgery, and obtaining audiobooks for diversion until visual acuity improves.

- Written and verbal discharge teaching should include eye care, activity restrictions, medications, follow-up visit schedule, and signs of possible complications (Table 22).
- Patients may have difficulty with self-care activities, especially if vision in the unoperated eye is poor. Include the patient's caregiver in your teaching. Provide an opportunity for the patient and caregiver to do return demonstrations of any self-care activities.

CELIAC DISEASE

Description

Celiac disease is an autoimmune disease that causes damage to the small intestinal mucosa. It is triggered by ingesting gluten, a protein in wheat, barley, and rye.

Celiac disease is not the same as the disease *tropical sprue,* a chronic disorder occurring primarily in tropical areas. Tropical sprue causes disruption of jejunal and ileal tissue, resulting in malnutrition. It is treated with folic acid and tetracycline.

Celiac disease affects about 1 in 100 people worldwide. First-degree relatives of someone with celiac disease have a 4%–10% chance of developing the disorder. It is associated with other autoimmune diseases, particularly rheumatoid arthritis and type 1 diabetes. It is slightly more common in women. Symptoms often begin in childhood. Many people seek treatment for nonspecific complaints for years before celiac disease is diagnosed.

Pathophysiology

Three factors necessary for the development of celiac disease are a genetic predisposition, gluten ingestion, and an immune-mediated response.

- About 95% of people with celiac disease have human leukocyte antigen (HLA) allele HLA-DQ2, and the other 5% have HLA-DQ8. Not everyone with these genetic markers develops the disease.
- Tissue destruction is the result of chronic inflammation activated by the ingestion of gluten found in wheat, rye, and barley.
- Damage is most severe in the duodenum, probably because it has more exposure to gluten. The inflammation lasts as long as gluten ingestion continues.

Clinical Manifestations

Classic manifestations of celiac disease include foul-smelling diarrhea, abdominal pain, flatulence, and abdominal distention. Atypical signs and symptoms include joint pain, liver problems, fatigue, peripheral neuropathy, and reproductive problems.

- A pruritic, vesicular skin lesion called *dermatitis herpetiformis* may be present as a rash on the buttocks, scalp, face, elbows, and knees.
- Weight loss, muscle wasting, and other signs of malnutrition may be present.
- Patients may have lactose intolerance.
- Iron deficiency anemia is common.

Diagnostic Studies

Celiac disease is confirmed by findings from the history and physical examination and serologic testing. Histologic analysis of small intestine biopsy specimens can confirm the diagnosis.

Interprofessional and Nursing Management

A strict gluten-free diet is the only effective treatment for celiac disease. Most patients need to maintain a gluten-free diet for the rest of their lives.

Periodic nutrition evaluations and laboratory monitoring are done to monitor for anemia and malnutrition. The patient should undergo bone density screening every 2–3 years. They often require a daily vitamin and mineral supplement.

- Refer all patients for a dietary consultation. Reinforce that continued gluten consumption will result in chronic inflammation, which can lead to anemia and osteoporosis.
- Dietary gluten comes from wheat, barley, rye, and oats (oats do not contain gluten but can become contaminated with gluten during milling). Gluten is also found in some medications, food additives, preservatives, and stabilizers.
- Many restaurants indicate gluten-free menu options.
- The Celiac Disease Foundation (www.celiac.org) provides suggestions for maintaining a gluten-free diet and living with celiac disease.

CERVICAL CANCER

Description and Etiology

Cervical cancer was once a common cause of cancer death. However, with early detection (Pap test, human papilloma virus [HPV] testing), the mortality rate from cervical cancer has significantly declined.

- Risk factors for cervical cancer include infection with high-risk strains of HPV 16 and 18, immunosuppression, using oral contraceptive pills (OCPs) for a long period of time, being exposed to the drug diethylstilbestrol (DES), and smoking.

The progression from normal cervical cells to dysplasia and on to cervical cancer occurs over years. There is a strong relationship between sexual exposure to HPV and cervical dysplasia. A vaccine can protect against cervical cancer that is caused by HPV types 16 and 18.

Clinical Manifestations

Early cervical cancer often has no symptoms. Unusual discharge, abnormal uterine bleeding, or postcoital bleeding eventually occurs.

- Vaginal discharge is thin and watery but becomes dark and foul-smelling as the disease advances.
- Vaginal bleeding is initially spotting, but becomes heavier and more frequent.
- Pain is a late symptom and is followed by weight loss, anemia, and cachexia.

Diagnostic Studies

- Pap test, colposcopy, and biopsy
- HPV testing can identify high-risk HPV types 16 and 18, of which 80% are associated with cervical cancer.

Interprofessional Management

Vaccination against HPV provides an opportunity for primary prevention of cervical cancer. Inform both parents and patients about the need to complete the HPV vaccination series at age 11–12 years, when the immune system has a good response to the vaccine. HPV vaccination is not recommended for everyone older than age 26 years, but adults age 27 through 45 years with high risk may decide to get the vaccine.

- Gardasil 9 protects against HPV types 6, 11, 16, 18, and five other HPV types. These vaccines are given in 2–3 IM doses (depending on the patient's age) over a 6-month period. They have few side effects.

Treatment depends on the stage of the cancer and if fertility is a concern.

- Cryotherapy, loop electrosurgical excision procedure (LEEP), laser therapy, or cone biopsy can remove abnormal cells and prevent progression to cervical cancer.
- The main treatment for early cancer is surgery or radiation therapy.
- Care for more advanced cancer can include a combination of surgery, chemotherapy, and radiation.
- Surgical procedures include hysterectomy, radical hysterectomy, and, rarely, pelvic exenteration (Table 23).

Nursing Management: Cervical Cancer and Other Cancers of the Female Reproductive System

In addition to cervical cancer, malignant tumors of the female reproductive system can be found in the endometrium, ovaries, vagina,

TABLE 23 Common Gynecological Surgical Procedures

Type of surgical procedure	Description
Dilation and Curettage (D and C)	Opening (dilation) of cervix and removal (scraping) of endometrial tissue
Endometrial Ablation	Destruction of endometrial lining using heat, cold, or electrical energy
Hysterectomy	Removal of the uterus Several different types: • Vaginal: Uterus is removed through an incision in the vagina • Abdominal: Uterus is removed through an incision in the abdomen • Laparoscopic: Uses a laparoscope and instrument inserted through abdominal incisions • Robotic-assisted laparoscopy: Uses a surgical robot to manipulate surgical instruments
Hysteroscopy	Examination uterine cavity using a hysteroscope (lighted, flexible viewing instrument), inserted through the cervix
Myomectomy	Removal of fibroids from the uterus, leaving the uterus in place
Oophorectomy	Removal of the ovary, can be unilateral or bilateral
Salpingectomy	Removal of the fallopian tube, can be unilateral or bilateral
Uterine artery embolization	Minimally invasive surgery to inject embolic agents into uterine arteries to block blood supply to uterine fibroids
Vaginectomy	Removal of vagina, may be partial or total
Vulvectomy	Removal of part or all the vulva

and vulva. Management of the patient with any cancer of the female reproductive system includes many similar interventions.

Goals

The overall goals of nursing care are that the patient will take part in treatment decisions, achieve satisfactory pain and symptom management, recognize and report complications, maintain quality of life, and practice cancer detection. Key concerns for the patient with gynecologic cancer include pain, disturbed body image, and impaired sexual functioning.

Interventions

Teach women the importance of routine screening for cancers of the reproductive system. Cancer can be prevented when screening reveals precancerous conditions of the vulva, cervix, endometrium, and rarely, the ovaries. Assist women to view routine cancer screening as an important self-care activity.

- Teach women about risk factors for cancers of the reproductive system. Limiting sexual activity during adolescence, HPV vaccination against cervical cancer, using condoms, having fewer sexual partners, and not smoking reduce the risk of cervical cancer.

All patients have a degree of anxiety while waiting for cancer surgery. The prospect of major gynecologic surgery increases these concerns. Some women may focus on the effect the surgery will have on their appearance and sexual functions.

- Discuss the woman's feelings and concerns about the surgery. Assess each patient individually. Be willing to listen since this can provide considerable support.

Standard preoperative care includes perineal or abdominal preparation and urinary catheter insertion.

After surgery, pain management, bowel and bladder care, and encouraging ambulation and exercise are important. Initiate venous thromboembolism (VTE) prophylaxis.

- Teach the patient about postoperative care and expectations for recovery.

CHLAMYDIAL INFECTIONS

Description

Chlamydia trachomatis infection is the most common reportable sexually transmitted infection (STI) in the United States. *Chlamydia,* a gram-negative bacterium, is transmitted through exposure to sexual fluids during vaginal, anal, or oral sex. Ejaculation does not have to occur for it to be transmitted.

High-risk groups and risk factors include women and adolescents, new or multiple sexual partners, sexual partners who have had multiple partners, history of STIs and cervical ectopy, coexisting STIs, and inconsistent or incorrect use of a condom.

- The incubation period for chlamydia is 1–3 weeks. Infection with chlamydia does not provide protection from reinfection, so people treated for chlamydia can be reinfected.

Clinical Manifestations

Patients with chlamydia often have no symptoms.

- Men may have pain with urination or a urethral discharge. Rarely, men have testicular pain or swelling caused by infection of the epididymis.
- In women, manifestations of cervicitis include mucopurulent vaginal discharge (mucus with pus), bleeding, dysuria, and pain with intercourse.

Symptoms of rectal chlamydia include anorectal pain, discharge, bleeding, anal pruritus, tenesmus, mucus-coated stools, or painful bowel movements.

Complications

Complications often develop from poorly managed, inaccurately diagnosed, or undiagnosed *chlamydia*.

- In men, rare complications may result in epididymitis with possible infertility.
- In women, infection may result in pelvic inflammatory disease, which damages fallopian tubes and increases the risk for ectopic pregnancy (pregnancy outside of uterus), infertility, and chronic pelvic pain.

Diagnostic Studies

Chlamydia can be diagnosed by collecting urine or swab specimens from the endocervix or vagina (women), urethra (men), oropharynx, or rectum. The most common test is the nucleic acid amplification test (NAAT).

Interprofessional and Nursing Management

Doxycycline (Vibramycin) is used to treat patients and their partners.

- All sexual contacts within 60 days should be evaluated and treated to prevent reinfection and further transmission.
- Teach patients to abstain from sexual contact for 7 days after treatment is completed, or until all partners have been treated and have also abstained from sexual contact for 7 days.
- Review the ways to reduce risk of acquiring a repeat or new STI in the future.

See Sexually Transmitted Infections: Nursing Management.

CHOLELITHIASIS/CHOLECYSTITIS

Description

The most common disorder of the biliary system is *cholelithiasis* (stones in the gallbladder). The stones may lodge in the neck of the gallbladder or in the cystic duct. *Cholecystitis* (inflammation of the gallbladder) may be acute or chronic, and it is usually associated with gallstones. Up to 10% of American adults in the United States have cholelithiasis.

- Gallstones are more common in women, especially multiparous women and those over 40 years of age. Postmenopausal women on estrogen replacement therapy and younger women on oral contraceptives are at an increased risk.
- Other factors that seem to increase the incidence of gallbladder disease are sedentary lifestyle, familial tendency, and obesity.
- The incidence of gallbladder disease is especially high in Native Americans.

Pathophysiology

The cause of gallstones is unknown. They develop when the balance of cholesterol, bile salts, and calcium in solution changes so that these substances precipitate. Conditions that upset this balance include infection and changes in cholesterol metabolism. Mixed cholesterol stones, which are mainly cholesterol, are the most common.

The stones may stay in the gallbladder or migrate to the cystic duct or common bile duct. They cause pain as they pass through the ducts and may lodge in the ducts and cause obstruction. Stasis of bile in the gallbladder can lead to cholecystitis.

Cholecystitis is most often associated with obstruction from gallstones or biliary sludge. Cholecystitis without obstruction occurs most often in those who are older or critically ill. Secondary infection with enteric pathogens, including *Escherichia coli*, *Enterococcus faecalis*, *Klebsiella*, *Pseudomonas*, and *Proteus*, is common. Perforation occurs in severe cases.

- During an acute attack of cholecystitis, the edematous and hyperemic gallbladder may be distended with bile or pus. The cystic duct may become occluded.
- The wall of the gallbladder becomes scarred after an acute attack. Decreased functioning occurs if large amounts of tissue become fibrotic.

Clinical Manifestations

Severity of symptoms from cholelithiasis depends on whether the stones are stationary or mobile and whether obstruction is present.

- A stone lodged in the ducts or moving through the ducts may produce severe pain, termed *biliary colic*. The severe pain may last up to 1 h, with residual tenderness in the right upper quadrant. The pain can be accompanied by tachycardia, diaphoresis, and prostration.
- The attacks of pain frequently occur 3–6 h after a high-fat meal or when the patient lies down.
- When total obstruction occurs, symptoms related to bile blockage occur. These include steatorrhea, pruritus, dark amber urine, bleeding tendencies, and jaundice.

   Manifestations of cholecystitis vary from indigestion to moderate to severe pain, fever, and jaundice. Initial symptoms include indigestion and acute pain and tenderness in the right upper quadrant. Pain may be referred to the right shoulder and scapula and be accompanied by restlessness, diaphoresis, and nausea and vomiting. Inflammation results in leukocytosis and fever. Physical findings include RUQ or epigastrium tenderness and abdominal rigidity.

- Symptoms of chronic cholecystitis include a history of fat intolerance, dyspepsia, heartburn, and flatulence.

Complications

Complications of cholecystitis include gangrenous cholecystitis, subphrenic abscess, pancreatitis, *cholangitis* (inflammation of biliary ducts), biliary cirrhosis, fistulas, and rupture of the gallbladder, which can cause bile peritonitis.

Diagnostic Studies

- Ultrasonography is used to diagnose gallstones.
- Endoscopic retrograde cholangiopancreatography (ERCP) allows for visualization of the gallbladder, cystic duct, common hepatic duct, and common bile duct. Bile taken during ERCP is sent for culture to identify any possible infecting organism.
- Percutaneous transhepatic cholangiography may locate stones in the bile ducts.
- Laboratory tests reveal increased serum enzymes and pancreatic enzymes, increased white blood cell (WBC) count, increased direct and indirect bilirubin levels, and urinary bilirubin.

Interprofessional Management

The treatment of gallstones in cholelithiasis depends on the stage of disease. Bile acids are used to dissolve stones, but the stones may recur. ERCP with sphincterotomy (papillotomy) may be used for stone removal and placement of stents.

Extracorporeal shock-wave lithotripsy (ESWL) uses high-energy shock waves to disintegrate gallstones.

During an acute episode of cholecystitis, treatment focuses on pain control, control of possible infection with antibiotics, and maintenance of fluid and electrolyte balance. Treatment is mainly supportive and symptomatic. Drug therapy for gallbladder disease includes analgesics, anticholinergics (antispasmodics), fat-soluble vitamins, and bile salts. Opioids may be used initially for pain management.

- If nausea and vomiting are severe, nasogastric (NG) tube insertion and gastric decompression may prevent further gallbladder stimulation.
- Anticholinergics may be administered to decrease secretions and counteract smooth muscle spasms.

Laparoscopic cholecystectomy is the preferred surgical procedure for symptomatic gallstones. The gallbladder is removed through one of four small punctures in the abdomen. Most patients have minimal postoperative pain and are discharged the day of surgery or the day after. In most cases, they can resume normal activities and return to work within 1 week.

An incisional (open) cholecystectomy involves removing the gallbladder through a right subcostal incision. A T tube may be placed in the common bile duct to keep the duct patent until the edema subsides.

Nursing Management

Goals

The overall goals are that the patient with gallbladder disease will have relief of pain and discomfort, no complications, and no recurrent attacks of cholecystitis or gallstones.

Nursing Interventions

Nursing actions for the patient undergoing conservative therapy include relieving pain, relieving nausea and vomiting, providing comfort and emotional support, maintaining fluid and electrolyte balance and nutrition, and observing for complications.

The patient with acute cholecystitis or gallstones often has severe pain. Give the drugs ordered to relieve the pain as needed. Observe for signs of obstruction of the ducts by stones, including jaundice;

clay-colored stools; dark, foamy urine; steatorrhea; fever; and increased WBC count.

Postoperative nursing care after a laparoscopic cholecystectomy includes monitoring for complications, such as bleeding, making the patient comfortable, and preparing the patient for discharge.

- Patients may report referred pain to the shoulder because of the CO_2 used to inflate the abdominal cavity during surgery. CO_2 can irritate the phrenic nerve and diaphragm, causing some difficulty breathing. Placing the patient in Sims' position (left side with right knee flexed) helps move the gas pocket away from the diaphragm. Encourage deep breathing, movement, and ambulation.

Postoperative nursing care for incisional cholecystectomy focuses on promoting ventilation and preventing respiratory complications.

- If the patient has a T tube, maintain the system drainage and observe for bile drainage.

▼ **Patient and Caregiver Teaching**
- When the patient has conservative therapy, teach about a low-fat diet. If needed, review a weight-reduction diet. The patient may need to take fat-soluble vitamin supplements.
- Teach the patient indications of biliary obstruction (stool and urine changes, jaundice, and pruritus).
- The patient who undergoes a laparoscopic cholecystectomy is discharged soon after the surgery, so home care and teaching are important (Table 24).

TABLE 24 Patient and Caregiver Teaching: Postoperative Laparoscopic Cholecystectomy

Include the following instructions in the patient's postoperative teaching plan.

1. Remove the bandages on the puncture sites the day after surgery and you can shower.
2. Notify your HCP if any of the following signs and symptoms occurs:
   - Redness, swelling, bile-colored drainage, or pus from any incision
   - Severe abdominal pain, nausea, vomiting, fever, chills
3. You can gradually resume normal activities.
4. Return to work within 1 week of surgery.
5. You can resume your usual diet. Many tolerate a low-fat diet better for several weeks after surgery.

CHRONIC OBSTRUCTIVE PULMONARY DISEASE

Description

Chronic obstructive pulmonary disease (COPD) is a progressive disease characterized by persistent airflow limitation. COPD is associated with an enhanced chronic inflammatory response in the airways and lungs. The main causes are cigarette smoking and other noxious particles and gases. Exacerbations and other coexisting problems may contribute to the severity of the disease.

Previous definitions of COPD have included such terms as chronic bronchitis and emphysema. Each condition has features of COPD, but neither by itself is COPD. Chronic bronchitis is the presence of cough and sputum production for at least three months in each of two consecutive years. It is an independent disease that may precede or follow the development of airflow limitation. Emphysema, the destruction of alveoli without fibrosis, describes one of several structural abnormalities in COPD (Fig. 4).

- Around 16 million adults in the United States have COPD. The number of people with COPD is underestimated because the disease is usually not diagnosed until it is moderately advanced. COPD is the third leading cause of death in the United States, causing more than 140,000 deaths each year.

Etiology

Many factors influence the development and progression of COPD.

- Cigarette smoking is the major risk factor for developing COPD. The irritating effect of cigarette smoke causes hyperplasia of cells, which increases mucus production. Hyperplasia reduces airway diameter and makes it harder to clear secretions. Smoking reduces ciliary activity and destroys alveolar walls.
- *Environmental tobacco smoke* (ETS) or secondhand smoke is associated with decreased pulmonary function, increased respiratory symptoms, and severe lower respiratory tract infections (e.g., pneumonia). ETS is associated with increased risk for nasal sinus cancer and lung cancer.
- Severe recurring respiratory tract infections in childhood are associated with reduced lung function and increased respiratory symptoms in adulthood. We are not sure if COPD is related to recurrent infections in adults.
- High levels of urban air pollution are harmful to people with existing lung disease.
- With intense or prolonged exposure to various dusts, vapors, irritants, or fumes in the workplace, symptoms of lung impairment

Figure 4 (A) Normal lungs showing bronchioles and alveoli. (B) Changes in the bronchioles and alveoli in the lungs of a patient with COPD.

consistent with COPD can develop. If a person has occupational exposure and smokes, the risk of COPD increases.

- Another risk factor is exposure to coal and other biomass fuels for indoor heating and cooking.
- Asthma may be a risk factor for COPD development. There is a considerable overlap between asthma and COPD, especially among older adults, who may have components of both.
- Genetic factors influence which smokers get the disease. α_1-*Antitrypsin (AAT) deficiency* is a genetic risk factor for COPD.

Pathophysiology

COPD is characterized by chronic inflammation of the airways, lung parenchyma (respiratory bronchioles and alveoli), and pulmonary blood vessels. The defining feature of COPD is airflow limitation not fully reversible during forced exhalation. The main cause is loss of elastic recoil and airflow obstruction from mucus hypersecretion, mucosal edema, and bronchospasm.

The inflammatory process starts with inhalation of noxious particles (e.g., cigarette smoke) and gases. With repeated exposure, chronic inflammation causes tissue destruction and disrupts the normal defense mechanisms and repair process of the lung.

- The predominant inflammatory cells are neutrophils, macrophages, and lymphocytes. These cells attract other inflammatory mediators (e.g., leukotrienes) and proinflammatory cytokines (e.g., tumor necrosis factor).
- After inhaling oxidants in tobacco or air pollution, protease activity (which breaks down the connective tissue of the lungs) increases and antiproteases (which protect against the breakdown) are inhibited.
- Inability to expire air is the main characteristic of COPD. As the peripheral airways become obstructed, air is progressively trapped during expiration. The chest hyperexpands and becomes barrel-shaped since the respiratory muscles are not able to function effectively.
- Gas exchange abnormalities result in hypoxemia and hypercapnia (increased CO_2) as the disease worsens. As air trapping increases and alveoli are destroyed, bullae (large air spaces in the parenchyma) and blebs (air spaces adjacent to pleurae) form. There is a significant ventilation-perfusion (V/Q) mismatch and hypoxemia results.
- Excess mucus production, resulting in a chronic productive cough, is caused by an increased number of mucus-secreting goblet cells, enlarged submucosal glands, dysfunction of cilia, and stimulation from inflammatory mediators.

- Pulmonary vascular changes result in mild to moderate pulmonary hypertension.

Clinical Manifestations

COPD typically develops slowly.

- A chronic intermittent cough, often the first symptom to develop, may later be present every day.
- Dyspnea with exertion is often progressive. In the late stages, dyspnea may be present at rest. Wheezing and chest tightness vary by time of the day or from day to day.
- The patient with advanced COPD often has fatigue, anorexia, and weight loss.
- During physical examination, a prolonged expiratory phase, wheezes, or decreased breath sounds are noted in all lung fields. The anterior-posterior diameter of the chest is increased *(barrel chest)* from chronic air trapping. The patient may assume a tripod position and use pursed-lip breathing.
- Over time, hypoxemia may develop with hypercapnia. The bluish-red color of the skin results from polycythemia and cyanosis. Polycythemia develops from increased production of red blood cells as the body tries to compensate for chronic hypoxemia.

Complications

Cor pulmonale results from pulmonary hypertension caused mainly by constriction of pulmonary vessels in response to alveolar hypoxia. When pulmonary hypertension develops, the pressure on the right side of the heart must increase to push blood into the lungs. Eventually right-sided heart failure develops (see Cor Pulmonale).

A *COPD exacerbation* is the acute worsening of the patient's usual patterns of dyspnea, cough, and/or sputum production. Respiratory infections are a common cause. Exacerbations are common and increase in frequency (averaging one to two per year) as the disease progresses.

- Teach the patient and caregiver early recognition of the cardinal symptoms of exacerbations (increase in dyspnea, sputum volume, or sputum purulence) to promote early treatment and thus prevent hospitalization and possible acute respiratory failure.
- Exacerbations are managed with short-acting bronchodilators, oral systemic corticosteroids, and antibiotics.

Acute respiratory failure may occur in patients with severe COPD who have exacerbations. Be alert for signs of increasing severity, such as use of accessory muscles, central cyanosis, edema in the lower extremities, unstable BP, right-sided heart failure, and altered alertness. Often, patients with COPD wait too long to contact a health care provider (HCP) after first experiencing symptoms. Stopping bronchodilator or corticosteroid medications may also precipitate respiratory failure. See Acute Respiratory Failure.

Diagnostic Studies

- A forced expiratory volume in 1 min/forced vital capacity ratio (FEV_1/FVC) < 70% along with the symptoms can help diagnose COPD. A lower value of FEV_1 indicates more severe COPD.
- A history and physical examination are important.
- Chest X-rays may show a flat diaphragm because of hyperinflation of lungs.
- Electrocardiogram (ECG) can be used to determine right- and left-sided ventricular failure.
- Sputum culture and sensitivity are done during an acute exacerbation.
- Arterial blood gases (ABGs) in later stages usually indicate low partial pressure of oxygen in arterial blood (PaO_2), elevated partial pressure of carbon dioxide in arterial blood ($PaCO_2$), decreased or low normal pH, and increased bicarbonate (HCO_3^-) levels.

Interprofessional Management

Most patients with COPD are treated as outpatients. They are hospitalized for an acute exacerbation or a complication, such as pneumonia, heart failure, or acute respiratory failure.

- Stopping cigarette smoking can have the biggest impact on reducing the risk of developing COPD and on decreasing progression of the disease.

O2 therapy is often part of the treatment of COPD. It is the only treatment linked to improved survival. For most patients, the goal of O2 therapy is to keep the SaO2 greater than 90% during rest, sleep, and exertion or the PaO2 greater than 60 mm Hg (see Oxygen Therapy).

- These goals may be modified for the patient with moderate to severe COPD. For example, based upon the patient's condition, the HCP may accept an SaO_2 and PaO_2 greater than 88%.

Drugs for COPD can reduce symptoms, increase exercise capacity, improve overall health, and reduce the number and severity of exacerbations.

- Bronchodilator therapy is the first line treatment for most patients. Bronchodilator drug therapy relaxes bronchial smooth muscle in the airway and improves the ventilation of the lungs, thus reducing the degree of breathlessness. Bronchodilator drugs commonly used are β2-adrenergic agonists, anticholinergics agents, and, to a much lesser extent, methylxanthines.

- A short-acting β2-adrenergic agonist (SABA) remains a mainstay of COPD treatment. The most common SABA is albuterol. Long-acting β2-adrenergic agonists (LABAs) are often used as monotherapy. Salmeterol and formoterol are widely used LABAs.

- Anticholinergics block the action of acetylcholine on the muscarinic receptors in the smooth muscle of the bronchiotracheal tree. The most common short-acting muscarinic agent (SAMA) is ipratropium bromide. For the patient who needs a drug with a more prolonged effect, long-acting muscarinic agents (LAMAs) such as tiotropium are an option.

- Combining short-acting bronchodilators with anticholinergic medications into a "combination" drug may help improve bronchodilation of the airways and potentially decrease the risk for side effects. Albuterol and ipratropium can be nebulized together or delivered by inhalation spray (Combivent Respimat).

- Regular treatment with inhaled corticosteroids (ICS) may be prescribed. However, unlike asthma, an ICS is not used as monotherapy in COPD because of the side effects. An ICS is often combined with a LABA for enhanced effect. Examples of combinations of ICSs with LABAs are fluticasone/salmeterol (Advair) and budesonide/formoterol (Symbicort). Oral corticosteroids are not used for long-term therapy in COPD but are effective for short-term use to treat acute exacerbations.

- Methylxanthines such as theophylline have serious side effects. Careful monitoring is needed. Theophylline interacts with many drugs and has a very narrow therapeutic window. A low dose of theophylline with an ICS may help a few patients who do not respond to other inhaled medications.

- Roflumilast (Daliresp) is an oral antiinflammatory agent used to decrease exacerbations in patients with severe COPD and chronic bronchitis. It is a drug used for long-term therapy but does not treat acute problems.

- Mucolytic agents, such as N-acetylcysteine (NAC), may be used for COPD patients who have an acute exacerbation. They have antiinflammatory and mucolytic properties. NAC may help improve overall health and quality of life in some patients. The main types of breathing exercises commonly taught are pursed-lip breathing and diaphragmatic breathing. Diaphragmatic breathing in some patients with COPD may increase the WOB and dyspnea.

Airway clearance techniques (ACTs) loosen mucus and secretions so they can be cleared by coughing. Typically, the patient receives bronchodilator therapy through an inhaled device (e.g., nebulization) before ACT. Then the ACT is used, followed by effective coughing (e.g., huff coughing). Airway clearance devices can also help mobilize secretions. Weight loss and muscle wasting are common in the patient with severe COPD. To decrease dyspnea and conserve energy, the patient should rest at least 30 min before eating and use a bronchodilator before meals.

- A diet high in calories and protein, moderate in carbohydrates, and moderate to high in fat is recommended. Food can be divided into five or six small meals a day.

Surgical Therapy

Four different surgical procedures have been used in severe COPD. One type of surgery is *lung volume reduction surgery*, which is done to reduce the size of the lungs by removing the most diseased lung tissue so that the remaining healthy lung tissue can perform better. A second procedure, *bronchoscopic lung volume reduction surgery*, involves placing one-way valves in the airways. The valves let air out of diseased parts of the lung, but not in. Another surgical procedure is a *bullectomy*, which is used for patients with emphysematous COPD who have large bullae (>1 cm). The bullae are usually resected via thoracoscope. A fourth surgical procedure is *lung transplantation*, which helps a few patients with advanced COPD.

Nursing Management

Goals

The overall goals are that the patient with COPD will have relief from symptoms, ability to perform activities of daily living (ADLs) and improved exercise tolerance, no complications related to COPD, knowledge and ability to implement a long-term treatment plan, prevention of disease progression, and overall improved quality of life.

Interventions

Counsel the patient who smokes regarding smoking cessation, because it is the only way to slow the progression of COPD. Avoiding or controlling exposure to occupational and environmental pollutants and irritants is another preventive measure to maintain healthy lungs. Early diagnosis and treatment of respiratory tract infections and COPD exacerbations help prevent progression of the disease.

- Patients with COPD should avoid people who are sick, practice good hand-washing techniques, take drugs as prescribed, exercise regularly, and maintain a healthy weight. Influenza and pneumococcal vaccines are recommended.

- The patient with COPD needs acute intervention for exacerbations of COPD, pneumonia, cor pulmonale, and acute respiratory failure.

▼ **Patient and Caregiver Teaching**

Teaching is the most important aspect of long-term care of the patient with COPD (Table 25). In pulmonary rehabilitation (PR),

---

TABLE 25 Patient and Caregiver Teaching: Chronic Obstructive Pulmonary Disease (COPD)

Include the following information in the teaching plan to assist the patient with COPD and the caregiver to improve quality of life through promoting lifestyle practices that support successful living with COPD.

What is COPD?

- Basic anatomy and physiology of lung
- Basic pathophysiology of COPD
- Signs and symptoms of COPD, exacerbation
- How to tell COPD from the common cold, flu, pneumonia
- Tests to assess breathing

Breathing and airway clearance exercises

- Pursed-lip breathing
- Airway clearance technique—huff cough

Energy conservation techniques

- Daily activities (e.g., bathing, grooming, shopping, traveling)
- Consultation with physical therapist and occupational therapist

Medications

- Types (include class, mechanism of action, and devices)
- Establishing medication schedule
- Correct use of inhalers, spacer, and nebulizer
- Reason for use of O_2 equipment
- Guide for home O_2 use and equipment

Psychosocial/emotional issues
Open discussion (sharing with patient, caregiver, and family)

- Concerns about interpersonal relationships (e.g., intimacy)
- Problems with emotions (e.g., depression, anxiety, panic)
- Dependency

TABLE 25 Patient and Caregiver Teaching: Chronic Obstructive Pulmonary Disease (COPD)—cont'd

Include the following information in the teaching plan to assist the patient with COPD and the caregiver to improve quality of life through promoting lifestyle practices that support successful living with COPD.

Treatment decisions

Support and rehabilitation groups

COPD management plan

Nurse and patient develop and write up COPD management plan that meets individual needs.

- Focus on self-management
- Need to report changes
- Cause of acute exacerbations
- Recognition of signs and symptoms of respiratory infection, heart failure
- Reduce risk factors, especially smoking cessation
- Exercise program of walking and arm strengthening
- Yearly follow-up evaluations

Nutrition support

- Ways to lose or gain weight, as needed
- Consultation with dietitian

For more information, see American Lung Association at *www.lung.org/lung-disease/copd.*

an interprofessional team works to individualize the treatment plan for the patient with COPD.

- Components of PR vary but usually include exercise training, smoking cessation, nutrition counseling, and teaching.

Energy conservation is an important component in COPD rehabilitation. Exercise training of the upper extremities may improve muscle function and reduce dyspnea. Plan alternative energy-saving practices for ADLs and scheduled rest periods.

- Teach the patient coordinated walking with slow, pursed-lip breathing. Encourage the patient to walk 15–20 min/day at least 3 times a week, with gradual increases.
- Modifying sexual activity can contribute to a healthy psychologic well-being. Using an inhaled bronchodilator before sexual activity can help ventilation.

- Adequate sleep is extremely important. The patient who is a restless sleeper, snores, stops breathing while asleep, and has a tendency to fall asleep during the day may need to be tested for sleep apnea.
- Healthy coping is a challenge for the patient and family. As the disease progresses, patients with COPD frequently have to deal with lifestyle changes that may involve decreased ability to care for themselves, decreased energy for social activities, and loss of a job. Support groups at local chapters of the American Lung Association, hospitals, and clinics may be helpful.
- End-of-life issues and advance directives are important topics for discussion in the latter stages of COPD. This may be hard for the patient and family to consider because of the uncertainty of the disease.

See eNursing Care Plan 31-2 (available on the website) for care of the patient with COPD.

CIRRHOSIS

Description

Cirrhosis, the end stage of liver disease, is characterized by extensive degeneration and destruction of liver cells. The most common causes of cirrhosis in the United States are chronic hepatitis C infection, nonalcoholic steatohepatitis (NASH), and alcohol-induced liver disease.

- In patients with alcohol-induced liver disease, malnutrition adds to the damage caused by the alcohol itself.
- Some cases of nutrition-related cirrhosis have resulted from extreme dieting, malabsorption, and obesity. Environmental factors and genetic predisposition may lead to the development of cirrhosis.
- Right-sided heart failure, primary biliary cirrhosis, and primary sclerosing cholangitis can also cause cirrhosis.

Pathophysiology

Damaged liver cells try to regenerate, but a disorganized process results in abnormal blood vessel and bile duct architecture. The overgrowth of new and fibrous connective tissue distorts the liver's normal structure, resulting in lobules of irregular size and shape with impeded blood flow and poor function.

Clinical Manifestations

The few symptoms in early-stage disease may include fatigue or an enlarged liver. Later manifestations may be severe and result from liver failure and portal hypertension. Jaundice, peripheral edema, and ascites develop gradually. Other late signs and symptoms include skin lesions, hematologic and endocrine problems, and peripheral neuropathies. In advanced stages, the liver becomes small and nodular. (See Fig. 5 for systemic clinical manifestations of cirrhosis.)

- *Jaundice* occurs because of the decreased ability of the liver to conjugate and excrete bilirubin.
- *Skin lesions*, such as *spider angiomas*, that occur on the nose, cheeks, upper trunk, and neck and a redness of the palms of

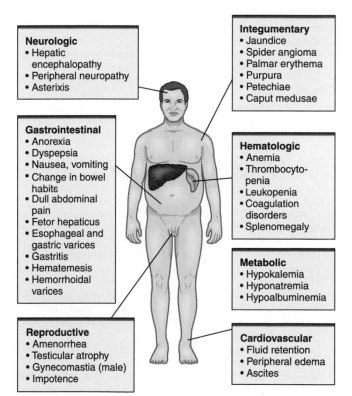

Neurologic
- Hepatic encephalopathy
- Peripheral neuropathy
- Asterixis

Integumentary
- Jaundice
- Spider angioma
- Palmar erythema
- Purpura
- Petechiae
- Caput medusae

Gastrointestinal
- Anorexia
- Dyspepsia
- Nausea, vomiting
- Change in bowel habits
- Dull abdominal pain
- Fetor hepaticus
- Esophageal and gastric varices
- Gastritis
- Hematemesis
- Hemorrhoidal varices

Hematologic
- Anemia
- Thrombocytopenia
- Leukopenia
- Coagulation disorders
- Splenomegaly

Metabolic
- Hypokalemia
- Hyponatremia
- Hypoalbuminemia

Reproductive
- Amenorrhea
- Testicular atrophy
- Gynecomastia (male)
- Impotence

Cardiovascular
- Fluid retention
- Peripheral edema
- Ascites

Figure 5 Systemic clinical manifestations of liver cirrhosis.

the hands, *palmar erythema*, are from an increase in circulating estrogen because the liver cannot metabolize steroid hormones.

- *Hematologic disorders*, such as anemia, leukopenia, and thrombocytopenia, may be caused by splenomegaly that results from backup of blood from the portal vein into the spleen (portal hypertension). Coagulation problems result from the liver's inability to make prothrombin and other clotting factors.
- *Endocrine problems* result because adrenocortical hormones, estrogen, and testosterone cannot be metabolized by a damaged liver. In men with cirrhosis, gynecomastia, loss of axillary and pubic hair, testicular atrophy, and impotence with loss of libido may occur because of increased estrogen levels. Younger women with cirrhosis may develop amenorrhea. Older women may have vaginal bleeding. Hyperaldosteronism causes sodium and water retention and potassium loss.
- *Peripheral neuropathy* is probably caused by a dietary deficiency of thiamine, folic acid, and cobalamin.

Complications

Major complications of cirrhosis are portal hypertension with resultant esophageal and/or gastric varices, peripheral edema, abdominal ascites, hepatic encephalopathy (coma), and hepatorenal syndrome.

Structural changes from cirrhosis obstruct blood flow in and out of the liver, causing *portal hypertension*, an increased pressure within the liver's circulatory system, and *esophageal* and *gastric varices*.

- Collateral channels often form in the lower esophagus, anterior abdominal wall, parietal peritoneum, and rectum. Varicosities (distended veins) develop where collateral and systemic circulations join, resulting in esophageal and gastric varices, *caput medusae* (ring of varices around the umbilicus), and hemorrhoids.
- *Esophageal varices* are a complex of tortuous veins at the end of the esophagus. *Gastric varices* are found in the upper part of the stomach. These fragile collateral vessels tolerate high pressure poorly and bleed easily.
- Bleeding esophageal varices are the most life-threatening complication of cirrhosis and are a medical emergency.

Peripheral edema occurs in the lower extremities and presacral area. Edema results from decreased colloidal osmotic pressure from impaired liver synthesis of albumin and increased portacaval pressure from portal hypertension.

Ascites is the accumulation of serous fluid in the peritoneal or abdominal cavity by several mechanisms. Portal hypertension causes proteins to move from the blood vessels into the lymph space and then leak into the peritoneal cavity. The liver's inability to make albumin leads to hypoalbuminemia, decreased colloidal oncotic pressure, and fluid shifting. The liver's inability to metabolize aldosterone leads to hyperaldosteronism, causing increased renal reabsorption of sodium and water.

- Ascites is manifested by abdominal distention with weight gain. In severe ascites, the umbilicus may be everted. Abdominal striae with distended abdominal wall veins may be present.
- Patients may have signs of dehydration (e.g., dry tongue and skin, sunken eyeballs, muscle weakness) and decreased urinary output.
- Hypokalemia is common due to an excessive loss of potassium from hyperaldosteronism and the use of diuretic therapy to treat ascites.

Hepatic encephalopathy is a neuropsychiatric manifestation of liver disease. When blood is shunted past the liver by way of collateral vessels or the liver is unable to convert ammonia to urea, the levels of ammonia in the systemic circulation rise. Ammonia crosses the blood-brain barrier and produces neurologic manifestations.

- Factors that increase ammonia in the circulation include GI hemorrhage, constipation, infection, hypokalemia, hypovolemia, dehydration, and metabolic alkalosis.
- Hepatic encephalopathy causes changes in neurologic and mental responsiveness, ranging from sleep problems to trouble concentrating to deep coma. *Asterixis* (flapping tremors) is a rapid flexion and extension movement of the hands when the arms and hands are held stretched out.

Hepatorenal syndrome is a type of renal failure with advancing azotemia, oliguria, and intractable ascites. There is no structural abnormality of the kidneys. Portal hypertension along with liver decompensation results in decreased arterial blood volume, renal vasoconstriction, and renal failure. In the patient with cirrhosis, this syndrome frequently follows diuretic therapy, GI hemorrhage, or paracentesis.

Diagnostic Studies

- Liver function studies demonstrate an elevation in alkaline phosphatase, aspartate aminotransferase (AST), alanine aminotransferase (ALT), and γ-glutamyl transferase (GGT) are initially high due to their release from inflamed liver cells. However, in end-stage liver disease, AST and ALT levels may be normal due to the death and loss of hepatocytes.

- Prothrombin time is prolonged. Serum albumin and protein levels are decreased and bilirubin and globulin levels are increased. Low cholesterol levels reflect changes in fat metabolism.
- Ultrasound elastography and biopsy (percutaneous needle) can help determine severity of cirrhosis.

Interprofessional Management

The goal of treatment is to slow the progression of cirrhosis and prevent and treat any complications. Management of ascites focuses on sodium restriction (2 g/day), diuretic therapy (e.g., a potassium-sparing diuretic combined with a loop diuretic), and fluid removal (paracentesis) for those patients with impaired respiration or abdominal pain.

The main goal related to esophageal varices is to prevent bleeding. The patient who has esophageal varices should avoid ingesting alcohol, aspirin, and nonsteroidal antiinflammatory drugs (NSAIDs). Patients with varices may take a nonselective β-adrenergic blocker (nadolol or propranolol) to decrease portal pressure.

- When variceal bleeding occurs, the first step is to stabilize the patient and manage the airway. IV therapy may include blood products. A combination of drug therapy and endoscopic therapy is more successful than either approach alone. Drug therapy may include somatostatin analog octreotide (Sandostatin) or vasopressin.
- At the time of endoscopy, band ligation or sclerotherapy may be used to prevent varices from rebleeding. Balloon tamponade may be used to control hemorrhage that cannot be controlled on initial endoscopy.
- Supportive measures during an acute variceal bleed include giving fresh frozen plasma and packed red blood cells (RBCs), vitamin K, and proton pump inhibitors (e.g., pantoprazole [Protonix]). Lactulose and rifaximin (Xifaxan) may be given to prevent hepatic encephalopathy from breakdown of blood and the release of ammonia in the intestine. Antibiotics are given to prevent bacterial infection.

Various surgical shunting procedures can decrease portal hypertension by diverting some of the portal blood flow while allowing adequate liver perfusion. The surgical shunts most often used are the portacaval shunt and the distal splenorenal shunt. Transjugular intrahepatic portosystemic shunt (TIPS) is a procedure where a catheter is placed in the jugular vein to create a tract (shunt) between the systemic and portal venous systems. TIPS reduces portal hypertension by diverting blood flow around the liver.

- Hepatic encephalopathy can occur after placement of a TIPS.

The goal of managing hepatic encephalopathy is to reduce ammonia formation. Lactulose, a drug that traps ammonia in the gut, reduces ammonia formation in the intestines. We can give it orally, as an enema, or through a nasogastric (NG) tube. The drug's laxative effect expels the ammonia from the colon. Antibiotics such as rifaximin may be given when patients do not respond to lactulose.

Specific nutrition therapy varies with the degree of liver damage and the danger of encephalopathy. The diet is high in calories (3000 cal/day) and carbohydrates. Sodium is restricted for patients with ascites and edema. A patient with alcoholic cirrhosis often needs protein supplements that the liver can easily metabolize.

Nursing Management
Goals
The patient with cirrhosis will have relief of discomfort, have minimal to no complications, and return to as normal a lifestyle as possible.
Interventions
Prevention and early treatment of cirrhosis focus on reducing or eliminating risk factors.

- Urge patients to abstain from alcohol. Encourage those with a history of chronic alcohol use to enroll in support programs that help them maintain sobriety.
- Adequate nutrition promotes liver regeneration.
- Identify and treat acute hepatitis before it progresses to chronic hepatitis and cirrhosis.

Nursing care for the patient with cirrhosis focuses on conserving the patient's strength while maintaining muscle strength. Modify the activity and rest schedule according to signs of clinical improvement (e.g., decreasing jaundice, improvement in liver function studies).

- Anorexia, nausea and vomiting, pressure from ascites, and poor eating habits all interfere with adequate intake of nutrients. Make between-meal snacks available. Offer preferred foods when possible.

- Assess the patient for jaundice and pruritus. Check urine and stool color.
- Record intake and output, daily weights, and measurements of extremities and abdominal girth to help monitor edema.
- A semi-Fowler's or Fowler's position allows for maximal respiratory efficiency when dyspnea is a problem. Use pillows to support arms and chest.
- When the patient is taking diuretics, monitor serum electrolyte levels.
- Meticulous skin care is needed because edematous tissues are subject to breakdown. Use an alternating air pressure mattress or other special mattress. Adhere to a turning schedule (minimum of every 2 h). Support the abdomen with pillows.
- Have the patient void immediately before a paracentesis to prevent bladder puncture. After the procedure, monitor for hypovolemia and electrolyte changes. Check the dressing for bleeding and leakage.
- Observe for signs of bleeding from esophageal or gastric varices, such as hematemesis and melena. If hematemesis occurs, assess the patient for hemorrhage, call the health care provider (HCP), and be ready to assist with treatments to control bleeding.

▼ **Patient and Caregiver Teaching**

Explain that cirrhosis is a chronic illness and requires continual health care. Teach the symptoms of complications and when to seek medical attention to enable prompt treatment.

- Teach the patient to avoid potentially hepatotoxic over-the-counter drugs, because the diseased liver is unable to metabolize them.
- Encourage abstinence from alcohol because continued use increases the rate of liver disease progression and risk of liver complications.
- Instruct the patient with esophageal or gastric varices to avoid aspirin and NSAIDs to prevent hemorrhage.
- Teach the patient with portal hypertension and varices that straining at stool, coughing, sneezing, retching, and vomiting may increase the risk of variceal hemorrhage.

COLORECTAL CANCER

Description

Colorectal cancer (CRC) is the second leading cause of cancer-related deaths in men and women combined. The risk of CRC increases with age and is higher in men. While about 85% of new CRC cases are detected in people older than 50, the rate among younger people is rising.

Pathophysiology

No single risk factor accounts for most cases of CRC. The risk is the highest in people with first-degree relatives with CRC and people with inflammatory bowel disease (IBD). About 20% of cases occur in patients with a family history of CRC.

About 30%–50% of people with CRC have an abnormal *KRAS* gene. The *KRAS* gene, which is primarily involved in regulating cell division, belongs to a class of genes known as *oncogenes*. When mutated, oncogenes have the potential to cause normal cells to become cancerous.

- Maintaining a healthy weight, being physically active, limiting alcohol use, not smoking, and eating a diet with large amounts of fruits, vegetables, and grains may decrease the risk of CRC.

CRC usually starts as a polyp on the inner lining of the colon or rectum that grows over a period of 10–20 years. Most polyps are adenomas, which arise from the cells that make mucus. As the tumor grows, the cancer invades and penetrates the wall of colon or rectum. Eventually cancer cells gain access to the lymph nodes and vascular system and spread to distant sites. Since venous blood leaving the colon and rectum flows through the portal vein and the inferior rectal vein, the liver is a common site of metastasis. The cancer spreads from the liver to other sites, including the lungs, bones, brain, and adjacent structures.

Clinical Manifestations and Complications

CRC develops slowly. Symptoms do not appear until the disease is advanced (See Fig. 6).

- Early disease: no findings or nonspecific findings (fatigue, weight loss).
- More advanced disease: abdominal pain or tenderness with a change in bowel habits, palpable abdominal mass, hepatomegaly, ascites.

Bleeding on the right side is more common than the left side. It is often unrecognized and an early manifestation is often anemia.

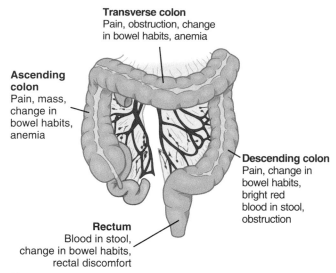

Transverse colon
Pain, obstruction, change
in bowel habits, anemia

**Ascending
colon**
Pain, mass,
change in
bowel habits,
anemia

Descending colon
Pain, change in
bowel habits,
bright red
blood in stool,
obstruction

Rectum
Blood in stool,
change in bowel habits,
rectal discomfort

Figure 6 Signs and symptoms of colorectal cancer by location of primary cancer.

Hematochezia (fresh blood in the stool) is more often caused by left-sided CRC.

Right-sided cancers are more likely to cause diarrhea. Left-sided cancers are usually detected later and could present with bowel obstruction. Complications of CRC include obstruction, bleeding, perforation, peritonitis, and fistula formation.

Diagnostic Studies

Regular screening is advocated to detect and remove polyps before they become cancerous. Persons at risk should begin screening earlier and have screening done more often. From age 45–75 years, those at average risk for developing CRC should have screening tests based on one of these testing schedules:

- Flexible sigmoidoscopy (every 5 years)
- Colonoscopy (the gold standard for CRC screening; every 10 years)
- Double-contrast barium enema (every 5 years)
- CT colonography (virtual colonoscopy) (every 5 years)

  Tests that primarily find cancer include the following:
- High-sensitivity fecal occult blood test (FOBT) (every year)
- Fecal immunochemical test (FIT) (every year)
- Stool deoxyribonucleic acid (DNA) test (every 3 years)

Complete blood count (CBC), coagulation studies, and liver function tests are done when the diagnosis is confirmed by colonoscopy and biopsy.

- CT scan, PET scan, or MRI of abdomen and pelvis is used to detect liver metastases.
- Carcinoembryonic antigen (CEA) serum test is used as a baseline to follow the progress of the patient after surgery or chemotherapy.

Interprofessional Management

Prognosis and treatment correlate with the pathologic staging of the disease. The TNM staging system is the most commonly used method to stage the tumor (see TNM Classification System). Prognosis worsens with greater size and depth of tumor, lymph node involvement, and metastasis.

Surgical Therapy

Surgical goals include complete resection of the tumor, thorough exploration of the abdomen to detect spread, removal of all lymph nodes that drain the cancer area, and restoration of normal bowel function.

- Polypectomy during colonoscopy can be used to resect CRC in situ.
- The site of the tumor determines the site of the resection (e.g., right hemicolectomy, left hemicolectomy).
- Surgery for stage I cancer includes removal of the tumor, surrounding tissue, and nearby lymph nodes. The cancer-free ends are sewn back together when possible. Laparoscopic surgery is sometimes used, especially for tumors in the left colon.
- Chemotherapy is used after to surgery for high-risk stage II tumors.
- Stage III tumors are treated with surgery and chemotherapy.

In treating rectal cancer, options include: (1) local excision, (2) abdominal-perineal resection (APR) with a permanent colostomy, and (3) low anterior resection (LAR) to preserve sphincter function.

Chemotherapy and Targeted Therapy

Chemotherapy can be used to shrink the tumor before surgery, as adjuvant therapy after bowel resection, and as palliative treatment for nonresectable cancer (see Chemotherapy). Current protocols include varying doses of oxaliplatin (Eloxatin) with either fluorouracil (FU) and leucovorin (LV) or capecitabine (Xeloda). Irinotecan can be given with FU and LV alone or with oxaliplatin. Capecitabine or fluorouracil can be used alone in patients for whom oxaliplatin therapy is not inappropriate.

Several targeted therapies have a role in treating metastatic CRC. Angiogenesis inhibitors inhibit the blood supply to tumors. These include aflibercept (Zaltrap), bevacizumab (Avastin), and ramucirumab (Cyramza). Cetuximab (Erbitux) and panitumumab (Vectibix) block the epidermal growth factor receptor. These drugs are often given with a combination chemotherapy regimen.

Regorafenib (Stivarga) is a multikinase inhibitor that blocks several enzymes that promote cancer growth. It, or Lonsurf, a combination of trifluridine and tipiracil, is given to patients with metastatic CRC who are no longer responding to other therapies. Trifluridine impairs DNA function and angiogenesis. Tipiracil prevents the rapid metabolism of trifluridine, thus increasing its bioavailability.

Radiation Therapy

Radiation therapy may be used as an adjuvant to surgery and chemotherapy or as a palliative measure for patients with metastatic cancer. As a palliative measure, its primary goal is to reduce tumor size and provide symptomatic relief. See Radiation Therapy.

Management

Goals

The patient with CRC will have normal bowel elimination patterns, quality of life appropriate to disease progression, relief of pain, and feelings of comfort and well-being.

Interventions

Encourage patients older than 45 years to have regular screening for CRC. Help identify those at high risk who need screening at an earlier age.

- Endoscopic and radiographic procedures can only reveal polyps when the bowel has been adequately prepared. Provide teaching about bowel cleansing for outpatient diagnostic procedures, and give cleansing preparations to inpatients.

Preoperative Care

Nursing care for patients with a colon resection is similar to care for patients undergoing a laparotomy (see Abdominal Pain, Acute). Patients who have had an APR will have a permanent ostomy. Provide emotional support to cope with the diagnosis of cancer and the impending changes in body appearance and function.

Postoperative Care

Patients who have immediate reanastomosis of bowel require general postoperative care. Postoperative care of patients with more extensive surgery, such as an APR, includes sterile dressing changes, care of drains, and patient and caregiver teaching about the stoma. Consult with a wound, ostomy, and continence nurse (WOCN) before surgery to select the ostomy site on the abdomen, and then provide follow-up care and teaching.

- A patient who has an open wound with packing needs meticulous care. Reinforce dressings and change them often. The drainage is usually serosanguineous and likely to be profuse during the first several hours postoperatively. Carefully assess all drainage for amount, color, and consistency. Examine the wound regularly and record bleeding, excessive drainage, and unusual odor.

- The patient may have phantom rectal sensation because the sympathetic nerves responsible for rectal control are not severed during the surgery. Assess to distinguish phantom sensations from the pain of a developing perineal abscess.

- The likelihood of sexual problems as a possible complication of APR depends on the surgical technique used. The surgeon should discuss the possibility with the patient.

▼ **Patient and Caregiver Teaching**
- Patients with colostomies need to know how to care for them.
- Teach about diet, incontinence products, and strategies for managing bloating, diarrhea, and bowel evacuation.
- Patients undergoing sphincter-sparing surgery may need antidiarrheal drugs or bulking agents to control diarrhea. A dietitian should help the patient choose foods that are less likely to cause diarrhea.
- Patients may need information and support regarding changes in body image and options for sexual activity.
- Teach the patient and caregiver about community resources and services available for assistance.

CONJUNCTIVITIS

Conjunctivitis is an infection or inflammation of the conjunctiva. Conjunctivitis may be caused by bacteria or viruses. Inflammation can result from exposure to allergens or chemical irritants. See Table 26 for a comparison of clinical manifestations and management of the different types of conjunctivitis.

TABLE 26 Types of Conjunctivitis

Description	Clinical manifestations	Management
Bacterial		
• Acute bacterial conjunctivitis (pinkeye) • More common in children • *Staphylococcus aureus* is most common cause.	• Discomfort, pruritus, redness, mucopurulent drainage • Generally spreads to unaffected eye	• Usually self-limiting, but antibiotic drops will shorten course • Careful hand washing • Individual or disposable towels help prevent spread
Viral		
• Caused by many different viruses • Adenovirus conjunctivitis contracted by direct contact and in contaminated swimming pools	• Tearing, foreign body sensation, redness, mild photophobia • Usually mild and self-limiting but can be severe with increased discomfort and subconjunctival hemorrhaging	• Treatment is palliative: ice packs, artificial tears, and dark glasses • Topical corticosteroids for temporary relief
Chlamydial		
• *Chlamydia trachomatis* serotypes A–C cause trachoma, a major cause of blindness worldwide. • Adult inclusion conjunctivitis (AIC) caused by *C. trachomatis* serotypes D–K is increasing with rise in chlamydial infections. AIC does not lead to blindness.	• Mucopurulent ocular discharge, irritation, redness, lid swelling	• Antibiotic therapy • Patients with AIC have a high risk of concurrent chlamydial genital infection and other sexually transmitted infections (STI)s. Refer for STI testing and treatment.

TABLE 26 Types of Conjunctivitis—cont'd		
Description	Clinical manifestations	Management
Allergic		
• Conjunctivitis may develop after exposure to pollens, animal dander, ocular solutions, contact lenses, or other allergens.	• Itching (defining symptom), burning, redness, and tearing	• Artificial tears to dilute allergen and wash from eye • Topical antihistamines and corticosteroids • Teach to avoid known allergens

CONSTIPATION

Description

People with constipation have fewer than three stools per week, often accompanied by straining, a feeling of incomplete evacuation, a need for digital assistance to evacuate stool, bloating, and hard or lumpy stools. Constipation is a symptom, not a disease. It can be acute, usually lasting <1 week, or chronic, lasting over 3 months.

Risk factors associated with chronic constipation include a low-fiber diet, decreased physical activity, or ignoring the defecation urge. Ignoring the urge to defecate for a prolonged period can cause the muscles and mucosa of the rectum to become insensitive to the presence of feces. Prolonged retention of feces results in water absorption from the stool, making the feces harder to expel. Emotions, including anxiety, depression, and stress, affect the GI tract and can contribute to constipation.

Clinical Manifestations

Constipation varies from a mild discomfort to a more severe acute event mimicking an "acute abdomen." Stools are absent or hard, dry, and difficult to pass. Abdominal distention, bloating, increased flatus, and a sensation of increased rectal pressure may be present.

- Hemorrhoids are a common complication resulting from venous engorgement during repeated Valsalva maneuvers (straining) and venous compression from hard impacted stool (see Hemorrhoids).

- Rectal mucosal ulcers and fissures may occur from stool stasis or straining.
- In the presence of obstipation (severe constipation with no passage of gas or stool) or fecal impaction, colonic perforation may occur. Perforation, which is life-threatening, causes abdominal pain, nausea, vomiting, fever, and a high white blood cell (WBC) count.

Diagnostic Studies

In most patients, the diagnosis of constipation is based on findings from a thorough history and physical examination including a digital rectal examination (DRE).

- Diagnostic testing may include abdominal X-rays, barium enema, and colonoscopy or sigmoidoscopy. The patient with severe constipation may undergo anorectal manometry, GI tract transit studies, balloon expulsion test, or defecography.

Interprofessional Management

Increasing dietary fiber, fluid intake, and exercise can prevent many cases of constipation. Laxatives and enemas are an option to promote bowel movements, but each class works differently. Which one a patient receives depends on the severity and duration of the constipation and the patient's health.

- Daily bulk-forming laxatives (psyllium) can prevent constipation because they work like dietary fiber and do not cause dependence.
- Osmotic laxatives or stimulant laxatives are recommended for patients with chronic constipation who do not respond to diet and lifestyle modifications.
- Peripherally acting opioid receptor antagonists (e.g., methylnaltrexone, naldemedine, naloxegol) reduce constipation caused by opioid use.
- Enemas are fast-acting for immediate treatment of constipation but must be used cautiously.

Biofeedback therapy may benefit patients who are constipated as a result of anismus (uncoordinated contraction of the anal sphincter during straining). A patient with severe constipation related to a motility or mechanical disorder may require more intensive treatment, including surgery.

Nursing Management

Encourage patients to exercise the abdominal muscles and contract the abdominal muscles several times each day. Sit-ups and straight-leg raises can improve abdominal muscle tone.

- Teach the patient and caregiver the importance of a high-fiber diet, increased fluid intake, and a regular exercise program to prevent constipation.
- Teach the patient to establish a regular time to defecate and not suppress the urge.
- Discourage the patient from using laxatives and enemas.

Defecation is the easiest when the person is sitting on a commode with the knees higher than the hips. The sitting position allows gravity to aid defecation, and flexing the hips straightens the angle between the anal canal and the rectum so that stool is expelled more easily.

- Place a footstool in front of the toilet to promote flexion of the thighs.
- For a patient in bed sitting on a bedpan, elevate the head of the bed as high as tolerated.
- Provide as much privacy as possible and offer an odor eliminator.

COR PULMONALE

Description

Cor pulmonale is enlargement of the right ventricle (RV) caused by a primary disorder of the respiratory system. Overt heart failure (HF) may be present.

- The most common cause of cor pulmonale is chronic obstructive pulmonary disease (COPD).

Clinical Manifestations and Diagnostic Tests

- Manifestations are often masked by the symptoms of the pulmonary condition. Common symptoms include exertional dyspnea, tachypnea, cough, and fatigue.
- Physical signs include evidence of right ventricular hypertrophy on the electrocardiogram (ECG) and increased intensity of the second heart sound. Chronic hypoxemia leads to polycythemia and increased total blood volume and viscosity of the blood.
- If heart failure accompanies cor pulmonale, manifestations include peripheral edema, weight gain, distended neck veins, full bounding pulse, and enlarged liver.

Diagnostic tests may include arterial blood gases (ABGs), arterial O_2 saturation by pulse oximetry (SpO_2), b-type natriuretic peptide (BNP) level, ECG, chest X-ray, CT scan, MRI, and cardiac catheterization.

Interprofessional and Nursing Management

Early identification is essential before irreversible changes to the heart develop. Management is directed at treating the underlying pulmonary problem. Long-term O_2 therapy to correct the hypoxemia reduces vasoconstriction and pulmonary hypertension.

- Fluid, electrolyte, and acid-base imbalances must be corrected. Diuretics and a low-sodium diet decrease plasma volume and reduce the heart's workload. Diuretics must be used with extreme caution. In some cases, decreases in fluid volume from diuresis can worsen heart function.
- Bronchodilator therapy is needed if the underlying respiratory problem is caused by an obstructive disorder.
- Other treatments include those for pulmonary hypertension, such as vasodilator therapy, calcium-channel blockers, and anticoagulants.

Nursing management of cor pulmonale resulting from COPD is similar to that described for COPD (see Chronic Obstructive Pulmonary Disease).

CORONARY ARTERY DISEASE

Description

Coronary artery disease (CAD) is a type of blood vessel disorder that is included in the general category of atherosclerosis. *Atherosclerosis* is derived from two Greek words: *athero*, meaning "fatty mush," and *skleros*, meaning "hard." It can occur in any artery in the body. When the atheromas (fatty deposits) form in the coronary arteries, the disease is called *CAD*.

- The terms arteriosclerotic heart disease (ASHD), cardiovascular heart disease (CVHD), ischemic heart disease (IHD), and coronary heart disease (CHD) are other terms used to describe CAD.
- Cardiovascular disease (CVD) is the major cause of death worldwide. CAD is the most common type of CVD and the leading cause of death in the United States.
- Patients with CAD may be asymptomatic or develop chronic stable angina (chest pain).

CAD may evolve to the more serious conditions of unstable angina (UA) and myocardial infarction (MI), which are referred to as "acute coronary syndrome" (ACS) (See Acute Coronary Syndrome). Fig. 1 shows the relationship among the clinical manifestations of CAD. Risk factors for CAD are grouped as nonmodifiable or modifiable (Table 27).

Pathophysiology

Atherosclerosis is characterized by lipid deposits within the intima of the artery. Inflammation and endothelial injury play a key role in the

TABLE 27 Risk Factors for Coronary Artery Disease

Nonmodifiable risk factors	Modifiable risk factors

• Increasing age
• Ethnicity (white men have the highest incidence of CAD)
• Gender (women experience the onset of heart disease about 10 years later than men)
• Genetic predisposition and family history of heart disease
	Major
	• BP > 120/80 mm Hg
	• Diabetes
	• Lipid levels:
	  • Total cholesterol >200 mg/dL
	  • Triglycerides ≥150 mg/dL
	  • LDL cholesterol >130 mg/dL
	  • HDL cholesterol <40 mg/dL in men or <50 mg/dL in women
	• Metabolic syndrome
	• Obesity
	• Physical inactivity
	• Tobacco use
	Contributing risk factors
	• ↑ Homocysteine, CRP, lipoprotein(a) levels
	• Psychosocial risk factors (e.g., depression, hostility
	• Substance use

HDL, High-density lipoprotein; *LDL,* low-density lipoprotein.

C

development of atherosclerosis. Although elevation of any of these levels may increase the risk for development of CAD, they are not part of a routine risk assessment for CAD. They can be used in patients with an intermediate or high-risk suspicion of CAD.

- Damage to the endothelial lining can result from tobacco use, hyperlipidemia, hypertension, toxins, diabetes, inflammation, and infection.
- C-reactive protein (CRP), a protein produced by the liver, is a nonspecific marker of systemic inflammation. It is increased in many patients with CAD.
- Lipoprotein(a) is a type of low-density lipoprotein (LDL) attached to a protein called apo(a). Homocysteine is made by the breakdown of the essential amino acid methionine, found in dietary protein. High lipoprotein(a) and homocysteine levels may contribute to atherosclerosis by damaging the inner lining of blood vessels, promoting plaque buildup, and changing the clotting mechanism to make clots more likely to occur.

- CAD takes many years to develop. When the patient becomes symptomatic, the disease process is usually well advanced. Stages of development in atherosclerosis are: (1) fatty streak, (2) fibrous plaque resulting from smooth muscle cell proliferation, and (3) complicated lesion.

  Normally some arterial anastomoses or connections, called *collateral circulation*, exist within the coronary circulation (Fig. 7).

- When blockages in coronary arteries occur over a long period, there is a greater chance of collateral circulation developing, and the heart muscle may still receive adequate blood and oxygen.

- With rapid-onset CAD, there is not enough time to develop collateral circulation. Reduced blood flow results in more severe ischemia or infarction.

Clinical Manifestations

CAD is a progressive disease. Patients may be asymptomatic for many years or may develop chronic stable angina. When the demand for myocardial oxygen exceeds the ability of the coronary arteries to supply the heart with oxygen, myocardial ischemia occurs.

- *Angina*, or chest pain, is a symptom of reversible myocardial ischemia. The main reason for insufficient blood flow is narrowing of coronary arteries by atherosclerosis.

- Chronic stable angina refers to chest pain that occurs intermittently over a long period with the same pattern of onset, duration, and intensity of symptoms (see Angina, Chronic Stable).

Figure 7 Vessel occlusion with collateral circulation. (A) Open, functioning coronary artery. (B) Partial coronary artery closure, with collateral circulation being established. (C) Total coronary artery occlusion with collateral circulation bypassing the occlusion to supply blood to the myocardium.

When ischemia is prolonged and not immediately revers-
ible, ACS develops and encompasses the spectrum of UA, non-
ST-segment-elevation myocardial infarction (NSTEMI), and
ST-segment-elevation myocardial infarction (STEMI) (see Fig. 1).

Diagnostic Studies

- Chest X-ray to detect cardiac enlargement, cardiac calcifications, and pulmonary congestion.
- The 12-lead electrocardiogram (ECG) detects heart rhythm,
  pacemaker activity, conduction abnormalities, heart position,
  atrial and ventricular size, and ischemia/injury/infarction.
- Serum lipid levels to screen for risk factors.
- Exercise or stress testing to detect ST segment and T wave
  changes that indicate ischemia with exercise.
- Ambulatory 24–48-hr ECG monitoring to identify silent
  ischemia.
- Nuclear imaging studies to determine myocardial perfusion,
  contractility, and ejection fraction.
- Positron emission tomography (PET) to identify and quantify
  ischemia and infarction.
- Angiography studies to visualize coronary arteries and help
  determine treatment and prognosis.
- Echocardiography with exercise to diagnose coronary artery
  stenosis.

Interprofessional Management

Encourage people who have modifiable risk factors to make lifestyle changes to prevent, modify, or slow CAD progression.
Lifestyle changes, including a low-saturated-fat, high-fiber diet;
avoiding tobacco; and increase in physical activity, can help reduce
coronary events.

- Everyone should aim for at least 150 minutes (30 minutes at
  least 5 days per week) of moderate aerobic activity per week.
  Examples of moderate physical activity include brisk walking,
  biking, and recreational swimming. Another option is to do
  75 minutes of vigorous aerobic activity each week such as jog-
  ging, singles tennis, or swimming laps.
- Dietary recommendations focus on lowering LDL cholesterol.
  They emphasize a decrease in saturated fat and cholesterol
  intake and an increase in complex carbohydrates (e.g., whole
  grains, fruit, vegetables) and fiber. Fat intake should be about
  25%–35% of total calories, with most coming from monoun-
  saturated and polyunsaturated fats. Foods high in unsaturated
  fat include unsalted nuts (e.g., walnuts, peanuts, almonds) and

avocado. Examples of oils low in saturated fat include canola, olive, and avocado. With a high serum triglyceride level, the patient should reduce or eliminate alcohol and simple sugars.

- Omega-3 fatty acids reduce triglyceride levels and can slow the progression of CAD. They do not affect LDL levels. The AHA recommends eating fatty fish twice a week because they are high in omega-3 fatty acids. Examples of fatty fish include salmon, albacore tuna, and mackerel.

Drug Therapy

People with serum cholesterol levels higher than 200 mg/dL are at risk for CAD. Treatment usually begins with dietary caloric restriction (if overweight), decreased dietary fat and cholesterol intake, and increased physical activity. Serum lipid levels are reassessed after 6 weeks of diet therapy. If they remain elevated, additional dietary options and drug therapy may be considered. Drug therapy for hyperlipidemia often continues for a lifetime. Diet modification minimizes the need for drug therapy.

- The statin drugs are the most widely used lipid-lowering drugs. They inhibit the synthesis of cholesterol in the liver and increase the numbers of hepatic LDL receptors, removing more LDL from the blood. Statins also cause a minor increase in HDL. Rosuvastatin (Crestor) is the most potent statin currently available. Serious adverse effects are rare. They include liver damage and myalgia (muscle ache or weakness without breakdown of skeletal muscle) that can progress to rhabdomyolysis (breakdown of skeletal muscle).
- Niacin, a water-soluble B vitamin, is effective in lowering triglyceride levels and mildly lowering LDL levels. At high doses, niacin increases HDL levels, but it does not correlate to a decreased risk of CAD or MI. Unfortunately, common side effects include severe flushing, pruritus, gastrointestinal (GI) symptoms, and orthostatic hypotension.
- Fibric acid derivatives, such as gemfibrozil (Lopid), aid the removal of VLDLs. They lower triglyceride levels and increase HDL levels. There is no effect on LDLs. Although most patients tolerate the drugs well, GI irritability is common. They should be used with caution when combined with statins due to increased risk for myopathy.
- ATP-citrate lyase inhibitors such as bempedoic acid (Nexletol) help lower LDL in patients with heterozygous familial hypercholesterolemia or patients with CAD who do not have adequate LDL lowering. We should monitor uric acid levels as the drug increases the risk of gout. Tendon rupture may occur, so use in caution with patients who have had a previous tendon rupture.

- Bile-acid sequestrants increase conversion of cholesterol to bile acids in the liver. The primary effect is a decrease in total cholesterol and LDL levels. Bile-acid sequestrants decrease absorption of many other drugs (e.g., warfarin, thiazides, thyroid hormones, β-adrenergic blockers). Tell patients to take those drugs 1 hr before or 3–4 hr after bile-acid sequestrants to decrease this adverse effect.
- PCSK9 inhibitors reduce the number of receptors in the liver that remove LDL cholesterol from the blood. By blocking PCSK9's ability to work, more receptors are available and can get rid of LDL. This decreases circulating LDL levels. Evolocumab (Repatha) and alirocumab (Praluent) are PCSK9 inhibitors.
- Ezetimibe (Zetia) selectively inhibits the absorption of dietary and biliary cholesterol across the intestinal wall. When combined with a statin as a combination drug (e.g., ezetimibe and simvastatin [Vytorin]) or as two separate drugs (ezetimibe and a statin), even greater reductions in LDLs occur.

Low-dose aspirin (81 mg) may be used for primary prevention (people without known CAD) in adults 40–70 years of age who have higher risk of CAD but do not have an increased risk for bleeding. Adults over age 70 should only use low-dose aspirin for secondary prevention (people with known CAD). You can recommend taking coated aspirin to help with GI protection.

Nursing Management

Management of CAD risk factors in CAD may prevent, modify, or slow the disease progression. Risk screening involves obtaining a thorough health history. Question the patient about a family history of heart disease in parents and siblings. Note any cardiovascular symptoms.

Assess environmental factors, such as eating habits, type of diet, and level of exercise, to identify lifestyle patterns. Include a psychosocial history to determine tobacco use, alcohol intake, recent stressful events (e.g., loss of a spouse), and psychologic state (e.g., anxiety, depression, anger). The place and type of employment provide important information on the kind of activity performed, exposure to pollutants or noxious chemicals, and the degree of stress associated with work.

- Identify patient attitudes and beliefs about health and illness that may relate to misconceptions about risks and treatment of heart disease.
- Knowing the patient's educational background and health literacy is helpful for planning a teaching approach.
- Encourage the patient to make lifestyle choices that decrease cardiac risk factors.

CROHN'S DISEASE

Crohn's disease is an autoimmune disorder that, along with ulcerative colitis, is referred to as *inflammatory bowel disease* (IBD). See Inflammatory Bowel Disease for a discussion of the disorder.

CUSHING SYNDROME

Description

Cushing syndrome is a clinical condition that results from chronic exposure to excess corticosteroids, particularly glucocorticoids. The most common cause of Cushing syndrome is iatrogenic administration of *exogenous* corticosteroids (e.g., prednisone). About 85% of the cases of *endogenous* Cushing syndrome are caused by an adrenocorticotropic hormone (ACTH)-secreting pituitary tumor *(Cushing disease)*. Less common causes of Cushing syndrome include adrenal or other tumors.

Clinical Manifestations

Manifestations are seen in most body systems related to excess levels of corticosteroids. Although signs of glucocorticoid excess usually predominate, symptoms of mineralocorticoid and androgen excess can occur.

- Corticosteroid excess causes pronounced changes in appearance. Weight gain results from an accumulation of adipose tissue in the trunk (centripetal obesity), face ("moon face"), and cervical areas ("buffalo hump").
- Hyperglycemia occurs because of glucose intolerance associated with cortisol-induced insulin resistance and increased gluconeogenesis by the liver.
- Muscle wasting leads to muscle weakness, especially in the extremities.
- Loss of bone protein matrix leads to osteoporosis with pathologic fractures (e.g., vertebral compression fractures) and bone and back pain.
- Loss of collagen makes the skin weaker, thinner, and easier to bruise. Purplish-red striae appear on the abdomen, breast, or buttocks.
- Mineralocorticoid excess may cause hypokalemia from potassium excretion and hypertension. Adrenal androgen excess may cause severe acne, the development of male characteristics in women, and feminization in men.

Diagnostic Studies

- Plasma cortisol levels may be elevated.
- A 24-hr urine collection for free cortisol is done. Urine cortisol levels higher than 100 mcg/24 h in adults indicate Cushing syndrome. If these results are borderline, a low-dose dexamethasone suppression test is done.
- High or normal plasma ACTH levels indicate Cushing disease, while low or undetectable levels indicate an adrenal or medication cause.
- Other findings on diagnostic tests associated with Cushing syndrome include hyperglycemia, hypokalemia, glycosuria, hypercalciuria, and osteoporosis.
- CT scan and MRI of the pituitary and adrenal glands may be done.

Interprofessional Management

The primary goal is to normalize hormone secretion. The standard treatment for a pituitary adenoma is surgical removal of the pituitary tumor using the transsphenoidal approach. Radiation therapy is an option for patients who are not good surgical candidates. Adrenalectomy is indicated for adrenal tumors or hyperplasia. Patients with ectopic ACTH-secreting tumors (usually located in the lung or pancreas) are also treated surgically.

- When the patient is a poor candidate for surgery or prior surgery has failed, drug therapy is used to inhibit adrenal function (*medical adrenalectomy*). Drugs that inhibit corticosteroid synthesis include ketoconazole and mitotane.

If Cushing syndrome develops after prolonged administration of corticosteroids (e.g., prednisone), alternatives include gradually discontinuing corticosteroid therapy, reducing corticosteroid dose, and converting to alternate-day dosing.

Nursing Management

Goals

The patient with Cushing syndrome will have relief of symptoms, avoid serious complications, maintain a positive self-image, and actively take part in the therapeutic plan.

Interventions

Therapy for Cushing syndrome has many side effects. Assess for signs and symptoms of hormone and drug toxicity and complicating conditions (e.g., cardiovascular disease, diabetes, infection).

- Monitor vital signs, glucose, and daily weights.

- Assess for pain, loss of function, and purulent drainage. Signs and symptoms of inflammation (e.g., fever, redness) may be absent.
- Monitor for signs of thromboembolic phenomena, such as sudden chest pain, dyspnea, and tachypnea.

Provide emotional support regarding potentially distressing changes in appearance, such as truncal obesity, bruising, hirsutism in females, and gynecomastia in males. Reassure the patient that the physical changes and much of the emotional lability will resolve when hormone levels return to normal.

If treatment involves surgical removal of a pituitary adenoma, an adrenal tumor, or one or both adrenal glands, nursing care will include preoperative and postoperative care.

Preoperative Care

Before surgery, hypertension, hyperglycemia, and hypokalemia need to be controlled. A high-protein meal plan helps correct protein depletion. Teach about expected postoperative care including preventing venous thromboembolism.

Postoperative Care

Because of hormone fluctuations, the patient's BP, fluid balance, and electrolyte levels tend to be unstable after surgery. High doses of corticosteroids (hydrocortisone) are administered IV during surgery and for several days afterward to ensure adequate responses to the stress of the procedure.

- Report any rapid or significant changes in BP, respirations, or heart rate (HR).
- Carefully monitor fluid intake and output and assess for potential imbalance.
- If corticosteroid dosage is tapered too rapidly after surgery, acute adrenal insufficiency may develop. Vomiting, increased weakness, dehydration, and hypotension are signs of hypocortisolism. The patient may have painful joints, pruritus, or peeling skin and may have severe emotional problems.
- After surgery, the patient usually remains on bed rest until the BP stabilizes.
- Be alert for subtle signs of postoperative infections. Provide meticulous care during dressing changes and procedures that involve access to body cavities, circulation, or areas under skin.

▼ Patient and Caregiver Teaching

Emphasize discharge instructions about the patient's lack of endogenous cortisol and resulting inability to react physiologically to stressors. Many patients need lifetime hormone replacement therapy. It may take several months to satisfactorily adjust the dose.

- Teach patients to always wear a medical identification (Medic Alert) bracelet and carry instructions in a wallet or purse.
- Teach the patient to avoid exposure to extreme temperatures, infections, and emotional situations.
- Stress may precipitate acute adrenal insufficiency because the remaining adrenal tissue cannot meet an increased hormonal demand. Teach patients to adjust their corticosteroid replacement in accordance with stress levels. If the patient cannot adjust their own medication or if weakness, fainting, fever, or nausea and vomiting occur, the patient should contact the health care provider (HCP).

CYSTIC FIBROSIS

Description

Cystic fibrosis (CF) is an inherited, autosomal recessive genetic disorder characterized by altered transport of sodium and chloride ions in and out of epithelial cells. Airway obstruction occurs because of changes in exocrine glandular secretions, resulting in increased mucus production. This defect also affects the gastrointestinal (GI) system (pancreas and biliary tract) and reproductive organs.

There are about 30,000 people in the United States living with CF. More than 50% of the CF population are adults.

Pathophysiology

CF results from mutations in a gene found on chromosome 7 that produces a protein called CF transmembrane regulator (CFTR). CFTR regulates sodium and chloride channels in the epithelial surface of the airways, pancreatic ducts, and sweat gland ducts. Mutations in the *CFTR* gene alter the CFTR in such a way that the channel is blocked.

- Cells that line the passageways of the lungs, pancreas, and other organs make abnormally thick, sticky mucus that plugs up the ducts, ultimately resulting in organ failure.
- The disease progresses from the small airways *(chronic bronchiolitis)* to involving the larger airways and finally destroys lung tissue.
- With CF, there is a persistent, chronic airway infection that cannot be cured. Pseudomonas is the most common organism in adults. Antibiotic resistance can develop after multiple exposures to antibiotics. Lung inflammation is associated with

chronic infection. It can narrow airways and cause a decrease in lung function. An increase in inflammatory mediators (e.g., interleukins, oxidants, proteases released by neutrophils) contributes to disease progression. Lung disorders that initially occur are chronic bronchiolitis and bronchiectasis. Over a long period, pulmonary vascular remodeling occurs because of local hypoxia and arteriolar vasoconstriction. Enlarged pulmonary arteries, pulmonary hypertension, and cor pulmonale occur in the later phases of the disease.

- Mucous plugging of the pancreatic exocrine ducts causes pancreatic insufficiency. This results in atrophy and progressive fibrotic cyst formation. The pancreas's exocrine function may be completely lost. Because of this, the pancreas does not make enough pancreatic enzymes, such as lipase, amylase, and proteases (trypsin, chymotrypsin) to allow for absorption of nutrients. Malabsorption of fat, protein, and fat-soluble vitamins (A, D, E, and K) occurs. Fat malabsorption results in steatorrhea (large, oily, frequent bowel movements). Protein malabsorption results in failure to grow and gain weight. Osteopenia and osteoporosis are common. They are related to malnutrition, malabsorption of vitamin D, low testosterone levels, and chronic infections. Pancreatitis may occur.
- CF-related diabetes (CFRD) is caused by underdevelopment of pancreatic islet cells (in utero) and destruction of islet cells over the person's lifetime.

Clinical Manifestations

Manifestations vary depending on the disease severity. Carriers are not affected by the gene mutation.

- In the adult, a common symptom is frequent cough that becomes persistent and produces viscous, purulent sputum.
- Exacerbations (increased cough and sputum, weight loss) may ultimately lead to respiratory failure.
- Affected persons have delayed puberty and may be unable to conceive.
- Pneumothorax is an uncommon but serious complication caused by the formation of bullae and blebs. CF-related diabetes, bone disease, and liver disease are additional complications.

Diagnostic Studies

- Sweat chloride test (pilocarpine iontophoresis method) is the gold standard for diagnosing CF. Persons with CF excrete four times the normal amount of sodium and chloride in their sweat.

- A genetic test is often used if the results from a sweat test are uncertain.

Interprofessional and Nursing Management

A team should be involved in the care of a patient with CF, including a nurse, physician, respiratory and physical therapists, dietitian, and social worker. Goals for the patient with CF include adequate airway clearance, reduced risk factors associated with respiratory infections, adequate nutritional support, ability to perform activities of daily living (ADLs), recognition and treatment of complications, and active participation in a therapeutic regimen. Management is focused on relieving airway obstruction and controlling infection.

- Aerosol and nebulizer treatments promote drainage of thick bronchial mucus. The drugs we use dilate the airways, liquefy mucus, and promote clearance.
- The abnormal viscosity of secretions is increased by concentrated DNA from neutrophils involved in chronic infection. Drugs that degrade the DNA in CF sputum (e.g., inhaled dornase alfa [Pulmozyme]) increase airflow and reduce the number of acute exacerbations. Inhaled hypertonic saline (7%) increases osmolality, allowing water to collect on airway surfaces. It is effective in clearing mucus and decreases the frequency of exacerbations.
- Some patients need bronchodilators (e.g., β2-adrenergic agonists) to control bronchospasm.
- Airway clearance techniques (ACTs) are critical since the normal ciliary motion in CF airways is impaired. Postural drainage with percussion and vibration and high-frequency chest wall oscillation loosen mucus. Specialized expiratory techniques that use airflow to remove the loosened secretions help clear secretions. Examples include using devices, breathing exercises, pursed-lip breathing, and huff coughing. Patients may prefer a certain technique or device that works well for them in their daily routine.
- Aerobic exercise also seems to be effective in clearing airways.
- The use of antibiotics should be carefully guided by sputum culture results.

All patients with CF should have CFTR genotyping to see if they carry a mutation that is a target of CFTR modulator therapy.

- Drugs, such as ivacaftor/lumacaftor (Orkambi) and Ivacaftor (Kalydeco), are used to treat patients with specific CFTR gene mutations.

Management of pancreatic insufficiency includes pancreatic enzyme replacement (e.g., pancrelipase [Pancreaze, Creon, Zenpep]) before each meal and snack. Fat-soluble vitamins need to be supplemented. Hyperglycemia may need treatment with insulin.

- Extra salt is needed when sweating is increased, such as during hot weather, with a fever, or from intense physical activity.

There is a higher incidence of depression among persons with CF. Issues such as fertility, decreased life expectancy, costs of health care, and career choices may lead to depression.

▼ **Patient and Caregiver Teaching**

- Sexuality is an important issue to discuss. Delayed development of secondary sex characteristics and menses is common.
- Genetic counseling is appropriate for those considering having children.
- Living with a chronic disease can be emotionally overwhelming. Community resources and the Cystic Fibrosis Foundation may be helpful.

DEMENTIA

Description

Dementia is a disorder characterized by a decline from previous level of function in one or more cognitive domains: complex attention, executive function, language, learning and memory, perceptual motor, and social cognition. The cognitive decline interferes with ability to function and perform daily activities. This decline does not occur with onset of an acute state of confusion, such as delirium, or the onset of another major mental disorder, such as depression.

- There are many causes of dementia. Alzheimer disease (AD) is the most common form.

Pathophysiology

The most common causes are neurodegenerative conditions that cannot be reversed. Most of these are due to AD. Other causes include dementia with Lewy bodies (DLB), frontotemporal dementia (FTD), and Parkinson disease with dementia (PDD).

Vascular, or multi-infarct dementia (VaD), is a loss of cognitive function caused by vascular disease. VaD may be caused by a single infarct (stroke) or multiple strokes. It is more common in men.

- Subcortical dementia is the most common type of VaD. It occurs when small vessels deep in the brain develop thick walls and become stiff. This reduces blood flow, which damages the nerve fibers that carry signals to white matter. This process can cause infarcts near the base of the brain.

Clinical Manifestations

Dementia associated with neurologic degeneration is often gradual and progressive. Vascular dementia often results in a more abrupt onset and progression. Other clinical manifestations of dementia are discussed with AD (see Alzheimer Disease).

- An acute (days to weeks) or a subacute (weeks to months) pattern of change may indicate an infectious or metabolic cause of dementia, including encephalitis, meningitis, hypothyroidism, or drug-related dementia.

Dementia is often mistaken for acute delirium or depression, especially among older adults. Manifestations of depression, especially among older adults, may include sadness, difficulty concentrating, fatigue, apathy, feelings of despair, and inactivity. When depression is severe, poor concentration and inattention may result, causing memory and functional impairment. When dementia and depression occur together, there can be marked intellectual decline. Table 28 compares key features of dementia, delirium, and depression.

Diagnostic Studies

- Comprehensive medical, neurologic, and psychologic histories help in determining the presence and cause of dementia.
- Physical examination and neuroimaging techniques (CT or MRI) may be performed to rule out some causes of dementia.
- Dementia is often diagnosed when two or more brain functions, such as memory loss or language skills, are significantly impaired.

Interprofessional and Nursing Management

Management of dementia is similar to care of the patient with AD (see Alzheimer Disease). Preventive measures for VaD include treatment of risk factors, such as hypertension, diabetes, smoking, hypercholesterolemia, and dysrhythmias. Drugs used for patients with AD are also useful for patients with vascular dementia.

TABLE 28 Comparison of Dementia, Delirium, and Depression

Feature	Dementia	Delirium	Depression
Onset	Insidious	Abrupt, although initially can be subtle.	Often coincides with life changes. Often abrupt.
Progression	Slow	Abrupt. Can fluctuate from day to day.	Variable, rapid to slow but may be uneven.
Duration	Years (average of 8, can be longer).	Hours to days to weeks. Can be prolonged.	Can be several months to years, especially if not treated.
Thinking	Difficulty with abstract thinking, impaired judgment, words difficult to find.	Disorganized, distorted. Slow or accelerated incoherent speech.	Intact but with apathy, fatigue. May be indecisive. Feels sense of hopelessness. May not want to live.
Perception	Misperceptions often present. Delusions and hallucinations.	Distorted. Delusions and hallucinations.	May deny or be unaware of depression. May have feelings of guilt.
Psychomotor behavior	May pace or be hyperactive. As disease progresses, may not be able to perform tasks or movements when asked.	Variable. Can be hyperactive or hypoactive, or mixed.	Often withdrawn and hypoactive.
Sleep-wake cycle	Sleeps during day. Frequent awakenings at night. Fragmented sleep.	Disturbed sleep. Reversed sleep-wake cycle.	Disturbed, often with early morning awakening.

DIABETES INSIPIDUS

Description

Diabetes insipidus (DI) is caused by deficient production or secretion of antidiuretic hormone (ADH) or a decreased renal response to ADH. The decrease in ADH results in fluid and electrolyte imbalances caused by increased urine output and increased plasma osmolality. Depending on the cause, DI may be transient or a lifelong condition. There are several types of DI.

- *Central DI* (also known as *neurogenic DI*) results from an interference with ADH synthesis, transport, or release. Causes include brain tumor or surgery, central nervous system (CNS) infections, and head injury. It is the most common form of DI.
- *Nephrogenic DI* occurs when there is adequate ADH, but a decreased response to ADH in the kidney. Causes include drug therapy (especially lithium), renal damage, and hereditary renal disease.
- *Psychogenic DI* is associated with excessive water intake caused by a structural lesion in the thirst center or a psychologic disorder.

Clinical Manifestations

The main characteristic of DI is *polyuria*, large quantities of urine (2–20 L/day) with a very low specific gravity (<1.005) and urine osmolality (100 mOsm/kg). Serum osmolality is increased as a result of hypernatremia from pure water loss in the kidney.

- Most patients compensate for fluid loss by drinking great amounts of water (*polydipsia*) so that serum osmolality is normal or only moderately increased. The patient may be tired from nocturia and may have generalized weakness.
- Central DI is usually acute and accompanied by excess fluid loss.
- Although the clinical manifestations of nephrogenic DI are similar, the onset and amount of fluid losses are less dramatic than with central DI.
- Severe dehydration can result if oral intake cannot keep up with urinary losses. The patient will have hypotension, tachycardia, and hypovolemic shock.
- Uncorrected hypernatremia can cause brain shrinkage and intracranial bleeding. The patient may show CNS manifestations ranging from irritability and mental dullness to coma.

Diagnostic Studies

- Water deprivation test distinguishes central DI from nephrogenic DI. Patients with central DI exhibit a dramatic increase in urine osmolality with this test, from 100 to 600 mOsm/kg, and a

significant decrease in urine volume. The patient with nephrogenic DI is not able to increase urine osmolality to >300 mOsm/kg.
- Measuring ADH levels after an analog of ADH (e.g., desmopressin [DDAVP]) is given also distinguishes central DI from nephrogenic DI. If the cause is central DI, the kidneys will respond to the hormone by concentrating urine. If the kidneys do not respond in this way, the cause is nephrogenic.

Interprofessional and Nursing Management

Management of the patient with DI includes early detection, adequate hydration, and patient teaching for self-management. A therapeutic goal is maintaining fluid and electrolyte balance.

For central DI, fluid and hormone therapy are needed. Fluids are replaced orally or IV. Monitor serum glucose levels because hyperglycemia and glucosuria can lead to osmotic diuresis and fluid loss.
- Monitor level of consciousness, BP, heart rate, and urine output and specific gravity hourly in the acutely ill patient.
- Maintain an accurate record of intake and output and daily weights to determine fluid volume status.
- Desmopressin (DDAVP), a synthetic analog of ADH, is the hormone replacement of choice for central DI. Other ADH replacement drugs include aqueous vasopressin.
- Treatment for nephrogenic DI revolves around dietary measures (low-sodium diet) and thiazide diuretics. Limiting sodium intake to no more than 3 g/day often helps decrease urine output. Indomethacin, a nonsteroidal antiinflammatory drug (NSAID), may help increase renal responsiveness to ADH.

DIABETES MELLITUS

Description

Diabetes mellitus (DM), or diabetes, is a chronic multisystem disease characterized by hyperglycemia from abnormal insulin production, impaired insulin use, or both. In the United States, an estimated 34.2 million people, or 10.5% of the population, have DM. Prediabetes affects 88 million adults. About 7.3 million people with DM have not been diagnosed and are unaware that they have the disease. DM is the seventh leading cause of death in the United States.
- Diabetes is the leading cause of adult blindness, end-stage renal disease, and nontraumatic lower limb amputations.
- Adults with diabetes have heart disease death rates and risk for strokes that are 2–4 times higher than adults without diabetes.

The most common types of diabetes are type 1 DM and type 2 DM (Table 28).

Pathophysiology
Type 1 Diabetes Mellitus
Type 1 diabetes accounts for about 5%–10% of all people with DM. Type 1 DM generally affects people under 40 years of age, although it can occur at any age. Type 1 diabetes is an autoimmune

TABLE 28 Comparison of Type 1 and Type 2 Diabetes Mellitus

Factor	Type 1 DM	Type 2 DM
Age at onset	More common in young people but can occur at any age	More common in adults but can occur at any age. Incidence increasing in children
Type of onset	Signs and symptoms usually abrupt, although disease process may be present for several years	Gradual, may go undiagnosed for years
Prevalence	Accounts for 5%–10% of all types of DM	Accounts for 90%–95% of all types of DM
Endogenous insulin	Absent	Initially increased in response to insulin resistance. Secretion decreases over time.
Environmental factors	Virus, toxins	Higher weight, lack of exercise
Islet cell antibodies	Often present at onset	Absent
Primary defect	Absent or minimal insulin production	Insulin resistance, decreased insulin production over time, and changes in adipokines production
Symptoms	Polydipsia, polyuria, polyphagia, fatigue, weight loss without trying	Often none. Fatigue, recurrent infections. May also have polyuria, polydipsia, and polyphagia, blurred vision.

Continued

TABLE 28 Comparison of Type 1 and Type 2 Diabetes Mellitus—cont'd		
Factor	**Type 1 DM**	**Type 2 DM**
Ketosis	Present at onset or during insulin deficiency	Usually not present; can occur during infection or high stress
Insulin therapy	Required for all	Required for some. Progressive disease. Insulin may need to be added to treatment plan.
Body type	Thin, normal, or obese	Often overweight or obese with visceral adiposity ("apple shape"). May be normal.
Nutrition therapy	Essential	Essential
Vascular and neurologic complications	Frequent	Frequent

disorder in which the body develops antibodies against insulin and/ or the pancreatic β-cells that make insulin. This eventually results in not enough insulin for survival.

- A genetic predisposition and exposure to a virus are factors that may contribute to developing immune-related type 1 diabetes.

Once the pancreas can no longer make enough insulin to maintain normal glucose, the onset of symptoms is usually rapid.

- The patient usually has a history of recent and sudden weight loss and the classic symptoms of *polydipsia* (excessive thirst), *polyuria* (frequent urination), and *polyphagia* (excessive hunger).
- The person with type 1 diabetes requires a supply of insulin from an outside source (*exogenous insulin*) to sustain life. Without insulin, the patient develops *diabetes-related ketoacidosis* (DKA), a life-threatening condition resulting in metabolic acidosis.

Type 2 Diabetes Mellitus

Type 2 diabetes accounts for about 90%–95% of people with DM. Many risk factors contribute to developing type 2 DM. These include having a family history of type 2 DM, being overweight or obese, and being older. Although it occurs less often in children, the incidence is increasing due to the increasing prevalence of childhood obesity. Disease onset in type 2 diabetes is usually gradual, with signs and symptoms of hyperglycemia developing when about 50%–80% of β-cells no longer secrete insulin. Many people are diagnosed on routine laboratory testing or when they undergo treatment for other conditions and have high glucose or glycosylated hemoglobin (A1C) levels.

- In type 2 diabetes, the pancreas continues to produce some endogenous (self-made) insulin. However, the body either does not produce enough insulin or does not use it effectively, or both. The presence of endogenous insulin is the major difference between type 1 and type 2 diabetes.
- Genetic mutations that lead to insulin resistance and a higher risk for obesity have been found in many people with type 2 diabetes. Persons who have a first-degree relative with the disease are 10 times more likely to develop type 2 diabetes.

Four major metabolic abnormalities play a role in the development of type 2 diabetes.

- The first factor is *insulin resistance*, a condition in which body tissues do not respond to the action of insulin because insulin receptors are unresponsive, insufficient, or both. Entry of glucose into the cell is impeded, resulting in hyperglycemia.
- A second factor is a marked decrease in the ability of the pancreas to make insulin. The β-cells become fatigued from the compensatory overproduction of insulin or when β-cell mass is lost.
- A third factor is inappropriate glucose production by the liver. Instead of properly regulating the release of glucose in response to blood levels, the liver does so in a haphazard way that does not correspond to the body's needs at the time.
- A fourth factor is alteration in the production of hormones and cytokines by adipose tissue (adipokines). Adipokines play a role in glucose and fat metabolism.

Persons with metabolic syndrome are at an increased risk for the development of type 2 diabetes. Overweight persons with metabolic syndrome can reduce their risk for diabetes through a program of weight loss and regular physical activity (see Metabolic Syndrome).

Prediabetes

Persons diagnosed with prediabetes are at increased risk for the development of type 2 DM. *Prediabetes* is defined as impaired glucose tolerance (IGT), impaired fasting glucose (IFG), or both.

- A diagnosis of IGT is made if the 2-hr oral glucose tolerance test (OGTT) values are 140–199 mg/dL (7.8–11.0 mmol/L).

IFG is diagnosed when fasting glucose levels are 100–125 mg/dL (5.56–6.9 mmol/L).

People with prediabetes usually do not have symptoms. However, long-term damage to the body, especially the heart and blood vessels, may already be occurring. It is important for adults to undergo screening and understand risk factors for diabetes.

- Encourage those with prediabetes to have their blood glucose and A1C tested regularly and to self-monitor for symptoms of diabetes, such as polyuria, polyphagia, and polydipsia.
- Maintaining a healthy weight, exercising regularly, and eating a healthy diet reduce the risk of developing overt diabetes in people with prediabetes.

Gestational Diabetes

Gestational diabetes develops during pregnancy and occurs in about 2%–10% of pregnancies in the United States. Those at high risk include women who are obese, are of advanced maternal age, or have a family history of DM.

- Most women with gestational DM have normal glucose levels within 6 weeks' postpartum, but have up to a 63% risk of developing type 2 diabetes DM within 16 years.

Clinical Manifestations

Type 1 Diabetes

Because the onset of type 1 DM is rapid, the initial manifestations are usually acute. The osmotic effect of excess glucose produces polydipsia and polyuria. Polyphagia is a consequence of cellular malnourishment when insulin deficiency prevents use of glucose for energy. Weight loss, weakness, and fatigue may also occur.

Type 2 Diabetes

Manifestations of type 2 DM are often nonspecific, including fatigue, recurrent infections, prolonged wound healing, and vision problems. Polydipsia, polyuria, and polyphagia may also occur.

Acute Complications

Acute complications arise from events associated with hyperglycemia and hypoglycemia (also referred to as *insulin reaction*). Hypoglycemia worsens rapidly and constitutes a serious threat if action is not immediately taken. Table 29 compares hyperglycemia and hypoglycemia.

Diabetic Ketoacidosis

Diabetes-related ketoacidosis (DKA) is caused by a profound deficiency of insulin and is characterized by hyperglycemia, ketosis, acidosis, and dehydration. Precipitating factors include illness and

TABLE 29   Comparison of Hyperglycemia and Hypoglycemia

Hyperglycemia	Hypoglycemia
Manifestations	
• High glucose	• Glucose <70 mg/dL (3.9 mmol/L)
• ↑ Urination	• Cold, clammy skin
• ↑ Appetite followed by anorexia	• Numbness of fingers, toes, mouth
• Weakness, fatigue	• Tachycardia
• Blurred vision	• Emotional changes
• Headache	• Headache
• Glycosuria	• Nervousness, tremors
• Nausea and vomiting	• Faintness, dizziness
• Abdominal cramps	• Unsteady gait, slurred speech
• Progression to DKA or HHS	• Hunger
• Mood swings	• Changes in vision
	• Seizures, coma
Causes	
• Illness, infection	• Alcohol intake without food
• Corticosteroids	• Too little food—delayed, omitted, inadequate intake
• Too much food	
• Too little or no DM medication	• Too much DM medication
• Inactivity	• Too much exercise without adequate food intake
• Emotional, physical stress	• DM medication or food taken at wrong time
• Poor absorption of insulin	• Loss of weight without change in medication
	• Use of β-adrenergic blockers interfering with recognition of symptoms
Clinical course	
• More gradual onset	• More rapid onset
• Definition of high glucose varies by person, based on personal glucose targets	• Pattern of manifestations changes over time

D

Continued

TABLE 29   Comparison of Hyperglycemia and Hypoglycemia—cont'd

Hyperglycemia	Hypoglycemia

Treatment

- Get medical care
- Continue DM medication as prescribed
- Check glucose frequently and check urine for ketones. Record results.
- Drink fluids at least on an hourly basis
- Contact HCP about ketonuria

- Follow the Rule of 15 Conscious person: Give 15 g of a simple (fast-acting) carbohydrate (fruit juice or regular soft drink). Recheck the blood glucose 15 minutes later. If the value is still below 70 mg/dL, have the patient ingest 15 g more of carbohydrate and recheck the blood glucose in 15 minutes. Have the patient ingest a complex carbohydrate after recovery to prevent a rebound hypoglycemic attack. If no significant improvement occurs after 2 or 3 doses of 15 g of simple carbohydrate, contact the HCP.
- Worsening symptoms or unconscious patient: Subcutaneous or IM injection of 1 mg glucagon, or IV administration of 25–50 mL of 50% glucose.

Preventive measures

- Take prescribed dose of medication at proper time
- Accurately give insulin, noninsulin injectables, OA
- Make healthy food choices
- Follow sick-day rules when ill
- Check glucose routinely
- Wear or carry DM identification

- Take prescribed dose of medication at proper time
- Accurately give insulin, noninsulin injectables, OA
- Coordinate eating with medications
- Eat adequate food intake needed for calories for exercise
- Be able to recognize symptoms and treat them immediately
- Carry simple carbohydrates
- Teach family and caregiver about symptoms and treatment
- Check glucose routinely
- Wear or carry DM identification

DKA, Diabetic ketoacidosis; *HHS,* hyperosmolar hyperglycemic syndrome; *OA,* oral agent.

infection; inadequate insulin dosage; undiagnosed type 1 diabetes; lack of education, understanding, or resources; and neglect.

- DKA is most likely to occur in type 1 diabetes. It may be seen in type 2 during severe illness or stress when the pancreas cannot meet the extra demand for insulin. If left untreated, death is inevitable.
- When insulin is insufficient, glucose cannot be properly used for energy. The body compensates by breaking down fat into *ketones*, acidic by-products of fat metabolism.
- Manifestations of DKA include dehydration signs (e.g., poor skin turgor, dry mucous membranes), tachycardia, orthostatic hypotension with a weak and rapid pulse, vomiting, Kussmaul respirations, lethargy, weakness, and a sweet fruity odor of acetone on the breath.
- Laboratory findings include a blood glucose level of 250 mg/dL (13.9 mmol/L) or greater, arterial blood pH < 7.30, and serum bicarbonate level < 16 mEq/L (16 mmol/L). A moderate to large amount of ketones are found in the urine or serum.

Hyperosmolar Hyperglycemia Syndrome

Hyperosmolar hyperglycemia syndrome (HHS) is a life-threatening syndrome in the patient with DM who is able to make enough insulin to prevent DKA but not enough to prevent severe hyperglycemia, osmotic diuresis, and extracellular fluid depletion.

- The main difference between HHS and DKA is that the patient with HHS usually has enough circulating insulin to avoid ketoacidosis. Blood glucose levels can climb quite high before the problem is noted. The higher blood glucose levels increase serum osmolality and cause severe neurologic manifestations, such as somnolence, coma, seizures, hemiparesis, and aphasia.
- HHS is less common than DKA. It often occurs in patients >60 years of age who are newly diagnosed with type 2 diabetes. Common causes of HHS include urinary tract infections, pneumonia, sepsis, and acute illness.
- Laboratory values include a glucose level above 600 mg/dL (33.33 mmol/L) and a marked increase in serum osmolality. Ketone bodies are absent or minimal in both blood and urine.

Hypoglycemia

Hypoglycemia, or low blood glucose, occurs when there is too much insulin in proportion to available glucose in the blood. This causes the blood glucose level to drop below 70 mg/dL. Manifestations include shakiness, palpitations, nervousness, diaphoresis, anxiety, hunger, and pallor. Findings mimic alcohol intoxication. Untreated hypoglycemia can progress to loss of consciousness, seizures, coma, and death.

Chronic Complications

Chronic complications are primarily those of end-organ disease arising from damage to the blood vessels from chronic hyperglycemia. *Angiopathy,* or blood vessel disease, is one of the leading causes of diabetes-related deaths. These chronic blood vessel problems are divided into two categories: macrovascular complications and microvascular complications.

Macrovascular Complications

Macrovascular complications are diseases of the large and medium-sized blood vessels that occur with greater frequency and an earlier onset in people with diabetes. Women with DM have 4–6 times increased risk for cardiovascular disease (CVD). Men with DM have 2–3 times increased risk for CVD. Risk factors associated with macrovascular complications, such as obesity, smoking, hypertension, high fat intake, and sedentary lifestyle, can be reduced. Insulin resistance is implicated in the pathogenesis of essential hypertension and dyslipidemia.

Microvascular Complications

Microvascular complications result from thickening of the vessel membranes in the capillaries and arterioles (small vessels) in response to chronic hyperglycemia. The areas most noticeably affected are the eyes (retinopathy), kidneys (nephropathy), and nerves (neuropathy).

Diabetes-related retinopathy is the leading common cause of new cases of adult blindness.

- In *nonproliferative retinopathy*, the most common form, partial occlusion of the small blood vessels in the retina causes microaneurysms to develop in the capillary walls. Capillary fluid leaks out, causing retinal edema and eventually hard exudates or intraretinal hemorrhages. Vision may be affected if the macula is involved.
- *Proliferative retinopathy* is more severe and involves the retina and vitreous. When retinal capillaries are occluded, new, fragile blood vessels form. Eventually light does not reach the retina as vessels break and bleed. A tear or retinal detachment may occur. If the macula is involved, vision is lost. Treatment involves laser photocoagulation.

Diabetes-related nephropathy is associated with damage to the small blood vessels that supply the glomeruli of the kidney. It is the leading cause of end-stage renal disease in the United States and seen in 20%–40% of people with DM.

- Tight blood glucose control is critical to prevent or delay diabetes-related nephropathy.

- Hypertension significantly accelerates the progression of nephropathy, so aggressive BP management is indicated (See Hypertension).
- Patients with diabetes are screened for nephropathy annually to assess for albuminuria and measure the albumin-to-creatinine ratio. Serum creatinine is also measured to give an estimate glomerular filtration rate and the degree of kidney function.

Neuropathy is nerve damage associated with diabetes. About 60%–70% of patients with diabetes have some degree of neuropathy. More than 60% of nontraumatic amputations in the United States are done for people with diabetes. Screening for neuropathy should begin at the time of diagnosis in patients with type 2 diabetes and 5 years after diagnosis in patients with type 1 diabetes.

Two major categories of diabetes-related neuropathy are the more common *sensory neuropathy*, which affects the peripheral nervous system, and *autonomic neuropathy*, which can affect nearly all body systems.

- The most common form of sensory neuropathy is distal symmetric neuropathy, which affects the hands or feet. Findings include loss of sensation, abnormal sensations, pain, and paresthesias. The pain, which is often described as burning, cramping, crushing, or tearing, is usually worse at night. The paresthesias may be associated with tingling, burning, and itching sensations.
- Autonomic neuropathy can lead to hypoglycemia unawareness, bowel incontinence and diarrhea, and urinary retention. Delayed gastric emptying *(gastroparesis)*, a complication of autonomic neuropathy, can cause nausea, vomiting, gastroesophageal reflux, and persistent feelings of fullness. Cardiovascular abnormalities, such as postural hypotension, painless myocardial infarction, and resting tachycardia, can occur. Erectile dysfunction (ED) in men with diabetes is common and may be the first manifestation of autonomic neuropathy.

Control of blood glucose is the only treatment for diabetic neuropathy. It is effective in many but not all cases. Drug therapy may be used to treat neuropathic symptoms, particularly pain.

Diagnostic Studies

The diagnosis of diabetes can be made with one of the following four methods. Criteria 1–3 should be confirmed by repeat testing.

1. A1C level of 6.5% or greater.
2. Fasting plasma glucose (FPG) level at or above 126 mg/dL (7.0 mmol/L). Fasting is defined as no caloric intake for at least 8 hr.

3. Two-hour plasma glucose level at or above 200 mg/dL (11.1 mmol/L) during an OGTT, using a glucose load of 75 g.
4. In a patient with classic symptoms of hyperglycemia (polyuria, polydipsia, unexplained weight loss) or hyperglycemic crisis, a random plasma glucose of at least 200 mg/dL (11.1 mmol/L).

Interprofessional Management

The goals of diabetes management are to reduce symptoms, promote well-being, prevent acute complications related to hypo- or hyperglycemia, and prevent or delay the onset and progression of long-term complications. Nutritional therapy, drug therapy, exercise, and self-monitoring of blood glucose are used in the management of diabetes. The major types of glucose-lowering agents (GLAs) used in the treatment of diabetes are insulin, oral agents (OAs), and noninsulin injectable agents. For most patients, drug therapy is needed.

Drug Therapy: Insulin

Exogenous (injected) insulin is needed when someone has inadequate insulin to meet metabolic needs. People with type 1 diabetes require exogenous insulin to survive. People with type 2 diabetes may require exogenous insulin during periods of severe stress, such as illness or surgery.

Human insulin is derived from common bacteria (e.g., *Escherichia coli*) or yeast cells using recombinant DNA technology. Insulins are categorized as rapid-acting, short-acting, intermediate-acting, and long-acting. The regimens for insulin therapy vary. See Table 30.

- The insulin approach that most closely mimics endogenous insulin production is the basal-bolus plan (often called *intensive* or *physiologic insulin therapy*). It consists of multiple daily insulin injections or an insulin pump together with frequent self-monitoring of blood glucose (or a continuous glucose monitoring system).
- The timing of rapid- and short-acting insulin in relation to meals is crucial. Rapid-acting synthetic insulin analogs, which include aspart (NovoLog), glulisine (Apidra), and lispro (Humalog), have an onset of action of about 15 minutes. They should be injected within 15 minutes of mealtime. The rapid-acting analogs most closely mimic natural insulin secretion in response to a meal.
- A rapid-acting inhaled insulin (Afrezza) can be administered at the beginning of each meal or within 20 minutes after starting a meal. It is not a substitute for long-acting insulin.

TABLE 30   Types of Insulin

Classification	Examples
Rapid-acting insulin	Aspart (NovoLog, Fiasp)
	Glulisine (Apidra)
	Lispro (Humalog)
Short-acting insulin	Regular (Humulin R, Novolin R)
Intermediate-acting insulin	NPH (Humulin N, Novolin N)
Long-acting insulin	Degludec (Tresiba)
	Detemir (Levemir)
	Glargine (Basaglar, Lantus, Toujeo)
	Insulin glargine (Basaglar)
Combination therapy (premixed)	Aspart protamine/aspart 70/30[a] (NovoLog Mix 70/30)
	Degludec/aspart 70/30 (Ryzodeg)
	Lispro protamine/lispro 75/25[a] (Humalog Mix 75/25)
	Lispro protamine/lispro 50/50[a] (Humalog Mix 50/50)
	NPH/regular 70/30[a] (Humulin 70/30, Novolin 70/30)
	NPH/regular 50/50[a] (Humulin 50/50)
More concentrated insulin	Humulin R U-500
	Toujeo U-300 (Insulin glargine)
	Humolog U-200 (Insulin lispro)
Inhaled insulin	Afrezza

[a]These numbers refer to percentages of each type of insulin.

- In addition to mealtime insulin, people with type 1 diabetes use a long- or intermediate-acting (background) insulin to control glucose levels between meals and overnight.
- Combination insulin therapy involves mixing short- or rapid-acting insulin with intermediate-acting insulin to provide both mealtime and basal coverage with one injection. Premixed formulas are available for this regimen, but optimal glucose control is not as likely because there is less flexibility in dosing.

Routine doses of insulin are given by subcutaneous injection. Regular insulin can be given IV when immediate onset of action is desired.

- Continuous subcutaneous insulin infusion can be administered through an insulin pump, a small battery-operated device that resembles a standard pager in size and appearance. Every 2 or 3 days, the insertion site is changed. A major advantage of the pump is the potential for tight glucose control.

D

Nursing Care Related to Insulin Therapy. Nursing responsibilities for the patient receiving insulin include proper administration, assessment of patient's response to insulin therapy, and teaching the patient about administration of, adjustment to, and side effects of insulin.

- Assess the patient who is new to insulin and evaluate their ability to manage insulin therapy safely. This includes the ability to understand the interaction of insulin, diet, and activity and to recognize and appropriately treat the symptoms of hypoglycemia.
- The patient or the caregiver must be able to prepare and inject the insulin. If not able, additional resources will be needed.
- Follow-up assessment of the patient who has been using insulin therapy includes inspection of insulin sites for *lipodystrophy* (atrophy of subcutaneous tissue) and other reactions, a review of the insulin preparation and injection technique, a history pertaining to hypoglycemic episodes, and assessment of the patient's method for handling hypoglycemic episodes.

Drug Therapy: Oral and Noninsulin Injectable Agents

OAs and noninsulin injectable agents work to improve the mechanisms by which the body produces and uses insulin and glucose (Fig. 8). These drugs primarily work on three defects of type 2 DM: (1) insulin resistance, (2) decreased insulin production, and (3) increased liver glucose production. These drugs may be used in combination with agents from other classes or with insulin to achieve glucose goals.

Metformin, a biguanide, is the most effective first-line treatment for type 2 diabetes. Metformin reduces glucose production by the liver, but also enhances insulin sensitivity and improves glucose transport into cells. Many other types of OAs and noninsulin injectable agents (Table 31) are used in the treatment of type 2 diabetes.

Nursing Care Related to Oral and Noninsulin Injectable Agents. Your responsibilities for the patient taking oral and noninsulin injectable agents are similar to those for the patient taking insulin. Proper administration, assessment of the patient's use of and response to these drugs, and teaching the patient and family are all essential nursing actions.

- Your assessment is valuable in determining the most appropriate drug for a patient. This includes assessing the patient's mental status, eating habits, home environment, attitude toward diabetes, and medication history.

Nutrition Therapy

Patient-centered nutrition therapy, consisting of counseling, education, and ongoing monitoring, is a cornerstone of care for people with DM and prediabetes. Changing eating habits can be

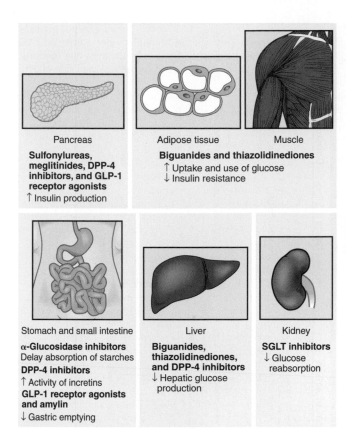

Figure 8 Sites and methods of action of type 2 diabetes drugs.

challenging for many people. Guidelines from the American Diabetes Association (ADA) indicate that within the context of an overall healthy eating plan, a person with DM can eat the same foods as a person who does not have diabetes. This means that the same principles of good nutrition that apply to the general population also apply to people with diabetes.

- *Type 1 diabetes.* People with type 1 diabetes base their meal planning on usual food intake and preferences balanced with insulin and exercise patterns. Day-to-day consistency in timing and amount of food eaten makes it much easier to manage

TABLE 31 Drug Therapy: Oral Agents and Noninsulin Injectable Agents

Type	Mechanism of action	Side effects	Considerations
Oral agents			
α-Glucosidase inhibitors			
Acarbose (Precose) Miglitol (Glyset)	Delays absorption of complex carbohydrates (starches) from GI tract.	Gas, abdominal pain, diarrhea	Take with the first bite of each main meal.
Biguanides			
Metformin (Fortamet Glucophage, Glucophage XR, Glumetza, Riomet)	↓ Liver glucose production. ↑ insulin sensitivity. Improves glucose uptake by tissues, especially muscles.	Diarrhea, lactic acidosis	Must be held 1–2 days before IV contrast media given and for 48 hr after. Take with food to minimize GI side effects.
Dipeptidyl peptidase-4 (DPP-4) inhibitors			
Alogliptin (Nesina) Linagliptin (Tradjenta) Saxagliptin (Onglyza) Sitagliptin (Januvia)	↑ Activity of incretins. ↑ Insulin release from pancreatic β-cells. ↓ liver glucose production.	Pancreatitis, allergic reactions	Take with or without food.

	Action	Side Effects	Nursing Considerations
Dopamine receptor agonists			
Bromocriptine (Cycloset)	Activates dopamine receptors in central nervous system. Unknown how it improves glucose levels.	Orthostatic hypotension, nausea, headache, fatigue	Take with food at the same time each day. Teach the patient to change positions slowly.
Meglitinides			
Nateglinide repaglinide	Stimulates a rapid and short-lived release of insulin from the pancreas.	Weight gain, hypoglycemia	Take any time from 30 minutes before each meal right up to the time of the meal. They should not be taken if a meal is skipped.
Sodium-glucose co-transporter 2 (SGLT2) inhibitors			
Canagliflozin (Invokana) Dapagliflozin (Farxiga) Empagliflozin (Jardiance) Ertugliflozin (Steglatro)	↓ Renal glucose reabsorption. ↑ Urinary glucose excretion.	Increased risk of genital and urinary tract infections. Hypoglycemia.	Take in the morning before the first meal of the day. Teach the patient to drink 1–2 glasses of water each day above their normal intake.

Continued

D

TABLE 31 Drug Therapy: Oral Agents and Noninsulin Injectable Agents—cont'd

Type	Mechanism of action	Side effects	Considerations
Sulfonylureas Glimepiride (Amaryl) Glipizide (Glucotrol, Glucotrol XL) Glyburide (DiaBeta, Glynase)	↑ Insulin release from pancreatic islets. ↓ Glycogenolysis and gluconeogenesis. Enhances cellular sensitivity to insulin.	Weight gain, hypoglycemia.	Take 30 minutes before meals. Avoid alcohol use.
Thiazolidinediones Pioglitazone (Actos) Rosiglitazone (Avandia)	↑ Glucose uptake in muscle. ↓ Endogenous glucose production.	Weight gain, edema. *Pioglitazone:* ↑ Risk for bladder cancer and worsen heart failure. *Rosiglitazone:* ↑ Risk for cardiovascular events (e.g., myocardial infarction, stroke).	Taken with or without food.
Combination oral therapy Actoplus Met, Actoplus Met XR	Same as for metformin and pioglitazone.	See side effects for individual drugs.	

Duetact	Same as for pioglitazone and glimepiride	Same as above
Glucovance	Same as for metformin and glyburide	Same as above
Glyxambi	Same as for empagliflozin and linagliptin	Same as above
Invokamet, Invokamet XR	Same as for canagliflozin and metformin	Same as above
Janumet, Janumet XR	Same as for metformin and sitagliptin	Same as above
Jentadueto, Jentadueto XR	Same as for linagliptin and metformin	Same as above
Kazano	Same as for alogliptin and metformin	Same as above
Kombiglyze	Same as for saxagliptin and metformin	Same as above
Oseni	Same as for alogliptin and pioglitazone	Same as above
PrandiMet	Same as for metformin and repaglinide	Same as above
Qtern	Same as for dapagliflozin and saxagliptin	Same as above
Qternmet XR	Same as for dapagliflozin, saxagliptin, and metformin XR	Same as above
Segluromet	Same as for metformin and ertugliflozin	Same as above
Steglujan	Same as for sitagliptin and ertugliflozin	Same as above
Synjardy, Synjardy XR	Same as metformin and empagliflozin	Same as above
Trijardy	Same as for empagliflozin, linagliptin, and metformin XR	Same as above
Xigduo	Same as for dapagliflozin and metformin	Same as above

Continued

D

TABLE 31 Drug Therapy: Oral Agents and Noninsulin Injectable Agents—cont'd

Type	Mechanism of action	Side effects	Considerations
Noninsulin injectable agents			
Amylin analogs			
Pramlintide (Symlin)	Slows gastric emptying. ↓ Glucagon secretion and endogenous glucose output from liver. ↑ Satiety.	Hypoglycemia, nausea, vomiting, decreased appetite, headache	Inject subcutaneously into the thigh or abdomen before meals. Do not inject into the arm because absorption from the arm is too variable.
Glucagon-like peptide-1 (GLP-1) receptor agonists			
Albiglutide (Tanzeum) Dulaglutide (Trulicity) Exenatide (Byetta) Exenatide extended-release (Bydureon) Liraglutide (Victoza) Lixisenatide (Adlyxin) Semaglutide (Ozempic)	↑ Insulin release. ↓ Glucagon secretion and slow gastric emptying. ↑ Satiety.	Nausea, vomiting, hypoglycemia, diarrhea, headache	The delayed gastric emptying may affect the absorption of other oral drugs. Tell patients to take fast-acting oral agents at least 1 hr before injecting a GLP-1 agonist drug.

blood glucose levels, especially for those persons using conventional, fixed insulin regimens. Rapid-acting insulin doses can be adjusted before the meal depending on current blood glucose level and the carbohydrate content of the meal. Multiple daily injections or the use of an insulin pump allows flexibility in food selection, and regimens can be adjusted for changes from usual eating and exercise habits.

- *Type 2 diabetes.* Nutrition therapy in type 2 diabetes emphasizes glucose, lipid, and BP goals. Modest weight loss may improve insulin resistance and glucose control.

Most often, a dietitian initially teaches the principles of nutrition as part of an interprofessional diabetes care team. When patients do not have access to a dietitian, you may need to assume responsibility for teaching basic dietary management of diabetes.

Exercise

Regular, consistent exercise is an essential part of diabetes and prediabetes management. Encourage patients to be active every day and to seek medical clearance before starting an intensive exercise program. The ADA recommends at least 150 minutes weekly (30 minutes, 5 days/week) of a moderate-intensity aerobic physical activity and resistance training 3 times a week unless contraindicated.

Exercise decreases insulin resistance and can have a direct effect on lowering blood glucose levels. It also contributes to weight loss, which further decreases insulin resistance, and in addition, it may help reduce triglyceride and low-density lipoprotein (LDL) cholesterol levels, increase high-density lipoprotein (HDL), reduce BP, and improve circulation.

- People who use insulin, sulfonylureas, or meglitinides are at increased risk for hypoglycemia when they increase physical activity. They should exercise about 1 hr after a meal or have a 10- to 15-g carbohydrate snack and check their blood glucose before exercising.

Blood Glucose Monitoring

Self-monitoring of blood glucose is a critical part of diabetes management. Providing a current blood glucose reading lets the patient make decisions about food intake, activity patterns, and medication dosages. Incorrect monitoring technique can cause errors in management strategies, so comprehensive patient teaching followed up with regular reassessment is essential.

Management of Acute Complications

Diabetic Ketoacidosis

If fluid and electrolyte imbalances are not severe and blood glucose levels can be safely monitored at home, DKA can be managed on an outpatient basis. Emergency management of DKA is needed when fluid imbalance is potentially life-threatening. The aim of fluid and electrolyte therapy is to replace extracellular and intracellular water and to correct deficits of sodium, chloride, bicarbonate, potassium, phosphate, magnesium, and nitrogen.

- A continuous IV infusion of insulin is directed toward correcting hyperglycemia and hyperketonemia.
- Although initial serum potassium may be normal or high, levels can rapidly decrease once therapy starts as insulin drives potassium into the cells, leading to life-threatening hypokalemia.

Hyperosmolar Hyperglycemic Syndrome

HHS is a medical emergency with a high mortality rate. Therapy is similar to that for DKA except that HHS requires more fluid replacement.

- Insulin is given immediately by IV infusion.
- Electrolytes are monitored and replaced. Assess vital signs, intake and output, tissue turgor, laboratory values, and cardiac monitoring to monitor the efficacy of fluid and electrolyte replacement.

Hypoglycemia

At the first sign of hypoglycemia, check the blood glucose if possible. If it is below 70 mg/dL (3.9 mmol/L), immediately begin treatment for hypoglycemia. If the patient has symptoms of hypoglycemia and monitoring equipment is not available, or if the patient has a history of chronic poor glucose control, assume it is hypoglycemia and begin treatment using the "Rule of 15."

- Hypoglycemia is treated by ingesting 15 g of a simple (fast-acting) carbohydrate, such as 4–6 ounces of fruit juice or regular soft drink. Avoid overtreatment with large quantities of quick-acting carbohydrates, such as candy bars, to avoid a rapid fluctuation to hyperglycemia.
- Recheck the blood glucose 15 minutes later. If the value is still below 70 mg/dL, have the patient ingest 15 g more of carbohydrate and recheck the blood glucose in 15 minutes. Because of the potential for rebound hypoglycemia after an acute episode, have the patient ingest a complex carbohydrate after recovery to prevent another hypoglycemic attack.
- If no significant improvement occurs after two or three doses of 15 g of simple carbohydrate, contact the HCP. For worsening symptoms or an unconscious patient, anticipate a subcutaneous or IM injection of 1 mg glucagon, or IV administration of 25–50 mL of 50% glucose.

Once acute hypoglycemia has been reversed, explore why the situation developed and provide additional patient teaching to avoid future episodes of hypoglycemia.

Nursing Management
Goals
The patient with diabetes will engage in self-care behaviors to actively manage their diabetes, have few or no episodes of acute hyperglycemic or hypoglycemic emergencies, maintain blood glucose levels at normal or near-normal levels, reduce the risk for chronic complications of diabetes, and adjust lifestyle to accommodate the diabetes regimen with a minimum of stress. The goal is for the patient with diabetes to safely and effectively fit diabetes into life, rather than living life around diabetes.

Nursing Interventions
Your role in health promotion is to identify, monitor, and teach the patient at risk for diabetes.

Management of Acute Illness and Surgery. Acute illness, injury, surgery, and emotional stress can increase blood glucose levels and result in hyperglycemia. When patients with diabetes are ill, they should check blood glucose at least every 4 hr. Teach acutely ill patients who have type 1 diabetes with a blood glucose level above 240 mg/dL (13.3 mmol/L) to test the urine for ketones every 3–4 hr.

- Persons with DM should contact the HCP when glucose levels are above 300 mg/dL for two tests in a row or urine ketone levels are moderate to high.
- Those persons who can eat normally should continue with the regular meal plan while increasing intake of noncaloric fluids, such as broth, water, dietary gelatin, and other decaffeinated beverages, and continue taking oral agents and insulin as prescribed.
- If illness causes the patient to eat less than normal, drug therapy should be continued while supplementing food intake with carbohydrate-containing fluids. Examples include low-sodium soups, juices, and regular, sugar-sweetened decaffeinated soft drinks. Notify the HCP if the patient is unable to keep down fluid or food.
- Adjustments in the diabetes plan during the intraoperative period can be made to ensure glycemic control. The patient is given IV fluids and insulin (if needed) immediately before, during, and after surgery when there is no oral intake.

D

- When caring for an unconscious surgical patient receiving insulin, be alert for hypoglycemic signs, such as sweating, tachycardia, and tremors.

Ambulatory Care. Successful diabetes management requires ongoing interaction among the patient, family, and interprofessional health care team. A certified diabetes educator (CDE) should be involved in the care of the patient and family.

Persons with diabetes face lifestyle choices that affect the food they eat, their activities, and demands on their time and energy. In addition, they face the challenge of preventing or dealing with the devastating complications of diabetes. Careful assessment of what it means to have diabetes is the starting point for patient teaching.

The potential for infection requires diligent skin care and dental hygiene. Routine care includes toothbrushing and flossing and regular bathing, with an emphasis on foot care. Skin injuries should be treated promptly. If the injury does not begin to heal within 24 hr or signs of infection develop, the HCP should be notified at once.

▼ **Patient and Caregiver Teaching**

The goals of diabetes self-management education are to match the level of self-management to the patient's ability so that they can become the most active participant possible. Those who actively manage their diabetes care have better outcomes than those who do not. Guidelines for patient and caregiver teaching for management of diabetes are listed in Table 32.

- Assess the patient's knowledge base frequently so that gaps in knowledge or inaccurate ideas can be quickly corrected.
- Tell the patient to carry medical identification at all times.

TABLE 32 Patient and Caregiver Teaching: Management of Diabetes Mellitus	
Component	**What to teach**
Disease process	• Introduce the pancreas and the islets of Langerhans.
	• Describe how insulin is made and what affects its production.
	• Discuss the relationship of insulin and glucose.
	• Explain the difference between type 1 and type 2 DM.

TABLE 32 **Patient and Caregiver Teaching: Management of Diabetes Mellitus—cont'd**	
Component	**What to teach**
Drug therapy	• Ensure that the patient understands the drug plan.
	• Account for a patient's physical or other limitations or inabilities for self-medication. If necessary, involve the family or caregiver in proper use of medication.
	• Discuss all side effects and safety issues.
Exercise	• Discuss the effect of regular exercise on managing glucose and improving cardiovascular function and general health.
Meal planning	• Stress the importance of a well-balanced diet as part of a DM management plan.
	• Explain the impact of carbohydrates on glucose levels.
Monitoring glucose	• Teach correct BGM.
	• Include when to check glucose levels, how to record them, and how to adjust insulin levels, if necessary.
Risk reduction	• Ensure that the patient understands and appropriately responds to the signs and symptoms of hypoglycemia and hyperglycemia.
	• Stress the importance of proper foot care, regular eye examinations, and consistent BGM.
	• Teach the patient about the effect that stress can have on glucose.
Psychosocial	• Help the patient identify resources that are available to help with the adjustment, and answer questions about living with a chronic condition such as DM.

D

DIARRHEA

Description

Diarrhea is the passage of at least three loose or liquid stools per day. It may be acute, lasting 14 days or less, or persistent, lasting >14 days. Chronic diarrhea lasts 30 days or longer.

Pathophysiology

The primary cause of acute diarrhea is ingesting infectious organisms. Viruses cause most cases of infectious diarrhea in the United States. Bacterial infections are also common. *Escherichia coli* O157:H7 is a common cause of bloody diarrhea in the United States. It is transmitted by undercooked beef or chicken contaminated with the bacteria or by fruits and vegetables exposed to contaminated manure. *Giardia lamblia* is the most common intestinal parasite that causes diarrhea in the United States.

Infectious organisms attack the intestines in different ways. Some organisms (e.g., *Rotavirus*, *Norovirus*, *G. lamblia*) change the secretion and/or absorption of the enterocytes of the small intestine without inflammation. Other organisms (e.g., *Clostridioides difficile*) impair absorption by destroying cells, causing inflammation in the colon, and producing toxins that cause damage.

Patients receiving broad-spectrum antibiotics (e.g., carbapenems, cephalosporins, piperacillin/tazobactam) are susceptible to infections with pathogenic strains of *C. difficile*. *C. difficile* infection (CDI) causes the most serious antibiotic-associated diarrhea and is a common cause of hospital-acquired GI illness in the United States.

Diarrhea is not always caused by infection. Drugs and food intolerances can also cause diarrhea. Diarrhea from celiac disease and short bowel syndrome results from malabsorption in the small intestine.

Clinical Manifestations

Infections that attack the upper GI tract (e.g., *Norovirus* organisms, *G. lamblia*) usually produce large-volume, watery stools; cramping; and periumbilical pain. Patients have either a low-grade or no fever and often have nausea and vomiting before the diarrhea begins. Infections of the colon and distal small bowel (e.g., *Shigella*, *Salmonella*, *C. difficile*) produce fever and frequent bloody diarrhea with a small volume.

Leukocytes, blood, and mucus may be present in the stool, depending on the causative agent. Severe diarrhea produces life-threatening dehydration, electrolyte problems (e.g., hypokalemia), and acid-base imbalances (metabolic acidosis). CDI can progress to severe colitis and intestinal perforation.

Diagnostic Studies

Most cases of diarrhea resolve quickly. Stool cultures are only indicated for patients who are very ill, have a significant fever, have diarrhea longer than 3 days, or were exposed during an outbreak. Those with travelers' diarrhea lasting 14 days or longer should be assessed for parasites.

- Stools are examined for blood, mucus, white blood cells (WBCs), and parasites. Cultures are done to identify infectious organisms.
- CDI is detected by enzyme immunoassay (EIA).
- In a patient with chronic diarrhea, measurement of stool electrolytes, pH, and osmolality may help determine whether diarrhea is related to decreased fluid absorption or increased fluid secretion.
- Measurement of stool fat and undigested muscle fibers may indicate fat and protein malabsorption conditions, including pancreatic insufficiency.
- Blood cultures are done in those with signs of sepsis or systemic infection (e.g., high fever) or who are immunocompromised.

D

Interprofessional Management

Treatment depends on the cause. Foods and drugs that cause diarrhea should be avoided. Acute infectious diarrhea is usually self-limiting. The major concerns are preventing transmission, replacing fluid and electrolytes, and protecting the skin.

Oral solutions containing glucose and electrolytes may replace losses from mild diarrhea. In severe diarrhea, IV fluids, electrolytes, vitamins, and nutrition may be needed.

Antidiarrheal agents may be given to coat and protect mucous membranes, absorb irritating substances, inhibit GI motility, decrease intestinal secretions, or decrease central nervous system (CNS) stimulation to the GI tract.

- Antidiarrheal agents have limited short-term use. They are used cautiously in inflammatory bowel disease because of the danger of *toxic megacolon.*
- Antibiotics are rarely used to treat infectious diarrhea.

CDI is a particularly hazardous health care-associated infection (HAI). The risk for contracting CDI is highest in patients receiving antimicrobial, chemotherapy, gastric acid-suppressing, or immunosuppressive agents. Its spores can survive for up to 70 days on objects including commodes, thermometers, bedside tables, and floors. Health care workers who do not adhere to infection control precautions can transmit CDI from patient to patient.

- CDI is treated with either oral vancomycin (125 mg, 4 times a day) or fidaxomicin (200 mg twice daily) for 10 days. Metronidazole is an option. All nonessential antibiotics, stool softeners, laxatives, and antidiarrheal agents should be stopped.

Nursing Management: Acute Infectious Diarrhea

Goals

The patient will have resumption of normal bowel pattern, normal fluid and electrolyte and acid-base balance, normal nutritional status, and no perianal skin breakdown.

Interventions

Consider all cases of acute diarrhea to be infectious until the cause is known.

- Use strict infection control precautions to prevent the illness from spreading to others. Wash your hands before and after contact with each patient and when handling any body fluids. Meticulous hand washing with soap and water is extremely important in limiting the spread of *C. difficile*.
- Provide private rooms for patients with CDI and ensure that visitors and health care providers (HCPs) wear gloves and gowns.
- Ensure surfaces and equipment are disinfected with a 10% bleach solution or a disinfectant labeled as *C. difficile* sporicidal.

▼ Patient and Caregiver Teaching

- Teach the patient and caregiver the principles of hygiene, infection control precautions, and potential dangers of an illness that is infectious to themselves and others.
- Discuss proper food handling, cooking, and storage.

DISSEMINATED INTRAVASCULAR COAGULATION

Description

Disseminated intravascular coagulation (DIC) is a serious bleeding and thrombotic disorder that results from abnormally initiated and accelerated clotting. Subsequent decreases in clotting factors and platelets may lead to uncontrollable hemorrhage. The term *DIC* can be misleading because it suggests that blood is only clotting. However, there is also profuse bleeding from depletion of platelets and clotting factors.

Pathophysiology

DIC is an abnormal response of the normal clotting cascade. DIC can occur as an acute, catastrophic condition, or it may exist at a subacute or chronic level.

- Diseases or disorders known to predispose patients to acute DIC include shock, septicemia, abruptio placentae, cancer, severe head injury, heatstroke, and pulmonary emboli. The underlying disease must be treated for DIC to resolve. The manifestations of DIC result from consumption and depletion of platelets and coagulation factors, as well as clot lysis and formation of fibrin split products (FSPs) that have anticoagulant properties. Tissue factor is released at the site of tissue injury and by some cancers, such as leukemia. It enhances normal coagulation mechanisms. Abundant intravascular thrombin, the most powerful coagulant, is made. It speeds the conversion of fibrinogen to fibrin and enhances platelet aggregation. There is widespread fibrin and platelet deposition in capillaries and arterioles, causing thrombosis. This process can lead to multiorgan failure. As FSPs accumulate and clotting factors are depleted, the blood loses its ability to clot. A stable clot cannot form at injury sites, which predisposes the patient to bleeding.

Clinical Manifestations

Question bleeding in a person with no previous history or obvious cause because it may be one of the first manifestations of acute DIC. Other manifestations include weakness, malaise, and fever. There are both bleeding and thrombotic manifestations in DIC (Fig. 9).

- *Bleeding manifestations* include petechiae, oozing blood, tachypnea, hemoptysis, tachycardia, hypotension, bloody stools, hematuria, dizziness, headache, changes in mental status, and bone and joint pain.
- *Thrombotic manifestations* are a result of fibrin or platelet deposition in the microvasculature. Manifestations include ischemic tissue necrosis, tachypnea, dyspnea, pulmonary emboli, cardiovascular and electrocardiogram (ECG) changes, kidney damage, and paralytic ileus.

Diagnostic Studies

Diagnostic findings include

- prolonged prothrombin time and partial thromboplastin time;
- prolonged activated partial thromboplastin time and thrombin time;
- reduced fibrinogen, antithrombin III (AT III), and platelets;
- elevated FSPs and elevated D-dimers (cross-linked fibrin fragments);
- reduced levels of factors V, VII, VIII, X, and XIII.

Interprofessional Management

It is important to diagnose DIC quickly, stabilize the patient (e.g., with oxygenation or volume replacement), treat the underlying

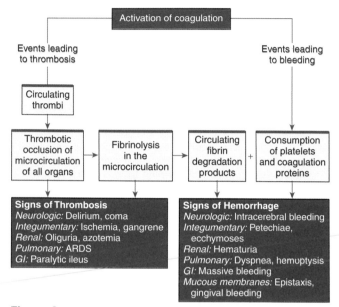

Figure 9 The sequence of events that occur during disseminated intravascular coagulation (DIC). *ARDS,* acute respiratory distress syndrome; *GI,* gastrointestinal.

causative disease or problem, and control the ongoing thrombosis and bleeding. Depending on its severity, a variety of measures are used to manage DIC.

- If chronic DIC is diagnosed in a patient who is not bleeding, treatment of the underlying disease may reverse DIC (e.g., chemotherapy when DIC is caused by cancer).
- Blood product support is usually reserved to stabilize the patient with life-threatening hemorrhage. Platelets are given to correct thrombocytopenia, and cryoprecipitate replaces factor VIII and fibrinogen. Fresh frozen plasma replaces all clotting factors except platelets and provides a source of antithrombin.
- A patient with thrombosis is often treated by anticoagulation with unfractionated heparin or low-molecular-weight heparin. Heparin is used in the treatment of DIC only when the benefit (reducing clotting) outweighs the risk of bleeding. Antithrombin III (AT III) (ATnativ) may be useful in fulminant DIC, although it increases the risk of bleeding.

- Chronic DIC does not respond to oral anticoagulants, but can be controlled with long-term use of heparin.

Nursing Management

Be alert to the possible development of DIC. The cause of DIC needs to be managed while you provide supportive care.

- Assess for signs of external bleeding (e.g., petechiae, oozing at IV or injection sites) and internal bleeding (e.g., changes in mental status, increasing abdominal girth, pain) and any indications that microthrombi may be causing clinically significant organ damage (e.g., decreased renal output).
- Handle the patient gently to minimize tissue damage and protect the patient from additional bleeding.
- Administer blood products and medications.

D

DIVERTICULOSIS/DIVERTICULITIS

Description

Diverticula are saccular dilations or outpouchings of the mucosa that develop in the colon. *Diverticulosis* is the presence of multiple noninflamed diverticula. *Diverticulitis* is inflammation of one or more diverticula, resulting in perforation into the peritoneum. Clinically, diverticular disease covers a spectrum from asymptomatic, uncomplicated diverticulosis to diverticulitis with complications, such as perforation, abscess, fistula, and bleeding. Diverticula are common, especially in older adults, but most people never develop diverticulitis.

Pathophysiology

Diverticula may occur anywhere in the GI tract but are most common in the left (descending, sigmoid) colon. They seem to occur at weak points in the intestinal wall, such as where the blood vessels pass through the muscle layer.

- The disease is more prevalent in populations with diets low in fiber, high in red meat, and high in refined carbohydrates. Diverticula are uncommon in vegetarians.
- Other risk factors for development of diverticula are obesity, inactivity, smoking, excessive alcohol use, and immunosuppression.

Clinical Manifestations and Complications

Most patients with diverticulosis have no symptoms. Some have abdominal pain, bloating, flatulence, and changes in bowel habits.

In more serious situations, the diverticula bleed or diverticulitis develops.

The most common signs and symptoms of diverticulitis are acute pain in the left lower quadrant, distension, decreased or absent bowel sounds, nausea, vomiting, and systemic symptoms of infection (fever, ↑ white blood cell [WBC] count). Older adults with diverticulitis may be afebrile, with a normal WBC count and little, if any, abdominal tenderness.

Diverticulitis can cause erosion of the bowel wall, perforation into the peritoneum, a localized abscess, peritonitis, or bleeding.

Diagnostic Studies

- History and physical examination
- Abdominal and chest X-rays to rule out other causes of acute abdominal pain
- Sigmoidoscopy or colonoscopy
- Diagnosis of diverticulitis is based on the physical assessment, complete blood count, and CT scan with contrast to confirm the diagnosis

Interprofessional and Nursing Management

A high fiber diet, mainly from fruits and vegetables with a decreased intake of fat and red meat, is the best way to prevent diverticular disease. High levels of physical activity seem to decrease the risk.

In acute diverticulitis, the goal of treatment is to let the colon rest and the inflammation subside. Some patients can be managed at home with a clear liquid diet, bed rest, and analgesics. Hospitalization is needed if symptoms are severe, the patient is unable to tolerate oral fluids, there are systemic manifestations of infection, or the patient has comorbid conditions (e.g., immunosuppression).

If hospitalized, the patient is kept on NPO status, placed on bed rest, and given IV fluids and antibiotics. Observe for signs of abscess, bleeding, and peritonitis, and monitor the WBC count. Give analgesics as needed. Maintain strict intake and output records. If needed, a nasogastric tube with low suction will provide decompression. When the acute attack subsides, give oral fluids first and then progress the diet to semisolids.

Patients with reoccurring diverticulitis or complications may need surgery. The usual surgical procedure involves resection of the involved colon with a primary anastomosis. If the health care provider is not able to anastomose the colon, the patient will have a temporary diverting colostomy.

Patient Teaching

Teach patients with diverticular disease to avoid increased intraabdominal pressure because it may precipitate an attack.

- Factors that increase intraabdominal pressure are straining at stool, vomiting, bending, lifting, and wearing tight, restrictive clothing.
- Teach about the importance of following a high-fiber diet. Encourage a fluid intake of at least 2 L/day. Explain that the patient does not have to avoid nuts, seeds, and corn.
- Weight reduction is important for the obese person with diverticular disease.

DYSMENORRHEA

Description

Dysmenorrhea is painful menses with abdominal cramping. The degree of pain and discomfort varies.

Pathophysiology

Primary dysmenorrhea is most common in adolescents around the time of menarche. It is thought to be caused by excess prostaglandin, a hormone secreted by the endometrium (uterine lining) during menstruation.

- Prostaglandin stimulates the uterus to contract. Uterine contractions and constriction of small endometrial blood vessels lead to tissue ischemia and increased sensitization of pain receptors. This results in painful menstrual cramps. As menstruation continues, prostaglandin levels decrease and menstrual cramping improves.

Secondary dysmenorrhea has similar symptoms of pain during menses but is caused by a uterine pathology. The most common causes of secondary dysmenorrhea are endometriosis, adenomyosis, or uterine fibroids. There may also be an association between dysmenorrhea and chronic pain conditions.

Clinical Manifestations

Both forms of dysmenorrhea present with painful uterine cramping at the start of menses. Symptoms often resolve spontaneously within 2 or 3 days after onset. Severe dysmenorrhea can impair patients' functioning and quality of life.

- Patients may also have back pain, nausea and vomiting, and symptoms of premenstrual disorders.

Depending on the cause, secondary dysmenorrhea may be associated with dyspareunia (painful intercourse), heavy or irregular vaginal bleeding, or infertility.

Diagnostic Studies

A diagnosis of primary dysmenorrhea can be made based on the presentation of symptoms in the absence of other suspected causes of pain.

- Pelvic examination may not be necessary for adolescents who are not at risk for sexually transmitted infections and present with classic symptoms of primary dysmenorrhea.
- Assessment for secondary dysmenorrhea includes pelvic examination and transvaginal or pelvic ultrasound imaging.

Interprofessional and Nursing Management

Treatment for primary dysmenorrhea includes drug and nonpharmacologic therapies. Validate the patient's pain and experience. Provide psychosocial support.

- Nonpharmacologic options include use of heat, exercise, and complementary and alternative therapy such as transcutaneous electrical nerve stimulation or acupuncture.
- First-line drug therapy includes nonsteroidal antiinflammatory drugs (NSAIDs). NSAIDs inhibit prostaglandins and decrease pain.
- If NSAIDs are ineffective or patients desire contraception, hormonal therapies such as oral contraceptive pills may help.

Treatment of secondary dysmenorrhea depends on the cause. Some patients' symptoms are improved by the same approaches used to treat primary dysmenorrhea.

- Common surgical treatments for dysmenorrhea include endometrial ablation (surgical destruction of the uterine lining) and hysterectomy (removal of the uterus).

DYSRHYTHMIAS

Description

Dysrhythmias are abnormal heart rhythms that result from disorders of impulse formation, impulse conduction, or both. Promptly assess abnormal cardiac rhythms and the patient's response to the rhythm.

Normally, the sinoatrial (SA) node is the natural pacemaker of the heart. A pacemaker from a site other than the SA node may be fired in two ways.

- If the SA node fires more slowly than a secondary pacemaker, the electrical signals from the secondary pacemaker may "escape."

The secondary pacemaker will then fire at its intrinsic rate: the atrioventricular (AV) node at a rate of 40–60 times per minute or the His-Purkinje system at a rate of 20–40 times per minute.

- Another way that secondary pacemakers can start is when they fire more rapidly than the normal pacemaker of the SA node. *Triggered beats* (early or late) may come from an *ectopic focus* (area outside the normal conduction pathway) in the atria, AV node, or ventricles. This results in a dysrhythmia, which replaces the normal sinus rhythm.

Dysrhythmias occur as the result of various abnormalities and disease states. The cause of a dysrhythmia influences the patient's treatment. Common causes of dysrhythmias are presented in Table 33. A systematic approach to assessing a cardiac rhythm is described in Table 34.

D

TABLE 33   Common Causes of Dysrhythmias[a]

Heart Conditions

- Accessory pathways
- Cardiomyopathy
- Conduction defects
- Heart failure
- Myocardial ischemia, infarction
- Valve disease

Other Conditions

- Acid-base imbalances
- Alcohol
- Caffeine, tobacco
- Connective tissue disorders
- Drowning
- Drug effects (e.g., antidysrhythmia drugs, stimulants, β-adrenergic blockers) or toxicity
- Electric shock
- Electrolyte imbalances (e.g., hyperkalemia, hypocalcemia)
- Emotional crisis
- Herbal supplements (e.g., areca nut, wahoo root bark, yerba maté)
- Hypoxia
- Metabolic conditions (e.g., thyroid problems)
- Sepsis, shock
- Toxins

[a]List is not all-inclusive.

TABLE 34 Approach to Assessing Heart Rhythm

When assessing a heart rhythm, use a consistent and systematic approach. One such approach includes the following:

1. Look for the P wave. Is it upright or inverted? Is there 1 for every QRS complex or more than 1? Are atrial fibrillatory or flutter waves present?
2. Evaluate the atrial rhythm. Is it regular or irregular?
3. Calculate the atrial rate.
4. Measure the duration of the PR interval. Is it normal duration or prolonged? Is it consistent in its duration before each QRS?
5. Evaluate the ventricular rhythm. Is it regular or irregular?
6. Calculate the ventricular rate.
7. Measure the duration of the QRS complex. Is it of normal duration or prolonged?
8. Assess the ST segment. Is it isoelectric (flat), elevated, or depressed?
9. Measure the duration of the QT interval. Correct for heart rate (cQT) to determine if it is normal or prolonged.[a]
10. Note the T wave. Is it upright or inverted?

Additional questions to consider include the following:

1. What is the dominant or underlying rhythm and/or dysrhythmia?
2. What is the clinical significance of your findings?
3. What is the treatment for the particular rhythm?

[a]A website for calculating the cQT interval for heart rate is available (www.mdcalc.com/corrected-qt-interval-qtc).

Types of Dysrhythmias

The characteristics of common dysrhythmias are described in Part Three (Reference Appendix). Examples of electrocardiogram (ECG) tracings of common dysrhythmias are presented in Chapter 39 of Harding et al., *Lewis' Medical-Surgical Nursing*, ed 12.

Sinus Bradycardia

Sinus bradycardia occurs when the SA node discharges at a rate <60 beats/minute. It may be a normal rhythm in aerobically trained athletes or in some people during sleep. It also occurs in response to carotid sinus massage, Valsalva maneuver, hypothermia, increased intraocular pressure, vagal stimulation, and the administration of certain drugs (e.g., β-adrenergic blockers, calcium channel blockers). Disease states associated with sinus bradycardia are hypothyroidism, increased intracranial pressure, hypoglycemia, and inferior wall myocardial infarction (MI).

- Symptomatic bradycardia refers to a heart rate (HR) that is <60 beats/minute and causes the patient to have symptoms of inadequate perfusion (e.g., fatigue, dizziness, chest pain, syncope).
- If bradycardia is caused by drugs, these may have to be held, discontinued, or reduced. For the patient with symptoms, treatment consists of giving IV atropine (anticholinergic drug). If atropine is ineffective, transcutaneous pacing or a dopamine or epinephrine infusion is an option. The patient may need a permanent pacemaker.

Sinus Tachycardia

Sinus tachycardia involves an HR of 101–180 beats/minute from the SA node due to vagal inhibition or sympathetic stimulation. This dysrhythmia is associated with many stressors. These include exercise, fever, pain, hypotension, hypovolemia, anemia, hypoglycemia, myocardial ischemia, heart failure (HF), hyperthyroidism, and anxiety. It can be an effect of drugs, such as epinephrine, norepinephrine, caffeine, theophylline, nifedipine, or hydralazine. Many over-the-counter cold remedies have active ingredients (e.g., pseudoephedrine) that can cause tachycardia.

- The clinical significance of sinus tachycardia depends on how the patient tolerates it. The patient may have dizziness, dyspnea, and hypotension because of decreased cardiac output (CO).
- An increased HR increases myocardial O_2 consumption. Angina or an increase in infarction size may occur with sinus tachycardia in those with coronary artery disease (CAD) or an acute MI.
- The underlying cause of tachycardia guides the treatment. If the patient has tachycardia from pain, effective pain management is important to treat the tachycardia. In clinically stable patients, vagal maneuvers can be tried. IV β-blockers (e.g., metoprolol), adenosine (Adenocard), or calcium-channel blockers (e.g., diltiazem) can reduce HR and decrease myocardial O_2 consumption. Clinically unstable patients may need synchronized cardioversion.

Premature Atrial Contraction

Premature atrial contraction (PAC) is a contraction starting from an ectopic focus in the atrium (in a location other than the SA node) sooner than the next expected sinus beat. The ectopic focus starts in the left or right atrium and travels across the atria by an abnormal pathway, creating a distorted P wave. At the AV node, it may be stopped (nonconducted PAC), delayed (lengthened PR interval), or conducted normally. If the impulse moves through the AV node, in most cases it is conducted normally through the ventricles.

In a normal heart, a PAC can result from emotional stress, fatigue, or from caffeine, tobacco, or alcohol use. A PAC can also result from hypoxia, electrolyte imbalances, hyperthyroidism, chronic obstructive pulmonary disease (COPD), and heart disease, including CAD and valvular disease.

- HR varies with the underlying rate and frequency of PACs, and the rhythm is irregular.
- In persons with healthy hearts, isolated PACs are not significant. Patients may report palpitations or a sense that the heart "skipped a beat."
- In persons with heart disease, frequent PACs may indicate enhanced automaticity of the atria or a reentry mechanism. Such PACs may warn of or start more serious dysrhythmias (e.g., supraventricular tachycardia).
- Treatment depends on the patient's symptoms. Withdrawal of sources of stimulation, such as caffeine or sympathomimetic drugs (e.g., epinephrine, dopamine), may be needed. β-Blockers may be used to decrease PACs.

Paroxysmal Supraventricular Tachycardia

Paroxysmal supraventricular tachycardia (PSVT), also known as *supraventricular tachycardia* (SVT) or *atrial tachycardia*, is a dysrhythmia starting in an ectopic focus anywhere above the bifurcation of the bundle of His. Identifying the ectopic focus requires recording the dysrhythmia as it starts.

PSVT occurs because of a reentrant phenomenon (reexcitation of the atria when there is a one-way block). Usually a PAC triggers a run of repeated premature beats. *Paroxysmal* refers to an abrupt onset and ending. A brief period of *asystole* (absence of all cardiac electrical activity) may follow the termination. AV block may prevent some of the impulses from being conducted to the ventricles. PSVT can occur with Wolff-Parkinson-White (WPW) syndrome or "preexcitation" with extra conduction or accessory pathways. HR is 151–220 beats/minute, and rhythm is regular. Some degree of AV block may be present.

- Clinical significance depends on the symptoms. A prolonged episode and HR above 180 beats/minute decreases CO, resulting in hypotension, dyspnea, and angina.
- Treatment for PSVT includes vagal stimulation and drug therapy. Common vagal maneuvers include Valsalva, carotid massage, and coughing. IV adenosine is the drug of choice to convert PSVT to a normal sinus rhythm. This drug has a short half-life (10 seconds) and is well tolerated. IV β-blockers and calcium-channel blockers (e.g., diltiazem, verapamil) are also options. The patient who becomes hemodynamically unstable undergoes synchronized cardioversion.

Atrial Flutter

Atrial flutter is an atrial tachydysrhythmia identified on the ECG by recurring, regular, sawtooth-shaped flutter waves that originate from a single ectopic focus in the right atrium. Atrial flutter is associated with CAD, hypertension, mitral valve disorders, pulmonary embolus, chronic lung disease, cor pulmonale, cardiomyopathy, hyperthyroidism, and the use of drugs, such as digoxin, quinidine, and epinephrine.

- The atrial rate is 250–350 beats/minute. The ventricular rate varies depending on the conduction ratio. In 2:1 conduction, the ventricular rate is typically about 150 beats/minute. Atrial and ventricular rhythms are usually regular.
- High ventricular rates (>100 beats/minute) can decrease CO and cause serious consequences, such as HF. The primary treatment goal is to slow ventricular response by increasing AV block. Drugs used to control the ventricular rate include calcium-channel blockers and β-blockers.
- Electrical cardioversion may be done to convert the atrial flutter to sinus rhythm in an emergency (i.e., when the patient is clinically unstable) and electively.
- Antidysrhythmic drugs can convert atrial flutter to sinus rhythm (e.g., ibutilide [Corvert]) or to maintain sinus rhythm (e.g., amiodarone, flecainide, dronedarone [Multaq]).
- Radiofrequency catheter ablation in an electrophysiologic (EPS) laboratory is the treatment of choice for atrial flutter.

Atrial Fibrillation

Atrial fibrillation is characterized by a total disorganization of atrial electrical activity because of multiple ectopic foci. It results in loss of effective atrial contraction. The dysrhythmia may be *paroxysmal* (beginning and ending spontaneously) or persistent (lasting longer than 7 days).

Atrial fibrillation is the most common clinically significant dysrhythmia. Its prevalence increases with age. Atrial fibrillation usually occurs with underlying heart disease. It often develops acutely with thyrotoxicosis, alcohol intoxication, caffeine use, electrolyte problems, stress, or after heart surgery.

- The atrial rate may be as high as 350–600 beats/minute. Chaotic, fibrillatory waves replace the P waves. The ventricular rate varies, and the rhythm is usually irregular.
- When the ventricular rate is between 60 and 100 beats/minute, atrial fibrillation has a *controlled ventricular response.*
- Atrial fibrillation decreases CO due to ineffective atrial contractions and/or rapid ventricular response. Thrombi may form in the atria because of blood stasis. An embolized clot may pass to the brain, causing a stroke.

D

The goals of treatment include a decrease in ventricular response to <100 beats/minute, prevention of cerebral embolic events, and conversion to sinus rhythm, if possible. Drugs used for rate control include calcium-channel blockers (e.g., diltiazem), β-blockers (e.g., metoprolol), amiodarone, and digoxin. Amiodarone is often used for maintenance of sinus rhythm after cardioversion.

Electrical cardioversion may convert atrial fibrillation to normal sinus rhythm.

- If a patient is in atrial fibrillation for longer than 48 hr, anticoagulation therapy is needed for 3–4 weeks before the cardioversion and for several weeks after successful cardioversion. Warfarin requires monitoring for therapeutic levels (e.g., international normalized ratio [INR]). Alternatives to warfarin that do not require routine laboratory testing include dabigatran (Pradaxa), apixaban (Eliquis), and rivaroxaban (Xarelto).
- For patients with drug-refractory atrial fibrillation or those who do not respond to electrical conversion, radiofrequency catheter ablation (similar to the procedure for atrial flutter) and the Maze procedure (surgical intervention that interrupts ectopic electrical signals) may be used.
- Left atrial appendage occlusion is a surgical strategy to prevent blood clot formation in patients who have atrial fibrillation but cannot use oral anticoagulants.

First-Degree Atrioventricular Block

In first-degree AV block, every impulse from the atria is conducted to the ventricles, but the time of AV conduction is prolonged. After the impulse moves through the AV node, the ventricles usually respond normally. First-degree AV block is associated with increasing age, MI, CAD, rheumatic fever, hyperthyroidism, vagal stimulation, and drugs such as digoxin, β-blockers, calcium-channel blockers, and flecainide.

- HR is normal and rhythm is regular.
- Patients with first-degree AV block are asymptomatic.
- There is no treatment for first-degree AV block. Associated conditions may be treated.

Second-Degree Atrioventricular Block, Type I (Mobitz I, Wenckebach)

A type I second-degree AV block is characterized by gradual lengthening of the PR interval. It occurs because of an AV conduction time that is increasingly prolonged until an atrial impulse is nonconducted and a QRS complex is blocked (missing). Type I AV block may result from use of digoxin or β-blockers. It may be caused by CAD, myocardial ischemia, or inferior MI. It is generally transient and well tolerated. However, it may be a warning signal of a more serious AV conduction disturbance (e.g., complete heart block).

- The rhythm appears on the ECG in a pattern of grouped beats.
- If the patient is symptomatic, atropine is used to increase HR. A temporary pacemaker may be needed, especially if the patient has had an MI.

Second-Degree Atrioventricular Block, Type II (Mobitz II)

In type II second-degree AV block, the P wave is nonconducted without progressive PR lengthening. This usually occurs when a bundle branch block is present. On conducted beats, the PR interval is constant. In a second-degree heart block, a certain number of impulses from the SA node are not conducted to the ventricles. This occurs in ratios of 2:1, 3:1, and so on when there are 2 P waves to 1 QRS complex, 3 P waves to 1 QRS complex, and so on. It may occur with varying ratios. Type II AV block is associated with rheumatic heart disease, CAD, anterior MI, and drug toxicity.

- The atrial rate is usually normal. The ventricular rate depends on the intrinsic rate and degree of AV block. The atrial rhythm is regular, but the ventricular rhythm may be irregular.
- Type II AV block often progresses to third-degree AV block and is associated with a poor prognosis.
- Reduced HR frequently results in decreased CO with subsequent hypotension and myocardial ischemia.
- Transcutaneous pacing or the insertion of a temporary pacemaker may be necessary before the insertion of a permanent pacemaker if the patient becomes symptomatic (e.g., hypotension, angina) (see Pacemakers). Atropine is not an effective drug for this dysrhythmia.

Third-Degree Atrioventricular Block (Complete Heart Block)

In third-degree AV block, no impulses from the atria are conducted to the ventricles. The atria are stimulated and contract independently of the ventricles. Ventricular rhythm is an escape rhythm from above or below the bifurcation of the bundle of His. This rhythm is associated with severe heart disease, including CAD, MI, myocarditis, cardiomyopathy, and some systemic diseases, such as amyloidosis and scleroderma. Drugs such as digoxin, β-blockers, and calcium-channel blockers can cause third-degree AV block.

- Atrial rate is usually a sinus rate of 60–100 beats/minute. Ventricular rate depends on the site of the block. If it is in the AV node, the rate is 40–60 beats/minute, and if it is in the Purkinje system, it is 20–40 beats/minute. Atrial and ventricular rhythms are regular but unrelated to each other.
- Third-degree AV block usually results in reduced CO with subsequent ischemia and heart failure.

■ Symptomatic patients need a temporary transcutaneous pacemaker until a permanent pacemaker can be inserted. Atropine
is not effective for this dysrhythmia. Epinephrine and dopamine
are temporary measures to increase HR and support BP before
pacemaker insertion (see Pacemakers).

Premature Ventricular Contractions

Premature ventricular contractions (PVCs) originate in an ectopic focus in the ventricles. PVCs are a premature occurrence
of the QRS complex, which is wide and distorted in shape.
PVCs that start from different foci appear different in shape
from each other and are termed *multifocal PVCs.* When every
other beat is a PVC, the condition is called *ventricular bigem-
iny.* When every third beat is a PVC, the condition is called
ventricular trigeminy. Two consecutive PVCs are called *cou-
plets. Ventricular tachycardia* (VT) appears as three or more
consecutive PVCs. A PVC falling on the T wave of a preceding
beat is termed the *R-on-T phenomenon* and is considered to be
dangerous because it may precipitate VT or ventricular fibrillation (VF).

PVCs are associated with stimulants such as caffeine, alcohol,
nicotine, epinephrine, and digoxin. They can occur with electrolyte
imbalances, hypoxia, fever, exercise, and emotional stress. Disease
states associated with PVCs include MI, cardiomyopathy, mitral
valve prolapse, HF, and CAD.

■ HR varies depending on the intrinsic rate and number of PVCs.
Rhythm is irregular because of premature beats.

■ PVCs are usually not harmful in the patient with a normal
heart. In heart disease, PVCs may reduce CO and precipitate
angina and HF. PVCs in CAD or acute MI represent ventricular
irritability.

■ Treatment relates to the cause of the PVCs (e.g., oxygen
therapy for hypoxia, electrolyte replacement). Assess the
patient's hemodynamic status to determine if drug therapy
is indicated. Drug therapy includes β-blockers, lidocaine, or
amiodarone.

Ventricular Tachycardia

VT is a run of three or more PVCs that occurs when an ectopic
focus or foci fire repetitively. VT is a life-threatening dysrhythmia
because of the decrease in CO and the possibility of the development of VF. VT is associated with MI, CAD, significant electrolyte
imbalances, hypoxemia, cardiomyopathy, mitral valve prolapse,
long QT syndrome, digitalis toxicity, and central nervous system
disorders. The dysrhythmia can be seen in patients who have no
evidence of cardiac disease.

- The ventricular rate is 150–250 beats/minute.
- VT can be stable (patient has a pulse) or unstable (patient is pulseless). Sustained VT causes a severe decrease in CO because of decreased ventricular diastolic filling times and loss of atrial contraction. This results in hypotension, pulmonary edema, decreased cerebral blood flow, and cardiopulmonary arrest.
- VT must be treated quickly, even if it occurs only briefly and stops abruptly. Episodes may recur if prophylactic treatment is not started.

Different forms of VT exist:

- If the patient is hemodynamically stable and has *monomorphic VT* (QRS complexes have same shape, size, and direction) with preserved left ventricular function, then IV procainamide, amiodarone, or lidocaine is used. These drugs can also be used if the VT is polymorphic with a normal baseline QT interval.
- *Polymorphic VT* with a prolonged baseline QT interval is treated with IV magnesium, isoproterenol, phenytoin, or antitachycardia pacing. Drugs that prolong the QT interval (e.g., dofetilide [Tikosyn]) should be stopped. Cardioversion is used when drug therapy is ineffective.
- VT without a pulse is lethal and is treated in the same way as VF.

Ventricular Fibrillation

VF is a severe derangement of the heart rhythm characterized on the ECG by irregular waveforms of various shapes and amplitudes. This pattern represents the firing of multiple ectopic foci in the ventricle. Mechanically, the ventricle is simply "quivering," and no effective contraction or CO occurs. This dysrhythmia is lethal. VF occurs in acute MI, myocardial ischemia, and in chronic diseases such as CAD and cardiomyopathy. It occurs during cardiac pacing or cardiac catheterization procedures because of catheter stimulation of the ventricle. It may happen with coronary reperfusion after thrombolytic therapy. Other causes are electrical shock, hyperkalemia, hypoxemia, acidosis, and drug toxicity.

- HR is not measurable. Rhythm is irregular and chaotic.
- VF results in an unresponsive, pulseless, and apneic state. If VF is not treated quickly, the patient will not recover.
- Treatment consists of immediate initiation of cardiopulmonary resuscitation (CPR) and advanced cardiac life support (ACLS) with the use of defibrillation and definitive drug therapy (e.g., epinephrine, amiodarone). There should be no delay in starting chest compressions and using a defibrillator once available.

Asystole. Asystole is the total absence of ventricular electrical activity. Occasionally, P waves are seen. No ventricular contraction occurs because depolarization does not occur.

- Patients are unresponsive, pulseless, and apneic. Asystole requires immediate treatment.
- Asystole is usually a result of advanced heart disease, a severe cardiac conduction system problem, or end-stage HF. Generally, the patient with asystole has end-stage heart disease or has had a prolonged cardiac arrest.
- Treatment consists of CPR with ACLS measures. These include epinephrine, intubation, and efforts to determine the underlying cause.

EATING DISORDERS

Description

Eating disorders are psychiatric conditions associated with physiologic alterations. Patients with eating disorders may be hospitalized for fluid and electrolyte problems; dysrhythmias; and nutrition, endocrine, and metabolic problems. Menstrual problems may occur in women of childbearing age. Risk factors for eating disorders involve a range of biological, psychologic, and sociocultural issues. Some persons report a history of anxiety, perfectionism, and social problems, such as bullying or a limited social network.

The three most common types of eating disorders are *anorexia nervosa* (AN), *bulimia nervosa*, and *binge-eating disorder*. Binge-eating disorder is less severe than bulimia nervosa and AN. Persons with binge-eating disorder do not have a distorted body image and are often overweight or obese.

Anorexia Nervosa

AN most often occurs in females between the ages of 13 and 19. AN is characterized by restricting energy intake, difficulties in maintaining an appropriate weight, an intense fear of gaining weight or being fat, and distorted body image. People with AN generally restrict the number of calories and the types of food they eat. Some people exercise compulsively, purge via vomiting and laxatives, and/or binge eat. There may be an unwillingness to maintain a healthy weight, refusal to eat, continuous dieting, detailed food rituals, and avoiding social situations. Common assessment findings include signs of malnutrition, significant weight loss or low BMI (under 17), hypothermia, and muscle weakness.

Diagnostic studies often show osteopenia or osteoporosis, iron-deficiency anemia, and a high blood urea nitrogen level from marked intravascular volume depletion and abnormal renal function.

- Lack of potassium in the diet and loss of potassium in the urine lead to potassium deficiency. Manifestations of potassium deficiency include muscle weakness, dysrhythmias, and renal failure.
- Leukopenia, hypoglycemia, and decreased sodium, magnesium, and phosphorus may be present.

Treatment involves a combination of nutrition support and psychiatric care. Nutrition care focuses on reaching and maintaining a healthy weight and normal eating patterns.

Hospitalization may be needed if the patient has complications that cannot be managed in an outpatient therapy program.

- Nutrition repletion must be closely supervised to ensure consistent and ongoing weight gain. Refeeding syndrome is a rare but serious complication of behavioral refeeding programs. The use of enteral or parenteral nutrition may be needed (see Enteral Nutrition and Parenteral Nutrition).

Improved nutrition is not a cure for AN. Family-based therapy is recommended in addition to behavior and emotion-focused therapy.

Bulimia Nervosa

Bulimia nervosa is characterized by episodes of binge eating. To prevent weight gain, the person then engages in inappropriate compensatory behaviors (vomiting, laxative or diuretic misuse, overexercise). The person with bulimia is concerned with body image. They may have normal weight for height or the weight may fluctuate with binging and purging.

- Signs of frequent vomiting include macerated knuckles, swollen salivary glands, broken blood vessels in the eyes, and dental problems.
- Abnormal laboratory values, including hypokalemia, metabolic alkalosis, and increased serum amylase, may occur from frequent vomiting.

Combination treatment with psychologic counseling and nutrition therapy is essential.

- Fluoxetine (Prozac) is the only U.S. Food and Drug Administration (FDA)-approved antidepressant for treating bulimia nervosa.
- Education and emotional support for the patient and the family are vital.

ENCEPHALITIS

Description

Encephalitis is a serious, sometimes fatal, acute inflammation of the brain. It is usually caused by a virus. Many different viruses have been implicated in encephalitis; some are associated with seasons of the year or geographic areas. Ticks and mosquitoes transmit epidemic encephalitis, whereas nonepidemic encephalitis may occur as a complication of measles, chickenpox, or mumps.

- Herpes simplex virus (HSV) encephalitis is the most common form of nonepidemic viral encephalitis.
- Cytomegalovirus encephalitis occurs in patients with acquired immunodeficiency syndrome.

Clinical Manifestations and Diagnostic Studies

Infection can be acute or subacute. The onset is typically nonspecific, with fever, headache, nausea, and vomiting. Signs of encephalitis appear on day 2 or 3 and may range from minimal changes in mental status to coma.

- Almost any central nervous system abnormality can occur, including hemiparesis, tremors, seizures, dysphasia, cranial nerve palsies, personality changes, memory impairment, and amnesia.
- Diagnostic findings related to viral encephalitis are shown in Table 35.
- Brain imaging techniques include CT, MRI, and positron emission tomography.
- Polymerase chain reaction tests can be used to detect HSV and West Nile encephalitis.

West Nile virus infection should be strongly considered in adults older than 50 years who develop encephalitis or meningitis in summer or early fall. The best diagnostic test to identify West Nile virus is a blood test that detects viral ribonucleic acid.

Interprofessional and Nursing Management

Mosquito control to prevent encephalitis includes cleaning rain gutters, removing old tires, draining bird baths, and removing water where mosquitoes can breed. Insect repellant should be used outdoors during mosquito season.

Management of encephalitis, including West Nile virus infection, is symptomatic and supportive. Initially, many patients require intensive care. Prophylactic treatment with antiseizure drugs may be used in severe cases of encephalitis.

- Acyclovir is used to treat HSV encephalitis. For maximal benefit, treatment should be started before the onset of coma.

TABLE 35 Comparison of Cerebral Inflammatory Conditions

Feature	Meningitis	Encephalitis	Brain abscess
Cause	Bacteria[a] (*Streptococcus pneumoniae*, *Neisseria meningitidis*, group B streptococci), viruses, fungi	Bacteria, fungi, parasites, herpes simplex virus (HSV), other viruses (e.g., West Nile virus)	Streptococci, staphylococci (acquired through bloodstream)
CSF (reference interval)			
• Pressure (70–150 mm H$_2$O)	Increased *Bacterial:* 200–500 mm H$_2$O *Viral:* ≤ 250 mm H$_2$O	Normal to slight increase	Increased
• WBC count (0–5 cells/µL)	*Bacterial:* > 1000/µL (mainly neutrophils) *Viral:* 25–500/µL (mainly lymphocytes)	500/µL, neutrophils (early), lymphocytes (later)	25–300/µL (neutrophils)
• Protein (15–45 mg/dL [0.15–0.45 g/L])	*Bacterial:* > 500 mg/dL *Viral:* 50–500 mg/dL	Slight increase	Normal
• Glucose (40–70 mg/dL [2.2–3.9 mmol/L])	*Bacterial:* decreased at 5–40 mg/dL *Viral:* normal or low at > 40 mg/dL	Normal	Low or absent
• Appearance	*Bacterial:* turbid, cloudy *Viral:* clear or cloudy	Clear	Clear
Diagnostic studies	CT scan, Gram stain, smear, culture, PCR assay[b]	CT scan, EEG, MRI, PET, PCR, IgM antibodies to virus in serum or CSF	CT scan
Treatment	Antibiotics, dexamethasone, supportive care, prevention of ↑ ICP	Supportive care, prevention of ↑ ICP, acyclovir (Zovirax) for HSV infection	Antibiotics, incision and drainage Supportive care

CSF, cerebrospinal fluid; *DNA*, deoxyribonucleic acid; *EEG*, electroencephalography; *ICP*, intracranial pressure; *IgM*, immunoglobulin M; *PCR*, polymerase chain reaction; *PET*, positron emission tomography; *RNA*, ribonucleic acid; *WBC*, white blood cell.

[a]See also Meningitis, Bacterial.

[b]PCR testing is used to detect viral RNA or DNA.

ENDOCARDITIS, INFECTIVE

Description

Infective endocarditis (IE) is an infection of the endocardial (innermost) surface of the heart and the heart valves. We often classify IE based on the cause (e.g., IV drug use IE [IVDA IE], fungal IE) or site of involvement (e.g., prosthetic valve endocarditis [PVE]).

- We also describe IE as subacute or acute. The subacute form affects those with preexisting valve disease over a period of months. In contrast, the acute form affects those with healthy valves and appears as a rapidly progressive illness.

Pathophysiology

IE occurs when blood flow allows organisms to contact and infect previously damaged heart valves or other endothelial surfaces. About 50% of cases of IE are caused by *Staphylococcus aureus.* Other bacterial causes include *Streptococcus viridans* and *Coagulase Negative Staphylococci* and the organisms that colonize the oropharynx.

- Principal risk factors include history of IE, IV drug use, having a prosthetic valve, health care-associated infection from use of an intravascular device (e.g., methicillin-resistant *S. aureus* [MRSA]), and renal dialysis. At one time, rheumatic heart disease was the most common cause of IE. Now, it accounts for <20% of cases.

IE typically develops in three stages: (1) bacteremia, (2) adhesion, and (3) vegetation.

Vegetations, the primary lesions of IE, consist of fibrin, leukocytes, platelets, and microbes, which adhere to the valve surface or endocardium. The loss of portions of this vegetation into the circulation results in embolization.

- Left-sided heart vegetations move to various organs (e.g., brain, kidney, spleen) and extremities. Right-sided heart lesions embolize to the lungs, resulting in pulmonary emboli.

The infection may spread locally to cause damage to valves or their supporting structures. This can result in dysrhythmias and valve dysfunction. Invasion of the myocardium leads to heart failure (HF), sepsis, and heart block.

Clinical Manifestations

Nonspecific clinical manifestations can involve multiple organ systems. Most patients have fever. Fever may be low grade or may be absent in older adults or those who are immunocompromised.

Other symptoms include chills, weakness, malaise, fatigue, and anorexia.

- Most patients with IE have a new or worsening systolic murmur. HF is common, occurring in up to 80% of patients with aortic valve IE and 50% of those with mitral valve IE.
- Patients may have arthralgias, myalgias, back pain, abdominal discomfort, weight loss, headache, and clubbing of fingers in subacute forms of IE.
- Vascular signs may include splinter hemorrhages (black longitudinal streaks) in the nail beds. Petechiae from fragmentation and microembolization of vegetative lesions are common on the conjunctivae, lips, buccal mucosa, and palate and over the ankles, feet, and antecubital and popliteal areas. *Osler's nodes* (painful, tender, red or purple, pea-size lesions) may be on the fingertips or toes. *Janeway's lesions* (flat, painless, small, red spots) may be found on the palms and soles. Eye examination may show hemorrhagic retinal lesions called *Roth's spots.*

Diagnostic Studies

A health history should be obtained with inquiry made regarding any recent dental, urologic, surgical, or gynecologic procedures including normal or abnormal obstetric delivery. Note any previous history of intravenous drug abuse (IVDA), heart disease, recent heart catheterization, heart surgery, intravascular device placement, renal dialysis, or infections (e.g., skin, respiratory, urinary tract).

- Blood culture of three samples drawn 1 hr apart from three different sites will be positive in more than 90% of patients.
- A mild leukocytosis occurs in acute IE.
- Erythrocyte sedimentation rate (ESR) and C-reactive protein (CRP) levels may be elevated.
- Chest X-ray can detect an enlarged heart.
- Echocardiography can visualize vegetations.
- Electrocardiogram (ECG) may show first- or second-degree heart block because the valves lie in close proximity to the atrioventricular (AV) node.
- Cardiac catheterization may be used to evaluate valve functioning.

Interprofessional Management
Prophylactic Treatment
Antibiotic prophylaxis is recommended for people with high cardiac risk conditions including congenital heart disease, history of IE, prosthetic heart valves, surgically constructed systemic-pulmonary shunts, and heart valve disease after heart transplantation. Specific antibiotic regimens are recommended for dental,

respiratory, and surgical procedures that involve infected skin, skin structures, or musculoskeletal tissue.

Drug Therapy

Accurate identification of the causative organism is the key to successful treatment. Complete removal of the organisms generally takes weeks, and relapses are common. IV antibiotic therapy is based on blood cultures.

- Blood cultures that stay positive indicate inadequate or inappropriate antibiotics, aortic root or myocardial abscess, or the wrong diagnosis (e.g., an infection elsewhere).
- It is reasonable to obtain two sets of blood cultures every 24–48 hr until the infection is cleared.
- Fever that persists is treated with aspirin, acetaminophen, fluids, and rest.
- Complete bed rest is usually not needed unless the temperature remains elevated or there are signs of HF.

Fungal IE and PVE respond poorly to antibiotic therapy alone. Valve replacement surgery is done for uncontrolled infection, for valve dysfunction causing HF, or to prevent embolization. Endocarditis coupled with HF responds poorly to antibiotic therapy and valve replacement, so it can be life-threatening.

Nursing Management

Goals

The patient with IE will have normal or baseline cardiac function, perform activities of daily living without fatigue, and understand the therapeutic regimen to prevent recurrence of endocarditis.

Interventions

Identify those at risk for the disease. Teach them to avoid people with infections, especially upper respiratory tract infections, and to report cold, flu, and cough symptoms. Stress the importance of avoiding excessive fatigue, planning rest periods, using good oral hygiene, and scheduling regular dental visits.

IE generally requires treatment with antibiotics for 4–6 weeks. After initial treatment in the hospital, the patient may continue treatment in the home setting.

- Teach the patient or caregiver about monitoring body temperature because persistent, prolonged temperature elevations may indicate ineffective drug therapy.
- Bed rest may be needed when fever is present or there are complications (e.g., heart damage). Otherwise, the patient may perform moderate activity.
- Monitor laboratory data, including blood cultures, to determine antibiotic effectiveness. Assess IV lines for patency and

any signs of complications (e.g., phlebitis). Give antibiotics as scheduled and monitor for adverse drug reactions.

- To prevent problems related to decreased mobility, teach the patient to wear elastic compression stockings, perform range-of-motion (ROM) exercises, and cough and deep breathe every 2 hr.
- The patient may have anxiety and fear. Implement strategies to help the patient cope with the illness.

▼ **Patient and Caregiver Teaching**
- Instruct the patient about symptoms that may indicate another infection, such as fever, fatigue, malaise, and chills.
- Teach the patient about the importance of prophylactic antibiotic therapy before invasive procedures.
- Explain the relationship of follow-up care, good nutrition, regular dental care, and early treatment of common infections (e.g., colds) to maintaining good health.

ENDOMETRIAL CANCER

E

Description

Endometrial cancer is the most common gynecologic cancer. If endometrial cancer is diagnosed in the early stage, it has a low mortality rate. The major risk factor for endometrial cancer is exposure to estrogen, especially unopposed estrogen therapy (without progesterone). Obesity is a risk factor because of increased estrogen in adipose tissue. Other risk factors include family history of cancer or Lynch syndrome, infertility, and use of tamoxifen.

- Protective factors associated with reduced risk include use of hormonal contraceptive pills, breastfeeding, increased number of pregnancies, and physical activity.

Pathophysiology

Endometrial cancer arises from the endometrial lining. Most tumors are adenocarcinomas. In later stages, endometrial cancer can invade the myometrium (muscle of the uterus) and the regional lymph nodes. If metastasis occurs, common sites include the lung, liver, bone, and brain.

Clinical Manifestations and Diagnostic Studies

Abnormal uterine bleeding (especially postmenopause) is the classic sign of endometrial cancer. Other exam findings are often normal.

- Late symptoms can include dysuria, dyspareunia, unintentional weight loss, and pelvic pain.

A thickened endometrium may be seen on ultrasound. Endometrial biopsy is the primary diagnostic procedure for endometrial cancer.

Interprofessional and Nursing Management

Most patients with endometrial cancer have a good prognosis due to early diagnosis. Surgery (total hysterectomy and bilateral salpingo-oophorectomy) is the main treatment for uterine cancer. For complex cases, chemotherapy, radiation, or hormone therapy may be a part of the treatment plan. See Cervical Cancer.

ENDOMETRIOSIS

Description

Endometriosis is an inflammatory condition in which endometrial tissue accumulates outside the uterus. The most frequent sites are in or near the ovaries, uterosacral ligaments, and uterovesical peritoneum (Fig. 10). Endometriosis is thought to be caused by a combination of hormonal, genetic, and immunological factors.

Clinical Manifestations and Diagnostic Studies

Endometriosis may be suspected based on infertility, heavy menstrual bleeding, and pain.

- Pain may be chronic or occur during menses, intercourse, urination, or defecation.

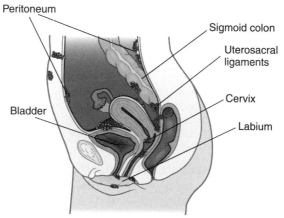

Figure 10 Common sites of endometriosis.

- Tenderness or nodules in the pelvic region may be noted on physical assessment.
- With menopause, the ovaries no longer make estrogen, and the symptoms may disappear.

Laparoscopy with biopsy is needed for a definitive diagnosis. Imaging such as ultrasound and MRI may aid in the diagnosis.

Interprofessional and Nursing Management

Management includes both medical and surgical approaches. The treatment depends on the patient's age, desire for pregnancy, severity of symptoms, and extent and location of the disease. Drug therapy is used to relieve pain, reduce inflammation, and suppress endometrial tissue growth.

- Common agents include NSAIDs, hormonal contraceptives, aromatase inhibitors, and gonadotropin-releasing hormone (GnRH) analogs (such as leuprolide [Lupron]).

The only cure for endometriosis is surgical removal of all endometrial tissue and adhesions. For women with infertility or who desire pregnancy, therapy may involve removing blockages in the fallopian tube and removing adhesions from the tubes, ovaries, and pelvic structures.

- Explore the patient's feelings about maintaining ovarian function. Actively involve the patient in making the decision about preserving ovaries if surgically possible.

If surgery is selected, nursing care is similar to general preoperative and postoperative care of a patient undergoing laparotomy (see Abdominal Pain, Acute).

E

ESOPHAGEAL CANCER

Description

Esophageal cancer is not common but the rates are increasing. The United States had 18,400 new cases diagnosed and 16,170 deaths occur from esophageal cancer in 2020. The overall 5-year survival rate is 20%. Risk factors include Barrett's esophagus, smoking, excessive alcohol intake, obesity, and occupational exposure to asbestos or cement dust.

Pathophysiology

Most tumors occur in the middle and lower portions of the esophagus. The tumor may penetrate the muscular layer and extend outside the esophageal wall. Many patients have advanced disease at the time of diagnosis.

- The tumor usually appears as an ulcerated lesion.
- Obstruction of the esophagus occurs in the later stages.
- Achalasia, a condition of slow esophageal emptying, is associated with squamous cell cancer.

Clinical Manifestations

By the time the patient has symptoms, the tumor is often advanced. The tumor may enlarge enough to cause esophageal obstruction, especially in the later stages.

- Progressive dysphagia is the most common symptom. It may be a substernal feeling that food is not passing. At first, dysphagia occurs with meat, then with soft foods, and eventually with liquids.
- Pain develops later in the substernal, epigastric, or back. The pain usually increases with swallowing and may radiate to the neck, jaw, ears, and shoulders.
- If the tumor is in the upper third of the esophagus, symptoms may include sore throat, choking, and hoarseness. Weight loss is common.
- When esophageal stenosis (narrowing) is severe, regurgitation of blood-flecked esophageal contents is common.

Bleeding occurs if the cancer erodes through the esophagus and into the aorta. Esophageal perforation with fistula formation into the lung or trachea sometimes develops.

Diagnostic Studies

- Esophagram (barium swallow) may detect narrowing at the tumor site.
- Endoscopic biopsy is required for diagnosis.
- Endoscopic ultrasonography (EUS) is important in staging esophageal cancer.

Interprofessional Management

Treatment depends on the tumor location and whether metastasis has occurred. The best results may be obtained with a combination of surgery, endoscopic ablation, chemotherapy, and radiation therapy.

- Surgical approaches may be open (thoracic or abdominal incision) or minimally invasive (e.g., laparoscopic vagal nerve-sparing surgery).

■ Endoscopic approaches use photodynamic therapy, endoscopic mucosal resection (EMR), or radiofrequency ablation.

Palliative therapy consists of restoring swallowing function and maintaining nutrition and hydration. Dilation and stent placement can relieve obstruction.

Nutritional Therapy

After esophageal surgery, parenteral fluids are given. A jejunostomy, gastrostomy, or esophagostomy tube may be placed to feed the patient. A swallowing study is often done before the patient takes oral fluids.

■ When fluids are permitted, water (30–60 mL) is given hourly, with gradual progression to small, frequent, bland meals. The patient should be in an upright position during and 2 hr after meals to prevent regurgitation.

Observe the patient for intolerance to the feeding or leakage into the mediastinum. Pain, increased temperature, and dyspnea may indicate leakage.

Nursing Management

Goals

The overall goals are that the patient with esophageal cancer will have relief of symptoms, including pain and dysphagia, achieve optimal nutrition, and experience a quality of life appropriate to stage of disease and prognosis.

Interventions

In addition to general preoperative teaching and preparation, pay attention to the patient's nutritional needs. Many patients are poorly nourished because of the inability to ingest adequate food and fluids. Teach about chest tubes (if a thoracic approach is used), IV lines, nasogastric (NG) and feeding tubes, turning, coughing, deep breathing, and meticulous oral care.

Postoperative care includes assessment of drainage; maintenance of the NG tube; oral and nasal care; and prevention of respiratory complications by turning, coughing, and deep breathing, with incentive spirometry every 2 hr, and placing the patient in a semi-Fowler's position to prevent gastric reflux and aspiration.

▼ Patient and Caregiver Teaching

■ Provide emotional and physical support, provide information, clarify test results, and maintain a positive attitude with respect to the patient's immediate recovery and long-term survival.

■ Refer the patient to a home health nurse as needed for continued care (e.g., gastrostomy teaching and follow-up wound care).

FIBROCYSTIC BREAST CHANGES

Description

Fibrocystic breast changes include the development of excess fibrous tissue, hyperplasia of the epithelial lining of the mammary ducts, proliferation of mammary ducts, and cyst formation. Fibrocystic changes are the most common breast disorder, occurring in more than 30%–60% of women of reproductive age. The changes occur most frequently in women between 30 and 50 years old but may begin earlier. They are not associated alone with increased breast cancer risk.

Fibrocystic changes most often occur in women with premenstrual abnormalities, early menarche or late menopause, or a history of spontaneous abortion. Others at risk include nulliparous women and nonusers of oral contraceptives.

Pathophysiology

Fibrocystic changes are thought to be heightened responsiveness of breast tissue to circulating estrogen and progesterone. These changes produce pain from chronic inflammation, edema, nerve irritation, and fibrosis.

- Masses or nodules are often found in the upper, outer quadrants bilaterally.
- Symptoms often worsen in the premenstrual phase and subside after menstruation.

Clinical Manifestations and Diagnostic Studies

Manifestations of fibrocystic breast changes include palpable lumps that are round, well delineated, and freely movable. Discomfort ranges from tenderness to pain.

- The lump usually increases in size and tenderness before menstruation. Cysts may enlarge or shrink rapidly.
- Nipple discharge is often green or dark brown, not bloody.

Mammography may help distinguishing fibrocystic changes from breast cancer. In some women the breast tissue is so dense that it is difficult to obtain a mammogram, and ultrasound may be more useful.

Interprofessional and Nursing Management

If the nodularity recurs, a wait of 7–10 days may reveal if changes are related to the menstrual cycle. With discovery of a discrete breast mass, aspiration or surgical biopsy may be indicated.

- An excisional biopsy should be done if no fluid is found on aspiration, the fluid is hemorrhagic, or a residual mass remains.

Many types of treatment have been suggested for a fibrocystic condition. Some relief for cyclic pain may occur by reducing intake of caffeine and fat, taking vitamin E or gamma-linolenic acid (evening primrose oil), and continually wearing a supportive bra. Compresses, ice, analgesics, and antiinflammatory drugs may help.

Tamoxifen may provide relief in up to 70% of women with few side effects. Bromocriptine, a prolactin inhibitor, may provide some with relief. It causes GI upset and light-headiness. Danazol is an FDA-approved treatment. The androgenic side effects (acne, edema, hirsutism) make this therapy unacceptable for many women.

▼ **Patient and Caregiver Teaching**

Your role in the care of the patient with fibrocystic breast changes is primarily one of teaching.

- Teach the patient to expect recurrences of the cysts until menopause and that cysts may enlarge or become painful just before menstruation. In addition, offer reassurance that cysts do not "turn into" cancer. Tell them that the HCP should examine any new lump that does not respond in a cyclic manner over 1–2 weeks.
- Encourage the patient with cystic changes to get regular follow-up care. Teach them breast self-examination (BSE) to self-monitor changes. Severe fibrocystic changes may make palpation of the breast more difficult. Teach them to report any changes in symptoms or changes found during the BSE so they can be evaluated.

FIBROMYALGIA

Description

Fibromyalgia syndrome (FMS) is a chronic central pain syndrome marked by widespread, nonarticular musculoskeletal pain and fatigue with multiple tender points. FMS affects about 4 million Americans. Women are twice as likely to get FMS. It is the most common cause of musculoskeletal pain in women of ages 20–55. FMS and systemic exertion intolerance disease (SEID) share many features (see Systemic Exertion Intolerance Disease).

Pathophysiology

FMS involves abnormal central processing of nociceptive pain input in the CNS. PET scans of the brains of people with FMS have shown widespread neuroinflammation. Spinal fluid can contain proteins linked to neuroinflammation. Pain inhibitory pathways do not work effectively. Genetic factors contribute to the development of FMS as a familial tendency exists. People with other

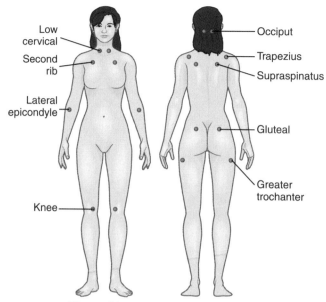

Figure 11 Tender points in fibromyalgia.

autoimmune diseases such as SLE or RA are at risk. Infection or trauma may be a trigger in susceptible people.

Clinical Manifestations

Widespread burning pain fluctuates through the course of a day. The patient often cannot determine whether pain occurs in the muscles, joints, or soft tissues.

- Head or facial pain often results from stiff or painful neck and shoulder muscles. This pain can accompany temporomandibular joint dysfunction.
- Assessment usually shows point tenderness at 11 or more of 18 identified tender points (nine pairs) (Fig. 11).
- Cognitive effects range from difficulty concentrating to memory lapses and a feeling of being overwhelmed when dealing with multiple tasks. Many persons report migraine headaches. Depression and anxiety often occur.
- Numbness or tingling in the hands or feet (paresthesia) often accompanies FMS. Restless legs syndrome is common.

- Women with FMS may have more difficult menstruation, with worse disease symptoms during this time.
- Increased urinary frequency and urgency or irritable bowel syndrome with diarrhea or constipation, abdominal pain, and bloating may occur.

Diagnostic Studies

Laboratory results may serve to rule out other suspected disorders. A definitive diagnosis is based on two elements: (1) pain in 11 of the 18 tender points on palpation, and (2) a history of widespread pain for at least 3 months.

Interprofessional and Nursing Management

Treatment is symptomatic. Because of the chronic nature of FMS, the patient needs consistent support from the health care team. Encourage the patient to be an active participant in treatment. Rest can help the pain, aching, and tenderness.

Drug therapy for the chronic widespread pain associated with fibromyalgia includes pregabalin (Lyrica), duloxetine (Cymbalta), and milnacipran (Savella). Low-dose tricyclic antidepressants (TCAs), selective serotonin reuptake inhibitors (SSRIs), or benzodiazepines (e.g., diazepam [Valium]) may be prescribed. If the TCA is not well tolerated, similar drugs can be substituted, such as doxepin, imipramine (Tofranil), or trazodone.

- In some patients, pain can be managed with OTC analgesics, such as acetaminophen, ibuprofen, or naproxen (Aleve). Nonopioids, such as tramadol (Ultram), may be used. Long-acting opioids are not used unless other therapies are not successful. Short-term use of zolpidem (Ambien) or trazodone can help patients with severe sleep problems. Antidepressants and muscle relaxants have sedative effects that can improve sleep. Regular, gentle exercise and stretching can help maintain muscle tone and decrease pain. Yoga and Tai Chi are often helpful. Low-impact aerobic exercise, such as walking, can help prevent muscle atrophy.
- Massage is often combined with ultrasound or use of alternating heat and cold packs to soothe tense, sore muscles and increase blood circulation. Suggest limiting intake of muscle irritants, such as sugar, caffeine, and alcohol.
- Pain and the related symptoms of FMS can cause significant stress. Effective relaxation strategies include biofeedback, guided imagery, and autogenic training. Counseling and a support group may be helpful.

FLAIL CHEST

Description

Flail chest results from the fracture of three or more consecutive ribs in two or more separate locations that cause an unstable segment. It can also be caused by fracture of the sternum and several consecutive ribs.

Pathophysiology

Instability of the chest wall causes paradoxical movement during breathing. During inspiration, the affected part is sucked in, and during expiration, it bulges out. In other words, the affected (flail) area moves in the opposite direction with respect to the intact part of the chest. This paradoxical chest movement may prevent adequate ventilation and increase the work of breathing. The underlying injured lung may be contused, worsening hypoxemia.

Clinical Manifestations and Diagnostic Studies

A flail chest is usually apparent on physical examination.

- The patient has rapid, shallow respirations and tachycardia.
- Movement of the thorax is asymmetrical and uncoordinated. The patient may ventilate poorly and try to splint the chest to assist with breathing. Observation of abnormal chest cavity movement, palpation for crepitus near the rib fractures, and chest X-ray all assist in the diagnosis.

Interprofessional and Nursing Management

Initial therapy consists of ensuring adequate ventilation and supplemental O_2 therapy. The goal is to promote lung expansion and ensure adequate oxygenation. Analgesia can help promote adequate respiration. Although many patients can be managed without mechanical ventilation, intubation and ventilation may be needed. In cases of extreme chest trauma, surgical fixation of the flail segment may be done.

FRACTURE

Description

A *fracture* is a disruption or break in the continuity of the structure of bone. Traumatic injuries cause most fractures. Other fractures are due to a disease process such as cancer or osteoporosis (pathologic fracture). Fractures are described as *open* or *closed* depending on communication with the external environment. In an open fracture, the skin is broken and bone exposed, causing soft tissue injury. In a closed fracture, the skin is intact over the site.

- Fractures are *complete* if the break goes completely through the bone and *incomplete* if the break is partly across a bone shaft but the bone is still intact. An incomplete fracture is often the result of bending or crushing forces applied to a bone.
- Fractures are also described according to the direction of the fracture line. Types include linear, oblique, transverse, longitudinal, and spiral fractures.
- In a *displaced* fracture, the ends of the broken bone are separated and out of their normal positions. Displaced fractures are often *comminuted* (more than two fragments) or oblique. In a nondisplaced fracture, the periosteum is intact and the bone is still in alignment. Nondisplaced fractures are usually transverse, spiral, or greenstick.

Clinical Manifestations

Manifestations include immediate localized pain, decreased function, and inability to bear weight on or use the affected part. Obvious bone deformity may be visible. The patient guards the extremity (protects it against movement).

Complications

The majority of fractures heal without complications.

- Direct complications include problems with bone infection, bone union, and avascular necrosis.
- Indirect complications include compartment syndrome, venous thromboembolism (VTE), fat embolism syndrome (FES), breakdown of skeletal muscle (rhabdomyolysis), and hypovolemic shock.
- Most musculoskeletal injuries are not life-threatening. Death after a fracture is usually caused by damage to underlying organs and vascular structures or complications of the fracture or immobility.
- Open fractures, fractures with severe blood loss, and fractures that damage vital organs (e.g., lung, heart) are medical emergencies requiring immediate attention.

Diagnostic Studies

- History and physical examination
- X-ray examination
- CT scan and MRI

Interprofessional Management

The goals of treatment are anatomic realignment of bone fragments through reduction of the fracture, immobilization to maintain realignment, and restoration of function of the injured part.

If a fracture is suspected, the extremity is immobilized in the position in which it is found. Unnecessary movement increases soft tissue damage and may convert a closed fracture to an open fracture or create further injury to adjacent nerves and blood vessels.

Fracture Reduction

Closed reduction is the nonsurgical, manual realignment of bones to their anatomic position. Traction and countertraction are applied to bone fragments to restore position, length, and alignment.

- Closed reduction is usually done under local or general anesthesia. After reduction, the injured part is immobilized by casting, traction, external fixation, splints, or orthoses (braces) to maintain alignment until healing occurs.

Open reduction is correction of alignment through surgery. It usually includes internal fixation of the fracture with the use of wires, screws, pins, plates, intramedullary rods, or nails.

- The main risks of open reduction are infection, complications associated with anesthesia, and effects of preexisting medical conditions (e.g., diabetes). However, open reduction with internal fixation (ORIF) facilitates early ambulation, which decreases the risk of complications related to prolonged immobility.

Traction devices apply a pulling force on the fractured extremity while countertraction pulls in the opposite direction. The two most common types of traction are skin traction and skeletal traction.

- *Skin traction* is generally used for short-term treatment (48–72 hours) until skeletal traction or surgery is possible. Tape, boots, or slings are applied directly to the skin to help decrease muscle spasms in the injured extremity. *Buck's traction* is a type of skin traction device sometimes used for the patient with a hip, knee, or femur fracture.

- *Skeletal traction* is used to align injured bones and joints or treat joint contractures and congenital hip dysplasia. It requires the insertion of a pin or wire into the bone. Fracture alignment depends on correct positioning of the patient while the traction forces remain constant. For extremity traction to be effective, forces must be pulling in the opposite direction *(countertraction)*.

- Countertraction is supplied by the patient's body weight or may be augmented by elevating the end of the bed.

Fracture Immobilization

A cast is a temporary immobilization device, which allows the patient to perform many normal activities of daily living (ADLs) while providing stability. A cast generally incorporates the joints above and below a fracture. Synthetic casting materials are light in weight and dry more quickly than plaster of Paris.

- Immobilization of an acute fracture or soft tissue injury of the upper extremity is often accomplished by use of the: (1) sugar-tong splint, (2) posterior splint, (3) short-arm cast, or (4) long-arm cast.
- Injuries to the lower extremity can be immobilized with a long leg cast, short leg cast, cylinder cast, or prefabricated splint or immobilizer.

An *external fixator* is composed of metal pins and wires that are inserted into the bone and attached to external rods to stabilize the fracture. It can be used to apply traction or to immobilize reduced fragments when the use of a cast or traction is not appropriate. Ongoing assessment for pin loosening and infection is needed. Infection signaled by exudate, redness, tenderness, and pain may require removal of the device.

Internal fixation devices (pins, plates, intramedullary rods, and metal and bioabsorbable screws) are surgically inserted to realign and maintain bony fragments. These metal devices are biologically inert and made from stainless steel, vitallium, or titanium. Proper alignment is evaluated by X-ray studies at regular intervals.

- Electrical bone growth stimulation can promote healing, especially with fracture nonunion or delayed union.

Nursing Management

Goals

The patient with a fracture will have healing with no associated complications, have acceptable pain relief, and achieve maximal rehabilitation potential.

Interventions

Patients with fractures may be treated in an emergency department or a physician's office and released to home care, or they may require hospitalization. Specific nursing measures depend on the type of treatment used and setting in which patients are placed.

Preoperative Care. If surgical intervention is needed, patients must be prepared. Review pain management strategies and teach patients about immobilization and assistive devices. Discuss expected activity limitations after surgery.

- Central and peripheral muscle relaxants, such as carisoprodol (Soma), cyclobenzaprine, or methocarbamol, may be used to manage pain associated with muscle spasms.
- Give tetanus and diphtheria toxoid or tetanus immunoglobulin to the patient with an open fracture when their immunization status cannot be confirmed.
- Bone-penetrating antibiotics, such as a cephalosporin (e.g., cefazolin), are given before surgery.

Postoperative Care. Perform frequent neurovascular assessments of the affected extremity. Monitor limitations of movement or activity related to turning, positioning, and extremity support.

- Minimize pain and discomfort through proper alignment and positioning.
- Frequently observe dressings, casts, and wound drainage systems for bleeding or drainage. Report increased or purulent drainage to the healthcare provider (HCP).
- Maintain the patency of any drainage system. Use aseptic technique to avoid contamination.
- When slings are used with traction, inspect exposed skin areas regularly.
- Observe skeletal traction pin sites for signs of infection. Pin site care often includes regularly cleansing with chlorhexidine, rinsing with sterile saline, and drying the area with sterile gauze.

Proper nutrition helps ensure optimal soft tissue and bone healing. Include ample protein (e.g., 1 g/kg body weight daily), vitamins (especially B, C, and D), and calcium, phosphorus, and magnesium. Plan care to prevent complications of immobility.

- Prevent constipation by increasing activity, maintaining a high fluid intake, and providing a diet high in bulk and roughage. Maintain a regular time for elimination. If these measures are not helpful, give stool softeners, laxatives, or suppositories as needed.
- Renal stones can develop because of bone demineralization related to reduced mobility. Unless contraindicated, maintain a fluid intake of 2500 mL/day.
- Rapid deconditioning of the cardiovascular system can occur from prolonged bed rest, resulting in orthostatic hypotension and decreased lung capacity. Unless contraindicated, have the patient sit on the side of the bed, and perform standing transfers.
- When the patient is allowed to increase activity, assess for orthostatic hypotension.
- Also assess patients for signs of VTE. They may wear compression gradient stockings (antiembolism hose) or use intermittent

pneumatic compression devices. Because of the high risk for VTE in the orthopedic surgical patient, prophylactic anticoagulant drugs may be given for 10–14 days.

▼ **Patient and Caregiver Teaching**

Teach the patient to recognize and promptly report tightness of the cast and areas of pressure or discomfort. Explain the importance of elevating the extremity above heart level to promote venous return and applying ice to control or prevent edema during the initial phase. In addition to specific instructions for cast, pin, or wound care and recognition of complications, encourage the patient to contact the HCP if questions arise. See Fracture, Hip; Fracture, Pelvis; and Fracture, Humerus.

FRACTURE, HIP

Description

Hip fractures are common in older adults, with 95% of these caused by a fall. More than 300,000 patients are admitted to hospitals each year because of a hip fracture. Up to 37% of those patients die within a year of injury. Many older adults develop disabilities that require long-term care. Hip fracture occurs more often in women than in men because of osteoporosis.

A fracture of the hip refers to a fracture of the proximal (upper) third of the femur, which extends up to 5 cm below the lesser trochanter.

- Fractures within the hip joint capsule are called *intracapsular fractures.* Intracapsular fractures (femoral neck) are identified by their specific locations: capital, subcapital, and transcervical. These fractures are associated with osteoporosis and minor trauma.
- *Extracapsular fractures* occur outside the joint capsule. They are *intertrochanteric* if they occur in a region between the greater and lesser trochanter or *subtrochanteric* if they occur below the lesser trochanter. Most are caused by severe direct trauma or a fall.

Clinical Manifestations

Manifestations of a hip fracture are external rotation, muscle spasm, shortening of the affected extremity, and severe pain and tenderness in the region of the fracture site. Displaced femoral neck fractures may disrupt the blood supply to the femoral head, which can result in avascular necrosis.

Interprofessional Management

Surgical treatment allows early mobilization and decreases the risk of major complications. The type of surgery depends on the location of the fracture, severity of the fracture, and person's age. Better outcomes are associated with surgery performed within 24 hours of injury.

- Surgical options include: (1) repair with internal fixation devices (e.g., hip compression screw, intramedullary devices), (2) replacement of part of the femoral head with a prosthesis (partial hip replacement), and (3) total hip replacement (involves both the femur and acetabulum).

The affected extremity may be immobilized by Buck's traction if the patient is too unstable for immediate surgery. Buck's traction can be used for 24–48 hours to relieve painful muscle spasms.

Nursing Management

Preoperative Management

Analgesics, muscle relaxants, comfortable positioning unless contraindicated, and properly adjusted traction can help manage severe muscle spasms.

- Plans for discharge begin as the patient enters the hospital, because the length of postoperative stay is only a few days.

Postoperative Management

Assess vital signs and intake and output and monitor respiratory activities such as deep breathing and coughing. Assess pain and give pain medication. Observe the dressing and incision for signs of bleeding and infection.

Neurovascular impairment is possible. Assess the patient's extremity for motor function, temperature and color, sensation, distal pulses, capillary refill, edema, and pain.

- Decrease edema by elevating the leg when the patient is in bed or a chair.
- Maintain limb alignment with pillows between the knees when turning the patient to the nonoperative side. Avoid turning patient to the affected side unless approved by the surgeon.
- The patient can exercise the unaffected leg and both arms. Encourage patient to use overhead trapeze bar and the opposite side rail to help in position changes. A physical therapist can teach the patient how to perform out-of-bed and chair transfers.
- If hemiarthroplasty or total joint replacement was done by a *posterior approach* (accessing the hip joint from the back), use measures to prevent dislocation. Tell the patient and caregiver about positions and activities that increase the patient's risk for

dislocation (>90 degrees of flexion, abduction, or internal rotation). Teach the patient to avoid putting on shoes and socks, crossing legs or feet while seated, assuming the side-lying position incorrectly, standing up or sitting down while the body is flexed more than 90 degrees relative to the chair, and sitting on low seats, especially low toilet seats, for at least 6 weeks.

- When the hip fracture is accessed during surgery with an *anterior approach* (joint reached from front of body), the hip muscles are left intact. This approach provides a more stable hip in the postoperative period and fewer complications. Patient precautions may include instructions to avoid hyperextension.

The patient is usually out of bed the first postoperative day. In collaboration with the physical therapist, monitor the patient's ambulation for proper crutch walking or use of the walker. Before discharge home, have the patient demonstrate the proper use of crutches or a walker, the ability to transfer into and from a chair and bed, and the ability to ascend and descend stairs.

- Hospitalization averages 3 or 4 days. Patients frequently require care in a subacute unit, skilled nursing facility, or rehabilitation facility before returning home.

Weight bearing after surgery may be restricted for 6–12 weeks. Limited weight bearing is typically the only restriction for the patient who had open reduction and internal fixation (ORIF) of the hip fracture.

▼ Patient and Caregiver Teaching

Inform the patient and caregiver about the patient's weight-bearing status after surgery. Remind the patient to keep hip in neutral, straight position when sitting, walking, or lying.

- Sudden severe pain, a lump in the buttock, limb shortening, or extreme external rotation indicates prosthesis dislocation. This requires a closed reduction or open reduction to realign the femoral head in the acetabulum. Teach the patient to notify surgeon immediately if severe pain, deformity, or loss of function occurs.
- Use a pillow between the legs for first 6 weeks when lying on nonoperative side or when supine.
- Use an elevated toilet seat.
- Place chair inside shower or tub and remain seated while washing.
- Inform the patient and caregivers about community referral services that can assist in the postdischarge rehabilitation phase.
- Discuss risk factors for prosthetic joint infection with surgeon and dentist before dental work.

FRACTURE, HUMERUS

Fractures involving the shaft of the humerus are common among young and middle-aged adults. Manifestations are obvious displacement of the humeral shaft, shortened extremity, abnormal mobility, and pain.

- Major complications are radial nerve injury and vascular injury to the brachial artery caused by laceration, transection, or muscle spasm.
- Skin or skeletal traction may be used for purposes of reduction and immobilization.

Treatment depends on the specific location and displacement of the fracture. Nonoperative treatment may include use of a hanging arm cast, shoulder immobilizer, the sling and swathe (which prevents shoulder movement), or the humeral cuff brace.

- When these devices are used, elevate the head of the bed to assist gravity in reducing the fracture. Allow the arm to hang freely when the patient is sitting and standing. Provide measures to protect the axilla and prevent skin maceration. Carefully place absorbable dressing pads in the axilla. Change them twice daily or as needed.

During the rehabilitative phase, an exercise program geared toward improving strength and motion of the injured extremity is important. This program should include assisted motion of the hands and fingers. If the fracture is stable, the shoulder can be exercised to prevent stiffness caused by frozen shoulder or fibrosis of the shoulder capsule.

FRACTURE, PELVIS

Pelvic fractures may be relatively minor or life-threatening, depending on the mechanism of injury and associated vascular damage. This type of injury is associated with a high mortality rate. Pelvic fractures may cause serious intraabdominal injury, including laceration and hemorrhage of the urethra, bladder, or colon. They can cause acute pelvic compartment syndrome and paralytic ileus. Patients may have complications such as sepsis, fat embolism syndrome, or venous thromboembolism.

- Pelvic fractures are diagnosed by X-ray and CT.
- Abdominal assessment may show local swelling, tenderness, deformity, unusual pelvic movement, and bruising. Because a pelvic fracture can damage other organs, assess bowel and urinary tract function, as well as distal neurovascular status.

Treatment depends on the severity of the injury.

- Stable, nondisplaced fractures require little intervention. Ambulation with weight bearing as tolerated is typically encouraged.
- Complex or displaced fractures (e.g., open book fracture) are often stabilized emergently with external fixation alone or combined with open reduction and internal fixation surgery. Use extreme care in handling or moving the patient to prevent further injury. Turn the patient only when approved by the healthcare provider. Provide back care with adequate help to turn the patient or while the patient is raised from the bed with use of the trapeze.

GASTRITIS

Description

Gastritis is an inflammation of the stomach mucosa. This common problem may be acute or chronic and diffuse or localized.

Pathophysiology

Gastritis occurs when breakdown in the normal gastric mucosal barrier allows hydrochloric acid (HCl) acid and pepsin to diffuse back into the mucosa. This back diffusion results in stomach tissue edema, disruption of capillary walls with plasma lost into the gastric lumen, and possible hemorrhage.

Drugs contribute to the development of acute and chronic gastritis. Corticosteroids and nonsteroidal antiinflammatory drugs (NSAIDs) inhibit the synthesis of prostaglandins that protect the gastric mucosa. This makes the mucosa more susceptible to injury. Factors that increase the risk for NSAID-induced gastritis include being female; being over age 60 years; having a history of ulcer disease; taking anticoagulants, other NSAIDs, or corticosteroids; and having a chronic debilitating disorder, such as cardiovascular disease. Some drugs, such as digoxin and alendronate, have direct irritating effects on the gastric mucosa.

There are a number of other causes of chronic gastritis.

- Eating large quantities of spicy, irritating foods can cause acute gastritis.
- A key cause of chronic gastritis is *Helicobacter pylori*. Other bacterial, viral, and fungal infections are also associated with chronic gastritis.
- Smoking, radiation exposure, and numerous chronic diseases also cause gastritis.

G

- Binge drinking alcohol can cause acute damage to the gastric mucosa. Prolonged damage from repeated alcohol use results in chronic gastritis.

Autoimmune metaplastic atrophic gastritis is an inherited condition. An immune response directed against parietal cells leads to malabsorption and pernicious anemia. Atrophic gastritis is associated with an increased risk of stomach cancer.

Clinical Manifestations

- *Acute gastritis* symptoms include anorexia, nausea and vomiting, epigastric tenderness, and a feeling of fullness. Acute gastritis is self-limiting, lasting from a few hours to a few days.
- *Chronic gastritis* symptoms are similar to those of acute gastritis. Some patients are asymptomatic. However, when parietal cells are lost from atrophy, the source of intrinsic factor is lost. Intrinsic factor is essential for cobalamin absorption. The lack of cobalamin results in pernicious anemia.

Diagnostic Studies

Diagnosis of acute gastritis is most often based on the patient's symptoms and history.

- Endoscopic examination with biopsy is used for definitive diagnosis.
- Breath, urine, serum, stool, and gastric tissue biopsy tests can help determine *H. pylori* infection.
- Complete blood count (CBC) may demonstrate anemia from blood loss or lack of intrinsic factor.
- Stools are tested for occult blood.
- Serum tests for antibodies to parietal cells and intrinsic factor are done.

Interprofessional and Nursing Management

Treatment of acute gastritis focuses on eliminating the cause and preventing or avoiding it in the future. The plan of care is supportive (see Nausea and Vomiting).

- If vomiting accompanies acute gastritis, rest, NPO status, and IV fluids may be prescribed. Antiemetics are given for nausea and vomiting. A nasogastric (NG) tube may be used to monitor for bleeding, lavage the precipitating agent from the stomach, or keep the stomach empty and free of noxious stimuli.
- Monitor for dehydration. It can occur rapidly in acute gastritis with vomiting.
- Resume clear liquids when acute symptoms subside. Gradually reintroduce solid, bland foods.

- Management strategies for upper gastrointestinal (GI) bleeding apply to the patient with severe gastritis (see Gastrointestinal Bleeding, Upper).

Drug therapy focuses on reducing irritation of the gastric mucosa and providing symptomatic relief. Histamine (H2)-receptor blockers (e.g., cimetidine) or proton pump inhibitors (PPIs) (e.g., omeprazole) reduce gastric HCl acid secretion.

- Antibiotic combinations are used to eradicate *H. pylori.*
- The patient with pernicious anemia needs lifelong administration of cobalamin.

Treatment of chronic gastritis focuses on evaluating and eliminating the specific cause. The patient may have to adapt to lifestyle changes and strictly adhere to a drug regimen. A team approach in which the healthcare provider (HCP), nurse, dietitian, and pharmacist provide consistent information and support may help patients make these changes.

GASTROESOPHAGEAL REFLUX DISEASE

Description

Gastroesophageal reflux disease (GERD) is a syndrome that results from mucosal damage caused by chronic reflux of stomach acid into the lower esophagus. GERD is the most common upper gastrointestinal (GI) problem. Approximately 15 million Americans have GERD symptoms each day.

Pathophysiology

GERD results when the reflux of acidic gastric contents into the esophagus overwhelms the esophageal defenses (Fig. 12). One of the primary factors in GERD is an incompetent lower esophageal sphincter (LES). Normally, the LES prevents reflux. An incompetent LES lets gastric contents move from the stomach to the esophagus when the patient is supine or has an increase in intraabdominal pressure. Gastric hydrochloric acid (HCl) acid and pepsin secretions that reflux cause esophageal irritation and inflammation (*esophagitis*).

- Decreased LES pressure can be caused by certain foods.
- Some drugs, such as nonsteroidal antiinflammatory drugs (NSAIDs) and potassium, can irritate the esophageal mucosa.
- Obesity increases intraabdominal pressure, which can worsen GERD.
- Cigarette and cigar smoking can contribute to GERD.
- See Hiatal Hernia, which often causes GERD.

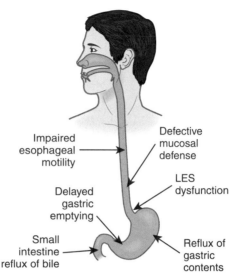

Fig. 12 Factors involved in the pathogenesis of gastroesophageal reflux disease. *LES,* Lower esophageal sphincter.

Clinical Manifestations

Persistent mild symptoms more than twice a week or moderate to severe symptoms that occur at least once a week indicate GERD.

- Heartburn (*pyrosis*), caused by irritation of the esophagus by secretions, is the most common manifestation. Heartburn is a burning, tight sensation that is felt intermittently beneath the lower sternum and spreads upward to the throat or jaw.
- *Dyspepsia* is pain or discomfort centered in the midline of the upper abdomen.
- *Regurgitation* is described as a hot, bitter, or sour liquid in the throat or mouth.

Respiratory findings may include wheezing, coughing, and dyspnea. Nighttime discomfort and coughing can result in disturbed sleep.

GERD-related chest pain (burning, squeezing, or radiating) can mimic angina. Unlike with angina, antacids relieve GERD-related chest pain.

Complications

Complications are due to the direct local effects of gastric acid secretion on the esophageal mucosa. Repeated esophagitis (inflammation of the esophagus) may cause scar tissue formation, stricture, and dysphagia. Barrett's esophagus, a precancerous lesion primarily due to GERD, increases the patient's risk for esophageal cancer.

- Gastric secretions irritating the upper airway cause cough, bronchospasm, laryngospasm, asthma, and chronic bronchitis.
- Acid reflux into the mouth may cause dental erosion.

Diagnostic Studies

GERD is often diagnosed based on symptoms and the patient's response to behavioral and drug therapies. Diagnostic studies help determine the cause of the GERD.

- Barium swallow determines if there is protrusion of the upper part of the stomach into the esophagus.
- Endoscopy is useful to assess LES competence, inflammation, potential scarring, and strictures.
- Biopsy and cytologic specimens can differentiate stomach and esophageal cancer from Barrett's esophagus (see Esophageal Cancer).
- Radionuclide tests can detect gastric reflux and the rate of esophageal clearance.

Interprofessional and Nursing Management

Most patients with GERD can successfully manage the condition through lifestyle modifications, nutrition therapy, and drug therapy. Encourage the patient to incorporate lifestyle changes (Table 36), including smoking cessation.

Teach patients to avoid foods that aggravate their symptoms, such as chocolate, peppermint, tomatoes, fatty foods, coffee, tea, orange juice, cola, and red wine. Small, frequent meals help prevent overdistention of the stomach. Late evening meals and snacking should be avoided. Weight reduction is recommended if the patient is overweight.

Drug Therapy

Drug therapy for GERD focuses on decreasing the volume and acidity of reflux, improving LES function, increasing esophageal clearance, and protecting the esophageal mucosa.

- The goal of HCl acid suppression treatment is to reduce the acidity of the gastric refluxate. Patients who are symptomatic with GERD but do not have esophagitis (nonerosive GERD) achieve symptom relief with PPIs and H2-receptor blockers.
- Antacids may be useful in patients with mild, intermittent heartburn.

G

TABLE 36 Patient and Caregiver Teaching: Gastroesophageal Reflux Disease (GERD)

Include the following instructions when teaching the patient and caregivers about management of GERD.

1. Explain the reason for a low-fat diet.
2. Encourage the patient to eat small, frequent meals to prevent gastric distention.
3. Explain the reason for avoiding alcohol, smoking (causes an almost immediate, marked decrease in lower esophageal sphincter pressure), and beverages that contain caffeine.
4. Advise the patient to not lie down for 2–3 hours after eating, wear tight clothing around the waist, or bend over (especially after eating).
5. Have the patient avoid eating within 3 hours of bedtime.
6. Encourage the patient to sleep with head of bed elevated on 4- to 6-inch blocks or 30-degree angle (gravity fosters esophageal emptying).
7. Provide information about drugs, including reasons for their use and common side effects.
8. Discuss strategies for weight reduction if appropriate.
9. Encourage patient and caregiver to share concerns about lifestyle changes and living with a chronic problem.

Surgical and Endoscopic Therapy

Surgical therapy is reserved for patients with complications of reflux, including esophagitis, intolerance of medications, stricture, Barrett's esophagus, and persistence of severe symptoms. Most surgical procedures are performed laparoscopically. Alternatives to surgery include endoscopic mucosal resection (EMR) and radiofrequency ablation.

GASTROINTESTINAL BLEEDING, UPPER

Description

In the United States, the incidence of acute upper GI (UGI) bleeding is 103 cases per 100,00 adults per year. The mortality rate in hospital admitted patients is 14% with 11% succumbing in the ED. Mortality from an UGI bleed increases with age.

Pathophysiology

Although the most serious loss of blood from the upper GI tract has a sudden onset, insidious occult bleeding can be a major problem.

TABLE 37   Causes of Upper Gastrointestinal Bleeding

Stomach and Duodenum
- Drug-induced
  - Corticosteroids
  - Nonsteroidal antiinflammatory drugs
  - Salicylates
- Erosive gastritis
- Peptic ulcer disease
- Polyps
- Stress-related mucosal disease
- Stomach cancer

Esophagus
- Esophageal varices
- Esophagitis
- Mallory–Weiss tear

Systemic Diseases
- Blood dyscrasias (e.g., leukemia, aplastic anemia)
- Renal failure

Bleeding from an arterial source is profuse and bright red. By contrast, "coffee ground" vomitus means that the blood has been in the stomach for some time. *Melena* (black, tarry stools) occurs with slow bleeding from an upper GI source.

The most common sites of GI bleeding are the esophagus, stomach, and duodenum. Table 37 lists common causes of upper GI bleeding.

- Peptic ulcers, caused by *Helicobacter pylori* infection and the use of nonsteroidal antiinflammatory drugs (NSAIDs), are the most common causes of upper GI bleeding. Aspirin and other NSAIDs and corticosteroids can cause disruption of the gastroduodenal mucosa and upper GI bleeding.
- Stress-related mucosal disease (SRMD), also called *physiologic stress ulcers*, describes mucosal damage in the GI tract ranging from small single lesions to multiple gastric ulcers and major bleeding. SRMD is most commonly seen in critically ill patients who have had severe burns, trauma, or major surgery.
- Bleeding from the esophagus is most likely caused by chronic esophagitis, Mallory–Weiss tear, or esophageal varices. Chronic

G

esophagitis can be caused by GERD, smoking, alcohol use, and ingestion of drugs that irritate the mucosa. Esophageal varices most often occur from cirrhosis of the liver (see Cirrhosis).

Diagnostic Studies

- Endoscopy is used to diagnose the source (e.g., peptic ulcer, esophageal varices, gastritis) of upper GI bleeding.
- Angiography is used to diagnose upper GI bleeding when endoscopy cannot be done or when bleeding persists.
- Laboratory studies include complete blood count (CBC), blood urea nitrogen (BUN), serum electrolytes, prothrombin time, partial thromboplastin time, liver enzymes, and arterial blood gases (ABGs).

Interprofessional Management

Endoscopy within the first 24 hours of bleeding is important for diagnosis and treatment. The goal of endoscopic hemostasis is to coagulate or thrombose the bleeding vessel. Mechanical therapy, injection therapy with epinephrine, or thermal cautery is used to achieve acute hemostasis. Surgical intervention is needed when bleeding continues from an identified site.

During the acute phase, drugs are used to decrease bleeding, decrease HCl secretion, and neutralize the HCl acid.

- Efforts are made to reduce acid secretion because the acidic environment can alter platelet function and interfere with clot stabilization. Proton pump inhibitors (PPIs) or H_2-receptor blockers are administered IV to decrease acid secretion.

Nursing Management

Goals

The overall goals are that the patient with upper GI bleeding will have no further GI bleeding, have the cause of the bleeding identified and treated, and return to a normal hemodynamic state.

Interventions

The patient with a history of chronic gastritis or peptic ulcer disease is at high risk for upper GI bleeding. Teach the at-risk patient to avoid known gastric irritants, such as alcohol and smoking, and to take only prescribed medications. Over-the-counter (OTC) drugs may contain ingredients (e.g., aspirin) that increase the risk of bleeding.

During acute GI bleeding, monitor for shock. Assess for complications of gut perforation and peritonitis indicated by a tense, rigid, board-like abdomen.

- IV lines, preferably two, with a 16- or 18-gauge needle are placed for fluid and blood replacement.
- Whole blood, packed red blood cells (RBCs), and fresh frozen plasma may be used for volume replacement in massive hemorrhage. When bleeding is less profuse, isotonic saline solution followed by packed RBCs restores the hematocrit more quickly.
- Supplemental O_2 delivered by face mask or nasal cannula may help increase blood oxygen saturation.
- An indwelling urinary catheter may be inserted so that output can be accurately assessed hourly.

Although room-temperature, cool, or iced gastric lavage is used in some institutions, its effectiveness as a treatment for upper GI bleeding is questionable. When lavage is used, approximately 50–100 mL of fluid is instilled at a time into the stomach. The lavage fluid may be aspirated from the stomach or drained by gravity.

- Monitor vital signs and ECG, especially in patients with cardiovascular disease, because dysrhythmias may occur.
- Keep the head of the bed elevated to provide comfort and prevent aspiration.
- Assess stools for blood. Black, tarry stools indicate prolonged upper GI bleeding.
- Monitor the patient's laboratory studies. The hemoglobin and hematocrit are usually evaluated about every 4–6 hours if the patient is actively bleeding.
- When oral nourishment is begun, observe the patient for symptoms of nausea and vomiting and a recurrence of bleeding. Feedings initially consist of hourly clear fluids. Gradually introduce food if the patient has no discomfort.
- When hemorrhage is the result of chronic alcohol use, closely observe the patient for delirium tremens as alcohol takes place. Symptoms indicating the onset of delirium tremens are agitation, uncontrolled shaking, sweating, and hallucinations.

▼ Patient and Caregiver Teaching

- Teach the patient and caregivers how to avoid future bleeding episodes. Emphasize adhering to prescribed drug therapy and avoiding aspirin and other NSAIDs.
- Encourage elimination of smoking and alcohol because they are sources of gastric irritation.
- Teach the patient and family what to do if an acute hemorrhage occurs.

G

GLAUCOMA

Description

Glaucoma is a group of disorders characterized by increased intra-ocular pressure (IOP) and its consequences of optic nerve atrophy and peripheral visual field loss. Many people with glaucoma are unaware of their condition.

- Glaucoma is the second leading cause of permanent blindness in the United States and the leading cause of blindness among blacks.
- Blindness from glaucoma is largely preventable with early detection and treatment.

Pathophysiology

Increased IOP results when the rate of aqueous production (inflow) is greater than aqueous reabsorption (outflow). If the pressure remains elevated, permanent vision loss may occur.

Primary open-angle glaucoma (POAG) is the most common type of primary glaucoma. In POAG, the aqueous outflow is decreased in the trabecular meshwork. The drainage channels become clogged and damage to the optic nerve can result.

Angle-closure glaucoma (ACG) is caused by reduced outflow of aqueous humor that results from angle closure. Usually this is from the lens bulging forward in the aging process. Angle closure may also occur due to pupil dilation in the patient with anatomically narrow angles. An acute attack may occur with drug-induced mydriasis, emotional excitement, or darkness. Check drug records and documentation before giving medications to the patient with angle-closure glaucoma. Teach the patient not to take any mydriatic medications.

Clinical Manifestations

- POAG develops slowly without symptoms of pain or pressure. The patient usually does not notice gradual visual field loss until peripheral vision is severely compromised (tunnel vision).
- Acute angle-closure glaucoma causes symptoms of sudden, severe pain in or around the eye that is often accompanied by nausea and vomiting. Visual symptoms include seeing colored halos around lights, blurred vision, and ocular redness.
- Symptoms of subacute or chronic angle-closure glaucoma appear gradually. The patient may report blurred vision, colored halos around lights, ocular redness, or eye or brow pain.

Diagnostic Studies

- IOP measurement with tonometry
- Visual acuity measurement and visual field perimetry
- Slit-lamp microscopy
- Ophthalmoscopy (direct and indirect)

Interprofessional Management

The primary focus of treatment is to keep the IOP low enough to prevent optic nerve damage. Treatment varies with the type of glaucoma.

- In chronic open-angle glaucoma, prostaglandin analogs are the preferred choice for initial treatment. Other drug therapy can include β-adrenergic receptor blocking agents, α-adrenergic agents, cholinergic agents (miotics), and carbonic anhydrase inhibitors (hyperosmotic agents).
- When prescribed medications are not effective or are not used as recommended, surgical options include argon laser trabeculoplasty (ALT) and trabeculectomy.
- Acute angle-closure glaucoma is an ocular emergency that requires immediate interventions, including carbonic anhydrase inhibitors and oral or IV hyperosmotic agents, including glycerin (Ophthalgan), isosorbide (Ismotic), and mannitol (Osmitrol). Laser peripheral iridotomy or surgical iridectomy is definitive treatment.

Nursing Management

Because glaucoma requires long-term management, assess the patient's ability to adhere to the plan. Also assess the patient's reaction to a potentially sight-threatening chronic disorder.

- Encourage adherence by helping the patient set up a medication schedule.
- Advocate for a change in treatment if the patient reports unacceptable side effects.

▼ **Patient and Caregiver Teaching**

See Table 22, Patient and Caregiver Teaching: After Eye Surgery.

Provide accurate information about the disease process and treatment options, including the rationale for each option. Teach about the purpose, frequency, and technique for administration of antiglaucoma drugs.

G

GLOMERULONEPHRITIS

Glomerulonephritis (inflammation of the glomeruli) is the third leading cause of end-stage renal disease in the United States. A variety of conditions can cause glomerulonephritis, ranging from kidney infections to systemic diseases.

- In *acute glomerulonephritis*, symptoms come on suddenly and may be temporary or reversible. *Chronic glomerulonephritis* is slowly progressive and generally leads to irreversible renal failure.
- Clinical manifestations of glomerulonephritis include hematuria and urinary excretion of various formed elements, including red blood cells (RBCs), white blood cells (WBCs), proteins, and casts.

Acute Poststreptococcal Glomerulonephritis

- *Acute poststreptococcal glomerulonephritis* (APSGN) develops 1–2 weeks after an infection of the tonsils, pharynx, or skin by nephrotoxic strains of group A β-hemolytic streptococci. The streptococcal antigen–antibody complex induces a process of glomerular inflammation and tissue injury.

  Manifestations include generalized body edema, hypertension, oliguria, hematuria with a smoky or rusty appearance, and proteinuria.■

Interprofessional and Nursing Management

Antibiotics are given if the streptococcal infection is still present. Rest is recommended until proteinuria, hematuria, and hypertension subside.

- Restricting sodium and fluid intake and giving diuretics can reduce edema. Severe hypertension is treated with antihypertensive drugs.
- We may restrict protein intake if there is evidence of an increase in nitrogenous wastes (e.g., increased BUN).

  One of the most important ways to prevent APSGN is to encourage early diagnosis and treatment of sore throats and skin lesions. If streptococci are found in the culture, encourage the patient to take the full course of antibiotics to ensure that the bacteria have been eradicated.

- Good personal hygiene is an important factor in preventing the spread of cutaneous streptococcal infections.

Chronic Glomerulonephritis

Chronic glomerulonephritis is a syndrome of permanent and progressive renal fibrosis involving the glomeruli. It is characterized by proteinuria, hematuria, and the slow development of uremia because of decreasing renal function. Chronic glomerulonephritis progresses insidiously to end-stage renal disease (ESRD). Treatment is supportive and symptomatic (see Kidney Disease, Chronic).

GONORRHEA

Description and Pathophysiology

Gonorrhea is the second most frequently occurring reportable sexually transmitted infection (STI) in the United States. It is caused by *Neisseria gonorrhoeae,* a Gram-negative diplococcus bacterium. Gonorrhea can be transmitted by exposure to sexual fluids during vaginal, anal, or oral sex. The incubation period is 1–14 days. The most common site of infection for men is the urethra and for women, the cervix. Men and women can get gonorrhea of the rectum from anal sex or of the oropharynx from oral sex. Prior infection does not provide protection from reinfection.

Clinical Manifestations

- Most men will be symptomatic within a few days. The most common symptoms are dysuria, purulent urethral discharge, and epididymitis.
- Most women are asymptomatic. Common symptoms are increased vaginal discharge, dysuria, frequency of urination, and bleeding after sex. Redness and swelling can occur at the cervix or urethra along with a purulent exudate.
- Symptoms and signs of rectal gonorrhea may include mucopurulent rectal discharge or bleeding, anorectal pain, pruritus, tenesmus, mucus-coated stools, and painful bowel movements.
- Most patients with gonorrheal infections in the throat have no symptoms. Some may have a sore throat.

Complications

Because men often seek treatment early, they are less likely to develop complications, such as prostatitis, urethral strictures, and sterility from orchitis or epididymitis.

Because women are likely to be asymptomatic and seldom seek early treatment, complications are more common. Untreated gonorrhea can cause an infection in the Bartholin's glands or Skene's glands or result in pelvic inflammatory disease (PID). PID increases risk for ectopic pregnancy, infertility, and chronic pelvic pain.

Neonates can develop *gonococcal conjunctivitis* (ophthalmia neonatorum) from exposure to an infected mother during delivery, which can result in permanent blindness. Almost all states have a law or health department regulation requiring prophylactic eye treatment of all newborns.

G

Diagnostic Studies

- For men, a presumptive diagnosis of gonorrhea is made if there is a history of sexual contact with a new or infected partner followed within a few days by a urethral discharge. Typical clinical manifestations combined with a positive finding in a Gram-stained smear of discharge from the penis give an almost certain diagnosis.
- For women, making a diagnosis of gonorrhea on the basis of symptoms is difficult. Most women are asymptomatic or have symptoms that may be confused with other conditions, such as a urinary tract infection. A culture may be performed to confirm the diagnosis.

Interprofessional and Nursing Management

Because of a short incubation period and high infectivity, treatment is instituted without waiting for culture results. The first-line treatment for gonorrhea is high-dose IM ceftriaxone. Patients who are treated but who have a positive test 7 days after treatment need antibiotic sensitivity testing.

- All sexual contacts within 60 days should be evaluated and treated to prevent reinfection and further transmission. Teach patients to abstain from sexual contact for 7 days after treatment, or until all partners have been treated and have also abstained from sexual contact for 7 days.
- Review the ways to reduce risk of acquiring a repeat or new STI in the future.
- See Nursing Management: Sexually Transmitted Infections.

GOUT

Description

Gout is a type of acute arthritis characterized by elevation of uric acid (hyperuricemia) and the deposit of uric acid crystals in joints. Sodium urate crystals may be found in articular, periarticular, and subcutaneous tissues. Gout is marked by painful flares lasting days to weeks followed by long periods without symptoms.

- More than 8 million Americans are affected by gout, with men affected three times as often as women. Black men and women are at increased risk of developing gout in middle and old age compared to whites. In particular, middle-aged black men have higher urate levels.

Pathophysiology

Uric acid is the major end product of purine catabolism and is primarily excreted by the kidneys. Gout is caused by an increase in uric acid production, reduced excretion of uric acid by the kidneys (the most common cause), or increased intake of foods containing purines (e.g., red and organ meat, shellfish, fructose drinks), which are metabolized to uric acid by the body. Increased uric acid production is most commonly linked to obesity. Excessive alcohol consumption is also a risk factor.

- High dietary intake of purine alone has relatively little effect on uric acid levels. Hyperuricemia may result from prolonged fasting or excessive alcohol drinking because of the increased production of keto acids, which then inhibit uric acid excretion. Reduced uric acid excretion can occur with chronic kidney disease or metabolic syndrome.

In *primary hyperuricemia*, a hereditary error of purine metabolism leads to the overproduction or retention of uric acid. *Secondary hyperuricemia* may be related to another acquired disorder or may be caused by drugs known to inhibit uric acid excretion (e.g., thiazide diuretics, β-adrenergic blockers, angiotensin-converting enzyme inhibitors). Postmenopausal women and organ transplant recipients taking immunosuppressive agents are also at risk for hyperuricemia.

Clinical Manifestations

Gouty arthritis may occur acutely in one or more joints. Affected joints may appear dusky or cyanotic and are extremely tender. Inflammation of the great toe *(podagra)* is the most common initial problem. Other joints affected may include the midfoot, ankle, knee, and wrist. The painful area is highly sensitive to light touch.

- Acute gouty arthritis is usually triggered by events such as trauma, surgery, alcohol ingestion, or systemic infection. Symptom onset is usually rapid. Swelling and pain peak within several hours, often accompanied by a low-grade fever.
- Individual attacks usually subside in 2–10 days. The affected joint returns to normal and patients have no symptoms between attacks.

Chronic gout is characterized by multiple joint involvement and visible deposits of sodium urate crystals *tophi* in the synovium, subchondral bone, olecranon bursa, and vertebrae; along tendons; and in the skin and cartilage.

Chronic inflammation may cause joint deformity. Large urate crystal deposits may pierce overlying skin, producing draining sinuses that often become infected. Excessive uric acid excretion may lead to urinary tract stone formation. Pyelonephritis related to intrarenal sodium urate deposits and obstruction may contribute to kidney disease.

The severity of gouty arthritis is variable. The clinical course may consist of infrequent mild attacks or multiple severe episodes and slowly progressive disability.

Diagnostic Studies

- Serum uric acid levels are usually elevated. However, hyperuricemia is not specifically diagnostic of gout because serum values may be normal during an acute gout attack.
- Twenty-four-hour urine uric acid levels help determine if the disease is caused by decreased renal excretion or overproduction of uric acid.
- X-rays appear normal in the early stages of gout. In chronic disease, tophi appear as eroded areas in the bone.
- Synovial fluid aspiration helps distinguish gout from septic arthritis and *pseudogout* (in which calcium phosphate crystals are formed). Affected fluid contains needle-like crystals of sodium urate.

Interprofessional Management

Goals for care include ending an acute attack with an antiinflammatory agent, such as colchicine. Drug therapy is the primary way to treat acute and chronic gout. Weight reduction (as needed) and possibly avoiding alcohol and foods high in purine (red and organ meats) are recommended.

Drug Therapy

Acute gouty arthritis is treated with colchicine, antiinflammatory, and analgesic nonsteroidal antiinflammatory drugs (NSAIDs). Future attacks are prevented with a xanthine oxidase inhibitor (allopurinol [Zyloprim]), or a drug that increases the urinary excretion of uric acid (probenecid [Probalan]). The angiotensin II receptor antagonist losartan (Cozaar) may be effective for treating older patients with gout and hypertension. Losartan promotes urate excretion and may normalize serum urate.

- Aspirin inactivates uricosuric drugs (e.g., probenecid). Acetaminophen can be used safely if analgesia is needed.
- Serious adverse effects limit the use of febuxostat (Uloric) to those not treated effectively or having severe side effects with allopurinol. Patients who cannot take or do not respond to drugs that lower uric acid in the blood may be given IV pegloticase (Krystexxa). This drug metabolizes uric acid into a harmless chemical excreted in the urine.

- Corticosteroids, either orally or by intraarticular injection, can be helpful in treating acute attacks.
- Adequate urine volume with normal renal function (2–3 L/day) must be maintained to prevent precipitation of uric acid in the renal tubules. Regardless of which drugs are used to treat gout, serum uric acid levels must be checked regularly to monitor treatment effectiveness.

Nutritional Therapy

Limiting alcohol and foods high in purine helps minimize uric acid production. Instruct obese patients in a carefully planned weight-reduction program.

Nursing Management

Nursing intervention is directed at supportive care of the inflamed joints.

- Bed rest may be appropriate, with affected joints properly immobilized. Use a bed cradle or footboard to protect a painful lower extremity from the weight of bed clothes.
- Assess the limitation of motion and degree of pain. Document treatment response.
- Explain the importance of drug therapy and the need for periodic determination of serum uric acid levels.
- Teach the patient about triggers for an attack, including purine-containing foods and alcohol, starvation (fasting), medication use (e.g., diuretics), and major medical events (e.g., surgery, heart attack).

GUILLAIN–BARRÉ SYNDROME

G

Description

Guillain–Barré syndrome (GBS) is an autoimmune process that occurs a few days or weeks after a viral or bacterial infection. The main features of GBS include acute, ascending, rapidly progressive, symmetric weakness of the limbs. Maximal weakness is reached in 4 weeks. Respiratory muscles may be affected. Some patients require mechanical ventilation.

GBS is rare, affecting about one person in every 100,000. It can occur at any age, but those over age 50 years are at greatest risk. The most common type of GBS is acute inflammatory demyelinating polyneuropathy (AIDP). Other types include acute motor axonal neuropathy (AMAN) and acute motor sensory axonal neuropathy (AMSAN). AMAN is more common in children.

- Although 80% of patients almost completely recover, the process may take months or years.

Pathophysiology

Following an infection, immune responses cause injury to either the myelin sheath (AIDP) or the nerve axon itself (AMAN). There is edema and inflammation of affected nerves. The result is segmental loss of the myelin sheath with exposed nerve membranes in nerve terminals and the nodes of Ranvier. Transmission of nerve impulses is stopped or slowed down. This leads to flaccid paralysis with muscle denervation and atrophy. In the recovery phase, remyelination occurs slowly. Neurologic function returns in a proximal-to-distal pattern. Most cases of GBS follow a viral or bacterial infection of the gastrointestinal or upper respiratory tract. Cytomegalovirus is the most common viral cause. *Campylobacter jejuni* gastroenteritis is the most common bacterial cause.

Clinical Manifestations

GBS symptoms range from mild to severe.

- The first symptoms are pain, paresthesia (numbness and tingling), and hypotonia (reduced muscle tone) of the limbs.
- Areflexia (lack of reflexes) and weakness or paralysis of the limbs usually peak within 4 weeks.
- Autonomic nervous system dysfunction manifests with orthostatic hypotension, hypertension, and abnormal vagal responses (bradycardia, heart block, asystole). Other autonomic dysfunctions include bowel and bladder dysfunction, facial flushing, and diaphoresis.
- Cranial nerve involvement is manifested as facial weakness and paresthesia, extraocular eye movement difficulties, and dysphagia.
- Pain is a common symptom including paresthesias, muscular aches and cramps, and hyperesthesias. Pain appears to be worse at night. Pain may lead to a decrease in appetite and interfere with sleep.

The most serious complication of GBS is respiratory failure, which occurs as paralysis progresses to the nerves that innervate the thoracic area. Respiratory infection or UTI may occur. Immobility from paralysis can cause paralytic ileus, muscle atrophy, VTE, PIs, orthostatic hypotension, and nutrition deficiencies.

Diagnostic Studies

Diagnosis is based primarily on patient history and clinical signs. Clinical features required for the diagnosis include progressive

weakness of more than one limb and diminished or absent reflexes.
- Cerebrospinal fluid (CSF) analysis is helpful in excluding other causes. In GBS, the CSF has more protein than normal.
- Results of electromyography (EMG) and nerve conduction studies are used to confirm the diagnosis.

Interprofessional and Nursing Management

Management of GBS is supportive. Ventilator support is critical during the acute phase. Immunomodulating treatments, such as plasma exchange (plasmapheresis) or high-dose IV immunoglobulin (IVIG), are most effective if used within the first 2 weeks of symptom onset.

- Plasmapheresis removes antibodies and other immune factors. It is used five times either daily or every other day in the first 2 weeks.
- IVIG interferes with antigen presentation and is given over 5 days. Because it is readily available, IVIG therapy has replaced plasmapheresis as the preferred treatment in many centers.
- Assess the respiratory system frequently by checking respiratory rate and depth to determine the need for immediate intervention, including intubation and mechanical ventilation (see Tracheostomy and Artificial Airways: Endotracheal Tubes). Monitor arterial blood gases (ABGs) and vital capacity.
- Evaluate motor and sensory function. Report changes in motor function (e.g., ascending paralysis), deep tendon reflexes, cranial nerve functions (e.g., swallowing, gag reflex, corneal reflex), and level of consciousness.
- Closely monitor BP and cardiac rate and rhythm during the acute phase because dysrhythmias, orthostatic hypotension, and increased or decreased BP and heart rate may occur. Vasopressors and volume expanders may be needed.
- If fever develops, obtain sputum and blood cultures to identify the pathogen. Appropriate antibiotic therapy is then started.
- Plan interventions to prevent muscle atrophy, venous thromboembolism (VTE), and pressure injuries.

Nutritional needs must be met in spite of possible problems associated with gastric dilation, paralytic ileus, and aspiration potential if the gag reflex is lost.

- Enteral feedings or parenteral nutrition may be used to ensure adequate caloric intake.

Coordinate early referrals for physical, occupational, and speech therapy. Counseling may help the patient adjust to the sudden disabling syndrome and dependence on others.

G

HEAD AND NECK CANCER

Description

Most head and neck cancers arise from squamous cells that line the mucosal surfaces of the head and neck. These cancers may involve the nasal cavity and paranasal sinuses, nasopharynx, oropharynx, larynx, oral cavity, and/or salivary glands. Most patients present with locally advanced disease. Disability from the disease and treatment includes the potential loss of voice, disfigurement, and social concerns.

- Head and neck cancer occurs most often in patients over age 50 years. Men are affected twice as often as women.
- Tobacco use causes most head and neck cancers. Excess alcohol consumption is also a major risk factor.
- Cancers in patients younger than 50 years are often related to human papillomavirus (HPV) infection. Other risk factors include exposure to the sun, asbestos, industrial carcinogens, marijuana use, radiation therapy, and poor oral hygiene.

Clinical Manifestations

Early signs of head and neck cancer vary with tumor location.

- Pharyngeal cancer may first be seen as a red or white patch in the mouth, an ulcer that does not heal, or a change in the fit of dentures.
- Hoarseness that lasts more than 2 weeks may be a symptom of early laryngeal cancer. Some patients have a change in voice quality or what feels like a lump in the throat.
- Other clinical manifestations may include a sore throat that does not get better, unilateral ear pain or ringing in the ears, swelling or lumps in the neck, constant coughing, and coughing up blood.
- Unintentional weight loss and difficulties with chewing, swallowing, moving the tongue, and breathing are typically late symptoms.

Diagnostic Studies

- The healthcare provider (HCP) may examine upper airways using indirect laryngoscopy or with a flexible nasopharyngoscope.
- A CT scan or MRI may show local and regional spread.
- Multiple biopsy specimens are obtained to determine the extent of the disease.

Interprofessional Management

Staging is slightly different for each type of cancer. In general, Stage 0 is in situ, or confined to where it began, progressing through Stage 4 with more advanced disease. Oral cancer staging considers a patient's HPV status. (See TNM staging.)

- Stage I and II cancers are potentially curable with radiation therapy or larynx-sparing surgery.
- Patients with advanced disease (stages III and IV) are treated with combinations of surgery, radiation, chemotherapy, and targeted therapy. Radiation can be delivered by either external-beam therapy or internal implants (brachytherapy).
- In a total laryngectomy, the entire larynx and preepiglottic region are removed and a permanent tracheostomy is created (see Tracheostomy). Radical neck dissection frequently accompanies total laryngectomy. Extensive dissection and reconstruction may be performed.
- Changes after a total laryngectomy include loss of speech, loss of the ability to taste and smell, inability to produce audible sounds (including laughing and crying), and a permanent tracheal stoma.
- Some patients refuse surgical intervention for advanced lesions because of the extent of the procedure and the potential risk. In this situation, external radiation therapy is used as the sole treatment or in combination with chemotherapy.
- Chemotherapy (e.g., cisplatin) and targeted therapy (e.g., cetuximab [Erbitux]) are used in combination with radiation therapy for patients with stage III or IV cancers.

Nutritional Therapy

After radical neck surgery, the patient may be unable to consume nutrients through the mouth. Parenteral fluids are given for the first 24–48 h.

- Because of swelling and difficulty swallowing after surgery, enteral nutrition is usually given through a nasogastric, nasointestinal, or gastrostomy tube that was placed during surgery.

When patients can successfully swallow with low or no risk of aspiration, they may have small amounts of thickened liquids or pureed foods while in high Fowler's position. Avoid thin, watery fluids because they are hard to swallow, increasing the risk of aspiration. Closely observe for choking. Oral suctioning can help prevent aspiration.

Nursing Management

Goals

The patient with head or neck cancer will have a patent airway, an acceptable body image, no complications related to treatment, adequate nutrition, minimal to no pain, and the ability to communicate.

Interventions

Include information about risk factors in health teaching. Continued use of tobacco and alcohol diminishes the chance of a cure. Encourage good oral hygiene. Teach patients about safe sex practices to prevent HPV infection.

For procedures that involve a laryngectomy, teaching should include information about expected changes in speech.

- Establish a means of communication to use postoperatively.
- After surgery, a laryngectomy (tracheostomy) tube will be in place. Keeping the airway patent is essential. Immediately after surgery, frequent suctioning is usually needed via the tracheostomy tube.
- Position the patient in semi-Fowler's position to decrease edema and tension on the suture lines.
- Monitor vital signs frequently because of the risk of hemorrhage and respiratory compromise.
- Encourage deep breathing and coughing and provide tracheostomy care as needed.
- Depression, changes in sexuality patterns, and altered body image are common after radical neck dissection. Help the patient regain an acceptable self concept.
- Schedule a speech therapist to meet with the patient who had a total laryngectomy to discuss voice restoration options.

▼ **Patient and Caregiver Teaching**

- Monitor patency of wound drainage tubes every hour in the first few hours after surgery, then every 4 h to ensure proper functioning. After drainage tubes are removed, closely monitor the area for swelling. If fluid accumulates, aspiration may be necessary.
- Teach the patient and caregivers how to manage tubes and whom to call if there are problems.
- Provide pictorial instructions for tracheostomy care, suctioning, stoma care, and tube feedings as appropriate.
- Teach the patient to cover the stoma before performing activities such as shaving and applying makeup, to avoid inhaling foreign materials.
- Encourage adequate humidity at home using a bedside humidifier and high oral fluid intake.
- Encourage preparation of food that is colorful, attractive, and nutritious. Taste may be diminished with loss of the sense of smell after surgery or radiation therapy.

HEAD INJURY

Description

Head injury includes any trauma to the scalp, skull, or brain. A serious form of head injury is *traumatic brain injury* (TBI). In US emergency departments, an estimated 2.8 million people with TBI are treated each year.

- Falls and motor vehicle crashes are the most common causes of head injury. Other causes of head injury include firearms, assaults, sports-related trauma, recreational injuries, and war-related injuries.
- Men are twice as likely to sustain a TBI as women.

Deaths from head trauma occur at three time points after injury: immediately after injury, within 2 h of injury, and about 3 weeks after injury.

- Most deaths occur immediately after the injury, either from the direct head trauma or massive hemorrhage and shock.
- Deaths occurring within a few hours of the trauma are caused by worsening of the head injury or internal bleeding. Immediately recognizing changes in neurologic status and rapid surgical intervention are critical in the prevention of deaths.
- Deaths occurring 3 weeks or more after the injury result from multisystem failure.

Types of Head Injuries

Scalp Laceration

Because the scalp contains many blood vessels with poor constrictive abilities, even relatively small wounds can bleed profusely. The major complications of scalp lesions are blood loss and infection.

Skull Fracture

Fractures often occur with head trauma. Fractures may be closed or open, depending on the presence of a scalp laceration or extension of the fracture into the air sinuses or dura.

- The type and severity of a skull fracture depend on the velocity, momentum, direction and shape of the injuring agent, and the site of impact. Specific manifestations of a skull fracture are generally associated with the location of the injury.

Major complications of skull fracture are intracranial infections and hematoma, as well as meningeal and brain tissue damage.

Head Trauma

Brain injuries are categorized as *diffuse* (generalized) or *focal* (localized). In Diffuse Injury (i.e., concussion, diffuse axonal), damage to the brain cannot be localized to one particular area, whereas a *focal injury* (e.g., contusion, hematoma) can be localized to a specific area.

H

Diffuse Injury. *Concussion* is a minor and diffuse head injury associated with a disruption in neural activity and a change in the level of consciousness (LOC). The patient may not lose total consciousness. A brief disruption in LOC, amnesia for the event (retrograde amnesia), and headache are generally of short duration.

- *Postconcussion syndrome* may develop in some patients, usually from 2 weeks to 2 months after the injury. Typical findings include persistent headache, lethargy, behavior changes, decreased short-term memory, and changes in intellectual ability.

Concussion is generally considered benign and resolves spontaneously. For some, the signs and symptoms are the beginning of a more serious, progressive problem.

- At the time of discharge, it is important to give the patient and caregiver instructions for observation and accurate reporting of symptoms or changes in neurologic status.

Diffuse axonal injury (DAI) is widespread axonal damage occurring after a TBI. Clinical signs of DAI include decreased LOC, increased intracranial pressure (ICP), decortication or decerebration, and global cerebral edema. Patients with severe injury have a poor functional prognosis

- Patients are rapidly triaged to an intensive care unit (ICU) and vigilantly watched and treated for signs of increased ICP (see Increased Intracranial Pressure).

Focal Injury. Focal injury can be minor to severe and localized to an area of injury. Focal injuries include lacerations, contusions, hematomas, and cranial nerve injuries.

Lacerations involve tearing of brain tissue. They often occur in depressed and open fractures and penetrating injuries. Tissue damage is severe, and surgical repair of the laceration is impossible. Management consists of antibiotics (until meningitis is ruled out) and preventing secondary injury from increased ICP. If bleeding is deep into the brain tissue, focal and generalized signs develop.

A *contusion* is bruising of brain tissue within a focal area. It is usually associated with a closed head injury. There may be areas of hemorrhage, infarction, necrosis, and edema.

- Contusions or lacerations may occur both at the site of the direct impact of the brain on the skull *(coup)* and at a secondary area of damage on the opposite side away from injury *(contrecoup),* leading to multiple contused areas. Contrecoup injuries tend to be more severe.
- Neurologic assessment may reveal focal and generalized findings, depending on the size and location of the contusion. Seizures can occur.

Complications

Epidural Hematoma

An *epidural hematoma* results from bleeding between the dura and inner surface of the skull. An epidural hematoma is a neurologic emergency. It is usually associated with a linear fracture crossing a major artery or vein in the dura, causing a tear.

- With arterial hematomas, the middle meningeal artery lying under the temporal bone is often torn. Because this is an arterial hemorrhage, the hematoma develops rapidly.
- Venous epidural hematomas are associated with a tear of the dural venous sinus and develop slowly.

Classic signs include an initial period of unconsciousness at the scene, with a brief lucid interval followed by a decrease in LOC. Other symptoms may be headache, nausea and vomiting, or focal manifestations. Rapid surgical intervention to evacuate the hematoma and prevent cerebral herniation, along with treatment to decrease ICP, dramatically improves outcomes.

Subdural Hematoma

A *subdural hematoma* occurs from bleeding between the dura mater and arachnoid layer of the meninges. The hematoma usually results from injury to the brain tissue and its blood vessels. A subdural hematoma is usually venous in origin and develops slowly. However, an arterial hemorrhage can cause a subdural hematoma, in which case it develops more rapidly. Subdural hematomas may be acute, subacute, or chronic (Table 38).

- An *acute subdural hematoma* manifests within 24–48 h of the injury. Manifestations are similar to those associated with brain tissue compression in increased ICP (see Increased Intracranial Pressure). They include decreasing LOC and headache. The patient may be drowsy, confused, or unconscious. The ipsilateral pupil dilates and becomes fixed if ICP is significantly elevated.
- A *subacute subdural hematoma* usually occurs within 2–14 days of the injury. After the initial bleeding, this hematoma may appear to enlarge over time as the breakdown products of the blood draw fluid into the subdural space.
- A *chronic subdural hematoma* develops over weeks or months after a seemingly minor head injury. The presenting symptoms are focal rather than signs of increased ICP. Chronic subdural hematomas are more common in older adults because of a potentially larger subdural space secondary to brain atrophy.

There may be a delay in diagnosing a subdural hematoma in the older adult because symptoms mimic other health problems in this age group, such as confusion, lethargy, and memory loss. Manifestations of a subdural hematoma are often attributed to vascular disease (stroke, transient ischemic attack [TIA]) or dementia.

H

TABLE 38 Types of Subdural Hematomas		
Occurrence After Injury	**Progression of Symptoms**	**Treatment**
Acute		
24–48 h after severe trauma	Immediate deterioration	Craniotomy, evacuation and decompression
Subacute		
48 h–2 weeks after severe trauma	Decline in mental status as hematoma develops. Progression dependent on size and location of hematoma	Evacuation and decompression
Chronic		
Weeks or months, usually >20 days after injury Often injury seemed trivial or was forgotten by patient	Nonspecific, nonlocalizing progression. Progressive change in level of consciousness	Evacuation and decompression, membranectomy

Intracerebral Hematoma

An *intracerebral hematoma* occurs from bleeding in the brain tissue. It usually occurs in the frontal and temporal lobes, possibly from the rupture of intracerebral vessels at the time of injury.

Diagnostic Studies

- CT scan is the best diagnostic test to rapidly evaluate for craniocerebral trauma.
- MRI, positron emission tomography (PET), and evoked potential studies assist in diagnosis and differentiation of head injuries.
- Transcranial Doppler studies are used to measure cerebral blood flow velocity.
- Cervical spine X-ray series, CT scan, or MRI of the spine may be done to check for cervical spine trauma.

Interprofessional Management

The principal treatment of head injuries is timely diagnosis and surgery, if needed. For the patient with a concussion or contusion, observation for and management of increased ICP are the main strategies. (see Increased Intracranial Pressure)

- The treatment of skull fractures is usually conservative. For depressed fractures and fractures with loose fragments, a craniotomy is done to elevate depressed bone and remove free fragments. If large amounts of bone are destroyed, the bone may be removed (craniectomy) and a cranioplasty will be needed at a later time.
- In cases of large acute subdural and epidural hematomas with significant neurologic impairment, a craniotomy is generally done to see and control the bleeding vessels. Burr-hole openings may be used in an extreme emergency for rapid decompression before craniotomy. A drain may be placed postoperatively for several days to prevent blood from reaccumulating.

Nursing Management

Goals

The patient with an acute head injury will maintain adequate cerebral oxygenation and perfusion; stay afebrile; be free of discomfort; be free from infection; have adequate nutrition; and attain maximal cognitive, motor, and sensory function.

Interventions

One of the best ways to prevent head injuries is to prevent car and motorcycle crashes.

- Be active in campaigns that promote driving safety, and speak to driver education classes regarding the dangers of unsafe driving and driving after drinking alcohol and using drugs.
- Teach community members that using seat belts in cars and helmets for riding on motorcycles is the most effective measure for increasing survival after crashes.
- Protective helmets should also be worn by lumberjacks, construction workers, athletes who play contact sports, miners, horseback riders, bicycle riders, snowboarders, skiers, and skydivers.

Acute Care. The general goal of nursing management of the head-injured patient is to maintain cerebral oxygenation and perfusion and prevent secondary cerebral ischemia. Monitoring for changes in neurologic status is critically important because the patient's condition may deteriorate rapidly, requiring emergency surgery or other interventions.

- Explain the need for frequent neurologic assessments to both patient and caregiver.
- Behavioral manifestations associated with head injury can result in a frightened, disoriented patient who is combative and resists help. Your approach should be calm and gentle. A family

H

member may be available to stay with the patient to decrease their anxiety and fear.

- Nausea and vomiting can be alleviated by antiemetic drugs.
- Headache can usually be controlled with acetaminophen or small doses of codeine. The major focus of nursing care for the brain-injured patient relates to increased ICP (see Increased Intracranial Pressure). The Glasgow Coma Scale (GCS) is useful in assessing the LOC (see Glasgow Coma Scale). Report signs of a deteriorating neurologic state, such as decreasing LOC or motor strength, promptly to the healthcare provider (HCP).
- If cerebrospinal fluid (CSF) rhinorrhea or otorrhea occurs, inform the HCP at once. The head of the bed may be elevated to decrease the CSF pressure so that a tear can seal. A loose collection pad may be placed under the nose or over the ear. Tell the patient not to sneeze or blow the nose. Do not insert a gastric tube or suction catheter through the nose.
- If the patient's condition deteriorates, intracranial surgery may be needed. A burr-hole opening or craniotomy may be done, depending on the underlying injury. The patient is often unconscious before surgery, making it necessary for a family member to sign the consent form for surgery. This is a frightening time for the patient's caregiver and family and requires sensitive nursing management. The suddenness of the situation makes it especially hard for the family to cope.

Eye problems may include loss of the corneal reflex, periorbital bruising and edema, and diplopia.

- Loss of the corneal reflex may require administering lubricating eye drops or taping the eyes shut to prevent abrasion. Periorbital ecchymosis and edema disappear spontaneously, but cold and, later, warm compresses provide comfort and hasten the process. Diplopia can be relieved by use of an eye patch.

Hyperthermia can result in increased metabolism, cerebral blood flow, cerebral blood volume, and ICP. Increased metabolic waste also produces further cerebral vasodilation. Maintain the patient's body temperature at 36–37°C.

Rehabilitation. Once stabilized, the patient is usually transferred for acute rehabilitation. There may be chronic problems related to motor and sensory deficits, communication, memory, and intellectual functioning.

- Outward appearance is not a good indicator of how well the patient will function in the home or work environment, given recovery time and rehabilitation.
- The mental and emotional sequelae are often the most incapacitating problems. Many patients who have been comatose for more than 6h undergo some personality change. The patient's

behavior may indicate a loss of social restraint, judgment, tact, and emotional control.

Progressive recovery may continue for years. Nursing management depends on specific residual deficits. The family needs to understand what is happening and be taught appropriate interaction patterns.

- The family often has unrealistic expectations for the patient's full return to pretrauma status as the coma begins to recede. In reality, the patient usually has reduced awareness and ability to interpret stimuli.
- Prepare the family for the emergence of the patient from coma and explain that the process of awakening often takes several weeks. Arrange for social work and chaplain consultations for the family, in addition to providing open visitation and frequent status updates.
- Family members, particularly spouses, go through role transition to that of caregiver.

HEADACHE

Description

Headache is probably the most common type of pain. Most people have functional headaches, such as migraine or tension-type headaches. Others have organic headaches caused by intracranial or extracranial disease. A person may have more than one type of headache.

- *Primary headaches* include tension-type, migraine, and cluster headaches. They are not caused by a disease or another condition. Characteristics and management of tension-type, migraine, and cluster headaches are shown in Table 39.
- *Secondary headaches* are caused by another condition or disorder, such as sinus infection, neck injury, or brain tumor.

Nursing Interventions

Difficulty coping with daily stresses can cause headaches. Help the patient examine the daily routine, recognize stressful situations and factors that precipitate headache, and develop more effective coping strategies.

- Encourage a consistent daily routine with adequate sleep and regular well-balanced meals. Encourage daily exercise, relaxation periods, and socialization as ways to decrease headaches.
- Suggest meditation, yoga, biofeedback, and other ways to reduce stress and address headache pain.
- Encourage the patient with migraines to seek a quiet, dimly lit environment. Massage and cool or hot packs or cool packs to the neck and head can help.

H

TABLE 39   Interprofessional Care: Headaches

Tension-type headaches	Migraine headache	Cluster headache
Location		
Bilateral, band-like pressure at base of skull	Unilateral in 60%, may switch sides; often anterior location	Unilateral, radiating up or down from one eye
Quality		
Constant, squeezing, tightness	Throbbing, synchronous with pulse	Severe, bone crushing
Frequency		
Cycles for many years	Periodic, cycles of several months and years	May have months or years between attacks. Attacks occur in clusters over a period of 2–12 weeks
Duration		
30 min–7 days	4–72 h	5 min–3 h
Time and mode of onset		
Not related to time	May be preceded by prodromal symptoms or aura. Onset after awakening. Improves with sleep	Nocturnal, often awakens person from sleep
Associated symptoms		
Palpable neck and shoulder muscle tension. Stiff neck. Tenderness	Aura: Visual, sensory, aphasic. Irritability, sweating. Nausea, vomiting. Photophobia. Phonophobia. Prodromal symptoms: Sensory, motor, or psychic phenomena	Facial flushing or pallor. Unilateral lacrimation, ptosis, rhinitis

TABLE 39 Interprofessional Care: Headaches—cont'd

Tension-type headaches	Migraine headache	Cluster headache
Treatment: Abortive and symptomatic drugs		
Nonopioid analgesics: Aspirin, acetaminophen, NSAIDS 　Analgesic combinations 　　Butalbital/ acetaminophen/ caffeine 　　Butalbital/aspirin/ caffeine (Fiorinal) Muscle relaxants	α-Adrenergic blockers 　Ergotamine 　Dihydroergotamine NSAIDs Serotonin receptor agonists 　Almotriptan 　Eletriptan (Relpax) 　Frovatriptan (Frova) 　Naratriptan (Amerge) 　Rizatriptan (Maxalt) 　Sumatriptan (Imitrex) 　Zolmitriptan (Zomig) Combination 　Acetaminophen/ caffeine/aspirin 　Sumatriptan/naproxen (Treximet) CGRP antagonists Lasmiditan (Reyvow)	α-Adrenergic blockers Serotonin receptor agonists 　Almotriptan 　Eletriptan 　Frovatriptan 　Naratriptan 　Rizatriptan 　Sumatriptan 　Zolmitriptan High-flow 100% O_2
Treatment: Preventive		
Antiseizure drugs 　Topiramate (Topamax) 　Divalproex (Depakote) β-Adrenergic blockers Botulinum toxin A Mirtazapine (Remeron) Muscle relaxation training selective serotonin reuptake inhibitors 　Fluoxetine (Prozac) 　Paroxetine (Paxil) Tricyclic antidepressants 　Amitriptyline 　Doxepin 　Nortriptyline	Antiseizure drugs β-Adrenergic blockers Botulinum toxin A CGRP antagonists Tricyclic antidepressants	α-Adrenergic blockers 　Ergotamine tartrate Antiseizure drugs 　Gabapentin 　Topiramate Corticosteroids CGRP antagonists Lithium Verapamil

H

NSAIDs, Nonsteroidal antiinflammatory drugs.

- Massage and moist hot packs to the neck and head can help a patient with tension-type headaches.

▼ **Patient and Caregiver Teaching**

A teaching guide for the patient with a headache is provided in Table 40.

TABLE 40   Patient and Caregiver Teaching: Headaches

Include the following instructions when teaching the patient with headaches and the patient's caregiver.

1. Keep a diary or calendar of headaches and possible precipitating events.
2. Avoid possible headache triggers:
   Drugs such as ergot-containing preparations (ergotamine tartrate) and monoamine oxidase inhibitors
   Fatigue
   Foods
   - Alcohol (especially red wine)
   - Amines (cheese, chocolate)
   - Aspartame
   - Caffeine
   - Fermented or marinated foods, vinegar
   - Ice cream
   - Monosodium glutamate
   - Nitrites (meats, such as hot dogs)
   - Onions
   - Oranges
   - Tomatoes
   - Nicotine
3. Learn the purpose, action, dosage, and side effects of drugs taken.
4. Self-administer sumatriptan nasally or subcutaneously, if prescribed.
5. Use stress management techniques.
6. Take part in regular exercise.
7. Avoid smoking and exposure to environmental triggers, such as strong perfumes.
8. Contact HCP if any of the following occur:
   - Symptoms become more severe, last longer than usual, or are resistant to medication
   - Nausea and vomiting (if severe or not typical), change in vision, or fever occurs with the headache
   - Problems occur with any drugs

HEART FAILURE

Description

Heart failure (HF) is a complex clinical syndrome in response to myocardial insult. HF results in the inability to meet the oxygen (O_2) needs of tissues and organs. Decreased cardiac output (CO) leads to decreased tissue perfusion, impaired gas exchange, fluid volume imbalance, and decreased functional ability. The percentage of the total blood volume in the left ventricle (LV) at the end of diastole that is pumped out of the LV with the next systole is called *the left ventricular ejection fraction* (LVEF). Normal LVEF is 55%–65%. HF manifestations occur because of a defect in either ventricular systolic function/LV contraction (*heart failure with reduced ejection fraction* [HFrEF]) or a defect in ventricular diastolic function/filling (*heart failure with preserved ejection fraction* [HFpEF]).

HF is associated with diseases such as hypertension (HTN), coronary artery disease (CAD), and myocardial infarction (MI). HF is increasing in incidence and prevalence because of better survival after cardiac events and the aging population. HF is primarily a disease of older adults. The incidence is similar in men and women.

- HTN and CAD are the primary risk factors for HF. HTN is a modifiable risk factor that should be aggressively treated and managed. Long-term treatment of HTN reduces the incidence of HF by 50%.
- Comorbidities such as diabetes, metabolic syndrome, advanced age, tobacco use, and vascular disease contribute to the development of HF.

Blacks and Hispanic Americans develop HF at an earlier age, are admitted to the hospital more often, and have higher mortality rates related to HF as compared to whites.

Pathophysiology

Any interference with the normal mechanisms regulating CO may cause HF. CO depends on: (1) preload, (2) afterload, (3) myocardial contractility, and (4) heart rate (HR). These factors affect stroke volume (SV), which is the amount of blood pumped per heartbeat. Thus the equation: $CO = SV \times HR$. Any changes in these factors can lead to decreased ventricular function and HF.

The major causes of HF are divided into two subgroups: primary causes and precipitating causes. Precipitating causes often increase the workload of the heart, resulting in an acute condition and decreased heart function. See the complete listing of causes in Tables 38.1 and 38.2, Harding et al., *Lewis' Medical-Surgical Nursing*, ed. 12.

H

Left-Sided Heart Failure

The most common form of HF, left-sided HF, results either from the inability of the LV to empty adequately during systole or fill adequately during diastole. Left-sided HF can be further classified as HFrEF (systolic HF), HFpEF (diastolic HF), or a combination of the two.

Heart Failure With Reduced Ejection Fraction (Systolic Failure).

HFrEF results from an inability of the heart to pump blood effectively. Patients with HFrEF generally have an LVEF < 40%. It can be as low as 5%–10%.

- HFrEF is caused by impaired contractility (e.g., MI), increased afterload (e.g., HTN), cardiomyopathy, and mechanical problems (e.g., valvular disorders).

The LV in HFrEF loses the ability to generate enough pressure to eject blood forward through the aorta. Over time, the LV becomes dilated and hypertrophied. The weakened heart muscle cannot generate adequate stroke volume, which impairs CO. Because the LV cannot effectively push blood forward, end-diastolic volumes and pressures in the LV increase. When the LV fails, blood backs up into the left atrium (LA). This causes fluid accumulation in the lungs. The increased pulmonary hydrostatic pressure causes fluid leakage from the pulmonary capillary bed into the interstitium and then the alveoli. This results in pulmonary congestion and edema.

Heart Failure With Preserved Ejection Fraction (Diastolic Failure).

HFpEF results from the inability of the ventricles to relax and fill during diastole. About 50% of patients with HF have HFpEF. In HFpEF, the LV is stiff and noncompliant, causing high filling pressures. Decreased filling of the ventricles results in decreased SV. The eventual result of HFpEF is the same as that of HFrEF, a reduced CO leading to fluid congestion.

- HTN is the primary cause of HFpEF. Other risk factors include older age, female gender, diabetes, and obesity.
- The diagnosis of HFpEF is based on: (1) signs and symptoms of HF, (2) normal LVEF, and (3) evidence of LV diastolic dysfunction by echocardiography or cardiac catheterization.

Right-Sided Heart Failure

Right-sided HF occurs when the right ventricle (RV) does not pump effectively. When the RV fails, fluid backs up into the venous system. This causes movement of fluid into the tissues and organs (e.g., peripheral edema, abdominal ascites, hepatomegaly, jugular venous distention [JVD]).

The most common cause of right-sided HF is left-sided HF. As the LV fails, fluid backs up into the pulmonary system, increasing pressures in the lungs. The RV must work harder to push blood to the pulmonary system, and over time, the RV gradually fails. Other causes of right-sided HF (independent of the function of the LV) include RV infarction, pulmonary embolism, and cor pulmonale (RV dilation and hypertrophy caused by pulmonary disease).

Biventricular Failure

Biventricular failure includes both right and left ventricular dysfunction. Decreased contractility leads to fluid build-up and systemic venous engorgement. Inadequate CO decreases perfusion to vital organs.

Clinical Manifestations

Acute Decompensated Heart Failure

Acute decompensated HF (ADHF) is an increase (usually sudden) in symptoms of HF with a decrease in functional status, often requiring rapid escalation of therapy and hospital admission. ADHF is the most common cause of hospitalization for older Americans.

The clinical presentation of ADHF typically includes symptoms and signs related to pulmonary congestion and volume overload. ADHF can manifest as *pulmonary edema,* an acute, life-threatening situation in which the lung alveoli become filled with fluid. The most common cause of pulmonary edema is acute LV failure secondary to CAD.

- Manifestations of pulmonary edema include acute manifestations of left HF, such as dyspnea, respiratory rate >30 breaths/min, orthopnea, and paroxysmal nocturnal dyspnea (PND).
- JVD is the most sensitive and specific sign for elevated LV filling pressures.
- Auscultation of the lungs may reveal crackles and wheezes. Coughing may produce frothy, blood-tinged sputum.
- The patient's HR is often rapid. An abnormal S3 or S4 heart sound may be heard.
- BP may be high or low. Hypotension indicates severe LV systolic dysfunction and possible cardiogenic shock.

Chronic Heart Failure

Chronic HF is a progressive syndrome of reduced CO and increased venous pressure associated with the death of cardiac muscle cells. Neurohormonal and hemodynamic mechanisms to compensate for reduced CO include vasoconstriction and sympathetic nervous system (SNS) stimulation, an inflammatory response involving cytokines, and ventricular remodeling. These physiologic responses are responsible for the clinical manifestations of chronic HF. Table 41 lists manifestations of left-sided and right-sided chronic HF. The patient with chronic HF usually has manifestations of biventricular failure.

- Fatigue after usual daily activities is one of the earliest symptoms.

H

TABLE 41   Manifestations of Heart Failure

	Right-sided failure	Left-sided failure
Signs	• RV heaves • ↑ HR • Murmurs • Jugular venous distention • Edema (e.g., pedal, scrotum, sacrum) • Weight gain • Ascites • Anasarca (massive generalized body edema) • Hepatomegaly (liver enlargement)	• LV heaves • ↑ HR • Pulsus alternans (alternating pulses: strong, weak) • PMI displaced inferiorly and posteriorly (LV hypertrophy) • ↓ PaO_2, slight ↑ $PaCO_2$ (poor O_2 exchange) • Crackles (pulmonary edema) • S_3 and S_4 heart sounds • Pleural effusion • Changes in mental status • Restlessness, confusion • Shallow, rapid respirations • Dry, hacking cough • Frothy, pink-tinged sputum (advanced pulmonary edema)
Symptoms	• Anorexia and GI bloating • Anxiety, depression • Fatigue • Nausea • Right upper quadrant pain	• Anxiety, depression • Dyspnea • Fatigue, weakness • Nocturia • Orthopnea • Paroxysmal nocturnal dyspnea

GI, Gastrointestinal; *HR,* heart rate; *LV,* left ventricular; *PaCO₂,* partial pressure of CO_2 in arterial blood; *PaO₂,* partial pressure of O_2 in arterial blood; *PMI,* point of maximal impulse; *RV,* right ventricular.

- Dyspnea is common. Shortness of breath occurs when lying down (orthopnea).
- PND occurs when the patient is asleep. The patient awakens in a panic, has feelings of suffocation, and has a strong desire to sit or stand up.
- A dry, nonproductive cough may be an early sign.
- Other common signs include tachycardia; edema in the legs, liver, abdominal cavity, and lungs; nocturia; dusky skin; restlessness and confusion; chest pain; and weight changes.

Complications

- Pleural effusion results from increasing pressure in the pleural capillaries.
- Atrial fibrillation or ventricular dysrhythmias caused by enlargement of the heart chambers.
- Hepatomcgaly, impaired liver function, and cirrhosis can develop as the liver becomes congested with venous blood.
- Decreased perfusion to the kidneys can lead to anemia, renal insufficiency, or renal failure.

Diagnostic Studies

Diagnosing HF is often difficult because signs and symptoms mimic other medical conditions (e.g., anemia, lung disease). Diagnostic tests for ADHF and chronic HF are presented in Table 42.

A primary goal is to determine the cause of HF. An endomyocardial biopsy (EMB) may be done for unexplained, new-onset HF unresponsive to usual care. An echocardiogram provides information on the EF, which helps distinguish between HFpEF and HFrEF. In general, b-type natriuretic peptide (BNP) and N-terminal prohormone of BNP (NT-proBNP) levels correlate positively with the degree of LV failure.

Interprofessional and Nursing Management Acute Decompensated Heart Failure

Patients with ADHF need continuous monitoring and assessment. Stable patients may be managed in an emergency department or telemetry unit. Unstable patients are managed in an intensive care unit (ICU). In addition to continuous ECG and O_2 saturation monitoring, vital signs and urine output are assessed at least hourly. The patient may have continuous hemodynamic monitoring. Supplemental O_2 helps increase the percentage of O_2 in inspired air. In severe pulmonary edema, the patient may need noninvasive ventilatory support or intubation and mechanical ventilation. Table 42 summarizes interprofessional care of the patient with ADHF.

- Position the patient who has dyspnea in a high Fowler's position with the feet horizontal in the bed or dangling at the bedside. This position helps decrease venous return by pooling blood in the extremities and increases the thoracic capacity for improved breathing.
- Ultrafiltration can rapidly remove intravascular fluid volume while maintaining hemodynamic stability.

Circulatory assist devices are used to manage patients with worsening HF.

H

TABLE 42 Interprofessional Care: Heart Failure

Both ADHF and chronic HF	ADHF	Chronic HF
Diagnostic Assessment		
• History and physical assessment	• Measure LV function	• Cardiopulmonary exercise stress test
• Determine underlying cause	• Hemodynamic monitoring	• 6-minute walk test
• Serum chemistry panel, cardiac markers, BNP or NT-proBNP level, liver function tests, thyroid function tests, CBC, lipid profile, kidney function tests, urinalysis	• Endomyocardial biopsy in select patients	• Sleep studies in select patients
• Chest X-ray		
• 12-lead ECG		
• Two-dimensional echocardiogram		
• Nuclear imaging		
• Cardiac catheterization		

Management

- Treatment of underlying cause
- Drug therapy
- Circulatory assist devices (e.g., ventricular assist device)
- Daily weights
- O_2 by mask or nasal cannula if indicated
- Sodium- and possibly fluid-restricted diet
- High Fowler's position
- Noninvasive positive pressure ventilation
- Circulatory assist device: IABP, ECMO, LVAD
- Endotracheal intubation and mechanical ventilation
- Vital signs, urine output at least q1hr
- Continuous ECG and pulse oximetry monitoring
- Hemodynamic monitoring (e.g., intraarterial BP, PAWP, CO)
- Cardioversion (e.g., atrial fibrillation)
- Ultrafiltration
- Cardiac resynchronization therapy with biventricular pacing and implantable cardioverter-defibrillator (ICD)
- Heart transplantation
- Rest-activity periods
- Dietitian consult
- Physical/occupational therapy consult
- Cardiac rehabilitation
- Home health nursing care (e.g., telehealth monitoring)
- Palliative and end-of-life care

ADHF, Acute decompensated heart failure; *BNP,* b-type natriuretic peptide; *CBC,* complete blood count; *CO,* cardiac output; *ECMO,* extracorporeal membrane oxygenation; *ECG,* electrocardiogram; *HF,* heart failure; *LV,* left ventricular; *LVAD,* LV assist device; *NT-proBNP,* N-terminal prohormone of BNP; *PAWP,* pulmonary artery wedge pressure.

H

- The intraaortic balloon pump (IABP) increases coronary blood flow to the heart muscle and decreases the heart's workload.
- Ventricular assist devices (VADs) can be used to maintain the pumping action of the heart.
- Extracorporeal membrane oxygenation (ECMO) can offer short-term mechanical circulatory support for refractory HF and cardiogenic shock or as a bridge to heart transplant.

Drug Therapy

Drug therapy is essential in treating acute HF.

- *Diuretics.* Diuretics are the first line for treating patients with volume overload. They decrease sodium reabsorption in the kidneys, enhancing sodium and water loss. Decreasing intravascular volume reduces fluid returning to the LV (preload). This allows for more efficient LV pumping, decreased pulmonary vascular pressures, and improved alveolar gas exchange. IV administration of loop diuretics (e.g., furosemide) by bolus or infusion is preferred. Increased urine output, decreased symptoms, and fluid weight loss indicate effective diuretic therapy. Serum potassium and magnesium levels are continually monitored.
- *Vasodilators.* Patients with ADHF who are not hypotensive are treated with vasodilators. IV nitroglycerin is a primary venodilator that reduces blood return to the right side of the heart. It also improves coronary artery blood flow by dilating the coronary arteries. So, nitroglycerin reduces preload, slightly reduces afterload (in high doses), and increases myocardial O_2 supply. Sodium nitroprusside reduces both preload and afterload, thereby improving myocardial contraction, increasing CO, and reducing pulmonary congestion. IV nesiritide, a recombinant form of BNP, causes both arterial and venous dilation.
- *Morphine.* Morphine dilates pulmonary and systemic blood vessels, reducing preload and afterload. It is often given in small IV boluses to relieve dyspnea associated with ADHF. Monitor the patient closely. Morphine has serious adverse effects, including respiratory depression, which can require mechanical ventilation.
- *Positive inotropics.* Inotropic drugs increase myocardial contractility and are used for patients with evidence of cardiogenic shock or with low CO. Drugs include β-agonists (e.g., dopamine, dobutamine, norepinephrine [Levophed]) and phosphodiesterase inhibitors (milrinone) and digitalis. The β-agonists are used as a short-term treatment of ADHF. In addition to increasing myocardial contractility and systemic vascular resistance (SVR), dopamine dilates the renal blood vessels and enhances urine output. Unlike dopamine, dobutamine is a selective β-agonist that works mainly on the β1-receptors in the heart and

does not increase SVR. Improved CO, BP, urine output, and reduced filling pressures indicate effective inotrope therapy.

Interprofessional Management Chronic Heart Failure

The goals of chronic HF therapies include optimal symptom management; mortality and morbidity benefit; minimizing side effects; and monitoring responses to therapies. Specifically, these therapies treat the underlying cause and contributing factors, maximize CO, improve ventricular function, improve quality of life, and preserve target organ function.

Nondrug Therapy

Supplemental O_2 to meet tissue O_2 needs helps relieve patient dyspnea and fatigue. Physical and emotional rest conserves energy and decreases O_2 needs. A patient with severe HF may be on bed rest with limited activity. A patient with mild to moderate HF can be ambulatory with a restriction of strenuous activity.

Having normal simultaneous electrical conduction (synchrony) in the right and left ventricles increases left ventricular function and CO.

- Patients with an LVEF <35% may be candidates for an *implantable cardioverter-defibrillator* (ICD), recommended for primary prevention of sudden cardiac death.
- *Cardiac resynchronization therapy* (CRT) may be used to coordinate right and left ventricular contractility through biventricular pacing.

Implanted ICD and CRT devices can also be used for remotely monitoring HF patients. Other mechanical assist devices are available to sustain HF patients with deteriorating function and those awaiting cardiac transplant.

Drug Therapy

The cornerstone of drug therapy in chronic HF is neurohormonal blockade. The results of neurohormonal blockade include decreased plasma aldosterone levels, decreased SNS activity, vasodilation, and sodium and water excretion.

- *Angiotensin-converting enzyme (ACE) inhibitors.* ACE inhibitors (e.g., captopril, enalapril) are first-line drugs to decrease mortality, morbidity, hospitalizations, and symptoms in patients with HFrEF. ACE inhibitors block the renin-angiotensin-aldosterone system (RAAS) by inhibiting the conversion of angiotensin I to angiotensin II. They reduce afterload and SVR and slow ventricular remodeling by inhibiting ventricular hypertrophy.
- *Angiotensin II receptor blockers* (ARBs). For patients who are unable to tolerate ACE inhibitors, ARBs are recommended. They prevent the vasoconstrictor and aldosterone-secreting effects of angiotensin II by binding to the angiotensin II receptor sites. ARBs promote afterload reduction and vasodilation.

H

- *Neprilysin-angiotensin receptor inhibitors.* Sacubitril/valsartan (Entresto) is a combination of a neprilysin inhibitor (sacubitril) and an ARB (valsartan). This drug provides dual blockade of the RAAS and the natriuretic peptide system. Sacubitril, a recombinant form of BNP, inhibits neprilysin, an enzyme that degrades natriuretic peptides. Sacubitril inhibition allows for more available circulating BNP. This results in decreased SVR, afterload, and central venous pressure (CVP), and increased natriuresis and diuresis. This drug is an alternative to ACE inhibitors and ARBs in patients meeting criteria with symptomatic HFrEF.
- *Aldosterone antagonists.* Spironolactone (Aldactone) and eplerenone (Inspra) are potassium-sparing diuretics that inhibit aldosterone activation. These drugs bind to receptors at the aldosterone-dependent sodium–potassium exchange site in the distal renal tubule where they have a mild diuretic effect. Carefully monitor serum potassium levels and renal function.
- *Nitrates.* Nitrates (e.g., nitroglycerin) cause vasodilation by acting directly on the smooth muscle of the vessel wall. Nitrates are of particular benefit in the management of myocardial ischemia related to HF because they promote vasodilation of the coronary arteries.
- *β-Adrenergic blockers.* β-Blockers directly block the negative effects of the SNS (e.g., increased HR) on the failing heart. Three β-blockers have been shown to decrease mortality in patients with HFrEF: metoprolol succinate (Toprol XL), bisoprolol (Zebeta), and carvedilol (Coreg). They may also increase LVEF. However, because β-blockers can reduce myocardial contractility, care must be taken in patients with volume overload. They are usually started at low dose. Major side effects include worsening of HF symptoms, hypotension, fatigue, and bradycardia.
- *Hydralazine/isosorbide dinitrate combination (Bidil).* A fixed combination of the vasodilators hydralazine and isosorbide dinitrate can reduce mortality and improve LVEF and exercise tolerance. The drug is specifically effective in blacks with HFrEF already receiving optimal doses of other medications.
- *Digitalis.* Digitalis (digoxin), a weak positive inotrope, acts primarily as a neurohormonal modulator that reduces the effects of the SNS and suppresses renin secretion from the kidneys. Better outcomes occur with digoxin serum levels of <0.9 ng/mL. Higher levels are associated with increased mortality and digoxin toxicity. Monitor renal function and serum potassium levels
- *Sodium-glucose cotransporter-2 (SGLT-2) inhibitor.* Dapagliflozin (Farxiga) reduces the risk of CV death and hospitalization for patients with HFrEF. This medication was developed to treat type 2 diabetes by stopping absorption of extra glucose

from the urine. The drug's effects in HF appear to be related to the unique osmotic diuretic properties. Side effects include dehydration and serious urinary tract and yeast infections. Monitor volume status and kidney function.

■ *Diuretics.* Diuretics reduce edema, pulmonary venous pressure, and preload. In chronic HF, the lowest effective dose of diuretic should be used. Thiazide diuretics (e.g., hydrochlorothiazide) inhibit sodium reabsorption in the distal tubule, thus promoting excretion of sodium and water. Loop diuretics, such as furosemide (Lasix), bumetanide (Bumex), and torsemide (Demadex), are potent but can cause hypokalemia and ototoxicity.

Nutritional Therapy

Diet and weight management are essential to the patient's control of chronic HF. Take a detailed diet history to determine what foods the patient eats and also when, where, and how often the person dines out.

■ Excess sodium may worsen HF symptoms. The degree of sodium restriction depends on the severity of the HF and the effectiveness of diuretic therapy.

■ Sodium intake is usually restricted to 2 gms per day. Teach the patient which foods are low and high in sodium content and how to read labels. Teach ways to enhance food flavors without the use of salt (e.g., adding lemon juice, spices).

Fluid restrictions are not often prescribed for the patient with mild to moderate HF. However, fluid restrictions may be needed for stage D HF patients with persistent fluid retention despite appropriate sodium restriction.

■ Teach patients to weigh themselves at the same time each day, preferably before breakfast, while wearing the same type of clothing. Tell patients to call the healthcare provider (HCP) about a weight gain of 3 lb (1.4 kg) over 2 days or a 3–5-lb (2.3-kg) gain over a week.

Nursing Management: Chronic Heart Failure

Goals

Nursing care focuses on the priority problems of decreased CO, impaired oxygenation, fluid overload, intolerance of physical activity, and managing a complex medication regimen. The overall goals for the patient with HF include: (1) decrease in symptoms (e.g., shortness of breath, fatigue), (2) decrease in peripheral edema, (3) increase in exercise tolerance, (4) adherence with the treatment plan, including appropriate evidence-based medication and device therapies, and (5) no complications related to HF.

See care of the patient with HF in the eNursing Care Plan 34-1 on the website.

Interventions

Help aggressively identify and treat risk factors for HF to prevent or slow the disease progression. Recommended lifestyle modifications begin with weight management, diet, and regular exercise. Often, medications are needed. For example, teach the patient with HTN or hyperlipidemia measures to manage BP or cholesterol with medication, diet, and exercise. Patients with valve disease contributing to HF should be evaluated for valve repair or replacement.

Acute Care. Many people with HF will experience one or more episodes of ADHF. Successful HF care depends on several important principles: (1) HF is a progressive disease; (2) treatment plans are established with QOL goals; (3) symptom management depends heavily on adherence to self-management protocols (e.g., daily weights, diet, exercise, recognizing signs and symptoms of decompensation) and evidence-based therapy (EBT) regimens (drug and device therapies); (4) precipitating factors, etiologies, and contributing comorbid conditions must be addressed; (5) complex care needs often require care in multiple settings, increasing risk for fragmented care; and (6) support systems are essential to the success of the entire treatment plan.

Ambulatory Care. HF is a chronic and progressive condition that will require lifelong therapies. Intensive disease management programs that include extensive patient education on self-management and exercise and close home surveillance follow-up by nurses can reduce short-term readmission rates in the highest-risk patients.

- Assess patients with HF for depression and anxiety. Anxiety may increase the SNS response and increase myocardial workload. Reducing anxiety may be facilitated by a variety of nursing interventions and the use of sedatives (e.g., benzodiazepines, morphine sulfate).
- Exercise training for patients with HF, such as in a cardiac rehabilitation program, has been found to be safe, to improve overall sense of well-being, and has been associated with reduced mortality.

End-Stage Heart Failure Therapy. One in five persons with HF dies within a year of diagnosis. Repeated hospitalizations and ED visits for ADHF predict end-stage HF.

- Therapeutic options for stage D (end stage) HF patients include chronic inotropic therapy, mechanical circulatory support (MCS) devices, palliative care and hospice (with or without ICD deactivation), and heart transplant. Patients who are not eligible for heart transplant may be candidates for lifelong MCS. Morbidity and mortality are significantly reduced if MCS is started before onset of severe right HF and systemic organ failure.
- End-of-life discussions and management include advanced directives and information about advanced HF therapies (e.g., VADs, heart transplants), palliative care, and hospice.

A patient and caregiver teaching guide for HF is presented in Table 43.

TABLE 43 Patient and Caregiver Teaching: Heart Failure

Include the following instructions when teaching the patient and caregiver about the management of heart failure.

Diet therapy

- Consult the diet plan and list of permitted and restricted foods.
- Adhere to specific sodium restriction guidelines outlined by your healthcare provider (HCP).
- Read the labels to determine sodium content. Check the labels of over-the-counter drugs, such as laxatives, cough medicines, and antacids, for sodium content.
- Avoid using salt when preparing foods or adding salt to foods.
- Weigh yourself at the same time each day, preferably in the morning, using the same scale and wearing similar clothes.
- Eat small, frequent meals.

Activity program

- Increase walking and other activities gradually, provided that they do not cause fatigue or dyspnea.
- Consider a cardiac rehabilitation program.
- Avoid extremes of heat and cold.

Ongoing monitoring

- Know the signs and symptoms of worsening heart failure including dyspnea, cough, orthopnea, PND, weight gain, edema, fluid retention, fatigue, and tiredness with physical activity.
- Recall the symptoms when illness began. Reappearance of previous symptoms may indicate a recurrence.
- Report any of the following to the HCP at once:
  - weight gain of 3 lb (1.4 kg) in 2 days, or 3–5 lb (1.4–2.3 kg) in a week
  - difficulty breathing, especially with activity or when lying flat
  - waking up breathless at night
  - frequent dry, hacking cough, especially when lying down
  - fatigue, weakness
  - swelling of ankles, feet, or abdomen. Swelling of face or difficulty breathing (if taking ACE inhibitors)
  - nausea with abdominal swelling, pain, and tenderness
  - dizziness or fainting
- Follow up with HCP on a regular basis.
- Consider joining a local support group with your family members and caregivers.

H

Continued

TABLE 43   Patient and Caregiver Teaching: Heart Failure—cont'd

Health promotion

- Obtain annual influenza vaccination.
- Obtain pneumococcal vaccination.
- Develop plan to reduce risk factors (e.g., BP control, tobacco cessation, blood sugar/HGA1C control, weight reduction).

Rest

- Plan a regular daily rest and activity program.
- After exertion, such as exercise and ADLs, plan a rest period.
- Shorten working hours, or schedule a rest period during working hours.
- Avoid emotional upsets. Share any concerns, fears, feelings of depression, etc., with HCP.

Drug therapy

- Take each drug as prescribed.
- Develop a system (e.g., daily chart, weekly pillbox) to ensure that drugs have been taken.
- Count heart rate each day before taking drugs (if appropriate). Know the limits that your HCP wants for your heart rate.
- Take BP at determined intervals (if appropriate). Know your target BP limits.
- Know signs and symptoms of orthostatic hypotension and how to prevent them
- If taking anticoagulants, know signs and symptoms of internal bleeding (bleeding gums, increased bruises, blood in stool or urine) and actions to take.
- If taking warfarin (Coumadin), know INR results, target INR level, and how often to have INR checked.

ACE, Angiotensin-converting enzyme; *ADLS,* activities of daily living; *INR,* international normalized ratio; *PND,* paroxysmal nocturnal dyspnea.

HEMOPHILIA AND VON WILLEBRAND DISEASE

Description

Hemophilia is an X-linked recessive genetic disorder caused by a defective or deficient coagulation factor. The two major types of hemophilia that can occur in mild to severe forms are *hemophilia A* (classic hemophilia, factor VIII deficiency) and *hemophilia B* (Christmas disease, factor IX deficiency). *von Willebrand disease* is a related disorder involving a deficiency of the von Willebrand coagulation protein.

Hemophilia A is four times as common as hemophilia B. There are rare cases of acquired hemophilia A, which is caused by the development of antibodies against the body's own factor VIII. von Willebrand disease is the most common congenital bleeding disorder in humans.

Deficiency and inheritance patterns of these three forms of inherited coagulopathy are compared in Table 44.

TABLE 44	Types of Hemophilia	
Type	**Defect/deficiency**	**Inheritance pattern**
Hemophilia A	Factor VIII deficiency	Recessive sex-linked (transmitted by female carriers, displayed almost exclusively in men)
Hemophilia B	Factor IX deficiency	Recessive sex-linked (transmitted by female carriers, displayed almost exclusively in men)
von Willebrand disease	vWF, variable factor VIII deficiencies; platelet dysfunction	Autosomal dominant, seen in both genders Recessive (in severe forms of the disease)

vWF, von Willebrand factor.

Clinical Manifestations and Complications

Clinical manifestations and complications related to hemophilia include slow, persistent, prolonged bleeding from minor trauma and small cuts; delayed bleeding after minor injuries (the delay may be several hours or days); uncontrollable hemorrhage after dental extractions or irritation of the gingiva with a hard-bristle toothbrush; prolonged epistaxis, especially after a blow to the face; gastrointestinal (GI) bleeding from ulcers and gastritis; hematuria from genitourinary (GU) trauma and splenic rupture resulting from falls or abdominal trauma; ecchymoses, subcutaneous hematomas, and possible compartment syndrome. Neurologic signs such as pain, anesthesia, and paralysis may develop from nerve compression caused by hematoma formation, and hemarthrosis (bleeding into the joints) may lead to joint deformity severe enough to cause crippling (often in knees, elbows, shoulders, hips, and ankles).

Diagnostic Studies

Laboratory studies determine the type of hemophilia. Partial thromboplastin time is prolonged due to deficiency in intrinsic clotting system factor. Bleeding time is normal in hemophilia A and B but prolonged in von Willebrand disease due to structurally defective platelets.

Reductions in coagulation factors include factor VIII in hemophilia A, factor IX in hemophilia B, and vWF in von Willebrand disease.

Interprofessional Management

The goal of care is to prevent and treat bleeding. People with hemophilia or von Willebrand disease require preventive care, the use of replacement therapy during acute bleeding episodes and for prophylaxis, and treatment of complications of the disease and its therapy.

- Regular prophylaxis is preferred over on-demand treatment. The most common problem with acute management is starting factor replacement therapy too late and stopping it too soon. Minor bleeding episodes should be treated for at least 72 hours.
- The patient may need prophylactic replacement therapy before surgery and dental care.
- For mild hemophilia A or certain subtypes of von Willebrand disease, desmopressin acetate (DDAVP), a synthetic analog of vasopressin, may stimulate an increase in factor VIII.

Complications of treatment of hemophilia include development of inhibitors to factor VIII or IX, transfusion-transmitted infectious disorders, allergic reactions, and thrombotic complications with the use of factor IX because it contains activated coagulation factors. Eventually, a patient's development of inhibitors to the factor products requires individualized expert management.

Nursing Management

Because of the hereditary nature of hemophilia, refer affected people for genetic counseling.

Acute interventions are related to controlling the bleeding.

- Stop the topical bleeding as quickly as possible. Apply direct pressure or ice, pack the area with Gelfoam or fibrin foam, and apply topical hemostatic agents, like thrombin.
- Give the specific coagulation factor to raise the patient's level of the deficient coagulation factor. Monitor the patient for signs and symptoms of hypersensitivity.
- When joint bleeding occurs, in addition to giving replacement factors, it is important to use the "RICE" protocol. Rest the involved joint to prevent crippling deformities from hemarthrosis, ice the joint for 20 minutes every 3–4 hours, compress/wrap the joint, and elevate. Give analgesics to reduce severe pain. Do not use aspirin and aspirin-containing compounds. As soon as bleeding ceases, encourage mobilization of the affected area through range-of-motion exercises and physical therapy. Avoid weight bearing until all swelling has resolved and muscle strength has returned. Orthotics may be prescribed.
- Manage life-threatening complications that may develop because of hemorrhage. Examples are prevention or treatment of airway obstruction from hemorrhage into the neck and pharynx and early assessment and treatment of intracranial bleeding.

▼ Patient and Caregiver Teaching

Quality of life and survival are influenced by the patient's knowledge of the illness and how to manage it. Provide ongoing assessment of the patient's adaptation to the illness.

- Teach the patient with hemophilia to seek immediate medical attention for severe pain or swelling of a muscle or joint that restricts movement or inhibits sleep and for a head injury, swelling in the neck or mouth, abdominal pain, hematuria, melena, and skin wounds with continued bleeding.
- Teach the patient to perform daily oral hygiene without causing trauma.
- Advise the patient to only participate in noncontact sports (e.g., golf) and to wear gloves when doing household chores, to prevent cuts or abrasions from knives and other tools.

H

- The patient should wear a medical identification (Medic Alert) tag to ensure that healthcare providers (HCPs) know about the hemophilia in case of an accident.
- Refer the patient and caregiver to a local chapter of the National Hemophilia Foundation for additional information and support.
- Many patients or their caregivers can learn to self-administer the factor replacement therapies at home.

HEMORRHOIDS

Description

Hemorrhoids are abnormally dilated veins that may be internal (occurring above the internal sphincter) or external (occurring outside the external sphincter).

Pathophysiology

Hemorrhoids are thought to develop because of increased anal pressure and weakening of the connective tissue that supports the hemorrhoidal veins. Weakened supporting tissue allows for downward displacement of the hemorrhoidal veins, causing them to dilate. An intravascular clot in the venule results in a *thrombosed* external hemorrhoid.

Hemorrhoids are the most common reason for bleeding with defecation. They may be precipitated by pregnancy, obesity, constipation, diarrhea, straining to defecate, heavy lifting, prolonged standing and sitting, and ascites.

Clinical Manifestations

Classic findings include painless bright red bleeding, anal pruritus, prolapse, and pain.

- *Internal hemorrhoids* cause pain if they become constricted. Internal hemorrhoids can prolapse into the anal canal or externally, causing a sense of pressure with defecation and a protruding mass.
- *External hemorrhoids* are reddish blue and seldom bleed. There may be itching, burning, and edema. They cause pain and inflammation when a thrombosis (blood clot) is present. Thrombosed hemorrhoids are bluish purple masses palpable at the anal orifice. The clot can erode through the overlying stretched skin, causing bleeding with defecation. Constipation or diarrhea can worsen the symptoms.

Diagnostic Studies

- *Internal hemorrhoids* are diagnosed by digital examination, anoscopy, and sigmoidoscopy.
- *External hemorrhoids* can be diagnosed by visual inspection and digital examination.

Interprofessional Management

First-line therapy typically involves normalizing stool consistency by treating constipation or diarrhea. A high-fiber diet and increased fluid intake prevent constipation and reduce straining. Ointments, creams, suppositories, and pads containing anesthetics, corticosteroids, protectants, or antiseptics may shrink mucous membranes and relieve discomfort. Topical corticosteroids, such as hydrocortisone agents, should be limited to 1 week or less to prevent side effects such as contact dermatitis and mucosal atrophy. Stool softeners may ease defecation. Sitz baths and NSAIDs help relieve pain.

- Prolapsed or bleeding internal hemorrhoids or thrombosed external hemorrhoids may need medical treatment. For internal hemorrhoids, nonsurgical approaches (band ligation, infrared coagulation, cryotherapy, laser treatment) can be used.
- Surgery is needed when there is marked prolapse, excessive pain or bleeding, or large or multiple thrombosed hemorrhoids.

Nursing Management

Nursing care includes teaching measures to prevent constipation, avoiding prolonged standing or sitting, proper use of over-the-counter preparations, and instructions on when to seek medical care (e.g., excessive pain and bleeding, prolapsed hemorrhoids).

- Severe pain caused by sphincter spasm is common after a hemorrhoidectomy. Most patients initially receive an opioid and a nonsteroidal antiinflammatory drug (NSAID) in conjunction with topical preparations that provide anesthesia or reduce internal sphincter spasms, such as such as topical lidocaine, 2% diltiazem, and glyceryl trinitrate.
- Packing inserted into the rectum to absorb drainage is usually removed the first or second postoperative day. Provide privacy. Assess for rectal bleeding.
- Sitz baths are started 1 or 2 days after surgery. Initially, do not leave the patient alone because of the possibility of weakness or fainting.

H

- The patient usually dreads the first bowel movement and often resists the urge to defecate. Give pain medication before the bowel movement to reduce discomfort.
- Teach the importance of diet, sitz baths, symptoms of complications (especially bleeding), and avoiding constipation and straining.

HEPATITIS, VIRAL

Description

Hepatitis is an inflammation of the liver most often caused by viruses. The types of viral hepatitis are A, B, C, D, and E. The different types have similar manifestations. Their modes of transmission and disease course vary (Table 45). Other viruses known to damage the liver include cytomegalovirus, Epstein–Barr virus, herpesvirus, coxsackievirus, and rubella virus.

Hepatitis A

Hepatitis A is a self-limiting infection. It can cause a mild flu-like illness and jaundice. In more severe cases, it can cause acute liver failure. Hepatitis A virus (HAV) is a ribonucleic acid (RNA) virus. It is transmitted primarily through the fecal-oral route. It often occurs in small outbreaks caused by fecal contamination of food or drinking water.

Poor hygiene, improper food handling, homelessness, crowded situations, and poor sanitary conditions are risk factors.

- Hepatitis A vaccination and thorough hand washing are the best measures to prevent outbreaks.

Hepatitis B

Hepatitis B virus (HBV) is a blood-borne pathogen that can cause acute or chronic disease. HBV is a deoxyribonucleic acid (DNA) virus. It can be transmitted in several ways including perinatally to infants by mothers infected with HBV to their infants, percutaneously (e.g., IV drug use, accidental needlestick punctures), and via small cuts on mucosal surfaces and exposure to infectious blood, blood products, or other body fluids (e.g., semen, vaginal secretions, saliva).

- The incidence of HBV infection has decreased where there is widespread use of the HBV vaccine.

Hepatitis C

Infection with the hepatitis C virus (HCV) can result in both acute and chronic illness. HCV is a blood-borne RNA virus that is primarily transmitted percutaneously. The most common mode of transmission is the sharing of contaminated needles and equipment

TABLE 45 Characteristics of Hepatitis Viruses

Incubation period and mode of transmission	Sources of infection	Infectivity
Hepatitis A virus (HAV)		
Incubation: 15–50 days (average 28)	• Contaminated food, milk, water, shellfish	• most infectious during 2 wk before onset of symptoms
Fecal-oral (primarily fecal contamination and oral ingestion)	• Crowded conditions (e.g., day care, nursing home)	• infectious until 1–2 wk after the start of symptoms
	• Persons with subclinical infections, infected food handlers, sexual contact, IV drug users	
	• Poor personal hygiene	
	• Poor sanitation	
Hepatitis B virus (HBV)		
Incubation: 115–180 days (average 56–96 days)	• Contaminated needles, syringes, and blood products	• before and after symptoms appear
• Percutaneous (parenteral) or mucosal exposure to blood or blood products	• HBV-infected mother (perinatal transmission)	• infectious for months
• Sexual contact	• Sexual activity with infected partners.	• carriers continue to be infectious for life
• Perinatal transmission	• Asymptomatic carriers	
	• Tattoos or body piercing with contaminated needles	

Continued

H

TABLE 45 Characteristics of Hepatitis Viruses—cont'd

Incubation period and mode of transmission	Sources of infection	Infectivity
Hepatitis C virus (HCV) *Incubation:* 14–180 days (average 56 days) • Percutaneous (parenteral) or mucosal exposure to blood or blood products • High-risk sexual contact • Perinatal contact	• Blood and blood products • Needles and syringes • Sexual activity with infected partners, low risk	• 1–2 wk before symptoms appear • Continues during clinical course • 75%–85% go on to develop chronic HCV and remain infectious
Hepatitis D virus (HDV) *Incubation:* 2–26 wk • HBV must precede HDV • Chronic carriers of HBV always at risk	• Same as HBV • Can cause infection only when HBV is present	• Blood infectious at all stages of HDV infection
Hepatitis E virus (HEV) *Incubation:* 15–64 days (average 26–42 days) • Fecal-oral route	• Contaminated water, poor sanitation • Found in Asia, Africa, and Mexico • Not common in United States but is increasing in some areas	• Not known • May be similar to HAV

among injection IV drug users. High-risk sexual behavior especially among MSM is associated with increased risk of HCV.

- Hepatitis C is the most common cause of chronic liver disease and the most common indication for liver transplantation in the United States.

Hepatitis D

Hepatitis D virus (HDV), also called *delta virus,* cannot survive on its own and requires HBV to replicate. It can be acquired at the same time as HBV, or a person with HBV can be infected with HDV at a later time. HDV is transmitted percutaneously. HDV can cause a spectrum of illness ranging from an asymptomatic chronic carrier state to acute liver failure.

- There is no vaccine for HDV. However, vaccination against HBV reduces the risk of HDV coinfection.

Hepatitis E

Like hepatitis A, hepatitis E virus (HEV) is an RNA virus transmitted by the fecal-oral route. The usual mode of transmission is drinking contaminated water. HEV infection epidemics occur in the tropics, but it is widely circulating in the west. It is generally acute and self-resolving.

Pathophysiology

In viral hepatitis, hepatocytes become targets of the virus through direct action of the virus (as in HCV infection) or through a cell-mediated immune response to the virus (as in HBV and HCV infection). The destruction of hepatocytes leads to liver-related dysfunction in bile production, coagulation, blood glucose, and protein metabolism. Detoxification and processing of drugs, hormones, and metabolites may also be disrupted.

- Liver cells can regenerate and, if no complications occur, resume their normal appearance and function.
- Antigen–antibody complexes may form circulating immune complexes in the early phases of hepatitis and activate the complement system. Manifestations of this activation are rash, angioedema, arthritis, fever, and malaise.
- Chronic viral hepatitis can be insidious and silent, causing persistent and continual destruction of infected hepatocytes. Over time, scar tissue develops, leading to fibrosis, cirrhosis, and liver failure.

Clinical Manifestations

Many patients with acute hepatitis have no symptoms. Manifestations of viral hepatitis are classified into acute and chronic phases.

The *acute phase* usually lasts 1–6 months.

- During the incubation period, symptoms may include anorexia, lethargy, nausea, vomiting, skin rashes, diarrhea or constipation, malaise, fatigue, muscle pain, joint pain, other flu-like symptoms, and right upper quadrant tenderness.
- Physical examination may reveal hepatomegaly, lymphadenopathy, and sometimes splenomegaly. This is the period of maximal infectivity for hepatitis A.
- The acute phase may be *icteric* (jaundice) or anicteric. Jaundice, a yellowish discoloration of body tissues, results from a change in bilirubin metabolism or disrupted flow of bile into the hepatic or biliary duct systems. The urine may darken because of excess bilirubin excreted by the kidneys. If conjugated bilirubin cannot flow out of the liver because of bile duct obstruction, stools will be clay-colored. Pruritus, caused by bile salts beneath the skin, may result from cholestasis.
- Convalescence following the acute phase begins as jaundice is disappearing and lasts an average of 2–4 months. During this period, patients have malaise and fatigue.

In the *chronic phase,* patients may have malaise, fatigue, and hepatomegaly.

Complications

Complications of acute hepatitis include chronic hepatitis, cirrhosis, portal hypertension, and liver cancer. Sometimes, acute liver failure (fulminant hepatic failure) may occur with encephalopathy, coagulation problems, and jaundice. Liver transplantation is usually the cure for these patients.

Diagnostic Studies

The only definitive way to distinguish among the various types of viral hepatitis is by testing the patient's blood for the specific antigen or antibody. Table 46 presents the serologic tests for the different types of viral hepatitis. Liver function tests show significant abnormalities. Physical assessment may reveal hepatic tenderness, hepatomegaly, and splenomegaly. Noninvasive ultrasound assessment of liver fibrosis is increasingly replacing the need for liver biopsy.

Interprofessional Management

There is no specific treatment for acute viral hepatitis. Most patients are managed at home. Emphasis is on providing adequate nutrition and rest while the liver cells regenerate. The degree of rest depends on symptom severity.

TABLE 46   Diagnostic Tests for Viral Hepatitis

Virus	Tests	Significance
A (HAV)	HAV immunoglobulin M (IgM)	Acute infection
	HAV immunoglobulin G (IgG)	Previous infection or immunization Not routinely done in clinical practice
B (HBV)	HBsAg (hepatitis B surface antigen)	Marker of infectivity Present in acute or chronic infection Positive in chronic carriers
	Anti-HBs (hepatitis B surface antibody)	Indicates previous infection with HBV or immunization
	HBeAg (hepatitis B e antigen)	Indicates high infectivity Used to determine the clinical management of patients with chronic HBV
	Anti-HBe (hepatitis B e antibody)	Indicates previous infection In chronic HBV, indicates a low viral load and low degree of infectivity
	Anti-HBc (antibody to hepatitis B core antigen) IgM	Indicates acute infection Does not appear after vaccination
	Anti-HBc IgG	Indicates previous infection or ongoing infection with HBV Does not appear after vaccination
	HBV DNA quantitation	Indicates active ongoing viral replication Best indicator of viral replication and effectiveness of therapy in patient with chronic HBV
	HBV genotyping	Indicates the genotype of HBV
C (HCV)	Anti-HCV (antibody to HCV)	Marker for acute or chronic infection with HCV
	HCV RNA quantitation	Indicates active ongoing viral replication
	HCV genotyping	Indicates the genotype of HCV

H

Continued

TABLE 46   Diagnostic Tests for Viral Hepatitis—cont'd

Virus	Tests	Significance
D (HDV)	Anti-HDV	Present in past or current infection with HDV
	HDV Ag (hepatitis D antigen)	Present within a few days after infection
E (HEV)	Anti-HEV IgM and IgG	Present 1 wk–2 mo after illness onset
	HEV RNA quantitation	Indicates active ongoing viral replication

Drug Therapy

There are no specific drug therapies for the treatment of acute HAV. Supportive therapy may include antiemetics.

Treatment of acute hepatitis B is indicated in patients with severe hepatitis and liver failure. Drug therapy for chronic HBV infection is focused on decreasing the viral load and liver enzyme levels and on slowing the rate of disease progression.

- Nucleoside and nucleotide analogs suppress HBV replication by inhibiting viral DNA synthesis. Drugs such as lamivudine (Epivir), adefovir (Hepsera), entecavir (Baraclude), tenofovir (Viread), and telbivudine (Tyzeka) can reduce viral load and liver damage.

Treatment of chronic hepatitis C is based on the genotype of the HCV and the severity of liver disease. Drug therapy is directed at eradicating the virus through the use of direct-acting antivirals (DAAs) and preventing HCV-related complications.

Drug therapy is also used for prevention of HAV and HBV infection.

- Immune globulin (IG) provides temporary (1–2 months) passive immunity and is effective for preventing hepatitis A if given within 2 weeks after exposure
- IG and the HAV vaccine are recommended for people who do not have anti-HAV antibodies and are exposed because of close contact with people who have HAV or foodborne exposure.
- The traditional HBV vaccine of three doses is normally given in childhood.
- For postexposure prophylaxis, the vaccine and hepatitis B IG (HBIG) are used. HBIG contains antibodies to HBV and confers temporary passive immunity. HBIG is recommended in cases of

needlestick, mucous membrane contact, or sexual exposure and for infants born to mothers who are seropositive for hepatitis B surface antigen (HBsAg).

Nutrition Therapy

Emphasize a well-balanced diet that the patient can tolerate. During acute viral hepatitis, adequate calories are important because the patient usually loses weight. Vitamin supplements, particularly B-complex vitamins and vitamin K, are frequently used. If anorexia, nausea, and vomiting are severe, we may give IV glucose solutions or supplemental enteral nutrition (EN).

Nursing Management

Goals

The patient with viral hepatitis will have relief of discomfort, be able to resume normal activities, and return to normal liver function without complications.

Interventions

Viral hepatitis is a community health problem. Your role is important in the prevention and control of this disease. A suggested guideline for general practice to prevent you from contracting viral hepatitis from diagnosed and undiagnosed patients and carriers is for you to wear personal protective equipment (PPE) when fecal or blood contamination is likely in handling (1) soiled bedpans, urinals, and catheters and (2) when the patient's bed linens are soiled by body excreta or secretions.

Assess for the presence and degree of jaundice. Provide comfort measures to relieve pruritus, headache, and arthralgias.

- Small, frequent meals may be preferable to three large ones and may also help prevent nausea. Include measures to stimulate the appetite, such as mouth care, antiemetics, and attractively served meals in pleasant surroundings.
- Assess the patient's response to rest and activity, and modify plans as needed.
- Limited activity may produce anxiety and restlessness in some patients. Diversion activities, such as reading and hobbies, may help a patient cope with the plan of care and ensure adequate rest.

▼ Patient and Caregiver Teaching

- Teach the patient and caregivers how to prevent transmission.
- Caution the patient about overexertion.
- Assess the patient for manifestations of complications such as bleeding or encephalopathy.
- Teach the patient to have regular follow-up for at least 1 year.

H

- Teach the patient the symptoms of recurrent hepatitis B and C and the need for follow-up evaluations. All patients with chronic HBV or HCV infection should avoid alcohol because it can accelerate disease progression.
- Teach the patient who is receiving drug therapy for the treatment of hepatitis B or C about the drug(s).

HERNIA

Description

A *hernia* is a protrusion of tissue, such as the intestine, through an abnormal opening or a weakened area in the wall of the cavity in which it is normally contained. A hernia may occur in any part of the body, but usually occurs in the abdominal cavity.

- *Reducible* hernias easily return to the abdominal cavity. The hernia can be reduced manually or may reduce spontaneously when the person lies down.
- Irreducible, or incarcerated, hernias cannot be placed back into the abdominal cavity and have abdominal contents trapped in the opening. When the hernia is irreducible and intestinal flow and blood supply are obstructed, the hernia is *strangulated.* See Intestinal Obstruction.

Types

Types of hernias include hiatal, inguinal, femoral, umbilical, and ventral (incisional). See Hiatal Hernia.

- *Inguinal hernia* is the most common type of hernia. It occurs at the point of weakness in the abdominal wall where the spermatic cord in men or the round ligament in women emerges. Inguinal hernia is more common in men.
- *Femoral hernia* occurs when there is a protrusion through the femoral ring into the femoral canal. It easily becomes strangulated and occurs more frequently in women.
- *Umbilical hernia* occurs when the rectus muscle is weak (as with obesity) or the umbilical opening fails to close after birth.
- *Ventral* or *incisional hernia* is caused by a weakness of the abdominal wall at the site of a previous incision or stoma. They occur often in those who are obese, who have had multiple surgeries in the area, or who have had inadequate wound healing because of poor nutrition or infection.

Clinical Manifestations and Diagnosis

Pain is the classic symptom of a hernia. It may worsen with activities that increase intraabdominal pressure, such as lifting, coughing, and straining. A hernia may be readily visible, especially when the person tenses the abdominal muscles.

- A strangulated hernia causes severe pain with symptoms of a bowel obstruction, such as vomiting, cramping abdominal pain, and distention.
- Strangulated hernias or painful, inflamed hernias that cannot be reduced require emergency surgery.

Diagnosis is based on history and physical assessment findings. Ultrasound, CT, and MRI can assist in identifying a hernia and determining the contents.

Interprofessional and Nursing Management

Surgical repair of a hernia, known as a *herniorrhaphy*, is usually an outpatient procedure. Reinforcement of the weakened area with wire, fascia, or mesh is known as a *hernioplasty*. Surgery for strangulated hernias involves resecting the involved area with possible placement of a temporary colostomy.

After a hernia repair, the patient may have difficulty voiding. Measure intake and output and observe for a distended bladder.

- Encourage deep breathing, but not coughing. Teach patients to splint the incision and keep the mouth open when coughing or sneezing.
- Elevation of the scrotum with a scrotal support and application of an ice bag may help relieve pain and edema after an inguinal hernia repair.
- The patient may be restricted from heavy lifting (>10 lb) for 6–8 weeks.

HERPES, GENITAL

H

Description

Genital herpes is a common, lifelong, incurable infection. Two strains of herpes cause genital infections: herpes simplex virus type 1 (HSV-1) and herpes simplex virus type 2 (HSV-2). Most new infections are transmitted by someone who does not know they are infected.

Pathophysiology

The herpes simplex virus (HSV) enters through the mucous membranes or breaks in the skin during contact with an infected person.

HSV reproduces inside the cell and spreads to surrounding cells. The virus next enters the peripheral or autonomic nerve endings and ascends to the sensory or autonomic nerve ganglion, where it often becomes dormant. Viral reactivation (recurrence or outbreak) occurs when the virus travels down to the initial site of infection.

The virus persists within a person for life. Transmission occurs through direct contact with skin or mucous membranes when an infected person is symptomatic or through asymptomatic viral shedding.

Both HSV-1 and HSV-2 can cause either genital or orolabial infections. HSV-2 almost always infects sites "below the waist"— the genital tract, perineum, or anus.

Clinical Manifestations

A *primary (initial) episode* of genital herpes has an incubation of 2–12 days. Most people do not have any recognizable symptoms of primary HSV genital infection. If symptoms do occur, they follow a series of stages.

During the *prodromal* stage, the period before lesions appear, the patient may have burning, itching, or tingling at the site of inoculation. In the *vesicular* stage, a few to multiple small, often painful vesicles (blisters) may appear on the buttock, inner thigh, penis, scrotum, vulva, perineum, perianal region, vagina, or cervix. The vesicles contain large quantities of infectious viral particles. Urination may be painful from urine touching active lesions. Next, in the *ulcerative* stage, the lesions rupture and form shallow, moist ulcerations. Finally, crusting and epithelialization of the erosions occur.

- Local inflammation and pain, regional (inguinal node) lymphadenopathy, and systemic flu-like symptoms including fever, headache, malaise, and myalgia may occur with the primary episode.

Recurrent genital herpes occurs in many persons during the year after the primary episode. The symptoms of recurrent episodes are less severe, and the lesions usually heal more quickly. HSV-1 genital infections recur less often than HSV-2 genital infections. Over time, both are less frequent.

- Common triggers of recurrence include stress, fatigue, sunburn, general illness, immunosuppression, menses, or local trauma at the site of infection. Many patients can predict a recurrence by noticing early prodromal symptoms of tingling, burning, and itching at the site where lesions will eventually appear. Symptoms of recurrent episodes are less severe, and the lesions usually heal within 8–12 days. With time, the lesions will generally occur less often.

- The greatest risk for transmitting infection exists when active lesions are present. However, it is possible to transmit the virus when no visible lesions or symptoms are present.

Complications

- HSV-1 and HSV-2 can cause rare but serious complications such as blindness, encephalitis, and aseptic meningitis.
- Autoinoculation can result in lesions in the buttocks, groin, thighs, fingers, and eyes. Genital ulcers from HSV increase the risk of contracting human immunodeficiency virus (HIV).
- Pregnant women with HSV can transmit the virus to the baby if the virus is shed while the infant passes though the birth canal. Women with a primary episode of HSV near the time of delivery have the highest risk of transmitting genital herpes to the neonate. An active genital lesion at the time of delivery is an indication for cesarean delivery.

Diagnostic Studies

- Diagnosis is usually based on the patient's symptoms and history, then confirmed by visual examination.
- A viral culture of the active lesion can be used to isolate the virus and distinguish between HSV-1 and HSV-2.
- Highly accurate blood tests for antibodies are available for HSV-1 and HSV-2 but do not show the location of the infection. These antibodies usually appear by 12 weeks after exposure.

Interprofessional and Nursing Management

Three antiviral agents are available for treating HSV: acyclovir (Zovirax), famciclovir (Famvir), and valaciclovir (Valtrex). These drugs inhibit herpetic viral replication. They are prescribed for both primary and recurrent infections. Taken daily at a lower dose, they can be used as suppressive therapy to decrease frequent anogenital recurrences. IV acyclovir is reserved for severe or life-threatening infections.

The main goal is to keep eruptions clean and dry. Teach patients with active outbreaks to maintain good genital hygiene and wear loose-fitting cotton undergarments.

- Ways to reduce pain with urination include pouring water onto the perineal area while voiding to dilute the urine or voiding in the shower. Patients may need a local anesthetic such as lidocaine gel or analgesics such as ibuprofen, acetaminophen, acetaminophen with codeine, or aspirin.
- Ice packs to the affected area can provide some relief.
- See Sexually Transmitted Infections.

HIATAL HERNIA

Description

Hiatal hernia is herniation of a part of the stomach into the esophagus through an opening, or hiatus, in the diaphragm. It is also referred to as *diaphragmatic hernia* or *esophageal hernia*. Hiatal hernias are common among older adults and occur more often in women. Hiatal hernias are classified into two types (Fig. 13).

- A *sliding hernia* is the most common type. The junction of the stomach and esophagus is above the diaphragm. A part of the stomach slides through the hiatal opening in the diaphragm. This occurs when the patient is supine, and it usually goes back into the abdominal cavity when the patient is standing upright.

- A *paraesophageal* or *rolling hernia*. The fundus and greater curvature of the stomach roll up through the diaphragm, forming a pocket alongside the esophagus. The esophagogastric junction stays in the normal position. Acute paraesophageal hernia is a medical emergency.

Pathophysiology

Many factors contribute to the development of hiatal hernia. Structural changes, such as weakening of the muscles in the diaphragm around the esophagogastric opening, occur with aging. Factors that increase intraabdominal pressure predispose patients to developing a hiatal hernia. These include obesity, pregnancy, ascites, tumors, intense physical exertion, and frequent heavy lifting.

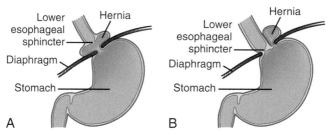

Fig. 13 (A) Sliding hiatal hernia. (B) Rolling or paraesophageal hernia.

Clinical Manifestations

Signs and symptoms of hiatal hernia are similar to those described for gastroesophageal reflux disease (GERD). Some people are asymptomatic.

- Heartburn is common, especially after a meal or after lying supine. Bending over, large meals, alcohol, and smoking may precipitate pain.
- Nocturnal attacks are common, especially if the person has eaten before lying down.

Complications may include GERD, esophagitis, hemorrhage from erosion, stenosis, ulcerations of the herniated part of the stomach, strangulation of the hernia, and regurgitation with tracheal aspiration.

Diagnostic Studies

- Barium swallow (esophagram) may show gastric mucosa protrusion through the esophageal hiatus. See GERD for other tests.

Interprofessional and Nursing Management

Conservative therapy for hiatal hernia is similar to that for GERD. Teach the patient to reduce intraabdominal pressure by eliminating constricting garments and avoiding lifting and straining.

Surgical approaches to hiatal hernias can include reduction of the herniated stomach into the abdomen, *herniotomy* (excision of the hernia sac), *herniorrhaphy* (closure of the hiatal defect), fundoplication, and *gastropexy* (attachment of the stomach below the diaphragm to prevent reherniation).

- Surgery to repair hiatal hernia is often done laparoscopically by Nissen or Toupet techniques.

HODGKIN'S LYMPHOMA

H

Description

Hodgkin's lymphoma, also called *Hodgkin's disease*, is a cancerous condition characterized by abnormal giant, multinucleated cells, called *Reed–Sternberg cells*, or its variant, Hodgkin cells (mononucleated), which proliferate in the lymph nodes. The disease accounts for 10% of all lymphomas, occurring most often in people 15–30 years of age and in those older than 55 years. About 85% of all patients are cured.

Pathophysiology

Several key factors are thought to play a role in the development of Hodgkin's lymphoma. The main interacting factors include infection with the Epstein–Barr virus, genetic predisposition, and exposure to occupational toxins. The incidence is increased in patients who have human immunodeficiency virus (HIV) infection.

The disease likely starts at a single location and spreads along adjacent lymphatics. It eventually infiltrates the lungs, spleen, and liver.

Clinical Manifestations

The initial sign is most often enlarged and nonpainful cervical, axillary, or inguinal lymph nodes.

- The patient may note weight loss, fatigue, weakness, fever, chills, tachycardia, or night sweats. A group of initial findings, including fever, night sweats, and weight loss (referred to as "B symptoms"), correlate with a worse prognosis.
- Generalized pruritus without skin lesions may develop. Cough, dyspnea, stridor, and dysphagia may reflect mediastinal node involvement.
- After having even small amounts of alcohol, patients with Hodgkin's lymphoma may have a rapid onset of pain at the site of disease. The cause for the alcohol-induced pain is unknown.
- In more advanced disease, there may be hepatomegaly and splenomegaly. Jaundice may result from liver involvement.
- Anemia results from increased destruction and decreased production of erythrocytes.
- Intrathoracic involvement may lead to superior vena cava syndrome.
- Enlarged retroperitoneal nodes may cause palpable abdominal masses or interfere with renal function.
- Jaundice may result from liver involvement.
- Spinal cord compression leading to paraplegia may occur with extradural involvement.
- Bone involvement may cause bone pain.

Diagnostic Studies

Peripheral blood analysis, excisional lymph node biopsy, bone marrow examination, and radiologic studies are important means of evaluating Hodgkin's lymphoma.

- Microcytic hypochromic anemia, leukopenia, and thrombocytopenia may develop, usually as a consequence of treatment, advanced disease, or hypersplenism (related to the disease process).

- Other blood studies may show increased erythrocyte sedimentation rate, high alkaline phosphatase from liver and bone involvement, hypercalcemia from bone involvement, and hypoalbuminemia from liver involvement.
- Positron emission tomography (PET) scans with or without CT scan are used to stage and then assess response to therapy.

Interprofessional Management

Treatment decisions are made based on the clinical stage of the disease. The standard for chemotherapy is the ABVD regimen: doxorubicin (formerly marketed as *A*driamycin), *b*leomycin, *v*inblastine, and *d*acarbazine, given for two to eight cycles of treatment, depending on disease stage and prognosis.

- Combination chemotherapy works well because the drugs have an additive antitumor effect without increasing side effects. As with leukemia, therapy must be aggressive. Therefore potentially life-threatening problems are encountered in an attempt to achieve a remission.

A variety of chemotherapy regimens and newer agents, such as brentuximab vedotin, nivolumab, bendamustine, and everolimus, are used to treat patients who have relapsed or refractory disease. Once remission is obtained, a curative option may be intensive chemotherapy and autologous or allogeneic hematopoietic stem cell transplantation.

The role of radiation as a supplement to chemotherapy varies depending on site of disease and the presence of resistant disease after chemotherapy.

Nursing Management

Nursing care for patients with Hodgkin's lymphoma is primarily based on managing problems related to the disease, such as pain; and side effects of therapy, such as pancytopenia (see Chemotherapy and Radiation Therapy).

- Because the survival of patients with Hodgkin's lymphoma depends on their response to treatment, support the patient through the consequences of treatment.
- Psychosocial, social, and spiritual considerations are as important as they are with leukemia (see Leukemia). However, the prognosis with Hodgkin's lymphoma is better than that with many forms of cancer.
- Delayed consequences of the disease and treatment, such as secondary cancers and long-term endocrine, cardiac, and pulmonary toxicities, may not be apparent for many years. The most common secondary cancers are lung and breast cancer. Encourage close follow-up and screening for early detection.

H

HUMAN IMMUNODEFICIENCY VIRUS INFECTION

Description

Human immunodeficiency virus (HIV) is a retrovirus that causes immunosuppression. More than 1.2 million people are living with HIV in the United States, with about 36,400 new infections occurring annually. Persons with HIV infection are more susceptible to other infections normally controlled through immune responses. With effective treatment, HIV is considered a chronic condition.

Pathophysiology

HIV is a ribonucleic acid (RNA) virus. HIV infects human cells that have CD4+ receptors on their surfaces. These include lymphocytes, monocytes/macrophages, astrocytes, and oligodendrocytes. Immune dysfunction in HIV disease is caused predominantly by destruction of *CD4+ cells (CD4 cell)*, a type of lymphocyte.

Over time, the ability of HIV to destroy CD4+ cells exceeds the body's ability to replace the cells. The decline in the CD4+ cells impairs immune function when the count drops below 500 CD4+ cells/μL. Severe problems develop with fewer than 200 CD4+ cells/μL. This allows opportunistic diseases (infections and cancers that occur in immunosuppressed patients) to develop. Opportunistic diseases are the main cause of disease, disability, and death in patients with HIV infection.

- HIV can be transmitted through contact with infected blood, semen, vaginal secretions, or breast milk. HIV transmission occurs through sexual intercourse with an infected partner; exposure to HIV-infected blood or blood products; and perinatal transmission during pregnancy, at delivery, or through breastfeeding. HIV is not spread through casual contact. In North America, HIV is most prevalent among men who have sex with men (MSM).
- The virus cannot be transmitted through hugging, dry kissing, shaking hands, sharing eating utensils, using toilet seats, or casual encounters in any setting. It is not spread by tears, saliva, urine, emesis, sputum, feces, sweat, respiratory droplets, or enteric routes. Healthcare personnel have a low risk for acquiring HIV at work, even after a needle-stick injury.

Clinical Manifestations

The typical course of untreated HIV infection follows the pattern shown in Fig. 14. Disease progression is highly individualized, however, and treatment can alter the pattern. HIV infections have acute and chronic stages.

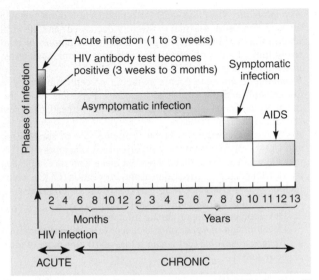

Fig. 14 Timeline for the spectrum of untreated HIV infection. The timeline represents the course of untreated illness from the time of infection to clinical manifestations of disease. *AIDS*, Acquired immunodeficiency syndrome; *HIV*, human immunodeficiency virus.

Acute Infection

During acute HIV infection, HIV-specific antibodies are produced (seroconversion) with a mononucleosis-like syndrome of fever, lymphadenopathy, pharyngitis, headache, malaise, nausea, and/or a diffuse rash.

- Symptoms begin 2–4 weeks after initial infection and last for 1–3 weeks.
- During this time, a high viral load is noted and CD4$^+$ cell counts fall temporarily but quickly return to baseline. Acute HIV symptoms may be taken for a bad case of the flu. People are most infectious during the acute infection stage because of the high amounts of circulating HIV.

Chronic Infection

There are three stages of chronic infection: asymptomatic infection, symptomatic infection, and acquired immunodeficiency syndrome (AIDS). The interval between untreated HIV infection and a diagnosis of AIDS is about 10 years.

H

- *Asymptomatic infection*—CD4+ lymphocyte counts remain above 500 cells/µL (normal or slightly decreased) and the viral load in the blood is low. The person has no symptoms or relatively limited signs of infection, so the risk of unknown transmission to others is high.
- *Symptomatic infection* occurs as the CD4+ cell count drops to 200 cells/µL and the viral load increases. Persistent fever, frequent night sweats, chronic diarrhea, recurrent headaches, and severe fatigue may develop.
- *AIDS* is characterized by severe immune system suppression and CD4+ cell counts below 200 cells/µL. A diagnosis of AIDS is made when an HIV-infected patient meets criteria established by the Centers for Disease Control and Prevention (CDC), which include the development of at least one of these conditions:
  1. CD4+ lymphocyte count <200/µL
  2. Development of opportunistic infection
  3. Development of opportunistic cancer (e.g., Kaposi sarcoma)
  4. *Wasting syndrome* (defined as a loss of 10% or more of ideal body mass)

Diagnostic Studies
Screening
The most useful screening tests detect HIV-specific antibodies or antigens in blood or saliva. There is a delay of several weeks (window period) after infection before antibodies can be detected.
Progression of Human Immunodeficiency Virus Infection
- CD4+ cell count and viral load monitor progression of infection.
- White blood cell (WBC) count, red blood cell count (RBC) count, and platelets decrease with progression of HIV.

Interprofessional Management
Care focuses on monitoring HIV disease progression and immune function, initiating and monitoring antiretroviral therapy (ART), preventing the development of opportunistic diseases, detecting and treating opportunistic diseases, managing symptoms, preventing or decreasing complications of treatment, and preventing further transmission of HIV.
Drug Therapy
Using drugs from different classes in combination therapy can inhibit viral replication and decrease the chance of drug resistance.
- Resistance tests can determine if a patient's HIV is resistant to drugs. Genotype and phenotype assays help HCPs know which medications can best control a patient's infection.

- The most effective means to suppress HIV replication is using at least three antiretroviral therapy (ART) drugs from different drug classes in optimum schedules and at full dosages (Table 47).
- Many ART agents cause potentially lethal interactions with other commonly used drugs.

Opportunistic diseases associated with HIV infection can be delayed or prevented with adequate ART, vaccines (including hepatitis B, influenza, and pneumococcal), and disease-specific prevention measures.

Nursing Management

Goals

Support the patient with HIV adhere to drug regimens; adopt a healthy lifestyle that includes avoiding exposure to other sexually transmitted infections and blood-borne diseases; protect others from HIV; maintain or develop healthy and supportive relationships; maintain activities and productivity; explore spiritual issues and come to terms with issues related to disease, disability, and death; and cope with symptoms caused by HIV and its treatments.

Interventions

Primary prevention and health promotion are the most effective healthcare strategies. HIV infection is preventable.

- Avoiding or modifying risky behaviors are the most effective prevention tools. Provide culturally sensitive, language-appropriate, and age-specific teaching and counseling.

Early intervention after detection of HIV infection can promote health and limit disability. Focus on early detection of symptoms, opportunistic diseases, and psychosocial problems. Interventions for patients with HIV infection include nutritional support; moderation or elimination of alcohol, tobacco, and drug use; keeping recommended vaccines up to date; adequate rest, exercise, and stress reduction; avoiding exposure to new infectious agents; mental health counseling; and attending support groups and community activities.

▼ Patient and Caregiver Teaching

Emphasize prevention and risk reduction. Teach safe sex options and the proper use and placement of male and female condoms. Recommend decreasing the number of sex partners. Refer patients to support services for substance use reduction and access to sterile drug equipment.

H

TABLE 47　Drug Therapy: Human Immunodeficiency Virus (HIV) Infection

Drug classification	Mechanism of action	Drug names
Attachment inhibitors	Interrupts the ability of HIV to attach to the CD4 cell	Fostemsavir (Rukobia) Ibalizumab-uiyk (Trogarzo)
Entry inhibitors	Prevent binding of HIV to cells, thus preventing entry of HIV into cells where replication would occur	Enfuvirtide (Fuzeon) Maraviroc (Selzentry)
Integrase inhibitors	Bind with integrase enzyme and prevent HIV from incorporating its genetic material into the host cell	Bictegravir[a] Dolutegravir (Tivicay) Elvitegravir[a] Raltegravir (Isentress)
Protease inhibitors (PIs)	Prevent the protease enzyme from cutting HIV proteins into the proper lengths needed to allow viable virions to assemble and bud out from the cell membrane	Atazanavir (Reyataz) Darunavir (Prezista) Fosamprenavir (Lexiva) Indinavir (Crixivan) Lopinavir + ritonavir (Kaletra) Nelfinavir (Viracept) Ritonavir (Norvir)[b] Saquinavir (Fortovase, Invirase) Tipranavir (Aptivus)

Reverse Transcriptase Inhibitors

Nonnucleoside reverse transcriptase inhibitors (NNRTIs)	Inhibit the action of reverse transcriptase	Efavirenz (Sustiva) Etravirine (Intelence) Delavirdine (Rescriptor) Nevirapine (Viramune XR) Rilpivirine (Edurant)

TABLE 47   Drug Therapy: Human Immunodeficiency Virus (HIV) Infection—cont'd

Drug classification	Mechanism of action	Drug names
Nucleoside reverse transcriptase inhibitors (NRTIs)	Insert a piece of DNA into the developing HIV DNA chain, blocking further development of the chain and leaving the production of the new strand of HIV DNA incomplete	Abacavir (Ziagen) Didanosine (Videx, Videx-EC) Doravarine (Pifeltro) Emtricitabine (Emtriva) Lamivudine (Epivir) Stavudine (Zerit) Zidovudine (retrovir)
Nucleotide reverse transcriptase inhibitor (NtRTI)	Combines with reverse transcriptase enzyme to block the process needed to convert HIV RNA into HIV DNA	Tenofovir (Viread)

DNA, deoxyribonucleic acid; RNA, ribonucleic acid.
[a]Elvitegravir and bictegravir are integrase inhibitors that are available only in fixed-dose combinations with tenofovir AF and emtricitabine.
[b]Most often used in low doses with other PIs to boost effect.

For a person infected wth HIV, direct teaching toward health promotion, managing the problems caused by HIV infection, and maximizing quality of life.

- Discuss infection control measures with the patient, caregivers, family, and visitors.
- Teach patients to recognize symptoms that may indicate disease progression and/or drug side effects and seek prompt medical care.
- Teach about new treatments, including drug therapy, dangers of nonadherence to therapy, how to take each medication, drug interactions to avoid, and side effects that need to be reported to the HCP.
- Symptomatic care includes teaching and treatment for diarrhea, pneumonia, fatigue, and wasting syndrome.
- Teach patients to conserve energy and maintain safety using assistive devices (e.g., shower chair).
- The focus of end-of-life care is on patient comfort, facilitating emotional and spiritual issues, and helping significant others deal with grief and loss.
- Provide information about support groups and community resources.

H

HUNTINGTON'S DISEASE

Description

Huntington's disease (HD) is a progressive, degenerative brain disorder causing deterioration of physical, emotional, and cognitive abilities. It is a genetically transmitted, autosomal dominant disorder. The onset of HD is usually between ages 30 and 55 years.

Pathophysiology

The pathologic process of HD involves the basal ganglia and extrapyramidal motor system. HD involves a deficiency of the neurotransmitters ACh and γ-aminobutyric acid (GABA). The net effect is an excess of DA, which leads to symptoms that are the opposite of those of parkinsonism.

- The offspring of a person with HD have a 50% risk of inheriting it. People who are asymptomatic but who have a positive family history of HD can decide if they want genetic testing. If the test is positive, the person will develop HD. However, we do not know when the disease will develop.

Clinical Manifestations

Manifestations include a movement disorder and cognitive and psychiatric problems. The movement disorder is marked by abnormal and excessive involuntary movements (chorea). These are writhing, twisting movements of the face, limbs, and body. The uncoordinated movements get worse as the disease progresses.

- Patients have difficulty with movement sequences (getting out of bed, getting out of a chair) and sustaining movement. The gait deteriorates, and ambulation eventually becomes impossible.
- Because facial movements involving speech, chewing, and swallowing are affected, aspiration and malnutrition are likely. Eventually all psychomotor processes, including the ability to eat and talk, are impaired.
- Psychiatric symptoms are often present in the early stage of HD, even before the onset of motor symptoms. Depression is common. Other psychiatric symptoms include anxiety, agitation, impulsivity, apathy, social withdrawal, obsessiveness, moodiness, and stubbornness.
- Cognitive deterioration is more variable. It involves perception, memory, attention, and learning. Cognitive problems progress to dementia.

The most common cause of death is pneumonia, followed by suicide. Other causes of death include injuries related to falls and other complications.

Diagnostic Studies

- The process begins with a review of family history and clinical symptoms.
- Genetic testing confirms excessive CAG protein repeats in the HTT gene.

Interprofessional and Nursing Management

Because HD has no cure, treatment is palliative. Drugs are available to control movements and behavioral problems.

- Tetrabenazine (Xenazine) and Deutetrabenazine (Austedo) are used to treat chorea. They decrease the amount of DA available at synapses of the nerves and reduce the involuntary movements. Other medications to lessen the chorea disorder include.
- Other medications used for the chorea disorder include neuroleptics and benzodiazepines.
- Cognitive disorders are treated as needed with nondrug therapies (e.g., counseling, memory books). Selective serotonin reuptake inhibitors, such as sertraline (Zoloft), are an option for depression. Antipsychotic medication, such as haloperidol or risperidone, may be needed.

The goal of nursing management is to provide the most comfortable environment possible for the patient and caregiver by maintaining physical safety, treating physical symptoms, and providing emotional and psychologic support.

- Because of the choreic movements, caloric requirements may be as high as 4000–5000 cal/day to maintain body weight. As HD progresses, meeting caloric needs becomes a greater challenge when the patient has difficulty swallowing and holding the head still. Depression and mental deterioration can also compromise nutritional intake. Enteral or parenteral nutrition may be indicated as the disease progresses.
- Discuss end-of-life issues with the patient and caregiver. These include care in the home or long-term care facility, artificial methods of feeding, advance directives, use of antibiotics to treat infections, and guardianship.

H

HYPERPARATHYROIDISM

Description

Hyperparathyroidism is a condition involving increased secretion of parathyroid hormone (PTH). PTH helps regulate serum calcium and phosphate levels by stimulating bone resorption of calcium, renal tubular reabsorption of calcium, and activation of vitamin D. Oversecretion of PTH causes increased serum calcium levels. Hyperparathyroidism is more common in women than in men.

Hyperparathyroidism is classified as primary, secondary, or tertiary.

- *Primary hyperparathyroidism* is caused by increased secretion of PTH leading to disorders of calcium, phosphate, and bone metabolism. The most common cause is a benign tumor (adenoma) in the parathyroid gland. Previous head and neck irradiation may be a risk factor for a parathyroid adenoma.
- *Secondary hyperparathyroidism* is a compensatory response to conditions that induce or cause hypocalcemia, the main stimulus of PTH secretion. These include vitamin D deficiencies, malabsorption, chronic kidney disease, and hyperphosphatemia.
- *Tertiary hyperparathyroidism* occurs when hyperplasia of the parathyroid glands causes autonomous secretion of PTH even with normal calcium levels. This may happen in patients who have a kidney transplant after a long period of dialysis treatment for chronic kidney disease.

Pathophysiology

High circulating PTH levels usually lead to hypercalcemia and hypophosphatemia. Multiple body systems are affected.

- Decreased bone density can occur as a result of the effect of PTH on osteoclastic (bone resorption) and osteoblastic (bone formation) activity.
- In the kidneys, excess calcium cannot be reabsorbed. Excess urinary calcium and phosphate can lead to stone formation.

Clinical Manifestations

Manifestations associated with hypercalcemia and range from no symptoms to overt symptoms. Loss of appetite, constipation, fatigue, emotional disorders, shortened attention span, and muscle weakness, especially in the proximal muscles of the lower extremities, often occur.

- Complications include osteoporosis, renal failure, kidney stones, pancreatitis, cardiac changes, and long bone, rib, and vertebral fractures.

Diagnostic Studies

- PTH levels are increased.
- Serum calcium levels are increased with decreased phosphorus levels.
- Urine calcium, serum chloride, serum uric acid, and serum creatinine are increased.
- Serum amylase (if pancreatitis is present) and alkaline phosphatase (if bone disease is present) are both increased.
- Bone density tests can detect bone loss.
- MRI, CT scan, and ultrasound can be used to localize adenoma.

Interprofessional Management

Treatment objectives are to relieve the symptoms and prevent complications caused by excess PTH.

- The most effective treatment of primary and secondary hyperparathyroidism is surgical removal of the parathyroid glands. The procedure most often involves outpatient endoscopy.
- Severe hypercalcemia is managed with IV sodium chloride solution and loop diuretics, such as furosemide, to increase the urinary excretion of calcium.
- IV bisphosphonates (e.g., pamidronate) can quickly lower serum calcium in patients with dangerously high levels.

A conservative approach is used in patients who are asymptomatic or have mild symptoms. This includes an annual examination with tests for serum PTH, calcium, phosphorus, and alkaline phosphatase levels and renal function; X-rays to assess for metabolic bone disease; and measurement of urinary calcium excretion. Dietary measures include high fluid and moderate calcium intake.

- X-rays and dual-energy X-ray absorptiometry (DXA) assess for metabolic bone loss.
- Bisphosphonates (e.g., alendronate [Fosamax]) inhibit osteoclastic bone resorption and improve bone mineral density. Phosphates are given if the patient has normal renal function and low serum phosphate levels.
- Calcimimetic agents (e.g., cinacalcet [Sensipar]) increase the sensitivity of the calcium receptor on the parathyroid gland, resulting in decreased PTH secretion and calcium blood levels.

Nursing Management

Nursing care after surgery is similar to that for the patient after thyroidectomy (see Hyperthyroidism). The major postoperative complications are hemorrhage and fluid and electrolyte problems. *Tetany,* a condition of neuromuscular hyperexcitability from a sudden decrease in calcium levels, is apparent early in the postoperative

H

period or may develop over several days. Mild tetany, character-ized by an unpleasant tingling of the hands and around the mouth, should resolve without problems. IV calcium gluconate should be readily available for use if tetany becomes severe (e.g., muscular spasms or laryngospasms).

- Assess calcium, potassium, phosphate, and magnesium levels frequently.
- Monitor for Chvostek's and Trousseau's signs.
- Monitor intake and output to evaluate fluid status.
- Encourage mobility to promote bone calcification.

▼ **Patient and Caregiver Teaching**
- Assist the patient to adapt the meal plan and consider referral to a dietitian.
- Because immobility can worsen bone loss, stress the impor-tance of an exercise program.
- Teach the patient the symptoms of hypocalcemia or hypercalce-mia and to contact the healthcare provider (HCP) if they occur.

HYPERTENSION

Description

About 45% of adults in the United States meet criteria for the gen-eral diagnosis of *hypertension,* or high BP. Hypertension is a major risk factors for cardiovascular disease (CVD). As BP increases, so does the risk of myocardial infarction (MI), heart failure (HF), stroke, and renal disease.

The classification of hypertension for adults is based on the aver-age of two or more properly measured BP readings on two or more office visits. Classification stages are described in Table 48.

Hypertension can be classified as primary (essential or idio-pathic) or secondary.

- *Primary hypertension* accounts for 90%–95% of all cases. The exact cause of primary hypertension is unknown, but there are several contributing factors. These include changes in endothe-lial function related to vasoconstricting or vasodilating agents, increased sympathetic nervous system (SNS) activity, over-production of sodium-retaining hormones, increased sodium intake, greater-than-ideal body weight, diabetes, tobacco use, and excess alcohol intake.
- *Secondary hypertension* is elevated BP with a specific cause that can often be corrected. This type accounts for 5%–10% of

TABLE 48	Classification of Hypertension		
Category	**SBP (mm Hg)**		**DBP (mm Hg)**
Normal	<120	and	<80
Elevated	120–129	and	<80
Hypertension, stage 1	130–139	or	80–89
Hypertension, stage 2	≥140	or	≥90

DBP, Diastolic blood pressure; *SBP*, systolic blood pressure.
Whelton PK, Carey RM, Aronow WS, et al: 2017 ACC/AHA/AAPA/ABC/ACPM/AGS/
APhA/ASH/ASPC/NMA/PCNA guideline for the prevention, detection, evaluation,
and management of high blood pressure in adults: a report of the American
College of Cardiology/AHA Task Force on Clinical Practice Guidelines, *J Am Coll
Cardiol* 71:e127, 2018.

hypertension cases. Causes of secondary hypertension include
coarctation or congenital narrowing of the aorta, renal artery stenosis, endocrine or neurologic problems, cirrhosis, sleep apnea,
and pregnancy-induced hypertension. Treatment of secondary
hypertension is directed at removing or treating the underlying
cause.

Pathophysiology of Primary Hypertension

The hemodynamic hallmark of hypertension is persistently
increased systemic vascular resistance (SVR). Table 49 shows factors that relate to the development of primary hypertension or contribute to its consequences.

Clinical Manifestations

Hypertension is called the "silent killer" because it is often asymptomatic until it becomes severe and target organ disease has
occurred. A patient with severe hypertension may have a variety
of symptoms secondary to effects on blood vessels in the various organs and tissues or to the increased workload of the heart.
These secondary symptoms include fatigue, dizziness, palpitations,
angina, and dyspnea.

The most common complications of hypertension are target
organ diseases occurring in the heart (hypertensive heart disease),
brain (cerebrovascular disease), peripheral vasculature (peripheral vascular disease), kidney (nephrosclerosis), and eyes (retinal
damage).

H

TABLE 49 Risk Factors for Primary Hypertension

Risk factor	Description
Age	• Systolic BP rises progressively with age • After age 50, SBP >140 mm Hg is a more important cardiovascular risk factor than diastolic BP
Alcohol	• Excess alcohol intake is associated with hypertension • Moderate intake of alcohol has cardioprotective properties; males should limit their daily intake of alcohol to two drinks per day, and one drink per day for females
Diabetes	• Hypertension is more common in patients with diabetes • When hypertension and diabetes coexist, complications (e.g., target organ disease) are more severe
Ethnicity	• Incidence of hypertension is two times higher in blacks than in whites

Excess dietary sodium	• High sodium intake can
	  ○ contribute to hypertension in salt-sensitive patients
	  ○ ↓Effectiveness of certain antihypertensive drugs

Family history	• History of a close blood relative (e.g., parents, sibling) with hypertension ↑ risk for developing hypertension
Gender	• More prevalent in men in young adulthood and early middle age • After age 64, hypertension is more prevalent in women
Increased serum lipids	• ↑ cholesterol and triglyceride levels are primary risk factors for atherosclerosis • Hyperlipidemia is more common in people with hypertension

TABLE 49 Risk Factors for Primary Hypertension—cont'd	
Risk factor	**Description**
Obesity	• Weight gain ↑ frequency of hypertension • Risk increases with central abdominal obesity
Sedentary lifestyle	• Regular physical activity can help control weight and reduce cardiovascular risk • Physical activity may ↓ BP
Socioeconomic status	• More prevalent in lower socioeconomic groups and among the less educated
Stress	• People exposed to repeated stress may develop hypertension more often • People who develop hypertension may respond differently to stress than those who do not develop hypertension
Tobacco use	• Smoking tobacco greatly↑ risk for CVD • People with hypertension who smoke tobacco are at even greater risk for CVD

Hypertensive Heart Disease

Hypertension is a major risk factor for coronary artery disease (CAD). The "response-to-injury" theory of atherogenesis suggests that hypertension disrupts the coronary artery endothelium. This results in a stiff arterial wall with a narrowed lumen and accounts for a high rate of CAD, angina, and MI. Sustained high BP also increases the cardiac workload and produces left ventricular hypertrophy (LVH).

Progressive LVH, especially in association with CAD, can cause *heart failure* (HF).

- The heart can no longer pump enough blood to meet the body's demands.

H

- The patient may have shortness of breath on exertion, paroxysmal nocturnal dyspnea, and fatigue.

Cerebrovascular Disease

Atherosclerosis is the most common cause of cerebrovascular disease. Atherosclerotic plaques or blood clots located at the bifurcation of the common carotid artery may break off and travel to intracerebral vessels, producing a thromboembolism. The patient may have transient ischemic attacks or a stroke. Adequate BP control decreases the risk of stroke.

Peripheral Vascular Disease

Hypertension speeds up the process of atherosclerosis in peripheral blood vessels. This leads to aortic aneurysm, aortic dissection, and peripheral vascular disease (PVD). *Intermittent claudication* (ischemic muscle pain precipitated by activity and relieved with rest) is a classic symptom of PVD.

Nephrosclerosis

Hypertension is one of the leading causes of chronic kidney disease (CKD). Some degree of renal disease is usually present even with mild hypertension. Ischemia causes narrowing of renal blood vessels and leads to the destruction of glomeruli, atrophy of tubules, eventual death of nephrons, and renal failure. Nocturia is an early symptom of renal disease.

Retinal Damage

Damage to the retinal vessels is seen with an ophthalmoscope indicates similar vessel damage in the heart, brain, and kidneys. Manifestations of severe retinal damage include blurred vision, retinal hemorrhage, and vision loss.

Diagnostic Studies

Accurate measurement of BP is essential in assessing and monitoring hypertension. Basic laboratory studies are performed to evaluate target organ disease, determine overall cardiovascular risk, or establish baseline levels before initiating therapy.

- Routine urinalysis
- Metabolic panel
- Fasting blood glucose level to assess for diabetes
- Lipid profile to assess for risk factors for atherosclerosis
- Electrocardiogram (ECG) for baseline cardiac status

Interprofessional Management

Treatment goals include achieving and maintaining goal BP and reducing cardiovascular risk and target organ disease. Lifestyle modifications are a part of therapy for all patients with prehypertension and hypertension. Assess as part of lifestyle modifications. The American Heart Association's "Life's Simple 7" steps support ways to modify and improve health. These are: (1) manage BP, (2) control cholesterol, (3) reduce blood sugar, (4) get active, (5) eat better, (6) lose weight, and (7) stop smoking. Other modifications by the task-force on hypertension address sodium restrictions and alcohol intake.

- Dietary therapy consists of restricting sodium intake to <2300 mg/day and following the Mediterranean diet or the DASH eating plan, which stresses fruits, vegetables, fat free or low-fat milk and milk products, whole grains, fish, poultry, beans, seeds, and nuts. Compared with the typical American diet, the plan contains less red meat, salt, sweets, added sugars, and sugar-containing beverages.
- For those who are overweight, weight loss can have a significant effect on lowering BP.
- Men should limit their intake of alcohol to no more than two drinks per day, and women and lighter-weight men to no more than one drink per day.
- Adults should perform a minimum of 150 min of moderate exercise or 75 min of vigorous exercise per week.
- Muscle-strengthening activities should also be performed using the major muscle groups at least twice a week. Flexibility and balance exercises are recommended at least twice a week for older adults, especially for those at risk for falls. Advise sedentary people to increase activity levels gradually.
- Screen for social determinants of health and psychosocial risk factors (e.g., low socioeconomic status, depression, social isolation), which can contribute to CVD. Make appropriate referrals (e.g., nutritional assistance, counseling) when indicated.
- Nicotine in tobacco causes vasoconstriction and increases BP in hypertensive people. Strongly encourage everyone to avoid tobacco use.

Drug Therapy

The following are recommendations for antihypertensive drug therapy from the Eighth Joint National Committee (JNC 8):

- In patients 60 years of age or older, start drug treatment for BP of 130 mm Hg or higher systolic or 90 mm Hg or higher diastolic, and treat to goal BP less than those thresholds.
- In patients younger than 60 years, treatment initiation and goals should be 130/80 mm Hg, the same threshold used in patients 18 years or older with either chronic kidney disease (CKD) or diabetes.

- In all other patients without CVD or other risk factors, a BP of <130/80 mm Hg may be reasonable.

The drugs currently available for treating hypertension have two main actions: reducing SVR and decreasing the volume of circulating blood. Most patients who have hypertension require two or more antihypertensive drugs to achieve their goal BP.

- Drugs used in the treatment of hypertension include diuretics, adrenergic (SNS) inhibitors, direct vasodilators, angiotensin-converting enzyme (ACE) inhibitors, A-II receptor blockers (ARBs), and calcium-channel blockers (Fig. 15). (See Table 36.6–36.8 in Harding et al., *Lewis' Medical-Surgical Nursing*, ed 12, for a description of antihypertensive drug therapy.)

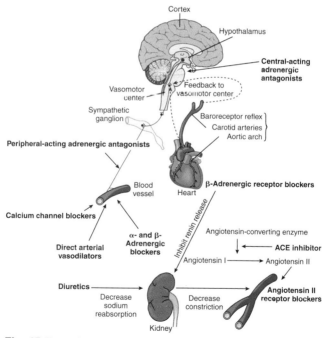

Fig. 15 Site and method of action of various antihypertensive drugs (bold type). (From US Department of Health and Human Services: *Seventh report of the Joint National Committee on Prevention, Detection, Evaluation, and Treatment of High Blood Pressure* [JNC 7], Washington, DC, 2003, National Institutes of Health.)

- Once antihypertensive therapy is started, patients should return for follow-up and adjustment of drug regimens often until the goal BP is reached.

Nursing Management
Goals
The overall goals for the patient with hypertension are that the patient will: (1) achieve and maintain the goal BP, (2) have minimal side effects of therapy, and (3) manage and cope with this condition.
Interventions
You are in an ideal position to assess for the presence of hypertension, identify risk factors for hypertension and CAD, and teach the patient about these conditions.

Initially, take the BP in both arms to note any differences. Atherosclerosis in the subclavian artery can cause a falsely low reading on the side where the narrowing occurs.

- Use the arm with the highest BP and take at least two readings, at least 1 min apart.
- Assess for orthostatic (or postural) changes in BP and pulse in older adults, people taking antihypertensive drugs, and patients who report symptoms consistent with reduced BP on standing (e.g., light-headedness, dizziness, syncope).

Your primary nursing responsibilities for long-term management of hypertension are to assist the patient in reducing BP and adhering to the treatment plan. Your nursing actions include evaluating effectiveness of therapy, detecting and reporting any adverse treatment effects, assessing and enhancing adherence, and teaching patients and caregivers.

▼ Patient and Caregiver Teaching
Help the patient and caregivers understand that hypertension is a chronic illness that cannot be cured. Stress that it can be controlled with drug therapy, diet changes, physical activity, periodic follow-up, and other relevant lifestyle modifications (Table 50).

H

TABLE 50 Patient and Caregiver Teaching: Hypertension

When teaching the patient and/or caregivers about hypertension, include the following:

General Instructions

1. Tell patient the BP reading and explain what it means (e.g., high, low, goal, borderline).
2. Encourage patient to monitor BP at home and teach the patient to call the HCP if BP exceeds high or low limits set by HCP.
3. Hypertension is usually asymptomatic, and symptoms (e.g., nosebleeds) do not reliably indicate BP levels.
4. Hypertension means high BP and does not relate to a "hyper" personality.
5. Long-term therapy and follow-up care are necessary to treat hypertension. Therapy involves lifestyle changes (e.g., weight management, sodium reduction, smoking cessation, regular physical activity) and, in most cases, drugs to regulate the blood pressure.
6. Therapy will not cure but should control hypertension.
7. Controlled hypertension usually results in an excellent prognosis.
8. Explain the potential dangers of uncontrolled hypertension (e.g., stroke, heart attack).

Instructions Related to Medication Therapy

1. Be specific about the names, actions, dosages, and side effects of prescribed drugs.
2. Help the patient plan regular and convenient times for taking medications and measuring BP.
3. Do not stop drugs abruptly, since withdrawal may cause a severe hypertensive reaction.
4. Do not double up on a dose when a dose is missed.
5. If BP increases or decreases, do not change the dose of the drug without consulting the HCP.
6. Do not take any drugs belonging to someone else.
7. Supplement diet with foods high in potassium (e.g., citrus fruits, green leafy vegetables) if taking potassium-wasting diuretics.
8. Avoid hot baths, excess amounts of alcohol, and strenuous exercise within 3 h of taking drugs that promote vasodilation.
9. Many drugs cause orthostatic hypotension. Reduce the effects of orthostatic hypotension by rising slowly from the bed, sitting on the side of the bed for a few minutes, standing slowly, and beginning to move if no symptoms develop (e.g., dizziness, lightheadedness).
10. Do not stand still for prolonged periods, do leg exercises to increase venous return, or sleep with the head of the bed raised. Do lie or sit down when dizziness occurs.

TABLE 50   Patient and Caregiver Teaching: Hypertension—cont'd
11. Some drugs cause sexual problems (e.g., erectile dysfunction, decreased libido). Consult with the HCP about changing drugs or dosages if sexual problems develop.
12. Some side effects may decrease with time (e.g., fatigue, diarrhea).
13. Be careful about taking potentially high-risk over-the-counter drugs such as high-sodium antacids, NSAIDs, appetite suppressants, and cold and sinus medications. Read warning labels and consult with a pharmacist.

HCP, Healthcare provider; *NSAIDs,* nonsteroidal antiinflammatory drugs.

HYPERTHYROIDISM

Description

Hyperthyroidism is hyperactivity of the thyroid gland with a sustained increase in synthesis and release of thyroid hormones. The most common form is Graves' disease. Other causes include toxic nodular goiter, thyroiditis, excess iodine intake, pituitary tumors, and thyroid cancer. Hyperthyroidism occurs in more women than in men, with the highest frequency in people 20–40 years old.

Thyrotoxicosis is hypermetabolism from excess circulating levels of thyroxine (T_4), triiodothyronine (T_3), or both. Hyperthyroidism and thyrotoxicosis usually occur together.

- Since hyperthyroidism may be caused by iodinated contrast media used in CT scans and other radiologic studies, monitor those at-risk closely after exposure.

Pathophysiology

Graves' disease is an autoimmune disease marked by diffuse thyroid enlargement and excess thyroid hormone secretion. Antibodies to the thyroid-stimulating hormone (TSH) receptor attach to receptors and stimulate the thyroid gland to release T_3, T_4, or both. The excess release of thyroid hormones leads to manifestations associated with thyrotoxicosis.

- Remissions and exacerbations may progress to destroying thyroid tissue, causing hypothyroidism.
- Risk factors, such as a lack of iodine, smoking, infection, and stress, may interact with genetic factors to cause Graves' disease.

H

Clinical Manifestations

Manifestations are related to the effect of excess thyroid hormones. A patient with advanced disease may have many symptoms, whereas a patient in the early stages of hyperthyroidism may only have weight loss and increased nervousness.

- Palpation of the thyroid gland may reveal a goiter. Auscultation of the thyroid gland may reveal bruits, a reflection of increased blood supply.
- *Exophthalmos,* or eyeball protrusion, is caused by impaired venous drainage from the orbit, leading to increased deposits of fat and edema fluid in the orbital tissues. When the eyelids do not close completely, exposed corneal surfaces become dry and irritated. Serious consequences, such as corneal ulcers and eventual loss of vision, can occur. Ocular muscle changes result in muscle weakness, causing diplopia.

See Table 51 for other manifestations.

Complications

Acute thyrotoxicosis (also called *thyrotoxic crisis, thyroid storm*) is an acute, severe, and rare condition that occurs when excess amounts of thyroid hormones are released into the circulation.

- Although this is a life-threatening emergency, death is rare when treatment is started early.

Thyrotoxicosis is thought to result from stressors (e.g., infection, trauma, surgery) in a patient with preexisting hyperthyroidism. Patients having a thyroidectomy are at risk because manipulation of the hyperactive thyroid gland results in an increased release of hormones.

In acute thyrotoxicosis, symptoms of hyperthyroidism are prominent and severe.

- Manifestations include severe tachycardia, heart failure, shock, hyperthermia (with temperatures up to 106°F [41.1°C]), agitation, delirium, seizures, abdominal pain, vomiting, diarrhea, and coma.
- Treatment is aimed at reducing circulating thyroid hormone levels by appropriate drug therapy, fever reduction, fluid replacement, and elimination or management of the initiating stressors.

Diagnostic Studies

Diagnosis is confirmed with findings of decreased serum TSH levels and elevated free thyroxine (T_4) levels.

- Radioactive iodine uptake (RAIU) differentiates Graves' disease from other forms of thyroiditis.

TABLE 51 Manifestations of Thyroid Hyperfunction

Cardiovascular system
- ↑ BP
- ↑ Rate and force of cardiac contractions
- Bounding, rapid pulse
- ↑ Cardiac output
- Systolic murmurs
- Dysrhythmias
- Palpitations
- Angina

GI system
- ↑ Appetite, thirst
- Weight loss
- ↑ Peristalsis
- Diarrhea, frequent defecation
- ↑ Bowel sounds
- Splenomegaly
- Hepatomegaly

Musculoskeletal system
- Fatigue
- Weakness
- Proximal muscle wasting
- Dependent edema
- Osteoporosis

Nervous system
- Hyperactive deep-tendon reflexes
- Depression
- Lack of ability to concentrate
- Rapid speech
- Insomnia
- Difficulty focusing eyes
- Nervousness
- Fine tremor of fingers and tongue
- Lability of mood, delirium
- Restlessness
- Personality changes of irritability, agitation
- Stupor, coma

H

Continued

TABLE 51 Manifestations of Thyroid Hyperfunction—cont'd

Reproductive system
- Menstrual irregularities
- Amenorrhea
- ↑ Libido
- ↑ Fertility
- Impotence and gynecomastia in men

Respiratory
- Dyspnea on mild exertion
- ↑ Respiratory rate

Skin
- Warm, smooth, moist skin
- Thin, brittle nails detached from nail bed (onycholysis)
- Hair loss (may be patchy)
- Clubbing of fingers (thyroid acropachy)
- Palmar erythema
- Fine, silky hair
- Premature graying (in men)
- Diaphoresis
- Vitiligo
- Pretibial myxedema (infiltrative dermopathy)

Other
- Goiter
- Intolerance to heat
- Lid lag, stare
- Eyelid retraction
- Exophthalmos
- ↑ Temperature

Interprofessional Management

The goal of management is to block the adverse effects of thyroid hormones, suppress oversecretion of thyroid hormone, and prevent complications. There are several treatment options including antithyroid medications, radioactive iodine therapy, and surgery.

Drug Therapy

Drugs used in the treatment of hyperthyroidism are useful in treating thyrotoxic states, but they are not curative.

- The first-line antithyroid drugs propylthiouracil and methimazole (Tapazole) inhibit the synthesis of thyroid hormones. Reasons for use include Graves' disease in the young patient, hyperthyroidism during pregnancy, or achieving a euthyroid state before surgery or radiation therapy. Propylthiouracil, which blocks the peripheral conversion of T4 to T3, is first-line treatment for thyrotoxic crisis.In large doses, iodine (e.g., Lugol's solution, saturated solution of potassium iodide [SSKI]) inhibits the synthesis of T3 and T4 and blocks the release of these hormones into circulation. Iodine decreases thyroid vascularity, making surgery safer and easier.
- β-Adrenergic blockers (e.g., propranolol [Inderal]) block the effects of sympathetic nervous stimulation, thereby decreasing tachycardia, nervousness, irritability, and tremors.
- Radioactive iodine (RAI) limits thyroid hormone secretion by damaging thyroid tissue. The full effect may not be seen for up to 3 months. Other drug therapy may be used until the effects of radiation become apparent. This treatment results in hypothyroidism for 80% of patients.

Surgical Therapy

Thyroidectomy is done for those who have a large goiter causing tracheal compression, are unresponsive to antithyroid therapy, or have thyroid cancer. A subtotal thyroidectomy involves the removal of a significant portion (90%) of the thyroid gland. A minimally invasive endoscopic or robotic thyroidectomy can be performed for patients with small nodules (<3 cm) without evidence of cancer.

Nutritional Therapy

Due to the increased metabolic rate, a high-calorie diet (4000–5000 cal/day) may be needed to satisfy hunger and prevent tissue breakdown. This can be achieved with six full meals each day and snacks high in protein, carbohydrates, minerals, and vitamins.

- Teach the patient to avoid highly seasoned and high-fiber foods, which can further stimulate the already hyperactive gastrointestinal (GI) tract. Provide substitutes for caffeine-containing liquids such as coffee, tea, and cola, because the stimulating effects of these fluids increase restlessness and sleep problems.
- Refer the patient to a dietitian for help in meeting nutritional needs.

Nursing Management

Goals

The patient with hyperthyroidism will have relief of symptoms, have no serious complications related to the disease or treatment, maintain nutritional balance, and cooperate with the therapeutic plan.

Interventions

Acute thyrotoxicosis requires aggressive treatment, often in an intensive care unit. Give medications (previously discussed) that block thyroid hormone production and the sympathetic nervous system. Monitor for dysrhythmias and decompensation, ensure adequate oxygenation, and give IV fluids to replace fluid and electrolytes. This is especially important in the patient who has fluid losses from vomiting and diarrhea.

- Adequate rest may be a challenge because of the patient's irritability and restlessness. Provide a calm, quiet room because increased metabolism and sensitivity of the sympathetic nervous system cause sleep problems.
- Use light bed coverings and change the linen frequently if the patient is diaphoretic.
- Encourage and assist with exercise involving large muscle groups (tremors can interfere with small-muscle coordination) to allow the release of nervous tension and restlessness.
- Establish a supportive, trusting relationship to promote coping by a patient who is irritable, restless, and anxious.

If exophthalmos is present, there is a risk for corneal injury related to irritation and dryness. Apply artificial tears to soothe and moisten conjunctival membranes.

- The patient should sit upright as much as possible to promote fluid drainage from the periorbital area. If the eyelids cannot be closed, lightly tape them shut for sleep. To maintain flexibility, teach the patient to exercise intraocular muscles several times each day by turning the eyes in the complete range of motion.

Nursing Management: Patient Having Thyroid Surgery

Preoperative teaching before subtotal thyroidectomy includes showing the patient how to support the head manually while turning in bed to minimize stress on the surgery suture line. The patient should practice neck range-of-motion exercises. Tell the patient that talking may be difficult for a short time after surgery.

Important nursing interventions after a thyroidectomy include the following:

- Assess the patient frequently for signs of hemorrhage or tracheal compression. The patient can expect hoarseness for 3 or 4 days after surgery because of edema.
- Respiration may become difficult because of excess swelling of the neck, hemorrhage, and hematoma formation.
- Laryngeal stridor (harsh, vibratory sound) may occur during respiration as a result of edema of the laryngeal nerve or because of tetany, which occurs if the parathyroid glands are removed or damaged during surgery.
- Recurrent laryngeal nerve damage is a potential complication that leads to vocal cord paralysis. If both cords are paralyzed, the patient needs an immediate tracheostomy.
- Place the patient in a semi-Fowler's position and support the head with pillows. Avoid flexion of the neck and any tension on the suture lines.
- Monitor vital signs and calcium levels. Check for signs of tetany secondary to hypoparathyroidism (e.g., tingling of toes, fingers, or around the mouth; muscular twitching; apprehension) and by evaluating any difficulty in speaking and hoarseness. To treat tetany, IV calcium salts, such as calcium gluconate, should be available.

▼ **Patient and Caregiver Teaching**

Follow-up care is important for the patient who has undergone thyroid surgery.

- Thyroid hormone balance should be monitored periodically to ensure that normal function has returned.
- To prevent weight gain, caloric intake must be substantially reduced below the amount that was required before surgery.
- Adequate iodine is needed to promote thyroid function, but excess inhibits the thyroid. Seafood once or twice per week or the normal use of iodized salt provides enough iodine intake.
- Encourage regular exercise to help stimulate the thyroid gland.
- Teach the patient to avoid high environmental temperatures because they inhibit thyroid regeneration.
- If a complete thyroidectomy was performed, teach the patient about the need for lifelong thyroid replacement. Teach the patient the signs and symptoms of thyroid failure and to contact the healthcare provider (HCP) if they develop.

HYPOPARATHYROIDISM

Description

Hypoparathyroidism is an uncommon condition of inadequate circulating parathyroid hormone (PTH) that results in hypocalcemia. PTH resistance at the cellular level may also occur (*pseudohypoparathyroidism*). This is caused by a genetic defect resulting in hypocalcemia despite normal or high PTH levels and is often associated with hypothyroidism and hypogonadism.

Pathophysiology

The most common cause of hypoparathyroidism is the accidental removal of parathyroids or damage to the vascular supply of the glands during neck surgery (e.g., thyroidectomy).

- Idiopathic hypoparathyroidism resulting from absence, fatty replacement, or atrophy of the glands is a rare disease associated with other endocrine disorders.
- Severe hypomagnesemia (e.g., malnutrition, alcohol use, renal failure) can also suppress PTH secretion.

Clinical Manifestations

Clinical manifestations of acute hypoparathyroidism are caused by hypocalcemia. Sudden decreases in calcium concentration cause tetany, characterized by lip tingling and extremity stiffness. Painful tonic spasms of smooth and skeletal muscles can cause dysphagia and laryngospasms that compromise breathing. Lethargy, anxiety, and personality changes may occur.

- Abnormal laboratory findings include decreased serum calcium and PTH levels and increased serum phosphate levels.

Interprofessional and Nursing Management

Treatment goals are to treat acute complications, such as tetany, maintain normal serum calcium levels, and prevent long-term complications. Emergency treatment of tetany after surgery requires IV calcium administration.

- Give IV calcium slowly. Use electrocardiogram (ECG) monitoring when giving calcium because high serum calcium levels can cause hypotension, serious dysrhythmias, or cardiac arrest.
- Assess IV patency. Calcium chloride can cause venous irritation and inflammation. Extravasation may cause cellulitis, necrosis, and tissue sloughing.
- Rebreathing may partially relieve acute symptoms associated with hypocalcemia, such as generalized muscle cramps or mild

tetany. Have the patient breathe into and out of a paper bag or breathing mask.

▼ **Patient and Caregiver Teaching**

The patient with hypoparathyroidism needs instruction in long-term nutrition and drug therapy.

- Most patients receive oral calcium supplements, magnesium supplements, and vitamin D. We usually do not recommend PTH replacement because of the expense and need for parenteral administration. Vitamin D (e.g., 1,25-dihydroxycholecalciferol, calcitriol) is used to enhance intestinal calcium absorption. It increases calcium levels rapidly and is quickly metabolized. A high-calcium meal plan includes foods such as dark green vegetables, soybeans, and tofu. Tell the patient to avoid foods containing oxalic acid (e.g., spinach, rhubarb), phytic acid (e.g., bran, whole grains), and phosphorus because they inhibit calcium absorption.

- Teach the patient about the need for lifelong treatment and follow-up care including monitoring of calcium levels several times a year.

HYPOTHYROIDISM

Description

Hypothyroidism is a deficiency of thyroid hormone that causes a general slowing of the metabolic rate. About 4% of the US population has mild hypothyroidism, with about 0.3% having more severe disease. Hypothyroidism is more common in women.

- Risk factors for hypothyroidism include being female, white ethnicity, advancing age or having type 1 diabetes, Down syndrome, family history of thyroid disease, goiter, previous hyperthyroidism, and external beam radiation in the head and neck area.

Pathophysiology

Hypothyroidism can be *primary* (related to destruction of thyroid tissue or defective hormone synthesis) or *secondary* (related to pituitary disease with decreased thyroid-stimulating hormone [TSH] secretion or hypothalamic dysfunction with decreased thyrotropin-releasing hormone [TRH] secretion). Hypothyroidism can be brief and related to thyroiditis or stopping thyroid hormone therapy.

- Iodine deficiency is the most common cause of hypothyroidism worldwide.

H

- In the United States, the most common cause of primary hypo-thyroidism is atrophy of the thyroid gland due to the autoim-mune diseases, Hashimoto's thyroiditis, or Graves' disease.
- Hypothyroidism can develop after treatment for hyperthyroid-ism, specifically thyroidectomy or radioactive iodine (RAI) therapy. Drugs such as amiodarone, which contains iodine, or lithium, which blocks thyroid hormone production, can cause hypothyroidism.
- Hypothyroidism that develops in infancy *(cretinism)* is caused by thyroid hormone deficiencies during fetal or early neonatal life.

Clinical Manifestations

Hypothyroidism is characterized by a slowing of body processes. The patient is often fatigued and lethargic. There may be personal-ity and mental changes including impaired memory, slowed speech, decreased initiative, and somnolence. Many appear depressed. Weight gain is a result of decreased metabolic rate.

- Hypothyroidism is associated with decreased cardiac output, decreased cardiac contractility, and coronary atherosclerosis. Anemia is common. High serum cholesterol and triglyceride lev-els and the accumulation of mucopolysaccharides in the intima of small blood vessels can result in coronary atherosclerosis.
- In the older adult, typical manifestations include fatigue, cold and dry skin, hair loss, hoarseness, cold intolerance, and consti-pation. Older adults who have confusion, lethargy, and depres-sion should be screened for thyroid disease.
- Long-standing hypothyroidism may cause *myxedema,* which alters the skin and subcutaneous tissues with puffiness, facial and periorbital edema, and a mask-like affect. Patients may have an altered self-image related to their altered appearance.

Complications

The mental sluggishness, drowsiness, and lethargy of hypothyroid-ism may progress gradually or suddenly to a notable impairment of consciousness or coma. This situation, termed *myxedema coma,* constitutes a medical emergency.

- Myxedema coma can be precipitated by infection, drugs (espe-cially opioids, tranquilizers, and barbiturates), exposure to cold, and trauma. Manifestations include low temperature, hypoten-sion, and hypoventilation.
- For the patient to survive myxedema coma, we must support vital functions and give IV thyroid hormone replacement.

Diagnostic Studies

- Serum TSH and free thyroxine (FT$_4$) are the most reliable indicators of thyroid function.
- If serum TSH level is high, the defect is in the thyroid; if low, it is in the pituitary or hypothalamus.
- The presence of thyroid antibodies suggests an autoimmune origin of the hypothyroidism.
- High cholesterol, triglycerides, and creatine kinase can occur, along with anemia.

Interprofessional Management

The treatment goal is the restoration of the euthyroid state as safely and rapidly as possible with hormone therapy.

Levothyroxine (Synthroid) is the drug of choice to treat hypothyroidism. In the young, otherwise healthy patient, the maintenance replacement dosage is adjusted according to the patient's response and laboratory findings. The initial dosages are low to avoid increases in resting heart rate and BP. Levothyroxine has a peak of action of 1–3 weeks. In the patient without side effects, the dose is increased at 4–6-week intervals.

- In the patient with compromised cardiac status, careful monitoring is needed when starting and adjusting the dosage because the usual dose may increase myocardial oxygen demand, causing angina and dysrhythmias.

Liotrix is a synthetic mix of levothyroxine (T$_4$) and liothyronine (T$_3$) in a 4:1 combination. Liotrix, with a fast onset of action and a peak of 2–3 days, can be used in acutely ill patients with hypothyroidism.

Nursing Management

Goals

The patient with hypothyroidism will have relief of symptoms, maintain a euthyroid state, maintain a positive self-image, and adhere to lifelong thyroid therapy.

Interventions

Most persons with hypothyroidism are treated on an outpatient basis. The patient who has myxedema coma requires acute nursing care, often in an intensive care unit (ICU). Mechanical respiratory support and cardiac monitoring are often needed. Give thyroid hormone therapy and other medications IV because severe gastric hypomotility may prevent the absorption of oral agents. Monitor core temperature because the patient with myxedema coma is often hypothermic.

H

- Use gentle soap and moisturize often to prevent skin breakdown. Frequent changes in patient positioning and a low-pressure mattress help maintain skin integrity.
- Monitor the patient's progress, vital signs, body weight, fluid intake and output, and visible edema. Cardiac assessment is especially important because the cardiovascular response to hormone therapy determines the medication regimen.
- Note energy level and mental alertness, which should increase within 2–14 days and continue to rise steadily to normal levels.

▼ **Patient and Caregiver Teaching**

At first the patient who is hypothyroid may have a hard time processing complex instructions. Provide written instructions, repeat the information often, and assess the patient's comprehension level.

- Stress the need for lifelong drug therapy and to avoid abruptly stopping the drugs. Explain the signs and symptoms that indicate hormone imbalance.
- Teach the patient to contact a healthcare provider (HCP) right away for signs of overdose, such as orthopnea, dyspnea, rapid pulse, chest pain, palpitations, nervousness, or insomnia.
- The patient with diabetes should test capillary blood glucose at least daily because a return to the euthyroid state often increases insulin requirements.
- Thyroid preparations increase the effects of other common drugs, such as anticoagulants, antidepressants, and digitalis compounds. Teach the patient the toxic signs and symptoms of these medications.
- Medication interactions are an important reason for patients to consult their HCP before switching brands of thyroid replacement medication. Switching brands may change bioavailability of the drug and physiologic response.

INCREASED INTRACRANIAL PRESSURE

Description

Increased intracranial pressure (ICP) is a potentially life-threatening situation that results from an increase in any or all three components within the skull: brain tissue, blood, and cerebrospinal fluid (CSF).

Pathophysiology

Common causes of increased ICP include a mass (e.g., hematoma, contusion, abscess, tumor) and cerebral edema (from tumors, hydrocephalus, head injury, or brain inflammation). These cerebral insults, which may result in hypercapnia, cerebral acidosis, impaired autoregulation, and systemic hypertension, worsen the cerebral edema. This edema distorts brain tissue, further increasing the ICP, and leads to even more tissue hypoxia and acidosis. Fig. 16 shows the progression of increased ICP.

There are three types of cerebral edema: vasogenic, cytotoxic, and interstitial. More than one type may occur in the same patient.

- *Vasogenic cerebral edema,* the most common type of edema, occurs mainly in the white matter. It is characterized by leakage of large molecules from capillaries into extracellular space. This edema may produce symptoms ranging from headache to a decrease in consciousness, including coma and focal neurologic deficits.
- *Cytotoxic cerebral edema* results from disruption of the integrity of the cell membranes. This type of edema develops from destructive lesions or brain trauma resulting in cerebral hypoxia or anoxia and syndrome of inappropriate antidiuretic hormone (SIADH) secretion.
- *Interstitial cerebral edema* is usually a result of hydrocephalus. It is caused by excess CSF production, obstruction of CSF flow, or an inability to reabsorb the CSF.

Clinical Manifestations

Manifestations of increased ICP can take many forms, depending on the cause, location, and rate of increase of ICP.

- *Change in level of consciousness* (LOC). LOC is a sensitive and reliable indicator of the patient's neurologic status. Changes in LOC may be dramatic, as in coma, or subtle, such as a flattening of affect, change in orientation, or a decrease in the level of attention.
- *Changes in vital signs. Cushing's triad* (systolic hypertension with widening pulse pressure, bradycardia with a full and bounding pulse, and irregular respirations) often does not appear until ICP has been increased for some time or is markedly increased (e.g., with head trauma). The effect of increased ICP on the hypothalamus can cause a change in body temperature.
- *Ocular signs.* Compression of the oculomotor nerve (cranial nerve [CN] III) results in dilation of the pupil on the same side (ipsilateral) as the mass lesion, sluggish or no response to light, an inability to adduct and move the eye upward, and ptosis of the eyelid. A fixed, unilaterally dilated pupil is a neurologic emergency that indicates brain herniation. Other cranial nerves may also be affected, with signs of blurred vision, diplopia, and changes in extraocular eye movements.

PATHOPHYSIOLOGY MAP

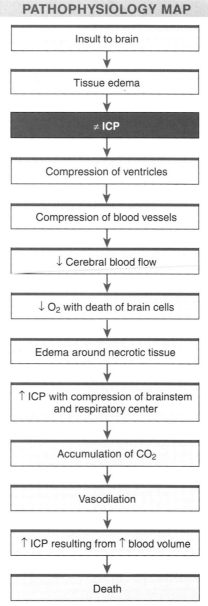

Insult to brain

Tissue edema

≠ ICP

Compression of ventricles

Compression of blood vessels

↓ Cerebral blood flow

↓ O_2 with death of brain cells

Edema around necrotic tissue

↑ ICP with compression of brainstem and respiratory center

Accumulation of CO_2

Vasodilation

↑ ICP resulting from ↑ blood volume

Death

Fig. 16 Progression of increased intracranial pressure (ICP).

- *Decrease in motor function.* As ICP rises, the patient shows changes in motor skills. A contralateral (opposite side of the mass lesion) hemiparesis or hemiplegia may develop. If a painful stimulus is used to elicit a motor response, the patient may localize to the stimulus or withdraw from it. *Decorticate* (flexor) and *decerebrate* (extensor) posturing may be elicited by noxious stimuli.
- *Headache.* Although the brain is not sensitive to pain, compression of other intracranial structures, such as the walls of arteries and veins and the cranial nerves, can produce headache. A nocturnal headache or a morning headache may indicate a tumor or other space-occupying lesion that is causing increased ICP. Straining, agitation, or movement may worsen the pain.
- *Vomiting.* Vomiting, usually without nausea, is often a nonspecific sign of increased ICP.

Sustained increases in ICP result in brainstem compression and brain herniation. Herniation occurs as the brain tissue is forcibly shifted from a compartment of greater pressure to a compartment of lesser pressure. Displacement and herniation of brain tissue can cause a potentially reversible process to become irreversible. Ischemia and edema are further increased, compounding the preexisting problem. Compression of the brainstem and cranial nerves may be fatal.

Diagnostic Studies

- MRI, CT scan, and positron emission tomography (PET) can be used to discern the cause of increased ICP.
- Other tests may include cerebral angiography, electroencephalography (EEG), ICP measurement, brain tissue oxygenation measurement via the LICOX catheter, transcranial Doppler studies, and evoked potential studies.

Interprofessional Management

The goals of management of increased ICP are to identify and treat the underlying cause of increased ICP, and support brain function. The earlier the condition is recognized and treated, the better the patient outcome.

- A careful history helps direct the search for the underlying cause.

Ensuring adequate oxygenation for brain function is important. Arterial blood gas (ABG) analysis guides the O_2 therapy. To meet the goal of maintaining the partial pressure of O_2 in arterial blood (PaO_2) at 100 mm Hg or greater and to keep the partial pressure of CO_2 in arterial blood ($PaCO_2$) in normal range at 35–45 mm Hg, an endotracheal tube or tracheostomy and mechanical ventilation may be needed.

- Surgical removal may be needed if the increased ICP is caused by a mass lesion, such as a tumor or hematoma (see Brain Tumors).

Drug Therapy

Drug therapy is an important part of the management of increased ICP.

- IV mannitol (Osmitrol) (25%) is an osmotic diuretic that decreases ICP in two ways: plasma expansion and osmotic effect. The immediate plasma-expanding effect reduces the hematocrit and blood viscosity. This increases cerebral blood flow and cerebral oxygenation. The osmotic effect causes fluid to move from the tissue into the blood vessels, which decreases total brain fluid content.
- IV hypertonic saline is used to manage increased ICP. It produces massive movement of water out of swollen brain cells and into the blood vessels.
- Corticosteroids (e.g., dexamethasone) are used to treat vasogenic edema surrounding tumors and abscesses. They are not recommended for traumatic brain injury. Corticosteroids stabilize the cell membrane and inhibit the synthesis of prostaglandins. These drugs also improve cerebral blood flow and restore autoregulation.
- Metabolic demands, such as fever (temperatures above 38°C), agitation/shivering, pain, and seizures, can increase ICP. The interprofessional team should plan to reduce these metabolic demands to lower the ICP.
- High-dose barbiturates (e.g., pentobarbital, thiopental) are used in patients with increased ICP refractory to other treatments. These drugs lower cerebral metabolism to decrease ICP.
- Patients with increased ICP who need mechanical ventilation may receive opiates, sedatives, and neuromuscular blocking agents by continuous infusion.
- Antiseizure prophylaxis against early seizures (within the first 7 days) may be prescribed for patients with severe brain injury.

Nutritional Therapy

The patient with increased ICP is in a hypermetabolic and hypercatabolic state that increases the need for glucose to provide the necessary fuel for metabolism of the injured brain. If the patient cannot maintain an adequate oral intake, enteral or parenteral nutrition should be started. Fluid therapy is directed at keeping patients normovolemic.

Nursing Management

Goals

The overall goals are that the patient with increased ICP will have ICP within normal limits, maintain a patent airway, demonstrate normal fluid and electrolyte balance, and have no complications from immobility and decreased LOC.

Interventions

Respiratory Function. Maintenance of a patent airway is critical in patients with increased ICP and is a major nursing responsibility. As the LOC decreases, the patient is at increased risk for airway obstruction.

- Be alert to altered breathing patterns. Snoring sounds indicate obstruction and require immediate intervention. An oral airway facilitates breathing and provides an easier suctioning route in the comatose patient.
- In general, any patient with a Glasgow Coma Scale score of 8 or less (see Glasgow Coma Scale) or an altered LOC who is unable to maintain a patent airway or effective ventilation needs intubation and mechanical ventilation.
- Careful monitoring is needed for the patient with increased ICP who requires mechanical ventilation and continuous sedation.
- Prevent hypoxia and hypercapnia. Frequently monitor and evaluate the ABG values. Take measures to maintain the levels within prescribed parameters. The appropriate ventilatory support can be ordered based on the PaO_2 and $PaCO_2$ values.
- Proper neutral positioning of the head is important. Elevating the head of the bed by 30 degrees enhances respiratory exchange and aids in decreasing cerebral edema.
- Suctioning and coughing can cause transient increases in ICP and decreases in PaO_2. Remove accumulated secretions by suctioning as needed.
- Try to prevent abdominal distention, which can interfere with respiratory function. Inserting a nasogastric tube to aspirate the stomach contents can prevent distention, vomiting, and possible aspiration. In patients with facial and skull fractures, a nasogastric tube is contraindicated because of risk of inadvertent intracranial placement. Oral insertion of a gastric tube is preferred.

Fluid and Electrolyte Balance. Fluid and electrolyte problems can have an adverse effect on ICP. Closely monitor IV fluids. Intake and output, accounting for insensible losses, and daily weights are important in the assessment of fluid balance.

- Monitor serum electrolytes, especially glucose, sodium, potassium, magnesium, and osmolality.
- Monitor urinary output for problems related to SIADH and diabetes insipidus (DI) (see Diabetes Insipidus).

Monitoring Intracranial Pressure

ICP monitoring is used with other parameters to guide care and assess the patient's response to care (see Intracranial Pressure Monitoring).

- The gold standard for monitoring ICP is the ventriculostomy, in which a specialized catheter is inserted into the lateral ventricle and coupled to an external transducer. This technique directly measures the pressure within the ventricles, facilitates removal and/or sampling of CSF, and allows for intraventricular drug administration. The transducer is external. We must ensure that the transducer is level with the foramen of Monro (interventricular foramen). The system must also be at the ideal height. A reference point for this foramen is the tragus of the ear. Every time the patient is repositioned, assess the system to ensure it is level.
- Infection is a serious complication with ICP monitoring. Factors that contribute to infection include ICP monitoring more than 5 days, use of a ventriculostomy, a CSF leak, and a concurrent systemic infection. Routinely assess the insertion site and use aseptic technique. Monitor the CSF for a change in drainage color or clarity.
- Fiberoptic catheters and air pouch/pneumatic technology can also be used to measure ICP.

Technology is available to measure cerebral oxygenation and assess perfusion. Three intracranial devices used in ICU settings are the LICOX catheter, Neurovent catheter, and jugular venous bulb catheter.

Body Position. Maintain the patient with increased ICP in the head-up position. Prevent extreme neck flexion, which can cause venous obstruction and increased ICP. Adjust the body position to decrease the ICP maximally and to improve cerebral perfusion pressure (CPP).

- Turn the patient with slow, gentle movements, because rapid changes in position, pain, and agitation may increase ICP. Avoid extreme hip flexion to decrease the risk of raising the intraabdominal pressure, which increases ICP.

Protection From Injury. The patient should be in a quiet, calm environment with minimal noise and interruptions. Observe the patient for signs of agitation, irritation, or frustration. Teach the caregiver and family about decreasing stimulation. Coordinate with the inter-professional team to minimize procedures that may cause agitation.

The patient with increased ICP and decreased LOC needs protection from self-injury. Confusion, agitation, and the possibility of seizures increase the risk of injury.

- Use restraints carefully in the agitated patient. If restraints are necessary to keep the patient from removing tubes or falling out of bed, they should be secure enough to be effective. Observe the skin area under the restraints regularly for irritation. Agitation may increase with the use of restraints, which indicates the need for other measures to protect the patient from injury.

Psychologic Considerations. Anxiety over the diagnosis and prognosis can be distressing to the patient, caregiver, family, and nursing staff. Provide support and short, simple explanations. Assess the family members' desire and need to assist in providing patient care and allow for their participation as appropriate.

- Touch and talk to the patient calmly, even the patient who is in a coma and may appear not to hear.

INFLAMMATORY BOWEL DISEASE

Description

Inflammatory bowel disease (IBD) is a chronic inflammation of the gastrointestinal (GI) tract characterized by periods of remission interspersed with periods of exacerbation. IBD is classified as either *Crohn's disease* or *ulcerative colitis* (UC) on the basis of clinical manifestations (Table 52). UC is usually limited to the colon. Crohn's disease can involve any segment of the GI tract from the mouth to the anus.

About 1.3 million Americans have IBD. It often begins during the teenage years and early adulthood and has a second peak in the sixth decade.

Pathophysiology

IBD is an autoimmune disease involving an immune reaction to a person's own intestinal tract. An overactive, inappropriate, or sustained immune response causes inflammation and widespread tissue destruction. The pattern of inflammation differs between Crohn's disease and UC.

The highest rates of IBD are in the Northern Hemisphere and industrialized nations. The risk for having IBD is greater in urban compared with rural areas and those of white and Ashkenazic

Jewish origin than in other racial and ethnic groups. The strongest risk factor is family history. IBD occurs more often in family members of people with IBD.

Lifestyle factors, such as diet, smoking, and stress, increase susceptibility by changing the environment of the GI microbial flora.

TABLE 52 Comparison of Ulcerative Colitis and Crohn's Disease

Characteristic	Ulcerative colitis	Crohn's disease
Clinical		
Usual age at onset	Teens to mid-30s. After 60 yrs	Teens to mid-30s. After 60 yrs
Abdominal pain	Common, severe constant	Common, cramping
Diarrhea	Common	Common
Fever (intermittent)	During acute attacks	Common
Malabsorption and nutritional deficiencies	Minimal incidence	Common
Rectal bleeding	Common	Sometimes
Tenesmus	Common	Rare
Weight loss	Rare	Common, may be severe
Pathologic		
Location	Usually starts in rectum and spreads in a continuous pattern up the colon	Occurs anywhere along GI tract. Most common site is distal ileum
Cobblestoning of mucosa	Rare	Common
Depth of involvement	Mucosa	Entire thickness of bowel wall (transmural)
Distribution	Continuous areas of inflammation	Healthy tissue interspersed with areas of inflammation (skip lesions)
Pseudopolyps	Common	Rare
Small bowel involvement	Minimal	Common

TABLE 52 Comparison of Ulcerative Colitis and Crohn's Disease—cont'd

Characteristic	Ulcerative colitis	Crohn's disease
Complications		
Cancer	Increased incidence of colorectal cancer after 10 year of disease	Increased incidence of small intestinal cancer. Increased incidence of colorectal cancer but less than with ulcerative colitis
C. difficile infection	Increased incidence and severity	Increased incidence and severity
Perforation	Common (because of toxic megacolon)	Common (because inflammation involves entire bowel wall)
Perianal abscess and fistulas	Rare	Common
Strictures	Occasional	Common
Toxic megacolon	More common	Rare

High intake of refined sugar, total fats, polyunsaturated fatty acid (PUFA), and omega-6 fatty acids seems to increase the risk of IBD. Nonsteroidal antiinflammatory drugs (NSAIDs), antibiotics, and oral contraceptives also increase the risk.

Crohn's Disease

The inflammation in Crohn's disease involves all layers of the bowel wall. It can occur anywhere in the GI tract from the mouth to the anus but often involves the distal ileum and proximal colon. Segments of normal bowel between diseased portions are called "skip lesions."

- Typically, deep and longitudinal ulcerations penetrate between islands of inflamed edematous mucosa, causing the classic cobblestone appearance.
- Strictures at the areas of inflammation can cause bowel obstruction.
- Microscopic leaks in the bowel wall can allow bowel contents to enter the peritoneal cavity and cause abscesses or peritonitis.
- Fistulas are common between adjacent areas of bowel, between bowel and bladder, and between bowel and vagina.

Ulcerative Colitis

UC is a disease of the colon and rectum. It usually starts in the rectum and moves in a continual fashion toward the cecum.

- Inflammation and ulcerations occur in the mucosal layer, the innermost layer of the bowel wall. Inflammation does not extend through all of the bowel layers, so fistulas and abscesses are rare.
- Inflamed mucosa forms pseudopolyps, which are tongue-like projections into the bowel lumen.

Clinical Manifestations

Manifestations are often the same (diarrhea, bloody stools, weight loss, abdominal pain, fever, and fatigue) in both conditions. Bloody stools are more common with UC, and weight loss is more common in Crohn's disease. Both forms of IBD are chronic disorders with mild to severe acute exacerbations that occur at unpredictable intervals over many years.

Crohn's Disease

Diarrhea and colicky abdominal pain are common symptoms of Crohn's disease.

- If the small intestine is inflamed, weight loss occurs from malabsorption.
- Rectal bleeding occurs less often with Crohn's disease than with UC.

Ulcerative Colitis

The primary symptoms of UC are bloody diarrhea and abdominal pain. Pain may range from the mild, lower abdominal cramping with diarrhea to the severe, constant abdominal pain from acute perforation.

- With *mild disease,* diarrhea may consist of up to four semi-formed stools daily that contain small amounts of blood. The patient may have no other manifestations.
- In *moderate disease,* there is increased stool output (up to 10 stools/day), increased bleeding, and systemic signs and symptoms (fever, malaise, mild anemia, anorexia).
- In *severe disease,* diarrhea is bloody, with mucus in the stool, and occurs 10–20 times a day. In addition, fever, weight loss (more than 10% of total body weight), anemia, tachycardia, and dehydration are present.

Complications

Patients with IBD have both local GI tract and systemic complications.

- GI tract complications include hemorrhage, strictures, perforation (with possible peritonitis), abscesses, fistulas, *Clostridium difficile* infection, and toxic megacolon.

- Toxic megacolon is more common with UC, while abscesses and perianal fistulas occur more often with Crohn's disease.
- Hemorrhage may lead to anemia. It is corrected with blood transfusions and iron supplements.
- People with a history of IBD are at increased risk for colorectal cancer. Those with Crohn's disease are at increased risk for small intestine cancer.

People with IBD may have systemic complications, such as multiple sclerosis and ankylosing spondylitis. Some are related to the inflammatory activity in the bowel, and they improve when the IBD improves. Other complications include malabsorption, liver disease (primary sclerosing cholangitis), and osteoporosis. Routine liver function tests are important because primary sclerosing cholangitis can lead to liver failure. Both men and women with IBD are at risk for osteoporosis. They need a bone density scan at baseline and every 2 years.

Diagnostic Studies

Diagnosis of IBD includes ruling out diseases with similar symptoms and then determining whether the patient has Crohn's disease or UC.

- Laboratory studies may indicate electrolyte problems, anemia, leukocytosis, hypoalbuminemia, and a high erythrocyte sedimentation rate.
- Stool is examined for blood, pus, and mucus and cultured to rule out infectious diarrhea.
- Double-contrast barium enema, small bowel series, transabdominal ultrasound, CT scan, MRI, and capsule endoscopy are useful for IBD diagnosis.
- Colonoscopy allows examination of the large intestine and sometimes the distal ileum.

Interprofessional Management

The goals of treatment are to rest the bowel, control inflammation, correct malnutrition, provide symptomatic relief, and improve quality of life. Hospitalization is indicated if the patient does not respond to drug therapy, the disease is severe, or complications are suspected.

Drug Therapy

Drugs are used to induce and maintain a remission of IBD. Drugs are chosen on the basis of the location and severity of inflammation. Five major classes of medications used to treat IBD are aminosalicylates, antimicrobials, corticosteroids, immunosuppressants, and biologic therapies (Table 53).

TABLE 53   Drug Therapy: Inflammatory Bowel Disease

Class	Action	Examples
5-Aminosalicylates (5-ASA)	Decrease inflammation by suppressing proinflammatory cytokines and other inflammatory mediators	*Systemic:* Balsalazide (Colazal), mesalamine (Asacol, Apriso, Delzicol, Lialda, Pentasa), olsalazine (Dipentum), sulfasalazine (Azulfidine) *Topical:* 5-ASA enema, foam, suppositories
Antimicrobials	Prevent or treat secondary infection	Ciprofloxacin (Cipro), clarithromycin (Biaxin), metronidazole (Flagyl)
Biologic therapies	*Anti-TNF agents:* Inhibit the cytokine tumor necrosis factor (TNF)	Adalimumab (Humira), certolizumab pegol (Cimzia), golimumab (Simponi), infliximab (Remicade)
	Integrin receptor antagonists: Prevent migration of leukocytes from bloodstream to inflamed tissue	Natalizumab (Tysabri), vedolizumab (Entyvio)
	IL-12/23 antagonists: Bind IL-12 and IL-23, preventing the activation of T-helper and natural killer cells	Risankizumab (Skyrizi), ustekinumab (Stelara)
	JAK inhibitors: Block the JAK enzyme, preventing it from activating immune cells that cause inflammation	Tofacitinib (Xeljanz)
Corticosteroids	Decrease inflammation	*Systemic:* Corticosteroids (prednisone, budesonide); hydrocortisone, methylprednisolone (IV for severe IBD) *Topical:* Hydrocortisone suppository, foam (Cortifoam), enema (Cortenema)
Immunomodulators	Suppress immune response	Azathioprine, cyclosporine, methotrexate, 6-mercaptopurine

Surgical Therapy

Many patients with Crohn's disease will eventually require surgery for complications such as strictures, bleeding, obstructions, or fistulas.

- The most common surgery involves resecting the diseased segments with reanastomosis of the remaining intestine. Unfortunately, the disease often recurs at the anastomosis site.
- Repeated removal of sections of small intestine can lead to *short bowel syndrome* (SBS). SBS occurs when either surgery or disease leaves too little small intestine surface area to maintain normal nutrition and hydration. Lifetime fluid boluses and parenteral nutrition (PN) may be needed.

In UC, surgical procedures used include total proctocolectomy with ileal pouch/anal anastomosis (IPAA) and total proctocolectomy with permanent ileostomy.

- Since UC affects only the colon, a total proctocolectomy is curative.

Nutritional Therapy

Many patients with IBD are malnourished. The goals of diet management are to provide adequate nutrition without exacerbating symptoms, correct and prevent malnutrition, replace fluid and electrolyte losses, and prevent weight loss. Consult a dietitian regarding dietary recommendations.

- Nutritional problems are caused by decreased oral intake, blood loss, and, depending on the location of the inflammation, impaired absorption.
- Patients with an IBD exacerbation may not be able to tolerate a regular diet. Liquid enteral feedings are preferred over parenteral nutrition because atrophy of the gut and bacterial overgrowth occur when the GI tract is not used.
- There are no universal food triggers for IBD, but some people may find that certain foods initiate diarrhea. A food diary helps identify problem foods to avoid.

Nursing Management

Goals

The patient with IBD will have fewer and less severe exacerbations, maintain normal fluid and electrolyte balance, be free from pain or discomfort, adhere to medical regimens, maintain nutritional balance, and have an improved quality of life.

Interventions

During the acute phase, focus your attention on hemodynamic stability, pain control, fluid and electrolyte balance, and nutritional support. Maintain accurate intake and output records and monitor the number and appearance of stools.

- Establish rapport and encourage the patient to talk about self-care strategies. Explain procedures and treatment to help build trust and allay apprehension.
- Talk with those who have Crohn's disease about smoking cessation because smoking can cause more severe disease.
- Given the chronicity and uncertainty related to the frequency and severity of flares, the patient may have frustration, depression, and anxiety. Psychotherapy, behavioral therapies, and support groups may help patients deal with feelings and manage their symptoms.
- Patients may lose sleep because of frequent episodes of diarrhea and abdominal pain. Nutritional deficiencies and anemia may leave the patient feeling weak and listless. Discuss managing fatigue and schedule activities around rest periods.
- Help the patient stay clean, dry, and free of odor. Meticulous perianal skin care using plain water (no harsh soap) together with a skin barrier prevents skin breakdown. Dibucaine (Nupercainal), witch hazel, sitz baths, and other soothing compresses or prescribed ointments may reduce perianal irritation. Place a deodorizer in the room.

▼ Patient and Caregiver Teaching

The patient and caregivers may need help in setting realistic short- and long-term goals.

- Your teaching should include: (1) the importance of rest and diet management, (2) perianal care, (3) drug action and side effects, (4) symptoms of disease recurrence, (5) when to seek medical care, and (6) use of diversional activities to reduce stress.
- Excellent teaching resources are available from the Crohn's and Colitis Foundation of America.

INTERSTITIAL CYSTITIS/PAINFUL BLADDER SYNDROME

Description

Interstitial cystitis (IC) is a chronic, painful inflammatory disease of the bladder characterized by urgency, frequency, and pain in the bladder and/or pelvis. IC is also called *bladder pain syndrome* or *painful bladder syndrome* (PBS).

- The term *interstitial cystitis/painful bladder syndrome* (IC/PBS) refers to urinary pain that cannot be attributed to other causes such as urinary tract infection (UTI) or stones. It is more common in women.

The cause of IC/PBS is unknown. Possible causes include neurogenic hypersensitivity of the lower urinary tract, changes in mast cells in the muscle and/or mucosal layers of the bladder, bladder attacked by the immune system, or production of a toxic substance in the urine.

Clinical Manifestations

Two primary clinical manifestations of IC are pain and bothersome lower urinary tract symptoms (LUTS) such as frequency and urgency. Symptoms may disappear after a period of weeks to months or persist for years.

- The pain is usually in the suprapubic area but may involve the vagina, labia, or entire perineal region. It varies from moderate to severe and may get worse with bladder filling, postponed urination, physical exertion, pressure against the suprapubic area, certain foods, or prolonged sitting. Sexual intercourse or emotional stress can worsen pain. Voiding temporarily relieves pain.
- People with severe cases may void 60 times/day including nighttime urination.
- The patient may have periods of remission and exacerbation. Women often report pain that occurs before menstruation.

Diagnostic Studies

IC/PBS is a diagnosis of exclusion.

- History and physical examination are necessary to rule out other disorders that produce somewhat similar symptoms, such as cancer, UTI, or endometriosis.
- Cystoscopic examination may reveal a small bladder capacity, Hunner lesions (distinct inflammatory areas on the bladder wall), and glomerulations (superficial ulcerations with pinpoint bleeding). These findings are not always present.

Interprofessional and Nursing Management

No single treatment consistently reverses or relieves symptoms. People with IC/PBS do not respond to antibiotic therapy. They rarely need surgery.

- Elimination of foods and beverages that irritate the bladder may provide some relief from symptoms. Typical bladder irritants include caffeine, alcohol, citrus products, carbonated drinks, chocolate, foods containing vinegar, curries, or hot peppers, and foods or beverages likely to lower urinary pH, including fruits such as cranberries.

- An over-the-counter (OTC) dietary supplement, calcium glycerophosphate (Prelief), alkalinizes the urine and can provide relief from the irritating effects of certain foods.

Two tricyclic antidepressants, amitriptyline and nortriptyline, may reduce the burning and urinary frequency. Pentosan (Elmiron) is used to enhance the protective effects of the glycosaminoglycan layer of the bladder. These drugs provide relief over weeks to months, but immediate relief for an acute exacerbation of symptoms may require a short course of opioid analgesics. Several agents may be instilled directly into the bladder through a small catheter.

- Dimethyl sulfoxide (DMSO) acts by desensitizing pain receptors in the bladder wall.
- Heparin, lidocaine, or sodium bicarbonate can be instilled into the bladder to relieve acute IC/PBS symptoms.

Surgical procedures, such as urinary diversion with an ileal conduit or fulguration and resection of Hunner lesions, can be used in an attempt to relieve debilitating pain.

Patient Teaching

Teach the patient to keep a bladder log or voiding diary over a period of at least 3 days to determine voiding frequency and patterns of nocturia. Teach the patient to maintain good nutrition, particularly in light of the dietary restrictions often necessary to control IC-related pain.

- Advise the patient to take a multivitamin containing no more than the recommended dietary allowance for essential vitamins and to avoid high-potency vitamins that may irritate the bladder.
- Advise the patient to avoid clothing that creates suprapubic pressure, including pants with tight belts or restrictive waistlines.
- Because stress can exacerbate IC/PBS, relaxation techniques (e.g., relaxation breathing, imagery) may help.
- Using lubrication or altering positions may decrease pain associated with sexual intercourse.
- Written educational materials concerning diet, ways to cope with the need for frequent urination, and strategies for coping with the emotional burden of IC/PBS are available from the Interstitial Cystitis Association (www.ichelp.org).

INTERVERTEBRAL DISC DISEASE

Description

Intervertebral disc disease is a condition that involves the deterioration, herniation, or other dysfunction of the intervertebral discs. Disc disorders can affect the cervical, thoracic, and lumbar spine.

Pathophysiology

Intervertebral discs separate the vertebrae of the spinal column and provide shock absorption for the spine. *Degenerative disc disease* (DDD) results from increased wear and tear on the intervertebral discs with aging (Fig. 17). The discs lose their elasticity, flexibility, and shock-absorbing abilities. Unless it is accompanied by pain, this wear-and-tear condition is a normal process.

The discs become thinner as the nucleus pulposus (gelatinous center of the disc) starts to dry out and shrink. This change limits the disc's ability to distribute pressure between vertebrae. The pressure is then transferred to the annulus fibrosus (strong outside part of the disc), causing progressive destruction.

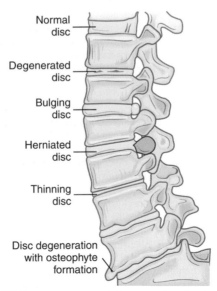

Normal disc

Degenerated disc

Bulging disc

Herniated disc

Thinning disc

Disc degeneration with osteophyte formation

Fig. 17 Common causes of degenerative disc damage.

- When the disc is damaged, the nucleus pulposus may seep through a torn or stretched annulus. This is called a *herniated disc* (slipped disc), a condition in which a spinal disc herniates and bulges outward between the vertebrae.

A herniated disc can result from natural degeneration with age, repeated stress, and trauma to the spine or spinal stenosis. The nucleus pulposus may first bulge, and then it can herniate, placing pressure on nearby nerves. The most common sites of rupture are the lumbosacral discs, specifically, L4-5 and L5-S1.

Clinical Manifestations

Lumbar Disc Disease

The most common manifestation is low back pain. Pain that radiates down the buttock and below the knee along the distribution of the sciatic nerve generally indicates disc herniation. The straight-leg raising test may be positive, indicating nerve root irritation. Back or leg pain may be reproduced by raising the leg.

- Reflexes may be depressed or absent, depending on the spinal nerve root involved. Paresthesia or muscle weakness in the legs, feet, or toes may occur.
- Multiple nerve root (cauda equina) compression may be marked by severe low back pain, progressive weakness, increased pain, or bowel/bladder incontinence. This is a medical emergency requiring surgery to reduce pressure on the nerves.

Cervical Disc Disease

Pain often radiates into the arms and hands, following the pattern of the involved nerve. Reflexes may not be present, and the handgrip is often weak.

Diagnostic Studies

- X-rays are done to detect any structural defects.
- A myelogram, MRI, or CT scan is helpful in localizing the damaged site.
- An epidural venogram or discogram may be necessary if other diagnostic studies are inconclusive.
- Electromyography (EMG) of the extremities can help to determine the severity of nerve irritation or to rule out conditions such as peripheral neuropathy.

Interprofessional Management

Conservative Therapy

Conservative therapy includes limitation of spinal movement (brace/corset/belt), local heat or ice, ultrasound and massage, traction, and transcutaneous electrical nerve stimulation (TENS). Drug therapy includes nonsteroidal antiinflammatory drugs (NSAIDs), short-term oral corticosteroids, opioid analgesics, muscle relaxants, antiseizure drugs, and antidepressants. Epidural corticosteroid injections may relieve acute pain.

- When symptoms subside, patients begin back-strengthening exercises twice per day. Teach the patient good body mechanics.
- Most patients heal with conservative treatment after 6 months.

Surgical Therapy

Surgery for a damaged disc is generally considered when the problem is not responding to conservative treatment and the patient is in consistent pain and/or has a persistent neurologic deficit.

- An *intradiscal electrothermoplasty* (IDET) is a minimally invasive outpatient procedure for treatment of back and sciatic pain. A needle is inserted into the affected disc with X-ray guidance. The heated wire threaded through the needle destroys the small nerve fibers that have grown into the disc.
- A similar outpatient technique is *radiofrequency discal nucleoplasty,* in which a special radiofrequency probe inserted into the disc is used to break up the molecular bonds of the gel in the nucleus.
- Implantable devices include *interspinous dynamic stabilizers* (ISDS) and *interspinous stabilizers* (ISS). *ISSs* reduce the degree of extension of the vertebrae with no effect on spinal stability. *ISDSs* stabilize the spinal segment and provide some spacer properties.
- *Diskectomy* can also be performed to decompress the nerve root. Microsurgical diskectomy is a version of the standard procedure.
- A *percutaneous diskectomy* uses instruments with a tiny camera and fluoroscopy guidance, then focuses a laser on the damaged part of the disc.
- Artificial disc replacement surgery may restore movement and eliminate pain. After removing the damaged disc, the device is surgically placed in the spine (usually through a small incision below the umbilicus).
- A *spinal fusion* may be needed if the spine is unstable. The spine is stabilized by creating an *ankylosis* (fusion) of adjacent vertebrae with a bone graft from the patient's fibula or iliac crest (autograft) or from donated cadaver bone (allograft). Metal fixation with rods, plates, or screws may be implanted. A posterior lumbar interbody fusion may be performed to give extra support for bone grafting or a prosthetic device. Bone morphogenetic protein (BMP), a genetically engineered protein, may be used to stimulate growth of the bone graft in spinal fusions.

- Artificial disc replacement surgery for patients with DDD includes the use of the Charité disc for lower disc damage and the Prestige cervical disc system.

Nursing Management: Spine Surgery

After spinal surgery, a key intervention is maintaining spinal alignment. The patient may be able to dangle the legs over the side of the bed, stand, or even ambulate the same day of surgery. After lumbar fusion, place pillows under the thighs when the patient is supine and between the legs when the patient is in the side-lying position to provide comfort and ensure alignment.

- The patient often fears turning or movement that increases pain. Reassure the patient that proper technique is being used to maintain body alignment. Have the patient logroll to turn in bed.
- After surgery, most patients will need opioids, such as morphine IV for 24–48 hours. Patient-controlled analgesia (PCA) allows for maintaining optimal analgesic levels. Diazepam (Valium) may be prescribed for muscle relaxation.

Frequently monitor the patient's peripheral neurologic condition. Movement of arms and legs and assessment of sensation should at least equal preoperative status. Paresthesias, such as numbness and tingling, may not be relieved immediately after surgery.

- Report any new muscle weakness or paresthesias to the surgeon at once and record the finding in the patient's medical record.

Because the spinal canal may be entered during surgery, there is potential for cerebrospinal fluid (CSF) leakage. Immediately report severe headache or CSF leakage on the dressing.

Paralytic ileus and interference with bowel function may occur for several days. Assess whether the patient is passing flatus, has bowel sounds, and has a flat, soft abdomen. Stool softeners (e.g., docusate sodium) and laxatives may prevent and relieve constipation.

- Emptying the bladder may be hard because of activity restrictions, opioids, or anesthesia. Encourage men to dangle their legs over the side of the bed or stand to urinate if allowed by the surgeon. Urge patients to use a bedside commode or ambulate to the bathroom, when allowed, to promote bladder emptying. Intermittent catheterization or an indwelling urinary catheter may be needed by patients with problems urinating.

After cervical spine surgery, be alert for signs of spinal cord edema, such as respiratory distress and a worsening neurologic status of the upper extremities. The patient's neck may be immobilized in either a soft or a hard cervical collar.

The healing time after a spinal fusion with bone graft is prolonged compared with that for a laminectomy. Activity may be limited for an extended time. A rigid orthosis (thoracic-lumbar-sacral orthosis or chairback brace) is often used.

■ Regularly assess the donor site for the bone graft, which usually causes greater postoperative pain than the fused area. If the donor site is the fibula, include neurovascular extremity assessments. Teach the patient to avoid sitting or standing for longed periods. Encourage walking and shifting weight from one foot to the other when standing.

■ Teach the patient to think through an activity before bending or stooping and avoiding any twisting movement. The thighs and knees, rather than the back, should be used to absorb the shock of activity and movement.

■ A firm mattress or bed board is essential.

INTESTINAL OBSTRUCTION

Description

Intestinal obstruction or bowel obstruction occurs when contents cannot pass through the gastrointestinal (GI) tract. An obstruction may be a small bowel obstruction (SBO) or large bowel/colon obstruction (LBO). The obstruction can be partial or complete, simple or strangulated. A partial obstruction usually resolves with conservative treatment, whereas a complete obstruction usually requires surgery. A simple obstruction has an intact blood supply, and a strangulated one does not.

Causes of intestinal obstruction are mechanical or nonmechanical (Fig. 18).

■ *Mechanical obstruction* is a physical blockage that most often occurs in the small intestine. Surgical adhesions are the most common cause of SBO. They can develop days or years after. Other causes of SBO are hernia, strictures from Crohn's disease, and intussusception after bariatric surgery. The most common cause of LBO is colorectal cancer. Other causes include adhesions, ischemia, volvulus, and Crohn's disease.

■ *Nonmechanical obstruction* occurs with reduced or absent peristalsis secondary to altered neuromuscular transmission of the parasympathetic innervation to the bowel. It may result from a neuromuscular or vascular disorder. *Paralytic ileus* (lack of intestinal peristalsis and bowel sounds), the most common form of nonmechanical obstruction, occurs to some degree after any abdominal surgery. Other causes of paralytic ileus include inflammatory reactions (e.g., acute pancreatitis, acute appendicitis), electrolyte imbalances (especially hypokalemia), and thoracic or lumbar spinal fractures.

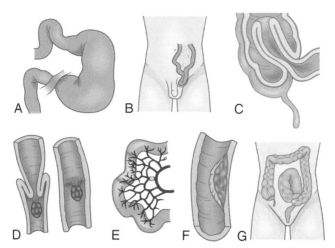

Fig. 18 Intestinal obstructions. (A) Adhesions. (B) Strangulated inguinal hernia. (C) Ileocecal intussusception. (D) Intussusception from polyps. (E) Mesenteric occlusion. (F) Neoplasm. (G) Volvulus of the sigmoid colon.

- *Vascular obstructions* are rare, caused by interference with the blood supply to a portion of the bowel. The most common causes are emboli and atherosclerosis of the mesenteric arteries.
- *Pseudoobstruction* is a GI motility disorder. Conditions associated with a pseudoobstruction include neurologic problems, drugs, endocrine and metabolic problems, lung disease, trauma, and burns.

Pathophysiology

When fluid, gas, and intestinal contents accumulate proximal to the obstruction, distention occurs and the distal bowel collapses. As the proximal bowel becomes increasingly distended, the intraluminal bowel pressure rises. The high pressure leads to an increase in capillary permeability and extravasation of fluids and electrolytes into the peritoneal cavity. Retention of fluid in the intestine and peritoneal cavity leads to a severe decrease in circulating blood volume and results in hypotension and hypovolemic shock.

- In *intestinal strangulation* or *intestinal infarction*, the bowel becomes so distended that the blood flow is stopped, causing edema, cyanosis, and gangrene of bowel segment. If it is not corrected quickly, the bowel will become necrotic and rupture, leading to infection, septic shock, and death.

Clinical Manifestations

- Manifestations vary depending on the location of the obstruction. The most important early manifestations of an SBO are colicky abdominal pain, nausea, vomiting, and abdominal distention.
- Patients with obstructions in the proximal small intestine rapidly develop nausea and vomiting, which is sometimes projectile and contains bile. Vomiting usually relieves pain in higher intestinal obstructions. Vomiting from more distal obstructions of the small intestine is gradual in onset and more fecal- and foul-smelling.
- Persistent, colicky abdominal pain, abdominal distention, constipation (new-onset), and lack of flatus are signs of lower intestinal obstruction.
- With mechanical obstruction, pain comes and goes in waves. By contrast, paralytic ileus produces a more constant, generalized discomfort. Strangulation causes rapid, severe, constant pain.
- Abdominal distention is usually minimal in proximal SBO and markedly increased in LBO. Abdominal tenderness and rigidity are present when there is strangulation or peritonitis.
- Bowel sounds are high-pitched above the area of obstruction. Bowel sounds may also be absent. *Borborygmi* (audible abdominal sounds caused by hyperactive intestinal motility) are often noted.

Diagnostic Studies

- CT scans and abdominal X-rays are used.
- Sigmoidoscopy or colonoscopy may provide direct visualization of an LBO.
- An elevated white blood cell (WBC) count may indicate strangulation or perforation.
- High hematocrit (Hct) values may reflect hemoconcentration.
- Low hemoglobin (Hgb) and Hct values may indicate bleeding from a neoplasm or strangulation with necrosis.
- Serum electrolytes, blood urea nitrogen (BUN), and serum creatinine are monitored frequently to assess the degree of dehydration.

Interprofessional Management

The treatment goal is to regain intestinal patency and resolve the obstruction. Treatment of a bowel obstruction depends on the cause. If a strangulated obstruction or perforation is present, the patient will need emergency surgery to relieve the obstruction and survive. In some, especially those due to surgical adhesions, an obstruction may resolve without surgery. If needed, the patient may have an NG tube for decompression. Some patients need PN to allow bowel rest and improve nutrition status before surgery.

- Stents can be placed via endoscopic or fluoroscopic procedures. They are used for palliative purposes or as "a bridge to surgery," allowing a patient to avoid emergency surgery. This gives the healthcare team time to correct fluid volume and other problems, thus improving surgical outcomes. Corticosteroids with antiemetic properties that decrease edema and inflammation may be used with stent placement.

Nursing Management

Goals

The patient with an intestinal obstruction will have relief and a return to normal bowel function, minimal to no discomfort, and normal fluid and electrolyte and acid–base status.

Interventions

Assess the patient regularly and notify the surgeon of changes in vital signs, changes in bowel sounds, decreased urine output, increased abdominal distention, and pain.

- Maintain a strict intake and output record including emesis and tube drainage.
- Monitor the patient closely for signs of dehydration and electrolyte imbalances. A patient with an SBO is more likely to have metabolic alkalosis. A patient with an LBO is at greater risk for metabolic acidosis.
- The patient is often restless, changing position to relieve the pain. Provide comfort measures and promote a restful environment.
- Vomiting leaves an unpleasant taste in the patient's mouth, and fecal odor may be present. With an NG tube in place, the patient will breathe through the mouth. Provide frequent oral care.
- Nursing care of the patient after surgery for an intestinal obstruction is similar to the care of the patient after a laparotomy (see Abdominal Pain, Acute).

IRRITABLE BOWEL SYNDROME

Description

Irritable bowel syndrome (IBS) is a disorder characterized by chronic abdominal pain and altered bowel patterns. Patients may have diarrhea, constipation, or both.

IBS has no known cause. Psychologic stressors (e.g., depression, anxiety, panic disorders, posttraumatic stress disorder) are associated with the development and exacerbation of IBS. Many people with IBS have a family member with the disorder. Patients often report a history of gastrointestinal (GI) infections and adverse reactions to food. Dietary intolerances that may contribute to symptoms include gluten and fermentable oligo-, di-, and monosaccharides and polyols (FODMAPs).

- Examples of oligosaccharides are wheat and rye products, some fruits and vegetables, onions, garlic, legumes, and nuts. The disaccharide lactose is found in milk and milk products. Fructose is a monosaccharide found in honey, apples, pears, and high-fructose corn syrup. Polyols are found in apples, pears, stone fruits, cauliflower, mushrooms, and artificial sweeteners, such as sorbitol.

The Rome IV criteria for diagnosing IBS require the presence of abdominal pain and/or discomfort at least 1 day per week for 3 months that is associated with two or more of the following: related to defecation, change in stool frequency, or change in the stool form. Depending on the stool patterns, IBS is categorized as IBS with constipation (IBS–C), IBS with diarrhea (IBS-D), IBS mixed, and IBS unsubtyped.

- Other common symptoms include abdominal distention, nausea, flatulence, bloating, urgency, mucus in the stool, and sensation of incomplete evacuation. Non-GI symptoms may include fatigue, headache, and sleep problems.

Ask patients to describe symptoms, health history (including psychosocial factors such as stress and anxiety), family history, and drug and diet history. Determine if and how IBS symptoms interfere with school, work, and social activities. Diagnostic tests are used to rule out other disorders, such as colorectal cancer, IBD, endometriosis, and malabsorption disorders (lactose intolerance, celiac disease).

Interprofessional and Nursing Management

No single therapy is effective for all patients with IBS. Treatment may include psychologic support, diet and lifestyle changes, and drugs to regulate stool output and reduce discomfort.

- Patients may keep a diary of symptoms, diet, and episodes of stress to help identify factors that trigger the IBS symptoms.

Cognitive behavior therapy and stress management techniques may help a patient cope.

- Regular exercise reduces bloating, constipation, and related symptoms.

Drug therapy focuses on the dominant bowel symptom and pain. All patients with IBS may benefit from antidepressants and antispasmodic agents (hyoscyamine, dicyclomine). Antispasmodics decrease GI motility and smooth muscle spasms, reducing pain and diarrhea.

- Treatment for IBS-D includes rifaximin, the opioid agonist eluxadoline (Viberzi), and the selective serotonin 5-HT$_3$ antagonist alosetron. Rifaximin is given as a 2-week course of treatment with repeated courses as needed. Loperamide may help some patients.

- Eluxadoline decreases colonic contractions to reduce diarrhea and pain. Alosetron is only given to women with severe IBS-D that did not respond to other therapy. Because of serious side effects (severe constipation, ischemic colitis), it is available only in a restricted access program. Eluxadoline and alosetron are taken daily.

- Besides laxative therapy, those with IBS-C may take linaclotide (Linzess). It is contraindicated in patients with a history of mechanical obstruction or prior bowel surgery.

- Women with IBS-C may benefit from lubiprostone (Amitiza).

Teach the patient foods that are high in FODMAPs and how to follow a low FODMAP diet.

- If dairy products tend to cause symptoms, yogurt may be the best option because of the lactobacillus bacteria it contains. Probiotics can improve symptoms.

- Tell the patient with flatulence to avoid common gas-producing foods, such as broccoli and cabbage.

- For those with constipation, encourage a high-fiber diet to produce soft, painless bowel movements.

KIDNEY CANCER

Kidney cancer arises from the renal cortex or pelvis and calyces. Adenocarcinoma (renal cell carcinoma), the most common type, occurs twice as often in men. Blacks have slightly higher rates of renal cell cancer.

- Smoking and obesity are significant risk factors. An increased incidence occurs in first-degree relatives of people who have or had renal cell cancer. Other risk factors include hypertension and exposure to certain chemicals such as trichloroethylene and cadmium.

Early-stage kidney cancer usually has no symptoms. The most common later manifestations are hematuria and flank pain. Other manifestations include weight loss, fever, anemia, fatigue, hypercalcemia, and/or a palpable mass in the flank or abdomen. Local extension of kidney cancer into the renal vein and vena cava is common. The most common sites of metastases are the lungs, lymph nodes, bone, and liver.

- Diagnosis is based on CT scan and ultrasound. Angiography, biopsy, and MRI are also used. Radionuclide scanning is used to detect metastases.

Interprofessional and Nursing Management

Preventive measures, including quitting smoking, maintaining a healthy weight, controlling BP, and reducing exposure to toxins, help reduce the incidence of kidney cancer. Patients in high-risk groups should be aware of their increased risk for kidney cancer. Teach them about early manifestations (e.g., hematuria, flank pain, hypertension). It is possible to cure kidney cancer if it is found and treated early.

- Partial nephrectomy or *simple total nephrectomy* (for smaller tumors) or a radical nephrectomy (for larger tumors) is the treatment for some renal cancers. *Radical nephrectomy* involves removal of the kidney, adrenal gland, surrounding fascia, part of the ureter, and draining lymph nodes. Nephrectomy can be performed by a conventional (open) approach or laparoscopically.
- Kidney cancer is resistant to most chemotherapy drugs and radiation therapy.
- Immunotherapy, with agents including α-interferon, interleukin-2 (IL-2), or nivolumab (Opdivo) without or with ipilimumab anti-CTLA-4 antibody, is an option in metastatic disease.
- Targeted therapy is another treatment for metastatic kidney cancer. Kinase inhibitors include sunitinib (Sutent), sorafenib (Nexavar), cabozantinib (Cabometyx), and axitinib (Inlyta). Bevacizumab (Avastin), sunitinib (Sutent), and pazopanib (Votrient) inhibit the formation of new blood vessel growth to the tumor. Temsirolimus (Torisel) and everolimus (Afinitor) inhibit a specific protein known as the *mechanistic target of rapamycin* (mTOR).

KIDNEY DISEASE, CHRONIC

Description

Chronic kidney disease (CKD) involves progressive, irreversible loss of kidney function. CKD can be defined as either the presence of kidney damage or a decreased glomerular filtration rate (GFR) to <60 mL/minutes/1.73 m^2 for more than 3 months. The classification of CKD is presented in Table 54. The last stage of kidney failure, termed *end-stage renal disease* (ESRD), occurs when the GFR is <15 mL/minutes. At this point, renal replacement therapy (dialysis or transplantation) is required.

The leading causes of CKD are diabetes (about 50%) and hypertension (about 25%). Less common causes include glomerulonephritis, cystic diseases, and urologic diseases. One of every nine Americans has CKD. Over half a million Americans are receiving treatment (dialysis, transplantation).

- CKD has a high incidence in minority populations, especially blacks and Native Americans, at increased risk for hypertension and diabetes.

Kidney disease is underdiagnosed and undertreated because patients are often asymptomatic until there is considerable nephron loss. About 70% of people with CKD may be unaware they have the disease. Prognosis and course of CKD are highly variable depending on the cause, patient's condition and age, and adequacy of healthcare follow-up.

Clinical Manifestations

As kidney function deteriorates, every body system is affected. Manifestations are a result of retained substances including urea, creatinine, phenols, hormones, water, and electrolytes. *Uremia* is a syndrome in which kidney function declines and symptoms develop in multiple body systems. It often occurs when the GFR is <15 mL/minutes.

- *Urinary system.* As CKD progresses, patients have increasing fluid retention and need diuretic therapy. After a period on dialysis, patients may develop anuria.
- *Metabolic disturbances.* As GFR decreases, blood urea nitrogen (BUN) and serum creatinine levels rise. Serum creatinine clearance determinations (calculated GFR) are considered more accurate indicators of kidney function. As BUN increases, patients have nausea, vomiting, lethargy, fatigue, impaired thought processes, and headaches.

TABLE 54	Stages of Chronic Kidney Disease	
Description	GFR (mL/minutes/1.73 m²)	Clinical action plan
Stage 1 Kidney damage with normal or ↑ GFR	≥90	Diagnosis and treatment CVD risk reduction Slow progression
Stage 2 Kidney damage with mild ↓ GFR	60–89	Estimation of progression
Stage 3A Moderate ↓ GFR	45–59	Evaluation and treatment of complications
Stage 3B Moderate ↓ GFR	30–44	More aggressive treatment of complications
Stage 4 Severe ↓ GFR	15–29	Preparation for renal replacement therapy (dialysis, kidney transplantation)
Stage 5 Kidney failure	<15 (or dialysis)	Renal replacement therapy (if uremia is present and patient desires treatment)

CVD, Cardiovascular disease; *GFR*, glomerular filtration rate.

- *Electrolyte and acid–base imbalances.* Hyperkalemia results from the kidneys excreting less potassium, the breakdown of cellular protein, bleeding, and metabolic acidosis. Potassium may come from foods, diet supplements, drugs, and IV infusions. Sodium retention contributes to edema, hypertension, and heart failure. Metabolic acidosis results from the kidneys' impaired ability to excrete excess acid and from the defective reabsorption and regeneration of bicarbonate.

- *Altered carbohydrate metabolism and elevated triglycerides.* Mild to moderate hyperglycemia and hyperinsulinemia occur. Insulin and glucose metabolism may improve after the initiation of dialysis. Patients with diabetes who develop uremia may require less insulin than before the onset of CKD. Insulin, which depends on the kidneys for excretion, remains in circulation longer.
- *Hematologic system.* Anemia results from a lack of erythropoietin. Bleeding tendencies occur because of a defect in platelet function. Cellular and humoral immune responses are suppressed, resulting in increased susceptibility to infection.
- *Cardiovascular system.* The most common cause of death in patients with CKD is cardiovascular disease (CVD). Vascular calcification and arterial stiffness are major contributors to CVD in CKD. Hypertension is highly prevalent among patients with CKD because hypertension is both a cause and a consequence of CKD. Hypertension is worsened by sodium retention and increased extracellular fluid volume. Patients with CKD are susceptible to dysrhythmias from hyperkalemia and decreased coronary artery perfusion.
- *Musculoskeletal system.* Low serum calcium, increased phosphate, and decreased vitamin D contribute to stimulation of the parathyroid gland and an accelerated rate of bone remodeling. CKD mineral and bone disorder results in skeletal complications, such as *osteomalacia* (bone demineralization from slow bone turnover and defective mineralization of newly formed bone) and *osteitis fibrosa* (decalcification of the bone and replacement of bone tissue with fibrous tissue), and increased risk for fractures.

Additional systemic signs include pulmonary edema, constipation, peripheral neuropathy, pruritus, infertility, and personality and behavior changes.

Diagnostic Studies

- Urinalysis detects red blood cells (RBCs), white blood cells (WBCs), casts, protein, and glucose. Persistent proteinuria is usually the first sign of kidney damage.
- BUN and serum creatinine are elevated.
- GFR, obtained from 24-hour urine creatinine clearance measures, is decreased.

- Hematocrit (Hct) and hemoglobin (Hgb) levels are decreased.
- Ultrasound can be used to detect obstructions and kidney size.
- Kidney biopsy provides a definitive diagnosis.

Interprofessional Management

The focus in CKD is to preserve existing kidney function, reduce the risks of CVD, prevent complications, and provide for the patient's comfort. It is important that patients with CKD receive appropriate follow-up care with referral to a nephrologist early in the course of the disease. The focus during stages 1 through 4 (see Table 54) before the need for dialysis (stage 5) includes the control of hypertension, hyperparathyroid disease, anemia, hyperglycemia, and dyslipidemia.

- Acute hyperkalemia may require treatment with IV glucose and insulin to move potassium into the cells, or IV 10% calcium gluconate. Sodium polystyrene sulfonate, a cation-exchange resin or patiromer (Veltassa), an oral suspension that binds potassium in the GI tract, are used to lower potassium levels in stage 4 CKD. Dialysis may be required to decrease potassium if dysrhythmias are present.
- Treatment of hypertension includes weight loss (if obese), therapeutic lifestyle changes (e.g., exercise, avoiding alcohol, smoking cessation), diet recommendations, and administration of antihypertensive agents. Drugs most commonly used include diuretics, β-adrenergic blockers, calcium-channel blockers, angiotensin-converting enzyme (ACE) inhibitors, and angiotensin receptor blockers. See Hypertension.
- Phosphate binders such as calcium carbonate and calcium acetate are used to bind phosphate in the bowel, which is then excreted in the stool. Phosphate binders that do not contain calcium include sevelamer (Renagel) and lanthanum (Fosrenol) or the iron-based, calcium-free phosphate binders, such as sucroferric oxyhydroxide (Velphoro) and ferric citrate (Auryxia).
- Exogenous erythropoietin (epoetin alfa [Epogen, Procrit]) is used to treat the anemia of CKD.

The kidneys partially or totally excrete many drugs. CKD causes decreased elimination, leading to drug accumulation and the potential for drug toxicity. Drugs of particular concern include digoxin, diabetic agents (metformin, glyburide), antibiotics (e.g., vancomycin, gentamicin), and opioids.

Nutritional Therapy

The diet for CKD is designed to maintain good nutrition. Refer patients with CKD to a dietitian for nutritional teaching. For CKD stages 1–4, many healthcare providers (HCPs) encourage a normal protein intake. However, teach patients to avoid high-protein diets and supplements, because they may overstress the diseased kidneys. During peritoneal dialysis (PD), protein intake must be high enough to compensate for the losses so that the nitrogen balance is maintained.

Fluids are not routinely restricted in patients with CKD stages 1–5 who are not receiving hemodialysis (HD).

- Patients on HD have a more restricted fluid intake than patients on PD. For those on HD, as their urine output decreases, fluids are restricted. Generally, 600 mL (from insensible loss) plus an amount equal to the previous day's urine output is allowed for a patient on HD.

Nutritional therapy also includes the restriction of sodium, potassium, and phosphate.

Nursing Management
Goals
The overall goals are that the patient with CKD will adhere to the therapeutic plan, have effective coping strategies, and continue with activities of daily living within limitations.

Additional information on nursing diagnoses for the patient with CKD is presented in eNursing Care Plan 51-1 (on the website).
Interventions
Identify people at risk for CKD including those diagnosed with diabetes, hypertension, a family history of kidney disease, or repeated urinary tract infections. Recommend regular checkups that include routine urinalysis and calculation of GFR.

- Those at risk need to take measures to prevent or delay the progression of CKD, including glycemic control for patients with diabetes; BP control; and lifestyle modifications, including smoking cessation.
- Because patients with CKD take many drugs, a pillbox organizer or a list of the drugs and the times of administration may be helpful. Teach the patient to avoid over-the-counter drugs such as nonsteroidal antiinflammatory drugs (NSAIDs) and aluminum- or magnesium-based laxatives and antacids.
- When potentially nephrotoxic drugs are prescribed, monitor the patient's renal function with serum creatinine, BUN, and GFR.
- Advise patients with diabetes to report any changes in urine appearance (color, odor), frequency, or volume to the HCP.

K

Even though transplantation offers the best therapeutic management for patients with kidney failure, the critical shortage of donor organs limits this option.

■ Inform the patient that if dialysis is chosen, transplantation is still an option. If a transplanted organ fails, the patient can return to dialysis.

Patients may initiate a conversation about palliative care. Respect the patient's choice to decline treatment.

■ Listen to the patient and caregivers, allowing them to do most of the talking, and pay special attention to their hopes and fears.

▼ **Patient and Caregiver Teaching**

Teach the patient and family about the diet, drugs, and follow-up medical care (Table 55).

TABLE 55 Patient and Caregiver Teaching: Chronic Kidney Disease

Include the following information in the teaching plan for the patient and caregiver.

1. Dietary (sodium, potassium, phosphate) and fluid restrictions.
2. Common problems patient will encounter in modifying diet and fluid intake.
3. Signs and symptoms of electrolyte imbalance, especially high potassium.
4. Alternative ways of reducing thirst, such as sucking on ice cubes, lemon, or hard candy.
5. Reasons for prescribed drugs and common side effects.
   Examples:
   • Phosphate binders (including calcium supplements used as phosphate barriers) should be taken with meals.
   • Take calcium supplements prescribed to treat hypocalcemia on an empty stomach, but not at the same time as iron supplements.
   • Iron supplements should be taken between meals.
6. The importance of reporting any of the following: Weight gain >4 lb (2 kg), increasing BP, shortness of breath, edema, increasing fatigue or weakness, or confusion or lethargy
7. Need for support and encouragement. Share concerns about lifestyle changes, living with a chronic illness, and decisions about type of dialysis or transplantation.

KIDNEY INJURY, ACUTE

Description

Acute kidney injury (AKI) is the term used to encompass the entire range of the syndrome ranging from a slight deterioration in kidney function to severe impairment. It is characterized by a rapid loss of kidney function with or without decreased urine output. This loss is accompanied by progressive increases in blood urea nitrogen (BUN), creatinine, and potassium.

- The severity of dysfunction can range from a small increase in serum creatinine or reduction in urine output to the development of azotemia, an accumulation of nitrogenous waste products (urea nitrogen, creatinine) in the blood.

Although AKI is potentially reversible, it has a high mortality rate. AKI usually affects people with other life-threatening problems. It often follows severe, prolonged hypotension or hypovolemia or exposure to a nephrotoxic agent.

Pathophysiology

AKI is categorized as prerenal, intrarenal (or intrinsic), or postrenal (Fig. 19).

- *Prerenal* causes of AKI involve factors external to the kidneys that reduce renal blood flow and lead to decreased glomerular perfusion and filtration. In prerenal *oliguria* (low urine volume), there is no damage to the kidney cells. The oliguria is caused by a decrease in circulating blood volume (e.g., severe dehydration, decreased cardiac output) and is reversible with treatment. Prolonged prerenal problems can lead to intrarenal disease.
- *Intrarenal* causes include problems that cause direct damage to the kidney tissue and impair nephron function. Intrarenal AKI is usually caused by prolonged ischemia, nephrotoxins (e.g., antibiotics), myoglobin released from necrotic muscle cells, or hemoglobin released from hemolyzed red blood cells (RBCs). Kidney diseases such as systemic lupus erythematosus and glomerulonephritis may also cause AKI. *Acute tubular necrosis* (ATN) is the most common cause of intrarenal AKI in hospitalized patients. Risk factors for developing ATN while in the hospital include major surgery, shock, blood transfusion reaction, muscle injury from trauma, and prolonged hypotension.
- *Postrenal* causes involve mechanical obstruction of urinary outflow and account for less than 10% of AKI cases. As the flow of urine is obstructed, urine refluxes into the renal pelvis, impairing kidney function. The most common causes are benign

Fig. 19 Prerenal, intrarenal, and postrenal causes of acute kidney injury (AKI).

prostatic hyperplasia (BPH), prostate cancer, stones, trauma, and extrarenal tumors. Bilateral ureteral obstruction leads to *hydronephrosis* (kidney dilation), increased hydrostatic pressure, and tubular blockage, resulting in a progressive decline in kidney function. If bilateral obstruction is relieved within 48 hours of onset, complete recovery is likely.

Clinical Manifestations

Clinically, AKI may progress through three phases: oliguric, diuretic, and recovery. In some situations, the patient does not recover from AKI, and chronic kidney disease (CKD) results (see Kidney Disease, Chronic).

The RIFLE classification describes the diagnostic criteria for stages of AKI (Table 56): *R*isk, the first stage of AKI, is followed by *I*njury, the second stage; AKI then increases in severity to the final or third stage, *F*ailure. The outcome variables are *L*oss and *E*nd-stage kidney disease.

TABLE 56   RIFLE Classification for Acute Kidney Injury

Stage	GFR criteria	Urine output criteria	Clinical example
Risk	Serum creatinine increased × 1.5 Or GFR decreased by 25%	Urine output <0.5 mL/kg/hr for 6 hours	• 68-year-old patient with type 2 diabetes, hypertension, CAD, CKD • Scheduled for emergency coronary artery bypass graft • Serum creatinine is 1.8 mg/dL (increased), weight 60 kg • Calculated GFR is 35 mL/minutes/1.73 m^2 • Has stage 3b CKD
Injury	Serum creatinine increased × 2 Or GFR decreased by 50%	Urine output <0.5 mL/kg/hr for 12 hours	• During surgery, hypotensive for a sustained period • Diagnosed with acute tubular necrosis • After surgery: Serum creatinine is 3.6 mg/dL, urine output reduced to 28 mL/hours
Failure	Serum creatinine increased × 3 Or GFR decreased by 75% Or Serum creatinine >4 mg/dL with acute rise ≥0.5 mg/dL	Urine output <0.3 mL/kg/hr for 24 ours (oliguria) Or Anuria for 12 hours	• 72 hours after surgery, develops ventilator-associated pneumonia and sepsis while in ICU • Serum creatinine rises to 5.2 mg/dL, urine output drops to 10 mL/hours • BP remains low despite dopamine therapy
Loss	Persistent acute kidney failure. Complete loss of kidney function >4 wk	—	• Starts on continuous venovenous hemodialysis • After 3 week of therapy has a cardiopulmonary arrest and does not survive
End-stage renal disease	Complete loss of kidney function >3 mo	—	—

CAD, Coronary artery disease; CKD, chronic kidney disease, GFR, glomerular filtration rate; ICU, intensive care unit.

Oliguric Phase

The most common initial manifestation of AKI is oliguria, a reduction in urine output to <400 mL/day. It usually occurs within 1–7 days of injury. If the cause is ischemia, oliguria often occurs within 24 hours. When nephrotoxic drugs are involved, onset may be delayed for a week. This phase lasts on average 10–14 days. It can last months. The longer the oliguric phase lasts, the poorer the prognosis for complete recovery of kidney function.

Nonoliguric AKI has a urine output >400 mL/day. About 50% of patients will be nonoliguric, making the initial diagnosis more difficult.

While changes in urine output do not correspond to changes in glomerular filtration rate (GFR), they can help in determining the cause of AKI. *Anuria* (no urine output) is usually seen with urinary tract obstruction. Oliguria is often seen with prerenal causes. Nonoliguric AKI is seen with acute interstitial nephritis and ATN.

- A urinalysis may show casts, red blood cells (RBCs), white blood cells (WBCs), a specific gravity fixed at around 1.010, and urine osmolality around 300 mOsm/kg (300 mmol/kg). This is the same specific gravity and osmolality as for plasma.
- Fluid retention occurs as urinary output decreases. Neck veins may be distended with a bounding pulse, and edema and hypertension may develop. Fluid overload can lead to heart failure, pulmonary edema, and pericardial and pleural effusions.
- Metabolic acidosis results when impaired kidneys cannot excrete hydrogen ions or the acid products of metabolism. The serum bicarbonate level decreases because bicarbonate is depleted in buffering hydrogen ions. The patient may develop Kussmaul (rapid, deep) respirations to excrete more carbon dioxide.
- Damaged tubules cannot conserve sodium. Urinary excretion of sodium may increase, resulting in normal or below-normal levels of serum sodium.
- In AKI, the serum potassium level increases because the kidney's normal ability to excrete potassium is impaired. Rapid development of hyperkalemia may result in clinical signs on an electrocardiogram (ECG). These changes include peaked T waves, widening of the QRS complex, and ST segment depression. Because cardiac muscle is intolerant of acute increases in potassium, emergency treatment of hyperkalemia is needed.
- Leukocytosis is often present. The most common cause of death in AKI is infection.
- BUN and serum creatinine levels are elevated in kidney failure. An increased BUN level also can be caused by dehydration, corticosteroids, or catabolism resulting from infections, fever,

severe injury, or GI bleeding. The best serum indicator of AKI is creatinine because it is not affected by other factors.

- Neurologic changes can occur as nitrogenous waste products accumulate in the brain and other nervous tissue. Manifestations can be as mild as fatigue and difficulty concentrating and can escalate to seizures, stupor, and coma.

Diuretic Phase

During the diuretic phase, daily urine output is 1–3 L/day but may reach 5 L/day or more. The kidneys recover the ability to excrete wastes but not to concentrate urine.

- The diuretic phase may last 1–3 weeks, with the patient's acid–base, electrolyte, and waste product values beginning to normalize. Monitor the patient for hyponatremia, hypokalemia, and dehydration.

Recovery Phase

The recovery phase begins when the GFR increases, allowing the BUN and serum creatinine levels to decrease. Kidney function may take up to 12 months to stabilize.

- The patient's overall health, severity of renal failure, and number and type of complications influence the outcome of AKI. Some patients progress to end-stage renal disease (ESRD). Patients who recover may achieve clinically normal kidney function but remain in an early stage of CKD.

Diagnostic Studies

- History is essential to determine the cause.
- Urine output and serum creatinine help make the diagnosis.
- Urinalysis is done to assess sediment, casts, hematuria, pyuria, and crystals.
- Urine osmolality, sodium content, and specific gravity help in differentiating the cause.
- Ultrasound and renal scan are used to assess renal blood flow, tubular function, and the collecting system.
- CT scan can identify lesions, masses, obstructions, and vascular abnormalities.
- An MRI or magnetic resonance angiography (MRA) with the contrast media gadolinium is not advised. Giving gadolinium to patients with kidney failure can be potentially fatal.

Interprofessional Management

The primary goals of treatment for AKI are to eliminate the cause, manage the signs and symptoms, and prevent complications while the kidneys recover. The first step is to determine if there is adequate intravascular volume and cardiac output (CO) to ensure adequate perfusion of the kidneys.

- Closely monitor fluid intake during the oliguric phase.
- Diuretic therapy usually includes loop diuretics (e.g., furosemide [Lasix], bumetanide) or an osmotic diuretic (e.g., mannitol). If AKI is established, forcing fluids and diuretics will not be effective.
- Hyperkalemia can cause dysrhythmias. Insulin or sodium bicarbonate can temporarily shift potassium into the cells. Calcium gluconate raises the threshold for dysrhythmias. Sodium polystyrene sulfonate (Kayexalate), patiromer (Veltassa), or dialysis actually removes potassium from the body.

If conservative therapy is not effective in treating AKI, renal replacement therapy (RRT) is used. The most common indications for RRT in AKI are: (1) volume overload, resulting in compromised cardiac and/or pulmonary status; (2) high serum potassium level; (3) metabolic acidosis (serum bicarbonate level <15 mEq/L [15 mmol/L]); (4) BUN level >120 mg/dL (43 mmol/L); (5) significant change in mental status; and (6) pericarditis, pericardial effusion, or cardiac tamponade.

- Peritoneal dialysis is an option for renal replacement. See Dialysis.
- Intermittent hemodialysis (HD) (4 hours daily, every other day, or three or four times per week) and continuous renal replacement therapy (CRRT) can be used effectively. CRRT is provided continuously over 24 hours through cannulation of an artery and a vein or of two veins.

Nutritional Therapy

The goal of nutritional management is to provide adequate calories to prevent catabolism despite the restrictions that prevent electrolyte and fluid problems and azotemia. Adequate energy should primarily be from carbohydrate and fat sources to prevent ketosis from endogenous fat breakdown and gluconeogenesis from muscle protein breakdown.

- 30–35 kcal/kg and 0.8–1.0 g protein/kg is recommended to prevent breakdown of body protein. Essential amino acid supplements can be given.
- Fat emulsion IV infusions provide a good source of nonprotein calories.
- Potassium and sodium are regulated per plasma levels. Sodium is restricted as needed to prevent edema, hypertension, and heart failure.

If a patient cannot maintain adequate oral intake, enteral nutrition is the preferred route for nutritional support (see Enteral Nutrition).

When the gastrointestinal tract is not functional, parenteral nutrition (PN) is needed (see Parenteral Nutrition). The patient treated with PN may need daily HD or CRRT to remove the excess fluid. Concentrated PN formulas are available to minimize fluid volume.

Nursing Management

Goals

The overall goals for the patient with AKI are to recover without loss of kidney function, maintain normal fluid and electrolyte balance, have decreased anxiety, and adhere to and understand the need for follow-up care.

Interventions

Prevention and early recognition of AKI are essential because of the high mortality rate. Prevention is directed toward identifying and monitoring high-risk populations, controlling exposure to nephrotoxic drugs and industrial chemicals, and preventing prolonged episodes of hypotension and hypovolemia. In the hospital, factors that increase the risk for developing AKI are preexisting CKD, older age, massive trauma, major surgery, extensive burns, HF, sepsis, and obstetric complications.

- Monitor renal function in persons taking potentially nephrotoxic drugs. Caution the patient about the use of over-the-counter analgesics (especially nonsteroidal antiinflammatory drugs [NSAIDs]), because these may worsen kidney function in the patient with mild CKD.
- Carefully monitor intake and output and electrolyte balance. Record extrarenal losses of fluid from vomiting, diarrhea, and hemorrhage.
- Prompt replacement of significant fluid losses helps prevent ischemic tubular damage associated with trauma, burns, and extensive surgery. Intake and output records and the patient's weight provide valuable indicators of fluid volume status.
- Angiotensin-converting enzyme (ACE) inhibitors can decrease perfusion pressure and cause hyperkalemia. If other measures, such as diet modification and diuretics, cannot control hyperkalemia, the ACE inhibitor may need to be reduced or stopped.

Contrast-induced nephropathy (CIN) can occur when contrast media for diagnostic studies causes nephrotoxic injury. In patients with diabetes receiving metformin, the drug should be held for 48 hours prior to and after the use of contrast media to decrease the risk for lactic acidosis.

- The best way to avoid CIN is to avoid exposure to contrast media by using other diagnostic tests, such as ultrasound. If contrast media is given to a high-risk patient, they should receive the lowest possible dose along with adequate fluid intake.

You have a key role in managing fluid and electrolyte balance during the oliguric and diuretic phases. Observe and record accurate intake and output.

- Assess for common signs and symptoms of hypervolemia (in the oliguric phase) or hypovolemia (in the diuretic phase), potassium and sodium changes, and other electrolyte imbalances that may occur in AKI.
- Because infection is the leading cause of death in AKI, use meticulous aseptic technique. A patient with renal failure who has an infection may not have an elevated temperature. Teach patients to avoid crowds and those with infections.
- If antibiotics are used to treat infection, the type, frequency, and dosage must be carefully considered. The kidneys are the primary route of excretion for many antibiotics.
- Perform good skin care. Mouth care is important to prevent stomatitis. Take measures to prevent pressure injuries, because mobility may be impaired.
- The long-term convalescence of 3–12 months may cause psychosocial and financial hardships for both the patient and family. Make appropriate referrals for counseling and resources.

Encourage the patient to schedule regular follow-up and evaluation of kidney function.

LACTASE DEFICIENCY

Description

Lactase deficiency is a condition in which the lactase enzyme that breaks down lactose into two simple sugars (glucose and galactose) is deficient or absent.

Primary lactase insufficiency is most often genetic. People in certain ethnic or racial groups, especially those with Asian or African ancestry, develop low lactase levels in childhood. Other causes include premature birth and congenital lactase deficiency. Lactose malabsorption can also occur when bacterial overgrowth promotes lactose fermentation in the small bowel and when intestinal mucosal damage interferes with absorption (e.g., inflammatory bowel disease, celiac disease).

Clinical Manifestations

Many do not have symptoms if they ingest lactose in small amounts. Manifestations of lactose intolerance include bloating, flatulence, crampy abdominal pain, and diarrhea. Symptoms generally occur within 30 minutes to several hours after ingesting lactose.

Diagnostic Studies

Many lactose-intolerant people are aware of their lactose intolerance and avoid milk products. Lactose intolerance is diagnosed by a lactose tolerance test, lactose hydrogen breath test, or genetic testing.

Nursing and Interprofessional Management

Treatment aims to improve patient symptoms and prevent malnutrition. Limiting dietary lactose generally results in symptom improvement. Teach the patient the importance of adherence to the diet.

- A lactose-free diet may be gradually advanced to a low-lactose diet.
- Avoiding milk and milk products can lead to calcium deficiency. Supplements may be necessary to prevent osteoporosis.
- A number of lactose-free milk products are readily available. Lactase tablets are available as an over-the-counter (OTC) product. They break down the lactose present in ingested milk.
- Some may see improvement through the use of prebiotics or probiotics that produce lactase in the gut.

LEIOMYOMAS

Leiomyomas (uterine fibroids) are noncancerous smooth-muscle tumors that appear most often in women of reproductive age. They are thought to be caused by hormonal and genetic factors.

- Many patients with fibroids have no symptoms. Others will have pelvic pain, abnormal uterine bleeding, or infertility.
- On physical assessment, the uterus may be enlarged or irregularly shaped. Pelvic ultrasound is used to confirm the diagnosis.

The approach to treatment depends on the patient's age, severity of symptoms, and desire for pregnancy. Most fibroids reduce in size after menopause.

- Drug therapy, such as hormonal contraception or GnRh agonists, can reduce heavy menstrual bleeding and pain.
- Surgical interventions such as removal of uterine fibroids (myomectomy), hysterectomy, or uterine artery embolization may be used for severe symptoms impacting quality of life or fertility.

LEUKEMIA

Description

Leukemia is a general term for a group of cancers affecting the blood and blood-forming tissues of the bone marrow, lymph system, and spleen. It results in an accumulation of dysfunctional cells due to a loss of regulation in cell division. Most types of leukemia result from a combination of factors including genetic and environmental influences. Chemical agents (e.g., benzene), chemotherapy drugs (e.g., alkylating agents, topoisomerase II inhibitors), viruses, radiation, and immunologic deficiencies increase the risk of leukemia. Depending on the type of leukemia, other potential causes are exposure to pesticides (farmworkers) and smoking.

Classification

Leukemia is classified as acute or chronic and by the type of white blood cell (WBC) involved. Table 57 summarizes the relative incidence and features of the four major types of leukemia.

Acute myelogenous leukemia (AML) represents only one-third of all leukemias, but it makes up about 80% of the acute leukemias in adults. Its onset is often abrupt and dramatic. A patient may have serious infections and abnormal bleeding from onset of the disease.

- AML is characterized by uncontrolled proliferation of myeloblasts, the precursors of granulocytes. There is bone marrow hyperplasia. Clinical manifestations are related to replacement of normal cells in the marrow by leukemic myeloblasts and to infiltration of other organs and tissue.

Acute lymphocytic leukemia (ALL) is the most common type of leukemia in children and accounts for about 20% of acute leukemias in adults. In ALL, immature lymphocytes proliferate in the bone marrow. Most are of B-cell origin. Most patients have fever at time of diagnosis. Signs and symptoms may appear abruptly with bleeding or fever, or their onset may be insidious, with progressive weakness, fatigue, and bleeding tendencies.

- Central nervous system (CNS) manifestations are especially common in ALL.

Chronic myelogenous leukemia (CML) is caused by excessive development of neoplastic granulocytes in the bone marrow. CML usually has a chronic stable phase that lasts for several years, followed by development of an acute aggressive phase (blastic phase).

- The Philadelphia chromosome, which is present in 90%–95% of patients with CML, is a diagnostic hallmark of CML. In addition, its presence is an important indicator of residual disease or relapse after treatment.

TABLE 57 Types of Leukemia

Type	Age at onset	Clinical manifestations	Diagnostic findings
Acute myelogenous leukemia (AML)	Accounts for 15%–20% of acute leukemia in children and 80% in adults Increase in incidence with advancing age after 60year	Fatigue and weakness, headache, mouth sores, anemia, bleeding, fever, infection, gingival hyperplasia, splenomegaly in some patients	Low RBC count, Hgb, Hct, platelet count Low to high WBC count with myeloblasts High LDH Hypercellular bone marrow with myeloblasts
Acute lymphocytic leukemia (ALL)	Accounts for 20% of acute leukemias in adults. Most adult patients older than 50 years of age.	Fever, pallor, bleeding, anorexia, fatigue, and weakness. Bone, joint, and abdominal pain. Generalized lymphadenopathy, infections, weight loss, hepatosplenomegaly, headache, mouth sores, neurologic manifestations: CNS involvement, increased intracranial pressure (nausea, vomiting, lethargy, cranial nerve dysfunction) from meningeal infiltration. Men may have painless enlargement of the scrotum	Low RBC, Hgb, Hct, platelet count. Low, normal, or high WBC count. High LDH. Hypercellular bone marrow with lymphoblasts. Lymphoblasts may be in cerebrospinal fluid. Presence of Philadelphia chromosome (up to 30% of patients).

Chronic myelogenous leukemia (CML)	Increase in incidence with advancing age. Median age at diagnosis of 67 year. Rare in children	No symptoms early in disease. Fatigue and weakness, fever, night sweats, sternal tenderness, weight loss, joint pain, bone pain, massive splenomegaly	Low RBC count, Hgb, Hct. High platelet count early, lower count later. High WBCs, including a wide variety of myeloid cells and basophils. Nucleated RBCs common. Philadelphia chromosome present in about 98% of patients.
Chronic lymphocytic leukemia (CLL)	Increase in incidence with advancing age after 65 year, with predominance in men	Frequently no symptoms. Detection of disease often during examination for unrelated condition, chronic fatigue, anorexia, splenomegaly and lymphadenopathy, hepatomegaly. May progress to fever, night sweats, weight loss, fatigue, and frequent infections	Mild anemia and thrombocytopenia with disease progression. Total WBC count >100,000/μL. Increase in peripheral lymphocytes and lymphocytes in bone marrow. May have autoimmune hemolytic anemia, idiopathic thrombocytopenic purpura, hypogammaglobulinemia

CNS, Central nervous system; Hct, hematocrit; Hgb, hemoglobin; LDH, lactate dehydrogenase; RBC, red blood cell; WBC, white blood cell.

L

Chronic lymphocytic leukemia (CLL) is the most common leukemia in adults in Western countries. It is characterized by the production and accumulation of functionally inactive but long-lived, small, mature-appearing lymphocytes. The B lymphocyte is usually involved. Lymph node enlargement (lymphadenopathy) is present throughout the body.

■ Because CLL is usually a disease of older adults, treatment decisions should consider disease progression and side effects. Many patients in the early stages of CLL require no treatment, but 30% require immediate intervention at time of diagnosis.

Clinical Manifestations

The manifestations of leukemia relate to problems caused by bone marrow failure and the formation of leukemic infiltrates (see Table 57). The patient is predisposed to development of anemia, thrombocytopenia, and decreased number and function of WBCs.

■ WBC infiltration into the organs leads splenomegaly, hepatomegaly, lymphadenopathy, bone pain, meningeal irritation, and oral lesions.

Diagnostic Studies

■ Peripheral blood evaluation and bone marrow examination are the primary methods of diagnosing and classifying the types of leukemia.
■ Morphologic, histochemical, immunologic, and cytogenetic methods are all used to identify leukemic cell types, stage of development, and significant genetic mutations.
■ Studies such as lumbar puncture and positron emission tomography (PET) or CT scans can detect leukemic cells outside the blood and bone marrow.

Interprofessional Management

Care first focuses on the goal of attaining remission. Combination chemotherapy is the mainstay of treatment for leukemia. The three purposes for using multiple drugs are to decrease drug resistance, minimize drug toxicity to the patient by using multiple drugs with varying toxicities, and interrupt cell growth at multiple points in the cell cycle. See Chemotherapy.

■ Corticosteroids and radiation therapy may have a role in therapy for the patient with leukemia.
■ Immunotherapy and targeted therapy, such as monoclonal antibodies and chimeric antigen receptor (CAR) T cells, may be indicated for specific leukemias.

- Total body radiation may be used to prepare a patient for bone marrow transplantation, or radiation may be restricted to certain areas (fields), such as the liver, spleen, or other organs affected by infiltrates.
- In ALL, prophylactic intrathecal methotrexate or cytarabine is given to decrease CNS involvement. When CNS leukemia occurs, cranial radiation may be used.
- In some cases, such as nonsymptomatic patients with CLL, watchful waiting with active supportive care may be appropriate.

Hematopoietic stem cell transplantation (HSCT) is another type of therapy used for patients with different forms of leukemia. The goal of HSCT is to totally eliminate leukemia cells from the body using combinations of chemotherapy with or without total body radiation. This treatment also eradicates the patient's hematopoietic stem cells, which are then replaced with those of a human leukocyte antigen (HLA)-matched sibling, with those of a volunteer donor (allogeneic) or an identical twin (syngeneic), or with the patient's own (autologous) stem cells that were removed (harvested) before the intensive therapy.

- The primary complications of patients with allogeneic HSCT are graft-versus-host disease (GVHD), relapse of leukemia, and infection or sepsis. The patient must weigh the significant risks of treatment-related death or treatment failure (relapse) against the hope of cure.

Nursing Management
Goals
The patient with leukemia will understand and adhere to the treatment plan, have minimal side effects and complications associated with both the disease and its treatment, establish realistic hope and goals, and feel hopeful and supported during periods of treatment, relapse, or remission.

See nursing care plans available on the website for anemia (eNursing Care Plan 34-1), thrombocytopenia (eNursing Care Plan 34-2), and neutropenia (eNursing Care Plan 34-3).

Interventions
The nursing role during acute phases of leukemia is challenging because the patient has many physical and psychosocial needs. The diagnosis of leukemia can evoke great fear and be equated with death. A patient may require protective isolation or may need to temporarily geographically relocate to an appropriate treatment center. This situation can lead a patient to feel deserted and isolated at a time when support is most needed.

- Help the patient realize that although the future may be uncertain, one can have a meaningful quality of life while in remission or with disease control, and that, in some cases, there is reasonable hope for cure.

- Families also need help in adjusting to the stress of the abrupt onset of serious illness and losses imposed by the sick role.

From a physical care perspective, you are challenged to make assessments and plan care to help the patient deal with the severe side effects of chemotherapy. The life-threatening results of bone marrow suppression (anemia, thrombocytopenia, neutropenia) require aggressive nursing interventions. Review all drugs being administered. Assess laboratory data reflecting the effects of the drugs. See Chemotherapy.

▼ **Patient and Caregiver Teaching**
Teach the patient and caregivers the importance of continued diligence in disease management and the need for follow-up care.

Involving the patient in survivor networks, support groups, or services may help the patient adapt to living after a life-threatening illness. Exploring national and community resources (e.g., American Cancer Society, Leukemia and Lymphoma Society Society) may reduce the financial burden and feelings of dependence. Provide resources for spiritual support.

LIVER CANCER

Description
Primary *liver cancer* (hepatocellular carcinoma [HCC]) is the fifth most common cancer in the world and the second most common cause of cancer death worldwide. It is the most common cause of death in patients with cirrhosis. Cirrhosis caused by hepatitis C virus (HCV) is the most common cause of HCC in the United States, followed by nonalcoholic fatty liver disease (NAFLD). Other primary liver tumors are cholangiomas or bile duct cancers. Primary liver tumors often metastasize to the lung.

Metastatic carcinoma of the liver is more common than primary carcinoma. The liver has a high rate of blood flow and extensive capillary network.

- Liver cancer grows rapidly. Without treatment, death may occur within 6–12 months from hepatic encephalopathy or massive gastrointestinal (GI) bleeding.

Clinical Manifestations
Liver cancer can be difficult to distinguish from cirrhosis because of similar clinical manifestations (e.g., hepatomegaly, splenomegaly, fatigue, jaundice, weight loss, peripheral edema, ascites, and other complications from portal hypertension).

- In late stages, patients will often have fever/chills, jaundice, anorexia, weight loss, palpable mass, and RUQ pain.

Diagnostic Studies

- Ultrasound, CT, and MRI are used to screen and diagnose liver cancer.
- A percutaneous biopsy is performed if imaging studies are inconclusive.
- Serum α-fetoprotein (AFP) is often elevated.

Interprofessional and Nursing Management

Treatment depends on the size and number of tumors, metastasis beyond the liver, and the patient's age and overall health. In general, management is similar to that for cirrhosis (see Cirrhosis).

- Surgical liver resection (partial hepatectomy) offers the best chance for a cure. However, only about 15% of patients have enough healthy liver tissue for this option.
- For those who have early-stage liver cancer, liver transplantation offers a good prognosis.
- Other options are percutaneous ablation, chemoembolization, radioembolization, and systemic therapies.
- Systemic therapy options include chemotherapy and immune-based therapy, such as monoclonal antibodies, tyrosine kinase inhibitors, and immune checkpoint inhibitors.

Nursing interventions focus on keeping the patient as comfortable as possible. Because liver cancer manifests the same problems as advanced liver disease, the nursing interventions for the patient with cirrhosis of the liver apply (see Cirrhosis).

LOW BACK PAIN, ACUTE

Description

Low back pain affects 80% of adults in the United States at least once during their lives. Risk factors include lack of muscle tone, obesity, trauma, poor posture, older age, smoking, pregnancy, prior compression fracture of the spine, spinal problems since birth, and a family history of back pain. Jobs that require repetitive heavy lifting, vibration (such as a jackhammer operator), and extended periods of sitting are associated with low back pain.

- Healthcare personnel who engage in direct patient care activities are at high risk for low back pain. Lifting and moving patients, excessive bending or leaning forward, and frequent twisting can result in low back pain.

Pathophysiology

Low back pain is a common problem because the lumbar region (1) bears most of the weight of the body, (2) is the most flexible region of the spinal column, (3) has nerve roots that are at risk for injury or disease, and (4) has a naturally unstable biomechanical structure. The causes of low back pain of musculoskeletal origin include acute lumbosacral strain, instability of lumbosacral bony mechanism, osteoarthritis of the lumbosacral vertebrae, degenerative disc disease, and herniation of the intervertebral disc.

Acute low back pain lasts 4 weeks or less. It is caused by trauma or activity that causes undue stress on the lower back. Often symptoms develop later because of swelling or a gradual increase in pressure on the nerve by an intervertebral disc.

- Symptoms may range from muscle ache to shooting or stabbing pain, limited flexibility or range of motion, or inability to stand upright.
- Few definitive diagnostic abnormalities are present with nerve irritation and muscle strain. One test is the straight-leg-raising test. MRI and CT scans are done if trauma or systemic disease (e.g., cancer, spinal infection) is suspected.

Interprofessional and Nursing Management

Most patients do better if they continue their regular activities. The patient may be treated on an outpatient basis with nonsteroidal antiinflammatory drugs (NSAIDs), muscle relaxants, massage and back manipulation, acupuncture, and use of alternating heat and cold compresses.

- Severe pain may require a brief course of corticosteroids or opioid analgesics. Some people may need a brief period (1–2 days) of rest, but prolonged bed rest should be avoided.

Patients should refrain from activities that increase the pain, including lifting, bending, twisting, and prolonged sitting. Most symptoms subside within 2 weeks.

Primary nursing responsibilities in acute low back pain are to assist the patient to maintain activity limitations, promote comfort, and teach the patient about the health problem and appropriate exercises.

- Consider referral to a physical therapist or personal trainer to address posture and core and abdomen strength.
- Safe patient handling devices to lift, transfer, and reposition patients are recommended for nurse and patient safety. Serve

as a role model by always using proper body mechanics. This includes raising the patient's bed height, bending at the knees, and asking for help in lifting and moving patients.

▼ **Patient and Caregiver Teaching**

Assess the patient's use of body mechanics and teach the patient how to avoid back strain (Table 58). Ensure that the patient understands the type and frequency of any exercise prescribed, as well as the rationale.

L

TABLE 58 Patient and Caregiver Teaching: Low Back Problems

Include the following instructions when teaching the patient and caregivers how to manage low back problems.

Do

- Maintain healthy body weight.
- Maintain a neutral pelvic position if standing. Place one foot on a low stool if standing for long periods.
- Choose a seat with good lower back support, armrests, and a swivel base. Place a pillow at the lumbar spine to maintain normal curvature. Keep knees and hips level.
- Sleep in a side-lying position with knees and hips bent, and a pillow between the knees for support.
- Sleep on back with a lift under knees and legs or on back with 10-inch-high pillow under knees to flex hips and knees.
- Use proper body mechanics when lifting heavy objects. Bend at the knees, not at the waist, and stand up slowly while holding object close to your body.
- Take part in regular strength and flexibility training and low-impact aerobic exercise.
- Use local heat and cold application to relieve muscle tension.

Do not

- Lean forward without bending knees.
- Lift anything above level of elbows.
- Stand unmoving for prolonged time.
- Sleep on abdomen or on back or side with legs out straight.
- Exercise without consulting healthcare provider (HCP) if having severe pain.
- Exceed prescribed amount and type of exercises without consulting HCP.
- Smoke or use tobacco products.

LOW BACK PAIN, CHRONIC

Description

Chronic low back pain lasts more than 3 months or involves repeated incapacitating episodes. It is often progressive. Causes include: (1) degenerative conditions such as arthritis or disc disease; (2) osteoporosis or other metabolic bone diseases; (3) weakness from the scar tissue of prior injury; (4) chronic strain on lower back muscles from obesity, pregnancy, or stressful postures on the job; and (5) congenital spine problems.

Spinal stenosis, a narrowing of the spinal canal, is a common cause of chronic low back pain. Spinal stenosis can be acquired or inherited.

- A common acquired cause is osteoarthritis in the spine. Arthritic changes (bone spurs, calcification of spinal ligaments, disc degeneration) narrow the space around the spinal canal and nerve roots, leading to compression. Inflammation caused by the compression results in pain, weakness, and numbness.
- Other acquired conditions that cause spinal stenosis include rheumatoid arthritis, spinal tumors, Paget's disease, and trauma to the vertebra.
- Inherited conditions that lead to spinal stenosis include congenital spinal stenosis and scoliosis.

The pain from lumbar spinal stenosis often starts in the low back and radiates to the buttock and leg. It is worse with walking and prolonged standing. Numbness, tingling, weakness, and sensation of heaviness in the legs and buttocks may be present. Decreased pain when the patient bends forward or sits down is often a sign of spinal stenosis.

Interprofessional and Nursing Management

Treatment regimens are similar to those for acute low back pain. Pain and stiffness are managed with nonsteroidal antiinflammatory drugs (NSAIDs). Antidepressants such as duloxetine (Cymbalta) may help with pain management and sleep problems. The antiseizure drug gabapentin (Neurontin) may improve walking and relieve leg symptoms.

Weight management, sufficient rest periods, local heat application, and exercise and activity throughout the day help keep the muscles and joints mobilized.

- Biofeedback, acupuncture, and yoga may help reduce the pain.
- Minimally invasive treatments, such as epidural corticosteroid injections and implanted devices that deliver pain medication, are options.

- Surgery may be indicated for those with severe chronic pain who receive no benefit from conservative care or have continued neurologic deficits. (See the Surgical Therapy section in Intervertebral Disc Disease.)

LUNG CANCER

Description

Lung cancer is the leading cause of cancer-related death in the United States and accounts for 25% of all cancer deaths. Smoking causes 80%–90% of all lung cancers.

- There is no safe form of tobacco or tobacco product. Tobacco smoke contains over 7000 chemicals, of which 250 are harmful. Exposure to tobacco smoke causes changes in the bronchial epithelium, which usually returns to normal when smoking is discontinued.

The risk of developing lung cancer is directly related to total exposure to tobacco smoke, measured by total number of cigarettes smoked in a lifetime, age at smoking onset, depth of inhalation, tar and nicotine content, and the use of unfiltered cigarettes. Sidestream smoke (smoke from burning cigarettes, cigars) has the same carcinogens found in mainstream smoke (smoke inhaled and exhaled by the smoker). This exposure to secondhand smoke creates a health risk for nonsmoking adults and children.

- Other causes of lung cancer include high levels of pollution, radiation (especially radon exposure), and asbestos. Heavy or prolonged exposure to industrial agents, such as radon, coal dust, asbestos, chromium, silica, arsenic, and diesel exhaust, increases risk, especially in smokers.
- Genetic, hormonal, and molecular influences may contribute to differences in lung cancer incidence, risk factors, and survival.

Pathophysiology

Most primary lung tumors are believed to arise from mutated epithelial cells. The growth of mutations that are caused by carcinogens is influenced by various genetic factors. Once started, tumor development is promoted by epidermal growth factor. These cells grow slowly, taking 8–10 years for a tumor to reach 1 cm in size, the smallest lesion detectable on an X-ray. Lung cancers occur primarily in the segmental bronchi or beyond and have a preference for the upper lobes of the lungs.

- Primary lung cancers are categorized into two broad types: *non-small-cell lung cancer* (NSCLC) (84%) and *small cell lung cancer* (SCLC) (13%). Lung cancers metastasize primarily by direct extension and through the blood and lymph system to the liver, brain, bones, and adrenal glands.

Clinical Manifestations

Manifestations are usually nonspecific and appear late in the disease process, depending on the type of primary lung cancer, its location, and extent of metastatic spread.

- Often the first sign is a persistent cough. Blood-tinged sputum may be present because of bleeding caused by the tumor.
- The patient may have dyspnea or wheezing. Chest pain, if present, may be localized or unilateral, ranging from mild to severe.

Later manifestations include nonspecific symptoms and signs, such as anorexia, nausea and vomiting, fatigue, and weight loss. Hoarseness may be present with laryngeal nerve involvement. Dysphagia, unilateral paralysis of the diaphragm, and superior vena cava obstruction may occur because of intrathoracic spread of the cancer. Lymph nodes are often palpable in the neck or axillae. Mediastinal involvement may lead to pericardial effusion, cardiac tamponade, and dysrhythmias.

Paraneoplastic syndrome is caused by *humoral* factors (*hormones, cytokines*) excreted by tumor cells or by an *immune response* against the tumor. SCLCs are most often associated with the paraneoplastic syndrome. Symptoms of paraneoplastic syndrome may manifest before the diagnosis of the cancer.

- Examples of paraneoplastic syndrome are hypercalcemia, syndrome of inappropriate antidiuretic hormone (SIADH) secretion, adrenal hypersecretion, polycythemia, and Cushing syndrome. These conditions may stabilize with treatment of the cancer.

Diagnostic Studies

- Chest X-ray is used for diagnosis and assessing for metastasis.
- Biopsy is needed for a definitive diagnosis. If thoracentesis is done to relieve a pleural effusion, the fluid is also analyzed for cancer cells.
- Additional tests include bone scans, CT scans, MRI, positron emission tomography (PET), blood tests, renal function tests, and pulmonary function tests.

Staging of NSCLC is performed according to the tumor-node-metastasis (TNM) staging system (see TNM Classification System).

Interprofessional Management

Surgical resection is the treatment of choice in NSCLC stages I and IIIA without mediastinal involvement. Resection gives the best chance for a cure. For other NSCLC stages, patients may have surgery along with radiation therapy and/or chemotherapy and targeted therapy. Surgical procedures may include segmental or wedge resection, lobectomy (removal of one or more lung lobes), and pneumonectomy (removal of an entire lung) procedures.

Radiation therapy may be used for both NSCLC and SCLC (see Radiation Therapy).

- Radiation relieves symptoms of dyspnea and hemoptysis from bronchial obstruction tumors and treats superior vena cava syndrome.
- Radiation can be used to treat the pain of metastatic bone lesions or cerebral metastasis, to reduce tumor mass preoperatively, or as an adjuvant measure postoperatively.
- Stereotactic body radiotherapy (SBRT) uses high doses of radiation delivered accurately to the tumor. SBRT is an option for patients with early-stage lung cancers who are not candidates for surgery.

Chemotherapy is the main treatment for SCLC. It is used for nonresectable tumors or as an adjuvant therapy to surgery in NSCLC. A variety of chemotherapy drugs and multidrug protocols have been used (see Chemotherapy).

One type of targeted therapy for patients with NSCLC is erlotinib (Tarceva), which blocks signals for growth in cancer cells. Other drugs, such as bevacizumab (Avastin), inhibit new blood vessel growth (angiogenesis). Drugs such as crizotinib (Xalkori), brigatinib (Alunbrig), and ceritinib (Zykadia) directly inhibit the kinase protein made by the *ALK* gene responsible for cancer development and growth.

Immunotherapy with nivolumab (Opdivo), atezolizumab (Tecentriq), or pembrolizumab (Keytruda) may be used to boost the immune response and can shrink some tumors or slow their growth.

Nursing Management
Goals
The patient with lung cancer will have a patent airway, adequate tissue oxygenation, minimal discomfort, understanding about the type of lung cancer, and a realistic outlook about treatment and prognosis.
Interventions
The best way to halt the epidemic of lung cancer is to prevent people from smoking, help smokers stop smoking, and decrease exposure to environmental pollutants. Using smokeless tobacco, pipes and cigars, hookah and waterpipe, bidis, and kreteks all pose significant risk for lung cancer. Modeling healthy behavior by not smoking, promoting smoking cessation programs, and actively supporting education and policy changes related to smoking are important nursing activities. You have a role in early detection of

lung cancer. Encourage adults aged 55–77 years with a history of smoking (30-pack year smoking history or currently smoke) or who quit smoking <15 years ago to consider annual screening for lung cancer using low-dose CT.

Care of the patient with lung cancer involves support and reassurance during the diagnostic evaluation. Individualized care depends on the plan for treatment.

- Assessment and symptom management are pivotal. Constant pain may become a major problem.
- Radiation therapy and chemotherapy can provide palliative relief from distressing symptoms.
- Provide patient comfort, monitor for side effects of prescribed medications, foster appropriate coping strategies, assess smoking cessation readiness, and help patients access resources.

▼ **Patient and Caregiver Teaching**
- Encourage the patient and family to provide a smoke-free environment. This may include smoking cessation for family members.
- If the treatment plan includes home oxygen, teach the patient and family about safe use.
- Teach the patient to recognize signs and symptoms that indicate cancer progression or recurrence.

LYME DISEASE

Description
Lyme disease is an infection caused by the spirochete *Borrelia burgdorferi* and transmitted through the bite of an infected deer tick. The tick typically feeds on mice, dogs, cats, cows, horses, deer, and humans. It is the most common vector-borne disease in the United States with an infection rate of 7.9 cases per 100,000 persons. Wild animals do not exhibit the illness, but clinical Lyme disease does occur in domestic animals. Person-to-person transmission does not occur.

- Human infection peaks in summer months. Most US cases occur in the northeastern states from Virginia to northern Maine and in Wisconsin and Minnesota. Reinfection is common.

Clinical Manifestations
The most characteristic sign is erythema migrans (EM), a skin lesion that occurs at the site of the tick bite within 1 month of exposure. The EM lesion begins as a central red macule or papule that slowly

expands to include a red outer ring of up to 12 inches, resembling a bull's-eye. It may be warm to the touch but is not itchy or painful.

- The rash is often accompanied by flu-like symptoms, such as low-grade fever, headache, neck stiffness, fatigue, loss of appetite, and migratory joint and muscle pain. Flu-like symptoms generally resolve over weeks or months, even if untreated.
- If not treated, the spirochete can disseminate within several weeks or months to the heart, joints, and central nervous system (CNS). Bell's palsy is the most common neurologic effect.
- Other complaints include short-term memory loss, cognitive impairment, shooting pains, and numbness and tingling in the feet.
- Cardiac symptoms such as heart block and pericarditis may require hospitalization.
- About 60% of persons with untreated infection develop chronic arthritic pain and swelling in the large joints, primarily the knee. Arthritis remains the second most common manifestation of Lyme disease.

Diagnostic Studies

Diagnosis is often based on clinical manifestations, in particular the EM lesion, and a history of exposure in an endemic area.

- Complete blood count (CBC) and erythrocyte sedimentation rate (ESR) are usually normal.
- A two-step laboratory testing process is recommended. The first step is the enzyme immunoassay (EIA), a test that will have positive results for most people with Lyme disease. If the EIA is positive or inconclusive, a Western blot test can confirm the infection.
- In those with neurologic involvement, cerebrospinal fluid should also be tested.

Interprofessional and Nursing Management

Doxycycline, cefuroxime, and amoxicillin are often effective in treating early-stage infection and preventing later stages of the disease. Doxycycline treats both Lyme disease and human granulocytic anaplasmosis, which can be transmitted as a coinfection with a single tick bite.

- A small percentage of people treated with antibiotics for Lyme disease may have lingering fatigue or joint and muscle pain. The International Lyme and Associated Diseases Society supports a diagnosis of chronic Lyme disease in these cases. Antibiotic treatment is extended as needed because the risks of untreated Lyme disease outweigh those of long-term antibiotic therapy.

Patient and caregiver teaching for the prevention of Lyme disease in endemic areas focuses on strategies for avoiding tick bites.

MACULAR DEGENERATION

Description

Age-related *macular degeneration* (AMD) is the leading cause of irreversible central vision loss. AMD is divided into two classic forms: *dry* (atrophic), which is more common; and *wet* (exudative), which is more severe. Wet AMD accounts for most cases of AMD-related blindness.

Pathophysiology

AMD is related to retinal aging. Other risk factors include family history, obesity, hypertension, and being white. Smoking significantly increases the risk of AMD.

- In *dry AMD,* yellowish extracellular deposits called *drusen* accumulate in the retinal pigment epithelium. Atrophy and degeneration of macular cells then lead to slowly progressive and painless vision loss.
- *Wet AMD* is characterized by the growth of new blood vessels in an abnormal location in the retinal epithelium. As the new blood vessels leak, scar tissue gradually forms.

Clinical Manifestations

The patient may have blurred and darkened vision, *scotomas* (blind spots in the visual fields), *metamorphopsia* (vision distortion), or acute vision loss.

Diagnostic Studies

- Visual acuity measurement
- Ophthalmoscopic examination for drusen and changes in the fundus
- Amsler grid test to define the involved area and provide a baseline for future comparison
- Fluorescein angiography to define the extent and type of AMD
- Optical coherence tomography (OCT) or scanning laser ophthalmoscopy to image retinal anatomy

Interprofessional and Nursing Management

Visual prognosis varies greatly for people with AMD. Limited treatment options for patients with wet AMD include several medications (i.e., ranibizumab [Lucentis], bevacizumab [Avastin], aflibercept [Eylea], and pegaptanib [Macugen]) injected directly into the vitreous cavity. These drugs inhibit endothelial growth factor and help slow vision loss.

- Photodynamic therapy with Verteporfin (Visudyne) IV is used in wet AMD to create blood clots that block the abnormal blood vessels and slow the vision loss. The patient must avoid direct exposure to sunlight and other intense light for 5 days after treatment to avoid a chemical burn.
- A supplement of antioxidant vitamins (e.g., vitamin C, vitamin E), lutein, zeaxanthin, and zinc may help slow the progression of AMD Teach the patient to eat dark green, leafy vegetables containing lutein (e.g., kale, broccoli, spinach) and foods such as beef, pork, dairy, and whole grains, which are high in zinc.
- Smoking cessation may help slow progression of dry AMD.
- Many patients with low-vision assistive devices can continue reading and keep a license to drive during the daytime at low speeds.

The permanent loss of central vision associated with AMD has significant psychosocial implications. Avoid giving patients the impression that "nothing can be done" about the problem. Although treatment will not recover lost vision, much can be done to augment the remaining vision.

MALNUTRITION

Description

Malnutrition or *undernutrition* occurs when nutrition reserves are depleted, and nutrient and energy intake is not sufficient to meet daily needs or added metabolic stress.

- Rates for malnutrition in the hospital setting range from 30% to 50%. The prevalence of malnutrition in older adults ranges from 6% (community-dwelling older adults) to 50% (rehabilitation settings).

The following terms indicate the interaction and importance of inflammation on nutritional status:

- *Starvation-related malnutrition*, or *primary protein-calorie malnutrition (PCM)*, occurs when nutritional needs are not met. It is a clinical state in which there is chronic starvation without inflammation (e.g., anorexia nervosa).
- *Chronic disease–related malnutrition*, or *secondary PCM*, is related to conditions that impose sustained inflammation of a mild to moderate degree. This occurs when diet intake does not meet tissue needs, although it would under normal conditions. Conditions associated with this type of malnutrition include organ failure, cancer, rheumatoid arthritis, and obesity.

- *Acute disease- or injury-related malnutrition* is related to a marked inflammatory response after major infection, burn, trauma, or surgery.

Many factors contribute to the development of malnutrition, including socioeconomic factors, physical illnesses, incomplete diets, and drug–nutrient interactions.

Pathophysiology of Starvation

Initially, the body selectively uses carbohydrates (glycogen), rather than fat and protein, to meet metabolic needs. This may deplete glycogen stores in the liver and muscles within 18 hours.

- When carbohydrate stores are depleted, skeletal protein is converted to glucose for energy, resulting in a negative nitrogen balance. Within 5–9 days, the body mobilizes fat to supply energy.
- In prolonged starvation, fat provides up to 97% of calories, conserving protein. Fat stores are generally used up in 4–6 weeks, then body proteins, including those in internal organs and plasma, are the only remaining source of energy.
- The liver is the organ that loses the most mass during protein deprivation. It gradually becomes infiltrated with fat due to decreased synthesis of lipoproteins.

Inflammatory states (e.g., major infection, burns, trauma, surgery) accelerate the process of starvation. Death will rapidly ensue if the person does not receive protein and necessary nutrients.

Clinical Manifestations

Manifestations of malnutrition range from mild to emaciation and death. The most obvious clinical manifestations on physical examination are apparent in the skin (dry and scaly skin, brittle nails, rashes, hair loss), mouth (crusting and ulceration, changes in tongue), muscles (decreased mass and weakness), and CNS (mental changes such as confusion, irritability).

- The person is more susceptible to infection. Both humoral and cell-mediated immunity are deficient. Leukocytes decrease in the peripheral blood. Phagocytosis is impaired due to lack of energy needed to drive the process. Many malnourished persons are also anemic.

Diagnostic Studies

- Decreased serum albumin and prealbumin levels indicate the presence of inflammation.
- C-reactive protein (CRP) and serum potassium are often elevated.
- Red blood cell (RBC) count and hemoglobin (Hgb) levels indicate the presence and degree of anemia.

- White blood cell (WBC) count and total lymphocyte count are decreased.
- Liver enzyme studies may be elevated.
- Body mass index (BMI), waist circumference, and waist-to-hip ratio help evaluate the response to therapy.

Interprofessional and Nursing Management

Goals

The patient with malnutrition will (1) achieve an appropriate weight, (2) consume a specified number of calories per day on an individualized diet, and (3) have no adverse consequences related to malnutrition or nutrition therapies.

Interventions

It is part of your role to teach and reinforce healthy eating habits. Use MyPlate, the Dietary Guidelines for Americans, and Nutrition Facts food labels to promote healthy nutrition. The MyPlate approach is a visual guide for sensible meal planning. It helps Americans eat healthfully and make good food choices. MyPlate focuses on the proportions of five food groups (grains, protein, fruits, vegetables, and dairy) that you should eat at each meal.

- At the health professionals' link at www.choosemyplate.gov, you can download daily food plans, sample menus, and tips for how to be physically active. These materials are valuable to use in patient teaching. MyPlate materials for older adults are available at https://hnrca.tufts.edu/myplate/.

Collaborate with the healthcare provider (HCP) and dietitian to identify patients with malnutrition and implement appropriate interventions to meet the patient's nutritional needs. Assess nutritional state during your assessment of the patient's other physical problems. Identify risk factors for malnutrition.

- Hospital-specific screening tools are based on common admission assessment criteria that typically include history of weight loss, intake before admission, use of nutritional support, chewing or swallowing issues, and skin breakdown.

Obtaining an accurate measure of body weight and height and recording this information are critical components of nutritional assessment. BMI is a measure of weight in proportion to height. BMIs outside the normal weight range are associated with increased morbidity and mortality.

- Daily weights provide an ongoing record of body weight change. To obtain an accurate weight, weigh the patient at the same time each day, using the same scale, with the patient wearing the same type or amount of clothing.

- You and the dietitian can assist the patient and caregiver in the selection of high-calorie and high-protein foods.
- If the patient is unable to consume enough nutrition with a high-calorie, high-protein diet, oral liquid nutritional supplements can be added.
- Encourage the family to bring the patient's favorite food while the patient is hospitalized.

Some patients may benefit from appetite stimulants, such as megestrol acetate or dronabinol (Marinol), to improve intake. If the patient is still unable to take in enough calories, enteral feedings may be considered (see Enteral Nutrition). Parenteral nutrition (PN) might be initiated if enteral feedings are not feasible (see Parenteral Nutrition).

▼ Patient and Caregiver Teaching
- Teach the patient and caregivers the importance of good nutrition and the rationale for recording the daily weight, intake, and output.
- Assess the ability of the patient and caregiver to follow dietary instructions related to past eating habits, religious and cultural preferences, age, income, other resources, and state of health.
- Discuss the availability and acceptability of community resources that provide meals, such as Meals on Wheels, senior congregate feeding sites, and the Supplemental Nutrition Assistance Program (SNAP). SNAP allows low-income households, regardless of age, to buy more food of a greater variety.
- Ensure follow-up through visits by the home health nurse and outpatient dietitian referrals.

MELANOMA

Description

Melanoma is a tumor arising from melanocytes, the cells that make melanin. The incidence of melanoma is steadily rising. Melanoma causes most skin cancer deaths. It can metastasize to any organ, including the brain and heart.

A combination of environmental and genetic factors is likely involved in the development of melanoma.
- Ultraviolet (UV) radiation from the sun is the main cause. Artificial sources of UV radiation, such as sunlamps and tanning booths, also play a role. UV radiation damages the deoxyribonucleic acid (DNA) in skin cells, causing mutations in their genetic code.

Although anyone can develop melanoma, the risk is greatest for people who have red or blond hair, blue or light-colored eyes, and light-colored skin that freckles easily. These people have less melanin and thus less protection from UV radiation. The use of immunosuppressive drugs and a history of dysplastic nevi also increase risk.

Clinical Manifestations

Melanoma often occurs on the lower legs in women and on the trunk and head in men. About 25% occur in existing nevi or moles. About 20% occur in dysplastic nevi.

- Because most melanoma cells continue to make melanin, melanoma tumors are often deep brown or black. Lesions showing any sudden or progressive change in the ABCDE rule need evaluated. These ABCDE signs include *a*symmetry, *b*order irregularity, *c*olor varied from one area of the lesion to another, *d*iameter > 6 mm, and *e*volving, changing appearance.

Melanoma in dark-skinned persons often goes unrecognized until the advanced stages.

Interprofessional Management

Suspicious lesions are biopsied using an excisional biopsy technique. The most important prognostic factor is tumor thickness.

- The *Breslow measurement* indicates tumor depth in millimeters. Melanomas less than 1 mm thick have a small chance of spreading. As the melanoma becomes thicker, it has a greater chance of spreading.

Treatment depends on the site of the original tumor and stage of the cancer. Initial treatment is wide surgical excision. Melanoma that has spread to the lymph nodes or nearby sites requires combinations of chemotherapy, immunotherapy, targeted therapy, and radiation.

- Immunotherapy can include cytokines (α-interferon, interleukin-2), programmed cell death protein 1 (PD-1) inhibitors, and cytotoxic T lymphocyte antigen 4 (CTLA-4) inhibitors. Cytokines enhance the production of many immune system cells, including T cells and B cells. Drugs that block PD-1 or CTLA-4 boost the immune response against melanoma cells. Anti PD-1 agents include nivolumab (Opdivo) and pembrolizumab (Keytruda). They block PD-1, a protein on T cells that keeps T cells from attacking other cells in the body. Atezolizumab (Tecentriq) targets PD-L1, a protein related to PD-1 that is found on some tumor cells. Ipilimumab (Yervoy) blocks the action of CTLA-4, another protein that normally suppresses the action of T cells.
- Targeted therapy for melanoma includes BRAF and MEK inhibitors. About half of all melanomas have mutations in the *BRAF* gene, which makes an altered BRAF protein that signals

melanoma cells to proliferate. Vemurafenib (Zelboraf), dabrafenib (Tafinlar), and encorafenib (Braftovi) directly target BRAF genes. MEK inhibitors include Trametinib (Mekinist), binimetinib (Mektovi), and cobimetinib (Cotellic).

Chemotherapy is not as effective for melanoma as it is for most other cancers. It is usually given only for advanced disease. Drugs used include dacarbazine and temozolomide. Radiation therapy is used in treating lymph node and brain metastases.

▼ **Patient and Caregiver Teaching**

Stress the importance of protection from the damaging effects of the sun, such as wearing a large-brimmed hat, sunglasses, and a long-sleeved shirt of a lightly woven fabric.

- Recommend avoiding direct sun during midday when rays of the sun are most dangerous.
- A broad-spectrum sunscreen with a minimum sun protection factor (SPF) of 15 should be reapplied every 2 hours while in the sun.
- Teach patients to self-examine their skin at least monthly to detect new or persistent skin lesions and to consult a healthcare provider (HCP) immediately if a mole or lesion shows a sudden or progressive size increase or changes in color or shape.

MÉNIÈRE'S DISEASE

Description

Ménière's disease is an inner ear problem characterized by episodic vertigo, tinnitus, sensation of aural fullness, and progressive hearing loss. Sudden, severe attacks of vertigo with nausea and vomiting are incapacitating. Symptoms usually begin between the ages of 40 and 60 years.

Pathophysiology and Clinical Manifestations

An accumulation of endolymph in the membranous labyrinth leads to hearing and balance problems.

- Attacks may occur without warning or be preceded by a sense of ear fullness, increasing tinnitus, and muffled hearing.
- The patient may report a whirling sensation and the feeling of being pulled to the ground ("drop attack").
- Autonomic signs and symptoms include pallor, nystagmus, nausea, and vomiting.
- An attack may last minutes to hours and occur several times per year.
- Hearing loss fluctuates and may progress to permanent hearing loss.

Diagnostic Studies

- Audiogram results demonstrate mild, low-frequency hearing loss.
- Vestibular tests may isolate the cause of vertigo.
- Glycerol test may show hearing improvement after oral glycerol dose.

Interprofessional and Nursing Management

During acute vertigo attacks, antihistamines (e.g., meclizine, diphenhydramine), anticholinergics (e.g., scopolamine), and benzodiazepines (e.g., lorazepam) can decrease vertigo and lessen nausea and vomiting. Those with severe vomiting may need IV hydration and antiemetics (e.g., ondansetron). Plan nursing interventions to minimize vertigo and maintain patient safety.

- Implement fall precautions.
- Reassure the patient that the condition is not life-threatening.
- Place the patient in a quiet, darkened room. Teach the patient to avoid sudden head movements or and position changes and to close the eyes until vertigo stops.
- Implement measures to address nausea and vomiting.
- Help the patient with ambulation as needed.
- Monitor intake and output and daily weights.

The overall goal is to treat symptoms and reduce the number of attacks. Careful management between attacks can slow the sensorineural hearing loss in many patients.

- Teach the patient to sit or lie down at the onset of dizziness to prevent falls.
- Teach the patient about diuretics and antihistamines.
- A low-salt diet with limited caffeine and alcohol intake often helps.
- Vestibular exercises may be recommended.

Surgical treatment including endolymphatic shunt, vestibular nerve resection, or labyrinth ablation is indicated for frequent attacks.

MENINGITIS, BACTERIAL

Description

Meningitis is an acute inflammation of the meningeal tissues surrounding the brain and spinal cord. Older adults and people who are debilitated are affected more often. College students living in dormitories and persons living in institutions (e.g., prisoners) are also at a high risk for contracting meningitis. Untreated bacterial meningitis has a high mortality rate.

Pathophysiology

Organisms usually gain entry to the central nervous system (CNS) through the upper respiratory tract or bloodstream. They also may enter from penetrating wounds of the skull or through fractured sinuses in basal skull fractures. *Streptococcus pneumoniae* and *Neisseria meningitidis* are the leading causes of bacterial meningitis. *N. meningitidis* has at least 13 different subtypes (serogroups), with five of them (A, B, C, Y, W) causing most cases.

- The use of *Haemophilus influenzae* vaccine has resulted in a significant decrease in meningitis from *H. influenzae*.

The inflammatory response to the infection tends to increase cerebrospinal fluid (CSF) production with a moderate increase in intracranial pressure (ICP). The purulent secretion produced by bacteria quickly spreads to other areas of the brain through the CSF.

- Observe patients with meningitis closely for signs of increased ICP, which is thought to result from swelling around the dura and increased CSF volume (see Increased Intracranial Pressure).

Clinical Manifestations

Fever, severe headache, nausea, vomiting, and *nuchal rigidity* (resistance to neck flexion) are key signs.

- Photophobia, a decreased level of consciousness (LOC), and signs of increased ICP may be present.
- If the infecting organism is the meningococcus, a nonblaching skin rash is common. Petechiae may be seen on the trunk, lower extremities, and mucous membranes.
- Seizures occur in one-third of all cases of meningitis.
- Coma is associated with a poor prognosis. It occurs in 5%–10% of patients with bacterial meningitis.

Complications

The most common acute complication of bacterial meningitis is increased ICP. Another complication is residual cranial nerve dysfunction.

- The optic nerve (CN II) is compressed by increased ICP. Papilledema is often present, and blindness may occur.
- When the oculomotor (CN III), trochlear (CN IV), and abducens (CN VI) nerves are irritated, ocular movements are affected. Ptosis, unequal pupils, and diplopia are common.

- Irritation of the trigeminal nerve (CN V) results in sensory losses and loss of the corneal reflex. Irritation of the facial nerve (CN VII) may produce facial paresis. Irritation of the vestibulo-cochlear nerve (CN VIII) causes tinnitus, vertigo, and deafness.
- Hemiparesis, dysphasia, and hemianopsia usually resolve over time.
- Acute cerebral edema may cause seizures, optic nerve palsy, bradycardia, hypertensive coma, and death.
- Headaches may occur for months until the irritation and inflammation have completely resolved.
- A noncommunicating hydrocephalus may occur if the exudate causes adhesions that prevent the normal flow of the CSF from the ventricles. CSF reabsorption by the arachnoid villi may be obstructed by the exudate. Surgical implantation of a shunt is the only treatment.
- A complication of meningococcal meningitis is *Waterhouse–Friderichsen syndrome*. The syndrome is manifested by petechiae, disseminated intravascular coagulation (DIC), and adrenal hemorrhage.

Diagnostic Studies

When a patient has manifestations suggesting bacterial meningitis, a blood culture and CT scan should be done. Diagnosis is usually verified by lumbar puncture with analysis of the CSF.

- CSF, sputum, and nasopharyngeal secretions are used to identify the causative organism.
- Skull X-rays may detect infected sinuses.
- CT scans may reveal increased ICP or hydrocephalus.

Interprofessional Management

Rapid diagnosis based on a history and physical examination is crucial because the patient is usually in a critical state when healthcare is sought.

- When meningitis is suspected, antibiotic therapy is instituted after collection of culture specimens, even before the diagnosis is confirmed. Ampicillin, penicillin, vancomycin, cefuroxime, ceftriaxone, and ceftazidime are commonly prescribed drugs for treating bacterial meningitis. Dexamethasone may also be prescribed before or with the first dose of antibiotics.

Nursing Management

Goals

The patient with meningitis will have a return to maximal neurologic functioning, resolution of infection, and control of pain and discomfort.

Interventions

Preventing respiratory infections through vaccination programs for pneumococcal pneumonia and influenza is important. Early and vigorous treatment of respiratory and ear infections that could spread to meningitis is important. People who have had close contact with someone who has meningitis should be given prophylactic antibiotics.

Meningitis generally requires respiratory isolation until the cultures are negative.

- Meningococcal meningitis is highly contagious, while other causes of meningitis may pose minimal to no infection risk with patient contact. Standard precautions are essential to protect the patient and nurse.

The patient with meningitis is acutely ill. The fever is high, and head pain is severe. Irritation of the cerebral cortex may result in seizures with changes in mental status and level of consciousness (LOC). The severity of manifestations is dependent on the level of ICP.

- Assess and record vital signs, neurologic status, fluid intake and output, skin, and lung fields regularly based on the patient's condition.
- Head and neck pain with movement require attention. Codeine provides some pain relief without undue sedation for most patients.
- A darkened room and cool cloth over the eyes relieve the discomfort of photophobia.
- All patients have some degree of mental distortion and hypersensitivity. They may be frightened and misinterpret the environment. Try to minimize environmental stimuli and prevent injury. For the delirious patient, additional low lighting may help decrease hallucinations.
- If seizures occur, take protective measures for patient safety. Administer antiseizure medications as ordered.

Manage problems associated with increased ICP (see Increased Intracranial Pressure).

- Treat fever vigorously because it increases cerebral edema and the risk of seizures. Aspirin or acetaminophen may reduce fever. If the fever is resistant to aspirin or acetaminophen, more vigorous means are needed, such as use of a cooling blanket. High fever greatly increases the metabolic rate, so assess the patient for dehydration and adequacy of intake. Enteral nutrition may be needed.
- After the acute period has passed, stress the importance of good nutrition with an emphasis on a high-protein, high-caloric diet in small, frequent feedings.

- Muscle rigidity may persist in the neck and backs of the legs. Progressive range-of-motion (ROM) exercises and warm baths are useful. Have the patient gradually increase activity as tolerated but encourage adequate rest and sleep.
- Residual effects can result in sequelae, such as dementia, seizures, deafness, hemiplegia, and hydrocephalus. Assess vision, hearing, cognitive skills, and motor and sensory abilities after recovery with appropriate referrals as indicated.
- Throughout the acute and convalescent periods, be aware of the anxiety and stress felt by the caregiver and other family members. Be calm and supportive. Provide accurate information.

METABOLIC SYNDROME

Description

Metabolic syndrome is a cluster of health problems, including obesity, hypertension, abnormal lipid levels, and high blood glucose. The syndrome increases a person's chance of developing cardiovascular disease, stroke, diabetes, renal disease, and polycystic ovary syndrome. One in three adults have metabolic syndrome.

- The prevalence is 50% for those 60 years of age and older. The number of persons aged 20–39 years with metabolic syndrome is steadily increasing.

Pathophysiology

Insulin resistance related to excessive visceral fat is the decreased ability of body cells to respond to the action of insulin. The pancreas compensates by secreting more insulin, resulting in hyperinsulinemia. Other characteristics of metabolic syndrome include hypertension, increased risk for clotting, and abnormal cholesterol levels (Fig. 20).

Clinical Manifestations

Signs of metabolic syndrome are impaired fasting blood glucose, hypertension, abnormal cholesterol levels, and obesity. Medical problems develop over time if the condition is not addressed.

Interprofessional and Nursing Management

There is no specific management of metabolic syndrome. The adoption of a healthy lifestyle is the cornerstone of treatment. Other

PATHOPHYSIOLOGY MAP

Fig. 20 Relationship among insulin resistance, obesity, diabetes, and cardiovascular disease. *HDL,* High-density lipoprotein.

interventions focus on weight loss and controlling risk factors for CVD and type 2 diabetes.

- Give patients information on healthy diets, exercise, and smoking cessation. The diet, which should be low in saturated fats, should promote weight loss. Weight loss and maintaining a lower weight are a priority in those with abdominal obesity and metabolic syndrome. Patients with obesity may be candidates for bariatric surgery.
- Increasing regular exercise will lower a patient's risk factors. In addition to helping with weight loss, regular exercise decreases triglyceride levels and increases HDL cholesterol levels in those with metabolic syndrome.

There are no specific medications for metabolic syndrome. Drugs to lower cholesterol and BP may be needed.

- Metformin (Glucophage) can lower glucose levels and enhance the cells' sensitivity to insulin.

MULTIPLE MYELOMA

Description

Multiple myeloma, or plasma cell myeloma, is a condition in which cancerous plasma cells proliferate and destroy the bones. The disease is more common in men than in women and usually develops between the ages of 65 and 74 years. Most patients need therapy off and on during the course of the disease.

Pathophysiology

The cause of multiple myeloma is unknown. Exposure to organic chemicals (such as benzene), herbicides, and insecticides may play a role. Viral infections, such as human immunodeficiency virus (HIV), may increase the risk.

Instead of plasma cells producing antibodies to fight different infections, myeloma tumors produce monoclonal antibodies (immunoglobulins). *Monoclonal* means they are all of one kind, making them ineffective and harmful. They do not fight infections, and they infiltrate the bone marrow. *Bence Jones proteins* show up in the urine of many patients with multiple myeloma.

The body's normal immune response is compromised by the reduction in number of normal plasma cells.

- Proliferation of cancerous plasma cells and the overproduction of immunoglobulin and proteins may result in the end-organ effects of myeloma on the bone marrow, bone, and kidneys and possibly the spleen, lymph nodes, liver, and heart.

Clinical Manifestations

Multiple myeloma develops slowly and insidiously. The patient often does not have symptoms until the disease is advanced.

- Skeletal pain is the major symptom. Pain in the pelvis, spine, and ribs is common.
- Diffuse osteoporosis develops as the myeloma protein destroys the bones. Osteolytic lesions develop on the skull, vertebrae, long bones, and ribs. Loss of bone integrity can lead to pathologic fractures and vertebral collapse with spinal cord compression.
- Degeneration causes calcium loss from bones, resulting in hypercalcemia. Hypercalcemia may cause renal, gastrointestinal (GI), or neurologic changes, such as polyuria, anorexia, confusion, and ultimately seizures, coma, and heart problems.
- The high levels of M protein can result in renal failure from renal tubular obstruction and interstitial nephritis.

- The patient may have anemia, thrombocytopenia, and granulocytopenia related to the replacement of normal bone marrow with plasma cells.

Diagnostic Studies

- Pancytopenia, hyperuricemia, hypercalcemia, and elevated creatinine may be found.
- Excessive production and secretion of monoclonal (M) protein are found in blood and urine.
- The light-chain part of the M protein (called *Bence Jones protein*) can be detected in the urine.
- Skeletal bone surveys, MRI, and/or positron emission tomography (PET) and CT scans show distinct areas of bone erosions; generalized thinning of the bones or fractures, especially in the vertebrae, ribs, pelvis, and bones of the thigh and upper arms.
- Higher blood levels of β_2-microglobulin and albumin are associated with a poorer prognosis.
- Bone marrow examination shows significantly increased numbers of plasma cells. Cytogenetic studies of the bone marrow play a role in prognostic stratification.

Interprofessional Management

The therapeutic approach involves managing both the disease and its symptoms. The current treatment options include corticosteroids, chemotherapy, immunotherapy, targeted therapy, and hematopoietic stem cell transplantation (HSCT). Multiple myeloma is seldom cured. Treatment can relieve symptoms, produce remission, and prolong life. Pain control of pain and preventing pathologic fractures are goals of management.

- Chemotherapy includes a corticosteroid plus two chemotherapy agents, such as bortezomib and lenalidomide or bortezomib and cyclophosphamide. The goal is to reduce the number of plasma cells. Initial treatment depends on whether the patient is a future stem cell transplant candidate and predicted tolerance of therapy (see Chemotherapy). High-dose chemotherapy followed by HSCT is the standard of care in eligible patients.
- Immunotherapy and targeted therapy are options. Immunomodulator drugs include thalidomide, lenalidomide, and pomalidomide. Proteosome inhibitors include bortezomib, carfilzomib, and ixazomib. Panobinostat is a drug that affects enzymes that promote cancer cell growth. Daratumumab is a monoclonal

antibody against CD38, a protein that is found on the surface of myeloma cells.

- Drugs may be used to treat the complications of multiple myeloma. For example, IV furosemide promotes renal excretion of calcium, and allopurinol may be given to reduce hyperuricemia.
- Zoledronic acid and denosumab inhibit bone breakdown. They are given for skeletal pain and hypercalcemia. They inhibit bone resorption without inhibiting bone formation and mineralization.
- Control of pain and prevention of pathologic fractures are other goals of interprofessional care. Analgesics, orthopedic supports, and localized radiation help reduce skeletal pain. Surgical procedures, such as vertebroplasty, may be done to support degenerative vertebrae.
- Assessment and prompt treatment of infection are important.

Nursing Management

Ambulation and adequate hydration are used to prevent hypercalcemia, dehydration, and potential renal damage. Weight bearing helps the bones reabsorb some calcium, and fluids dilute calcium and prevent protein precipitates from causing renal tubular obstruction. Fluids are administered to achieve a urine output of 1.5–2 L/day if the patient does not already have renal compromise. Because of the myeloma proteins, the patient is at additional risk for renal problems. Monitor electrolytes and fluid balance closely.

- Because of the potential for pathologic fractures, use caution when moving and ambulating the patient. A slight twist or strain on a weakened bone may cause a fracture.
- Peripheral neuropathy is common with several therapies for multiple myeloma. It contributes to discomfort, the inability to do basic activities of daily living, and the risk for injury from falling

Pain management requires innovative and knowledgeable nursing interventions.

- Analgesics, such as nonsteroidal antiinflammatory drugs (NSAIDs), acetaminophen, or acetaminophen with codeine, may be more effective than opioids alone in diminishing bone pain. Braces, especially for the spine, may also help prevent pain.

The patient's psychosocial needs require sensitive, skilled management. Help the patient and significant others adapt to changes and adjust to the losses related to the disease process, while helping maximize functioning and quality of life.

MULTIPLE SCLEROSIS

Description

Multiple sclerosis (MS) is a chronic, unpredictable, progressive, degenerative disorder of the central nervous system (CNS). It is characterized by demyelination of the nerve fibers of the brain and spinal cord.

- MS can affect people of any age. The onset is usually between ages 20 and 40 years. MS affects every patient differently, ranging from little permanent effect to severe disability. People diagnosed after age 50 often have more progressive disease. MS affects women two to three times more often. MS is more prevalent further away from the equator.

Pathophysiology

The cause of MS is likely due to a combination of genetic and environment factors. MS may develop in a genetically susceptible person after an environmental exposure, such as a viral infection. We believe viruses or other antigens activate T cells. The T cells cross the blood brain barrier and begin the inflammatory process, mistaking the myelin protein for the viral antigen.

MS is marked by three processes: chronic inflammation, demyelination, and gliosis in the CNS.

- The immune system attack on the myelin proteins causes damage to the myelin sheath. Transmission of nerve impulses still occurs, but it is slowed. The patient may have impaired function (e.g., weakness, numbness). Inflammation ceases and full recovery or partial recovery can occur. Symptoms all or partially disappear. At that point, the patient has a remission.
- As inflammation continues or recurs, nearby oligodendrocytes are affected. Myelin loses the ability to regenerate. Eventually damage occurs to the underlying axon. This disrupts nerve impulse transmission. Nerve function is lost permanently.
- White, gray, and axonal matter are all eventually effected. As inflammation subsides, glial scar tissue replaces damaged tissue. This leads to the formation of hard, rigid plaques throughout the white matter of the CNS. In late disease, cerebral cortex atrophy occurs.

Clinical Manifestations

The onset of MS is often slow and gradual. Vague symptoms occur periodically over months or years. For some patients, MS is marked by rapid, progressive deterioration. Others have remissions and exacerbations. With repeated exacerbations, the overall trend is progressive deterioration in neurologic function.

Because changes from MS have a spotty distribution in the CNS, symptoms vary based on the area of CNS involvement. Some patients have severe symptoms early in the disease. Some may have minimal symptoms for several years. The classification scheme of MS, with four primary patterns, is based on the clinical course (Table 59).

- Vision changes such as blurred or double vision, red-green color distortion, or blindness in one eye may be the first sign.
- Many patients describe extremity muscle weakness and problems with coordination and balance. Those symptoms may affect walking or standing. MS can cause partial or complete paralysis in the worst cases.
- Most have numbness and tingling. Lhermitte's sign is a temporary sensory symptom described as an electric shock going down the spine or into the limbs with neck flexion.
- Some patients report pain, especially around the low thoracic and abdominal regions. Labeled the "MS hug," this is from muscle spasm in intercostal and abdominal muscles.
- Other frequent problems include speech problems, hearing loss, tremors, and dizziness.
- Possible cerebellar signs include nystagmus, ataxia, dysarthria, and dysphagia.
- Many patients have severe, even disabling fatigue. Heat, humidity, deconditioning, and medication side effects worsen fatigue.
- Bowel problems usually involve constipation. Urinary problems include urgency and frequency, often with dribbling or incontinence, and urinary retention.
- Physiologic erectile dysfunction may result from spinal cord involvement in men.
- Women may have decreased libido, difficulty with orgasm, painful intercourse, and decreased vaginal lubrication. Some women with MS have remission or an improvement in symptoms during pregnancy.
- About half of people with MS have problems with cognitive function. Most involve problems with multitasking, concentration, short-term memory, speed of processing, and word finding. General intellect stays unchanged. There may be emotional changes, such as anger, depression, or euphoria.

MS reduces life expectancy by about 7 years. Death is usually caused by infection or complications of immobility (e.g., pneumonia).

M

TABLE 59	Patterns of Multiple Sclerosis
MS category	**Characteristics**
Relapsing-remitting	• Clearly defined attacks of worsening neurologic function (*relapses*) with partial or complete recovery (*remission*). • 85% of people first diagnosed with this type of multiple sclerosis (MS).
Primary-progressive	• Steadily worsening neurologic function from the beginning with minor improvements but no distinct relapses or remissions. • 10% of people first diagnosed with this type of MS.
Secondary-progressive	• A relapsing-remitting initial course, followed by progression with or without occasional relapses, minor remissions, and plateaus. • New treatments may slow progression. • Most people initially diagnosed with relapsing-remitting MS eventually transition to this type.
Progressive-relapsing	• Progressive disease from onset, with clear acute relapses, with or without full recovery. Periods between relapses are characterized by continuing progression. • 5% of people with MS.

Diagnostic Studies

No one specific diagnostic test for MS exists. The history and manifestations are important.
- MRI of the brain and spinal cord may show the presence of plaques, inflammation, atrophy, and tissue destruction.
- Cerebrospinal fluid (CSF) analysis may show an increase in immunoglobulin G (IgG) and the presence of oligoclonal banding.
- Evoked potential responses are often delayed as a result of decreased nerve conduction from the eye and ear to the brain.

To be diagnosed with MS, the patient must have: (1) evidence of at least two inflammatory demyelinating lesions in at least two different locations within the CNS, (2) damage or an attack occurring at different times (usually 1 month or more apart), and (3) all other possible diagnoses ruled out.

Interprofessional Management

No cure is currently known for MS. Care is aimed at treating the disease process and providing symptomatic relief.

Drug Therapy

Disease-modifying drugs (DMDs) suppress the immune system in order to modify disease progression and prevent relapses. DMDs are more effective when started early in the course of MS. DMDs include interferons, monoclonal antibodies, and synthetic agents. Treatment often begins with use of immunomodulator drugs. These drugs include interferon β-1a (Rebif, Plegridy, Avonex), interferon β-1b (Betaseron, Extavia), and glatiramer acetate (Copaxone, Glatopa).

- Teriflunomide (Aubagio) is an immunomodulatory agent with antiinflammatory properties.
- Fingolimod (Gilenya), ponesimod (Ponvory), and siponimod (Mayzent) reduce MS disease activity by preventing lymphocytes from reaching the CNS and causing damage.
- Cladribine (Mavenclad) is a cytotoxic agent taken orally in two cycles a year. Cancer risk increases with cladribine. Dimethyl fumarate (Tecfidera) helps the body defend itself against the inflammation and oxidative stress caused by MS. Dimethyl fumarate and fingolimod can cause a fatal viral brain infection, progressive multifocal leukoencephalopathy (PML).
- For more active forms of MS, IV monoclonal antibodies may suppress immunologic activity. These include natalizumab (Tysabri), alemtuzumab (Lemtrada), and ocrelizumab (Ocrevus). Due to the risk for PML and other side effects, these are only given to patients who had an inadequate response to other treatments. Ocrelizumab is approved for relapsing remitting and progressive forms of MS. It slows disease progression and improves symptoms. Ocrelizumab increases the risk for infection and breast cancer.
- IV corticosteroids (e.g., prednisone) can be used to treat acute MS exacerbations. They reduce edema and acute inflammation at the site of demyelination. They speed recovery but do not affect the residual neurologic impairment from the exacerbation. Therapeutic plasma exchange (plasmapheresis) and IV immunoglobulin G may be considered for a short time when treatment with corticosteroids alone does not achieve symptom improvement.

Many other drugs are used to treat the various MS symptoms. These may include drugs for spasticity, fatigue, tremor, vertigo or dizziness, depression, pain, bowel and bladder problems, sexual problems, and cognitive changes. For example, amantadine, modafinil (Provigil), and fluoxetine (Prozac) are used to treat fatigue. Anticholinergics (oxybutynin, propantheline) can treat bladder spasms. Tricyclic antidepressants and antiseizure drugs help with chronic pain. Dalfampridine (Ampyra) may improve walking speed. It is a selective potassium channel blocker that improves nerve conduction in damaged nerve segments. Use may cause seizures, especially at higher doses. Bethanechol is a common treatment for urinary retention.

Other Therapy

Severe muscle spasticity can be treated with stretching, physical therapy, baclofen, intrathecal pumps, or onabotulinumtoxin A (Botox). Other options include surgery (e.g., neurectomy, rhizotomy, cordotomy) or dorsal-column electrical stimulation. Tremors that become unmanageable with pharmacologic therapy can be treated with thalamotomy or deep brain stimulation.

- Neurologic problems sometimes improve with physical therapy. Exercise decreases spasticity, increases coordination, and retrains unaffected muscles to act for impaired ones. Water exercise is especially beneficial.

Nursing Management

Goals

The patient with MS will maximize neuromuscular function, maintain independence in activities of daily living for as long as possible, manage fatigue, optimize psychosocial well-being, adjust to the illness, and reduce factors that precipitate exacerbations.

Interventions

The patient with MS should be aware of triggers that may cause exacerbations or worsening of the disease. They include infection, trauma, live virus immunizations, childbirth, stress, and change in climate. Help the patient identify triggers and avoid or minimize their effects.

- The patient diagnosed with MS may need assistance with the grieving process.
- During an acute exacerbation, the patient may be immobile. Focus on preventing complications of immobility.
- Visual symptoms may make driving, reading, performing self-care, and even watching television difficult. Preparation for possible exacerbations can make coping with the physical changes easier.

▼ Patient and Caregiver Teaching

- Teach the patient about avoiding fatigue, extremes of heat and cold, and exposure to infection.
- Teach the patient to achieve a good balance of exercise and rest, eat nutritious and well-balanced meals, and minimize caffeine intake.
- Patients should know their treatment regimens, the side effects of drugs, and drug interactions with over-the-counter preparations.
- Bladder control is a concerning and potentially embarrassing problem. Drug therapy may help some patients. You may need to teach self-catheterization.

- Constipation is common. Stress a diet high in fiber and maintaining activity.

The National Multiple Sclerosis Society and its local chapters can offer a variety of services to meet the needs of MS patients and their families.

MYASTHENIA GRAVIS

Description

Myasthenia gravis (MG) is an autoimmune disease of the neuromuscular junction marked by fluctuating weakness of certain skeletal muscle groups that worsens with activity. In women, MG often starts between ages 20 and 30. Men usually develop MG in their 50s.

Pathophysiology

MG is caused by an autoimmune process in which antibodies attack and destroy ACh receptors. Fewer ACh receptor (AChR) sites at the neuromuscular junction prevents ACh molecules from attaching to receptors and stimulating muscle contraction. We think the thymus gives incorrect instructions to developing immune cells causing them to make ACh receptor antibodies.

Clinical Manifestations

The key feature of MG is fluctuating weakness of skeletal muscle. Muscles engaged in repetitive movements are affected the most: those used to move the eyes and eyelids, chew, swallow, speak, and breathe. Muscles are generally strongest in the morning and become exhausted with continued activity. A period of rest usually restores strength.

- In more than half of patients, the first muscles involved are the ocular muscles, causing ptosis (drooping of the eyelids) and double vision.
- Chewing, swallowing, and facial mobility and expression can be impaired. Speech is affected, and the voice often fades during conversation.
- There is no sensory loss. Reflexes are normal and muscle atrophy is rare.
- The course of MG is highly variable. Patients may have short-term remissions, stabilize, or have severe progressive disease.
- Fatigue, pregnancy, illness, trauma, temperature extremes, stress, and hypokalemia can exacerbate MG.
- Some drugs can worsen MG symptoms, including β-adrenergic blockers, calcium channel blockers, lithium, quinidine, and aminoglycoside antibiotics.

- The major complications of a *myasthenic crisis* result from muscle weakness in areas that affect swallowing and breathing. This can result in aspiration or respiratory insufficiency. The patient may need a ventilator or noninvasive respiratory support.

Diagnostic Studies

The diagnosis of MG can be made on the basis of history and physical examination.

- Single-fiber electromyography (EMG) may show a decreased response to repeated stimulation of the hand muscles, indicating muscle fatigue.
- A patient with MG has rapid improvement in muscle strength after receiving edrophonium.
- If MG is confirmed, a chest CT scan may be done to evaluate the thymus.

Interprofessional Management

Drug therapy for MG includes anticholinesterase drugs, alternate-day corticosteroids, and immunosuppressants.

- Acetylcholinesterase inhibitors prolong the action of ACh and facilitate transmission of impulses at the neuromuscular junction. Pyridostigmine (Mestinon) is the most successful drug in this group.
- Corticosteroids (prednisone) are used to suppress the immune response. Drugs such as azathioprine (Imuran), mycophenolate (CellCept), and cyclosporine (Sandimmune) may also be used for immunosuppression.
- Eculizumab (Soliris), an IV monoclonal antibody, stops the autoimmune response. Over time, it improves symptoms.
- Removal of the thymus gland results in improvement in most patients. A few patients achieve cure after thymectomy. Plasmapheresis and IV immunoglobulin G can provide short-term improvement for patients in crisis or in preparation for surgery.

Nursing Management

Goals

The patient with MG will have a return of normal muscle endurance, manage fatigue, avoid complications, and maintain a quality of life.

Interventions

The patient with MG who is admitted to the hospital usually has a respiratory tract infection or is in acute myasthenic crisis. Nursing care is aimed at maintaining adequate ventilation, continuing drug therapy, and watching for side effects of therapy. Be able to

TABLE 60 Comparison of Myasthenic and Cholinergic Crises	
Myasthenic crisis	**Cholinergic crisis**
Causes	
Exacerbation of myasthenia after precipitating factors or failure to take drug as prescribed or drug dose too low	Overdose of anticholinesterase drugs resulting in increased ACh at the receptor sites, remission (spontaneous or after thymectomy)
Differential diagnosis	
Improved strength after IV administration of anticholinesterase drugs	Weakness within 1 h after ingestion of anticholinesterase drugs
Increased weakness of skeletal muscles manifesting as ptosis, bulbar signs (e.g., difficulty swallowing, difficulty articulating words), or dyspnea	Increased weakness of skeletal muscles manifesting as ptosis, bulbar signs, dyspnea
	Effects on smooth muscle include pupillary miosis, salivation, diarrhea, nausea or vomiting, abdominal cramps, increased bronchial secretions, sweating, or lacrimation

ACh, Acetylcholine.

distinguish cholinergic from myasthenic crisis, because the causes and treatment differ greatly (Table 60).
- Care focuses on reducing the impact of MG on activities of daily living.
- Scheduling doses of medication so that peak action is reached at mealtime may make eating easier. Teach the patient about a balanced diet of foods that can be chewed and swallowed. Semi-solid foods may be easier to eat than solids or liquids.
- Recommend diversional activities that require little physical effort and match the patient's interests.

▼ **Patient and Caregiver Teaching**

Focus teaching on adherence to the treatment plan, complications, potential adverse reactions to specific drugs, complications of therapy (crisis conditions), and what to do about them. Help the patient and caregiver explore community resources, such as the Myasthenia Gravis Society and MG support groups.

MYOCARDIAL INFARCTION

Myocardial infarction is part of the spectrum referred to as "acute coronary syndrome." See Acute Coronary Syndrome for the discussion of this disorder.

MYOCARDITIS

Description

Myocarditis is a focal or diffuse inflammation of the myocardium. Causes include viruses, bacteria, fungi, radiation therapy, autoimmune disorders, and pharmacologic and chemical factors.

Pathophysiology

When the myocardium becomes infected, the causative agent invades the myocytes and causes cellular damage and necrosis. The immune response is activated, cytokines and oxygen free radicals are released, and an autoimmune response occurs, resulting in further destruction of myocytes and cardiac dysfunction.

Clinical Manifestations

The features of myocarditis vary from a benign course without overt symptoms to progressive heart failure (HF), dysrhythmias, or sudden cardiac death (SCD). Fever, fatigue, malaise, myalgias, pharyngitis, dyspnea, lymphadenopathy, and nausea and vomiting are early manifestations of the viral illness.

- *Early*: Cardiac signs appear 7–10 days after viral infection and include pericardial chest pain with a pericardial friction rub and effusion.
- *Late*: Cardiac signs relate to the development of HF and include S_3, crackles, jugular venous distention, syncope, peripheral edema, and angina.

Diagnostic Studies

- Electrocardiography (ECG) changes reflect pericardial involvement, including diffuse ST-segment abnormalities. Dysrhythmias and conduction problems may be present.
- Laboratory findings may include mild to moderate leukocytosis and atypical lymphocytes, elevated viral titers, increased erythrocyte sedimentation rate (ESR), C-reactive protein (CRP), and cardiac biomarkers such as troponin, and elevated viral titers. (Virus is generally present in tissue and fluid samples during the first 8–10 days of illness.)

- Endomyocardial biopsy is most diagnostic during the first 6 weeks of acute illness, when lymphocytic infiltration and myocyte damage are present.
- Echocardiography, radionuclide scans, and MRI are used to assess heart function.

Interprofessional Management

The treatment for myocarditis consists of managing symptoms.

- Angiotensin-converting enzyme (ACE) inhibitors and β-adrenergic blockers are used if the heart is enlarged or to treat HF.
- Diuretics reduce fluid volume and decrease preload.
- If the patient is not hypotensive, nitroprusside and milrinone may reduce afterload and improve cardiac output by decreasing systemic vascular resistance.
- Anticoagulation reduces the risk of clot formation from blood stasis in patients with a low ejection fraction (EF).
- Digoxin (Lanoxin) improves heart contractility and reduces heart rate. However, it is used cautiously in patients with myocarditis because of increased sensitivity to the adverse effects (e.g., dysrhythmias) and the potential toxicity.

Myocarditis with an autoimmune basis is treated with immunosuppressive agents to reduce heart inflammation and damage. However, the use of these drugs for the treatment of myocarditis is controversial because they may lead to recurrence. Antivirals may be used as adjunct therapy to treat myocarditis.

General supportive measures for management of myocarditis include O₂ therapy, bed rest, and restricted activity. In cases of severe HF, intraaortic balloon pump therapy and ventricular assist devices (VAD) may be needed.

Nursing Management

Focus interventions on improving cardiac output (CO) and managing the signs and symptoms of HF. Select nursing measures to decrease cardiac workload (e.g., semi-Fowler's position, spaced activity and rest, a quiet environment). Carefully monitor medications that increase the heart's contractility and decrease the preload or afterload.

- The patient may be anxious about the diagnosis of myocarditis. Assess the level of anxiety an institute measures to decrease anxiety. Keep the patient and caregivers informed.

The patient who receives immunosuppressive therapy is at an increased risk for infection. Monitor for complications and provide the patient with proper infection control procedures.

NAUSEA AND VOMITING

Description

Nausea and vomiting are the most common manifestations of gastrointestinal (GI) diseases. Although each manifestation can occur independently, they are closely related and usually treated as one problem. Nausea and vomiting occur in a wide variety of GI problems and in many conditions unrelated to GI disease. These include pregnancy, infection, central nervous system (CNS) problems (e.g., meningitis, tumor), and cardiovascular disease (CVD) (e.g., myocardial infarction, heart failure). They can occur with psychologic states (e.g., stress, fear) or when the GI tract becomes overly irritated, excited, or distended. Patients may have nausea and vomiting after surgery with general anesthesia or as a drug side effect (e.g., chemotherapy, opioids).

- *Nausea* is a feeling of discomfort in the epigastrium with a conscious desire to vomit. Anorexia usually accompanies nausea.
- *Vomiting* (*emesis*) is the forceful ejection of partially digested food and secretions from the upper GI tract. *Projectile vomiting* is a forceful expulsion of stomach contents without nausea.
- *Regurgitation* is an effortless process in which partially digested food slowly comes up from the stomach.

Pathophysiology

A vomiting center in the medulla coordinates the components involved in vomiting. Neural impulses reach the vomiting center by way of afferent pathways through branches of the autonomic nervous system. Receptors for these afferent fibers are in the GI tract, kidneys, heart, and uterus. When stimulated, these receptors relay information to the vomiting center, which initiates the vomiting reflex. In addition, the chemoreceptor trigger zone (CTZ) located in the brain responds to chemical stimuli of drugs and toxins. Once stimulated (e.g., in motion sickness), the CTZ transmits impulses directly to the vomiting center (Fig. 21).

Vomiting is a complex act. The simultaneous closure of the glottis, deep inspiration with contraction of the diaphragm in the inspiratory position, closure of the pylorus, relaxation of the stomach and lower esophageal sphincter, and contraction of the abdominal muscles with increasing intraabdominal pressure force stomach contents up and out of the mouth.

- Early morning vomiting is common in pregnancy.
- Emotional stressors may elicit vomiting during or right after eating.

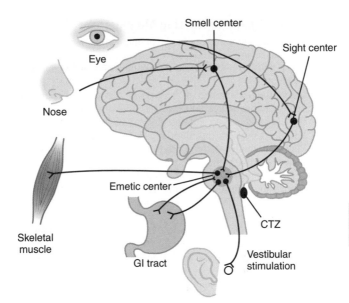

Figure 21 Stimuli involved in the act of vomiting. *CTZ*, Chemoreceptor trigger zone.

- Cyclic vomiting syndrome consists of recurring episodes of nausea, vomiting, and fatigue that last from a few hours up to 10 days.

Clinical Manifestations

When nausea and vomiting occur over a long period, dehydration can develop rapidly. Water and essential electrolytes (e.g., potassium, sodium, chloride) are lost. As vomiting persists, the patient may have severe electrolyte imbalances, extracellular fluid volume loss, decreased plasma volume, and eventually circulatory failure.

- Metabolic alkalosis may result from loss of gastric hydrochloric acid (HCl). Less often, metabolic acidosis can occur when vomiting small intestinal contents.
- Weight loss from fluid loss may occur quickly with severe vomiting.

The risk of pulmonary aspiration is a concern when vomiting occurs in older or unconscious patients or those with an impaired gag reflex. To prevent aspiration, put the patient who cannot adequately manage self-care in a semi-Fowler's or side-lying position.

Interprofessional and Nursing Management

The goals of management are that the patient will experience minimal or no nausea and vomiting, have normal electrolyte levels and hydration status, and return to a normal pattern of fluid balance and nutrient intake.

Document the appearance of the emesis. Assess the patient for precipitating factors. When the cause has not been determined, use drugs with caution. Using antiemetics before knowing the cause can mask the underlying problem and delay diagnosis and treatment. Many antiemetic drugs act to block the neurochemicals that trigger nausea and vomiting.

- $5-HT_3$ (Serotonin) receptor antagonists are effective in reducing chemotherapy-induced vomiting (CINV), postoperative nausea and vomiting (PONV), and nausea and vomiting related to migraine headache and anxiety.
- Dexamethasone is given with other antiemetics to manage acute and delayed CINV. Neurokinin-1 receptor antagonists (NK_1RAs) (e.g., aprepitant [Emend], rolapitant [Varubi]) can treat CINV and PONV.
- An oral cannabinoid (e.g., dronabinol) may be an option to manage CINV when other therapies are not effective.

The patient with severe vomiting requires IV fluid therapy with electrolyte and glucose replacement until able to tolerate oral intake. Some patients may need a nasogastric (NG) tube and suction to decompress the stomach. Secure the NG tube to prevent tube movement in the nose and throat that can stimulate nausea and vomiting. Record intake and output, position the patient to prevent aspiration, and monitor vital signs.

- Assess for dehydration, and observe for changes. Provide physical and emotional support and maintain a quiet, odor-free environment.

Once symptoms have subsided, offer clear liquids. Water is the initial fluid of choice for oral rehydration. Have the patient sip small amounts of fluid (5–15 mL) every 15–20 min. Other options include room temperature carbonated beverages with the carbonation removed and warm tea. Dry toast, crackers, and plain gelatin may be helpful. As the patient's condition improves, provide a diet high in carbohydrates and low in fat. Bland foods, such as pasta, rice, cereal, baked potato, or cooked chicken, are generally well tolerated in small amounts.

Some patients find that acupressure or acupuncture at specific points reduces PONV. Others use herbs, such as ginger and peppermint oil. Changes in body position or exercise may help some patients.

▼ **Patient and Caregiver Teaching**

- Provide explanations for diagnostic tests and procedures.
- Teach the patient and caregiver methods to prevent nausea and vomiting, and strategies to maintain fluid and food intake.
- Relaxation techniques, frequent rest periods, effective pain management strategies, and diversional tactics can prevent or reduce nausea and vomiting.
- Cleansing the face and hands with a cool washcloth and providing mouth care between episodes promote comfort.
- When food is identified as the precipitating cause of nausea and vomiting, help the patient identify the specific food and when it was eaten, prior history with that food, and whether anyone else who ate the food is sick.

NEPHROTIC SYNDROME

Description

Nephrotic syndrome results when the kidney glomerulus is excessively permeable to plasma protein, causing proteinuria and leading to low plasma albumin and edema. Common causes include primary glomerular disease, infections (e.g., hepatitis, streptococcal), cancers (e.g., Hodgkin's lymphoma), drugs (e.g., nonsteroidal antiinflammatory drugs [NSAIDs]), and multisystem diseases (e.g., diabetes, amyloidosis, systemic lupus erythematosus [SLE]).

Pathophysiology and Clinical Manifestations

The increased glomerular membrane permeability found in nephrotic syndrome is responsible for massive excretion of protein in the urine. This results in decreased total serum protein and subsequent edema formation, including ascites and anasarca.

- Diminished plasma oncotic pressure from the decrease in serum proteins stimulates hepatic lipoprotein synthesis, which results in hyperlipidemia. Fat bodies (fatty casts) in the urine cause urine to appear foamy.
- Immune responses are impaired. Infection is a major cause of morbidity and mortality.
- Calcium and skeletal abnormalities may occur, including hypocalcemia, blunted calcemic response to parathyroid hormone, hyperparathyroidism, and osteomalacia.
- Hypercoagulability from the urinary loss of anticoagulant proteins increases the risk for arterial and venous thromboembolism, including pulmonary embolism and deep vein or renal thrombus.

Characteristic manifestations of nephrotic syndrome include peripheral edema, massive proteinuria, hypertension, hyperlipidemia, hypoalbuminemia, and foamy urine.

Interprofessional and Nursing Management

The goals are to relieve the symptoms and cure or control the primary disease. Corticosteroids and cyclophosphamide may be used. Managing diabetes is important. Angiotensin-converting enzyme inhibitor or angiotensin receptor blocker drugs may reduce urine protein losses. The treatment of hyperlipidemia includes lipid-lowering agents.

The major focus of care is related to managing edema. Diuretics (typically loop diuretics) can improve edema.

- Management of edema includes low sodium intake (2–3 g/day), and a moderate-protein diet (1–2 g/kg per day). Patients have the potential to become malnourished from anorexia and the loss of protein in the urine. Serve small, frequent meals in a pleasant setting to encourage better dietary intake.
- Assess the edema by weighing the patient daily, accurately recording intake and output, and measuring abdominal girth or extremity size. Monitor effectiveness of diuretic therapy. Clean edematous areas carefully to avoid trauma to the skin.
- Support the patient in coping with an altered body image because embarrassment may be associated with the edematous appearance.
- Teach the patient to avoid exposure to people with known infections.

NON-HODGKIN'S LYMPHOMAS

Description

Non-Hodgkin's lymphomas (NHLs) are a broad group of cancers of primarily B-, T-, natural killer (NK), histiocytic, and dendritic cells. They affect persons of all ages. There are over 75 types categorized by the level of differentiation (maturity), cell of origin, immunophenotype (cell surface antigens, CD20, CD52), and genetic and clinical features. NHL is the most commonly occurring hematologic cancer.

Pathophysiology

The cause of NHL is usually unknown. NHLs may result from chromosomal translocations, infections, environmental factors, and immunodeficiency states. Chromosomal translocations have a key role in the pathogenesis of many NHLs. Viruses and bacteria implicated in the pathogenesis of NHL, include HTLV-1, EBV, human herpesvirus, hepatitis C, *H. pylori*, and *Chlamydia trachomatis*. Chemicals linked to NHL include pesticides, herbicides, solvents, and organic chemicals. NHL is more common in people who have inherited immunodeficiency syndromes, have used immunosuppressive agents (e.g., to prevent rejection after an organ transplant or to treat autoimmune disorders), or received chemotherapy or radiation therapy.

All NHLs involve lymphocytes arrested in various stages of development and may mimic a leukemia. *Diffuse large B cell lymphoma*, the most common aggressive lymphoma, starts in the lymph nodes, usually in the neck or abdomen. *Burkitt's lymphoma* is the most aggressive type of NHL.

Clinical Manifestations

A variety of presentations and courses occur, from indolent (slowly developing) to rapidly progressive disease. The method of spread can be unpredictable, and most patients have widespread disease at the time of diagnosis. The primary clinical manifestation is *lymphadenopathy*, painless lymph node enlargement. NHLs also can originate outside the lymph nodes.

- Symptoms and signs depend on where the disease is present (e.g., hepatomegaly with liver involvement, neurologic symptoms with central nervous system [CNS] disease).
- NHL can manifest in nonspecific ways, such as an airway obstruction, hyperuricemia and renal failure from tumor lysis syndrome, pericardial tamponade, and gastrointestinal (GI) symptoms.
- Patients with high-grade lymphomas may have lymphadenopathy, fever, night sweats, and weight loss.

Diagnostic Studies

Diagnostic studies for NHL resemble those used for Hodgkin's lymphoma. However, because NHL is more often found in extranodal sites, more diagnostic studies may be done. These include MRI or lumbar puncture to rule out CNS disease, a bone marrow biopsy to determine bone marrow infiltration, or a barium enema or upper endoscopy to look for GI involvement.

Interprofessional and Nursing Management

Treatment for NHL involves chemotherapy, biotherapy, radiation, and sometimes phototherapy and topical therapy (see Chemotherapy, Radiation Therapy, and Immunologic and Targeted Therapy). More aggressive lymphomas (diffuse large B cell) are generally more responsive to treatment. In contrast, indolent lymphomas (e.g., follicular lymphomas) have a naturally long course but are hard to treat effectively. Patients with low-grade (indolent) lymphoma may live 10 years or more without treatment. However, some early therapies can be well tolerated and may reduce the time to progression of the disease. Numerous chemotherapy combinations have been used to try to overcome the resistant nature of this disease.

- Rituximab, a monoclonal antibody against the CD20 antigen on the surface of normal and malignant B lymphocytes, is used to treat NHL in combination with other agents.
- An infectious cause, such as in *H. pylori* gastric lymphomas, may be treated with antibiotic or antiviral therapy.
- Hematopoietic stem cell transplantation may help in certain subtypes of NHL.
- Chimeric antigen receptor (CAR) T-cell immunotherapy may be used.
- Another therapy for some types of NHL is the monoclonal antibody ibritumomab tiuxetan (Zevalin). It contains a radioactive particle that can kill cancer cells.
- For more diffuse disease, treatment may include more aggressive combination therapies.

Nursing care for patients with NHL is similar to that for patients with Hodgkin's lymphoma. It is based on managing problems related to the disease (pain, spinal cord compression, tumor lysis syndrome), pancytopenia, and effects of therapy. However, NHL can be more extensive and involve specific organs, requiring additional interventions specific to effects on those organs.

- Psychosocial considerations are important. Help the patient and family understand the disease, treatment, and expected and potential side effects.
- Evaluation of patients with NHL for long-term effects of therapy is important because the consequences of disease and treatment may not become apparent for many years.

OBESITY

Description

Obesity is an excessively high amount of body fat or adipose tissue. Obesity is a global problem because it is a major risk factor for leading causes of death, including type 2 diabetes, heart disease, and certain cancers. Those who are overweight often have problems with mobility and sleeping that affect their health.

The consequences of obesity extend beyond the physical changes. Social stigma can take an emotional toll on a person's psychologic well-being. Many struggle with altered body image, depression, and low self-esteem and withdraw from social interaction.

- Obesity is a major public health issue in the United States. Currently, about 43% of adults in the United States are obese. Significant geographic, racial and ethnic, and income disparities exist. Obesity rates are highest in the South and Midwest, among blacks and Hispanics, and among lower-income, less educated Americans.
- Obesity in adulthood is often a problem that began in childhood or adolescence. One in 10 children becomes obese as early as age 2–5 years. Reversing the childhood obesity crisis is key to addressing the overall obesity epidemic.

The most common way we classify weight is the *body mass index* (BMI). BMI is calculated by dividing a person's weight (in kilograms) by the square of the height in meters. We combine other measures with the BMI for an accurate evaluation of a person's weight.

Persons with a BMI <18.5 kg/m² are considered underweight. A BMI between 18.5 and 24.9 kg/m² reflects a normal body weight. A BMI of 25–29.9 kg/m² is classified as being overweight, and people with values at 30 kg/m² or above are considered obese. The term *extreme obesity* (morbid or severe obesity) is used for those with a BMI >40 kg/m².

- The waist-to-hip ratio (WHR) ratio describes the distribution of both subcutaneous and visceral adipose tissue. The ratio is calculated by using the waist measurement divided by the hip measurement. In women, the ratio should be 0.8 or less, and in men, it should be 1.0 or less.
- Persons with fat located mainly in the abdominal area (*apple-shaped body*) are at greater risk for obesity-related complications than those whose fat is mainly located in the upper legs (*pear-shaped body*).

Pathophysiology

Obesity is a complex, multifactorial disease. It results from an energy imbalance where one takes in more calories than they need for the body's physical and metabolic functions. This results in an abnormal increase and accumulation of fat cells. Many factors, including genetic and environmental influences, contribute to obesity. Personal decisions about food choices, portion sizes, and exercise also are factors.

In obesity, there is an increase in the number of adipocytes, or fat cells, and an increase in their size (hypertrophy). When storage of existing fat cells is exceeded, preadipocytes are triggered to become adipocytes. This process occurs mainly in the visceral (intraabdominal) and subcutaneous tissues. The greatest increase in number of fat cells occurs from infancy through adolescence. Most obese people have *primary obesity*, which is excess calorie intake over energy expenditure for the body's metabolic demands. Others have *secondary obesity*, in which a medical problem caused the weight gain. These problems include some congenital conditions, endocrine disorders, central nervous system (CNS) lesions and disorders, or drugs (e.g., corticosteroids, antipsychotics).

- Environmental factors play a key role in obesity. People have greater access to high-calorie food and sweetened drinks. Eating outside of the home often means higher-calorie foods with large portion sizes.
- Lack of physical exercise contributes to weight gain and obesity.
- Socioeconomic status is a known risk factor for obesity in a variety of ways. People with low incomes may lack access to affordable and nutritious food or try to stretch their food dollars by buying less expensive foods that have poor nutritional quality. Low-income neighborhoods often lack locations for healthy exercise.

The association of food with comfort, reward, pleasure, and fun is a powerful incentive for overeating.

Diagnostic Studies

- History and physical examination are done to assess the extent and duration of obesity.
- Laboratory tests of liver function, fasting glucose level, triglyceride level, and low- and high-density lipoprotein cholesterol levels assist in evaluating the cause and effects of obesity.
- Classifications of body weight and obesity are defined by BMI, standardized height–weight charts, or WHR.

Interprofessional Management

A multifaceted approach includes attention to nutritional therapy, exercise, behavior modification, and, for some, medication or surgical intervention.

Drug Therapy

Drug therapy should be part of a holistic weight loss program that includes a reduced-calorie diet, exercise, and behavior therapy. Drugs are reserved for adults with a BMI of 30 kg/m^2 or greater (obese) or adults with a BMI of 27 kg/m^2 or greater (overweight) who have at least one weight-related condition such as hypertension, type 2 diabetes, or dyslipidemia. Drugs approved by the U.S. Food and Drug Administration (FDA) for treatment of obesity are presented in Table 61.

Surgical Therapy

Bariatric surgery on the stomach and/or intestines to help a person lose weight is currently the only treatment with a lasting impact of sustained weight loss for those with extreme obesity. Surgeries are categorized as restrictive, malabsorptive, or a combination of restrictive and malabsorptive. In restrictive procedures, the stomach is reduced in size or the amount if food allowed to enter the stomach is reduced. In malabsorptive procedures, the small intestine is shortened or bypassed (less food absorbed). Most procedures are performed laparoscopically.

- Common restrictive surgeries include adjustable gastric banding and sleeve gastrectomy. These surgeries are discussed further in Chapter 45 of Harding et al., *Lewis' Medical-Surgical Nursing*, ed 12.
- An intragastric balloon placed using an endoscope can help patients feel full, curb appetite, and reduce food intake.

The Roux-en-Y gastric bypass (RYGB) procedure is a combination of restrictive and malabsorptive surgery.

- This procedure involves creating a small gastric pouch and attaching it directly to the small intestine using a Y-shaped limb of the small bowel. After the procedure, food bypasses 90% of the stomach, the duodenum, and a small segment of jejunum.
- A complication of the RYGB is *dumping syndrome*, in which gastric contents empty too rapidly into the small intestine, overwhelming its ability to digest nutrients. Signs and symptoms can include vomiting, nausea, weakness, sweating, faintness, and diarrhea.

An alternative option is an implantable gastric stimulation device. It consists of a pacemaker-like electrical pulse generator,

TABLE 61 Drug Therapy: Obesity

Drug	Mechanism of action	Nursing considerations
Bupropion/naltrexone (Contrave)	• *Bupropion:* Antidepressant • *Naltrexone:* Opioid antagonist	• Side effects: Nausea, constipation, headache, dizziness, insomnia, dry mouth • Monitor for suicidal thoughts and behaviors and neuropsychiatric reactions • Can increase BP and heart rate. Should not be used in patients with uncontrolled hypertension • Can cause seizures. Must not be used in patients who have seizure disorder
Liraglutide (Saxenda)	• Glucagon-like peptide 1 (GLP-1) agonist • Induces satiety	• Used to treat type 2 diabetes • njected • Side effects: Nausea, diarrhea, headache, fatigue, dizziness • Monitor for suicidal ideation, pancreatitis
Orlistat (Xenical, Alli [low-dose form available over the counter])	• Inhibits gastrointestinal (GI) lipase • Blocks fat breakdown and absorption in intestine • Results in undigested fat excreted in feces	• Side effects: stool leakage, flatulence, diarrhea, abdominal bloating, especially if a high-fat diet is consumed • Liver injury, kidney stones may occur • May need daily multivitamin supplement • Taken with each main meal containing fat

TABLE 61 Drug Therapy: Obesity—Cont'd

Phentermine/topiramate ER (Qsmyia)	• *Phentermine*: Sympathomimetic • *Topiramate*: Decreases appetite	• Side effects: dizziness, insomnia, dry mouth, headache, high blood pressure • Do not use in patients with glaucoma or hyperthyroidism • Must avoid pregnancy • Can increase heart rate. Should not be used in patients with uncontrolled hypertension or heart disease
Plenity	• Gel pieces increase the volume of stomach and small intestine contents, • Induces satiety	• Side effects: Abdominal pain, constipation • Taken twice a day orally, 20 minutes before lunch and dinner, with 16 oz of water • Should not be used in patients with GI disease

wire leads, and electrodes implanted in the abdomen. Intermittent electrical pulses to the vagus nerve signal to the brain that the stomach feels empty or full.

Cosmetic surgeries may be used to reduce fatty tissue and skinfolds. These procedures include a *lipectomy* (adipectomy) to remove adipose folds and *liposuction* for cosmetic purposes.

Nursing Management

Goals

The overall goals are that the patient with obesity will modify eating patterns, take part in a regular exercise, achieve and maintain weight loss to a specified level, and minimize or prevent health problems related to obesity.

Interventions

Be sensitive and nonjudgmental in asking specific and leading questions about weight, diet, and exercise. Despite knowing benefits of weight loss, most people find the process tough. Successful weight management will be a hard, lifelong commitment. You can provide information and encouragement.

Restricting dietary intake so that it is below energy requirements is a cornerstone for any weight loss or maintenance program. Recommend a diet in which calorie restriction includes a variety of healthy foods.

- Achieving an "ideal" BMI may not be a realistic goal. Modest weight loss of even 5% of starting weight can have health benefits. Mutually agree on a realistic and healthy goal, such as losing 1–2 lb/wk, at the beginning of a weight loss program.
- Focusing on the reasons for wanting to lose weight may help patients develop strategies for a weight loss program. Direct the plan of care at two different processes: (1) successful weight loss, which requires a short-term energy deficit; and (2) successful weight control, which requires long-term behavior changes.
- During plateau periods, when no weight is lost for days to weeks, patients need encouragement and support.
- Exercise is an essential part of a weight control program. Patients should exercise daily, with a goal of more than 10,000 steps per day. Exercise is important in maintaining weight loss.
- People in behavior therapy programs are more successful in maintaining their weight losses over an extended time.
- Joining a support group with others having the same experiences may be useful.

Preoperative care for gastric surgery includes planning for the special needs of an obese patient, such as the availability of a larger-sized BP cuff, hospital gown, bed, chair, and commode. Consider how the patient will be weighed, transported through the hospital, and turned. Teach the patient the coughing technique, deep breathing, use of an incentive spirometer, and methods of turning and positioning to prevent pulmonary complications after surgery. Plan for venous thromboembolism (VTE) prevention.

Postoperative care focuses on careful assessment and immediate intervention for cardiopulmonary complications, VTE, anastomosis leaks, and electrolyte imbalances. Facilitate patient respiratory efforts (elevating the head of the bed, turning, coughing, deep breathing); monitor for wound infection, dehiscence, and delayed healing; and promote early ambulation. Patients have significant abdominal pain after surgery, so give pain medications as needed.

- Some patients express guilt feelings that the only way they could lose weight was by having surgery. Be ready to provide support.
- Stress the importance of long-term follow-up care to prevent and treat potential complications. Encourage patients to adhere to the prescribed diet and inform the health care provider of changes in their physical or emotional condition.

OBSTRUCTIVE SLEEP APNEA

Description

Obstructive sleep apnea (OSA), also called *obstructive sleep apnea–hypopnea syndrome* (*OSAHS*), is characterized by partial or complete upper airway obstruction during sleep. *Apnea* is the cessation of spontaneous respirations lasting longer than 10 seconds. *Hypopnea* is a condition characterized by shallow respirations (30%–50% reduction in airflow).

- Sleep apnea occurs in 25% of Americans. Risk increases with age >65 years, obesity (body mass index [BMI] greater than 30 kg/m^2), neck circumference greater than 16 inches, male sex, and postmenopausal status in women.

Pathophysiology

Airflow obstruction occurs when: (1) narrowing of the air passages with relaxation of muscle tone during sleep leads to apnea and hypopnea, and (2) the tongue and soft palate fall backward and partially or completely obstruct the pharynx.

- Each obstruction may last 10–90 seconds. During the apneic period, hypoxemia and hypercapnia may cause the person to arouse briefly and snort or gasp without fully awakening.
- Apnea and arousal cycles occur hundreds of times during one night of sleep.

Clinical Manifestations

Manifestations of sleep apnea include frequent arousals during sleep, insomnia, excessive daytime sleepiness, and witnessed apneic episodes. A bed partner may complain about the person's loud snoring. Other symptoms include morning headaches, personality changes, and irritability.

- Untreated sleep apnea may cause hypertension, right-sided heart failure from pulmonary hypertension, and dysrhythmias. Chronic sleep loss can lead to decreased ability to concentrate, impaired memory, failure to complete daily tasks, and interpersonal difficulties. Driving accidents may occur due to excessive daytime sleepiness.

Diagnostic Studies

- Sleep and medical history
- Polysomnography in a sleep lab or home sleep testing. OSA is defined as more than five apnea/hypopnea events per hour with a 3%–4% decrease in O_2 saturation.

Interprofessional and Nursing Management

Conservative Treatment

Conservative home treatment for mild sleep apnea (5–10 apnea/hypopnea events per hour) includes sleeping on the side rather than the back, elevating the head of the bed, and avoiding sedatives or alcoholic beverages 3–4 hours before sleep. Excessive weight worsens sleep apnea; refer patient to a weight loss program if needed.

- Continuous positive airway pressure (CPAP) is often used for patients with severe symptoms (more than 15 apnea/hypopnea events per hour). A nasal mask, nasal pillows, or full-face mask is worn attached to a high-flow blower.
- CPAP reduces apnea episodes, daytime sleepiness, and fatigue but benefits are dose-dependent. CPAP must be used at least 4 hours each night to reduce the negative cardiovascular effects of OSA.
- Bilevel positive airway pressure (BiPAP), which can deliver a higher inspiration pressure and a lower expiration pressure, may be better tolerated than CPAP.
- Oral appliances that bring the mandible and tongue forward, enlarging the airway space, may reduce OSA symptoms.
- Opioid analgesics and sedating medications may worsen OSA symptoms by depressing respiration.
- Teach patients with OSA who will be hospitalized to bring their home devices and continue CPAP use.

Surgery
Common surgical procedures are uvulopalatopharyngoplasty and genioglossal advancement and hyoid myotomy. Radiofrequency ablation may be used.
- Postoperative complications include airway obstruction or hemorrhage.
- Snoring may persist until inflammation subsides.
- Patients are usually discharged within 1 day after surgery.
- Tell patients to expect a sore throat and to reduce foul breath odor by rinsing with diluted mouthwash and then salt water for several days.

ORAL CANCER

Description
There are two types of *oral cancer*. *Oral cavity cancer* starts in the mouth. *Oropharyngeal cancer* develops in the part of the throat just behind the mouth. *Head and neck squamous cell carcinoma* (HNSCC) is a broad term for cancers of the oral cavity, pharynx, and larynx.
- Most oral cancer lesions occur on the lower lip. Cancer of the lip has a more favorable prognosis because the lesions are visible and are usually diagnosed earlier.
- Other common sites are the lateral border and undersurface of the tongue, labial commissure, and buccal mucosa.
- The 5-year survival rate is 84% for localized cancer and 65% for all stages of cancer of the oral cavity and pharynx combined.

Pathophysiology
Oral cancer has several predisposing factors including prolonged sun exposure, tobacco use (cigar, cigarette, pipe, snuff), and frequent alcohol consumption. Human papillomavirus (HPV) contributes to 25% of oral cancer cases.

Clinical Manifestations
Common manifestations include:
- *Leukoplakia*, called *smoker's patch*, is a whitish precancerous lesion on the mucosa of the mouth or tongue that results from chronic irritation, especially from smoking. The patch may become hard and leathery, called hyperkeratosis.
- *Erythroplakia* is a red velvety patch on the mouth or tongue. More than 50% of cases of erythroplakia progress to squamous cell carcinoma.

Patients may report chronic sore throat, sore mouth, and voice changes. Some patients with oral cancer have an asymptomatic neck mass. Later symptoms of oral cancer are pain, dysphagia (difficulty swallowing), and difficulty moving the jaw.

Lip cancer usually appears as an indurated, painless ulcer. The first sign of tongue cancer is an ulcer or area of thickening. Soreness or pain of the tongue may occur, especially on eating hot or highly seasoned foods.

- Later findings of tongue cancer include increased saliva, slurred speech, dysphagia, toothache, and earache.

Diagnostic Studies

- Biopsy of suspected lesion
- Oral exfoliative cytology and toluidine blue test are used to screen for oral cancer.
- CT scan, MRI, and positron emission tomography (PET) are used in staging cancer.

Interprofessional Management

Management usually consists of surgery, radiation therapy, and/or chemotherapy. Surgery remains the most effective treatment. Some patients with small tumors in the mouth and throat are candidates for minimally invasive robotic-assisted surgery. Many surgeries are radical procedures involving extensive resections. Examples are hemiglossectomy (removal of one-half of the tongue), glossectomy (removal of the entire tongue), and radical neck dissection (wide excision of the lymph nodes and their lymphatic channels). A tracheostomy (see Tracheostomy) is common with radical neck dissection.

Chemotherapy and radiation therapy are used together when there are positive margins, bone erosion, or positive lymph nodes (see Chemotherapy and Radiation Therapy). Chemotherapy agents used include fluorouracil, cisplatin, carboplatin, paclitaxel, docetaxel, and hydroxyurea.

Palliative treatment is used when the prognosis is poor, the cancer is inoperable, or the patient decides against surgery. If it becomes difficult for the patient to swallow, placing a gastrostomy allows for adequate nutrition. Frequent oral suctioning may be needed.

Nursing Management
Goals

The patient with carcinoma of the oral cavity will have a patent airway, be able to communicate, have adequate intake to maintain nutrition, and have relief of pain and discomfort.

Interventions
Identify patients at risk (users of tobacco products, alcoholics, those with poor dental hygiene, pipe smokers) and provide information regarding risk factors. Review information about smoking cessation with the patient who smokes or uses snuff or chewing tobacco.

- Refer any person with an ulcerative lesion that does not heal within 2–3 weeks to a health care provider.
- Teach the patient to report unexplained pain or soreness of the mouth, unusual bleeding, dysphagia, sore throat, voice changes, or swelling or lump in the neck.

See Head and Neck Cancer for the preoperative or postoperative care of patient who has a radical neck dissection.

OSTEOARTHRITIS

Description
Osteoarthritis (OA) is a slowly progressive noninflammatory disorder of the diarthrodial (synovial) joints. OA involves the gradual loss of articular cartilage with formation of bony outgrowths (spurs or osteophytes) at the joint margins. OA affects over 30 million adults in the United States. Numbers are expected to rise as the population ages (see Table 62).

- OA is not a normal part of the aging process, but aging is a risk factor for OA. Cartilage destruction likely begins between ages 20 and 30. Few patients have symptoms until after age 50. By age 65, almost 50% of adults report having arthritis.

Pathophysiology
OA may be caused by a known event or condition that directly damages cartilage or causes joint instability. However, we cannot identify a single cause for many persons with OA. Various genetic traits may contribute to the development of cartilage defects.

- Decreased estrogen at menopause may contribute to OA in aging women.
- Obesity contributes to hip and knee OA. It increases mechanical stress on the joints. Anterior cruciate ligament injury from quick stops and pivoting, as in football and soccer, increase risk for knee OA. Work that requires frequent kneeling and stooping also increases the risk for knee OA.
- Regular moderate exercise, which helps with weight, decreases the risk for OA development and progression.

TABLE 62 Comparison of Rheumatoid Arthritis and Osteoarthritis

Parameter	Rheumatoid arthritis	Osteoarthritis
Age at onset	Young to middle age	Usually >40 year
Gender	Female:male ratio is 2:1 or 3:1 Fewer marked sex differences after age 60 year	Female:male ratio 2:1 after age 60 year; except for traumatic arthritis, men less affected until age 70 or 80 year
Weight	Lost or maintained weight	Often overweight or obese
Disease	Systemic disease with exacerbations and remissions	Localized disease with variable, progressive course
Affected joints	Small joints typically affected first (PIPs, MCPs, MTPs), wrists, elbows, shoulders, knees Usually bilateral, symmetric joint involvement	Weight-bearing joints of knees and hips, small joints (MCPs, DIPs, PIPs), cervical and lumbar spine Often asymmetric
Pain characteristics	Stiffness lasts 1 hour to all day and may decrease with use. Pain is variable, may disrupt sleep.	Stiffness occurs on arising but usually subsides after 30 minutes. Pain gradually worsens with joint use and disease progression, relieved with joint rest but may disrupt sleep.
Effusions	Common	Uncommon
Nodules	Present, especially on extensor surfaces	Heberden's (DIPs) and Bouchard's (PIPs) nodes
Synovial fluid	WBC count 3000–25,000/µL with mostly neutrophils; decreased viscosity	WBC count <2000/µL (mild leukocytosis); normal viscosity

TABLE 62 Comparison of Rheumatoid Arthritis and Osteoarthritis—cont'd		
Parameter	**Rheumatoid arthritis**	**Osteoarthritis**
X-rays	Joint space narrowing and erosion with bony overgrowths, subluxation with advanced disease Osteoporosis related to decreased activity, corticosteroid use	Joint space narrowing, osteophytes, subchondral cysts, sclerosis
Laboratory findings	RF-positive in 70%–90% of patients; negative titers in early disease for about 25% of patients	RF-negative
	Increase in ANA titer likely.	ANA-negative
	Positive anti-CCP in 60%–80% of patients	Anti-CCP–negative
	Elevated ESR, CRP indicative of active inflammation	Transient elevation in ESR related to synovitis

ANA, Antinuclear antibodies; *anti-CCP*, anti-citrullinated peptide; *CRP*, C-reactive protein; *DIPs*, distal interphalangeals; *ESR*, erythrocyte sedimentation rate; *MCPs*, metacarpophalangeals; *MTPs*, metatarsophalangeals; *PIPs*, proximal interphalangeals; *RF*, rheumatoid factor.

Genetic, metabolic, and local factors interact to cause cartilage deterioration from damage at the level of the chondrocytes. Affected cartilage becomes softer, less elastic, and less able to resist wear. The body's attempts at cartilage repair cannot keep up with the destruction of OA. Articular surfaces become cracked and worn. Uneven joint surfaces reduce joint motion. Secondary synovitis may occur when phagocytes try to rid the joint of small pieces of cartilage torn from the joint surface. These changes cause the early pain and stiffness of OA. Pain in later disease occurs when articular cartilage is lost and bony joint surfaces rub on each other.

Clinical Manifestations

Manifestations of OA range from mild discomfort to significant disability. See Table 62 for distinctions between OA and rheumatoid arthritis.

Joints

Joint pain is the primary symptom and the typical reason the patient seeks medical attention. Pain generally gets worse with joint use. In early stages of OA, rest relieves the joint pain. However, the patient with advanced disease may report pain at rest or have trouble sleeping due to joint pain. Pain may also worsen as the barometric pressure falls before the onset of severe weather. The pain of OA may be referred to the groin, buttock, or side of the thigh or knee. Sitting down becomes difficult, as does rising from a chair when the hips are lower than the knees. As OA develops in intervertebral joints of the spine, localized pain and stiffness are common.

- Joint stiffness occurs after periods of rest or static position. Early-morning stiffness generally resolves within 30 minutes.
- Overactivity can temporarily increase stiffness. *Crepitation*, a grating sensation caused by loose cartilage particles in the joint cavity, can also contribute to stiffness.
- OA usually affects joints asymmetrically. The most commonly involved joints are the distal interphalangeal (DIP) and proximal interphalangeal (PIP) joints of the fingers, the metacarpophalangeal (MCP) joint of the thumb, the weight-bearing joints (hips, knees), the metatarsophalangeal (MTP) joint of the foot, and the cervical and lower lumbar vertebrae.

Deformity

Deformity or instability associated with OA is specific to the involved joint. For example, *Heberden's nodes* occur on the distal interphalangeal joints because of osteophyte formation and loss of joint space. *Bouchard's nodes* on the proximal interphalangeal joints indicate similar disease involvement. Heberden's and Bouchard's nodes are often red, swollen, and tender. These bony enlargements do not usually cause significant loss of function.

- Knee OA often leads to joint deformity as a result of cartilage loss. In advanced hip OA, one of the patient's legs may become shorter as the joint space narrows.

Diagnostic Studies

- X-rays confirm disease and monitor the progression of joint damage. However, these changes do not always reflect the degree of pain the patient experiences. A bone scan, CT scan, or MRI may be useful to diagnose OA.
- Synovial fluid analysis helps distinguish OA from types of inflammatory arthritis. In OA, fluid remains clear yellow with little or no sign of inflammation.
- No laboratory abnormalities or biomarkers are specific diagnostic indicators. The erythrocyte sedimentation rate (ESR) is normal except for slight elevations during acute inflammation.

Interprofessional Management

Management focuses on managing pain and inflammation, preventing disability, and maintaining and improving joint function. The affected joint should be rested during any periods of acute inflammation and maintained in a functional position with splints or braces if necessary. The patient may need to modify activities or use an assistive device to decrease stress on affected joints. Teach the patient with knee OA to avoid prolonged standing, kneeling, or squatting.

- Applications of heat and cold may help reduce pain and stiffness. Heat therapy is helpful for stiffness, including hot packs, whirlpool, ultrasound, and paraffin wax baths.
- If the patient is overweight, weight reduction is critical to the treatment plan. Help the patient evaluate the current diet to make needed changes.
- Exercise is an important part of OA management. Aerobic conditioning, range-of-motion exercises, and specific programs to strengthen muscles around the affected joint help many patients with knee OA.

Complementary and alternative therapies for OA symptom management are popular with patients who have not found relief through traditional medical care. Teach the patient to carefully research any alternative therapies. Acupuncture may reduce arthritis pain and improve joint mobility. Massage and Tai Chi may also reduce pain and improve function.

Drug Therapy

Nonsteroidal antiinflammatory drugs (NSAID) are first-line treatment for OA. If the patient is at risk for or develops GI side effects with an NSAID, a protective agent, such as misoprostol (Cytotec), may be needed. Arthrotec, a combination of misoprostol and the NSAID diclofenac, is available. Patients taking an anticoagulant (e.g., warfarin) and an oral NSAID are at high risk for bleeding.

Some patients start with a topical agent, such as capsaicin cream. It blocks pain by locally interfering with the transmission of pain impulses. A concentrated product is available by prescription.

- Creams of 0.025%–0.075% capsaicin are available over the counter (OTC). Diclofenac gel is another option. OTC products that contain camphor, eucalyptus oil, and menthol (e.g., Bengay, Arthricare) may provide temporary pain relief. Topical salicylates (e.g., Aspercreme) may be an option for some patients. Several applications may be needed daily because topical agents have short-acting effects.
- Teach the patient who is taking an oral NSAID to avoid use of a topical NSAID because of increased risk for adverse effects.

Intraarticular corticosteroid injections may be needed for those with local inflammation and swelling. Four or more injections without relief suggest the need for more intervention.

Surgical Therapy

Symptoms are often managed conservatively for many years. Loss of joint function, unmanaged pain, and increased dependence in self-care may lead to consideration of reconstructive surgery (e.g., hip and knee replacements).

Nursing Management

Goals

The patient with OA will maintain or improve joint function through a balance of rest and activity, use joint protection measures to improve activity tolerance, achieve independence in self-care and maintain optimal role function, and use drug and nondrug strategies to manage pain satisfactorily.

Interventions

Focus education on altering modifiable risk factors. For example, encourage the patient to lose weight and reduce occupational or recreational hazards. For athletic instruction and physical fitness programs, include safety measures that protect the joints. Traumatic joint injuries should be treated promptly to decrease the risk of developing OA.

The patient with OA is usually treated on an outpatient basis, often by an interprofessional team that includes a rheumatologist, a nurse, an occupational therapist, and a physical therapist.

- Drugs are used to treat pain and inflammation. Nondrug strategies may include massage, use of heat (thermal packs) or cold (ice packs), meditation, and yoga.
- Discuss home and work environment modification for patient safety, accessibility, and self-care. Measures include removing throw rugs, placing rails at the stairs and bathtub, using night lights, and wearing well-fitting supportive shoes. Assistive devices, such as canes, walkers, elevated toilet seats, and grab bars, reduce the load on an affected joint and promote safety. Sexual counseling may help the patient and their partner enjoy physical closeness by introducing the idea of alternate positions and timing for sexual activity.

▼ Patient and Caregiver Teaching

Provide information about the nature and treatment of the disease, pain management, posture and body mechanics, correct use of assistive devices such as a cane or walker, principles of joint protection and energy conservation, and an exercise program.

- Individualize home management goals to meet the patient's needs. Include the patient caregiver, family, and significant others in goal setting and teaching.
- Assure the patient that OA is a localized disease and that severe deforming arthritis is not the usual course. The patient may appreciate resources such as the Arthritis Foundation's Self-Help Course (www.arthritis.org).

OSTEOMALACIA

Osteomalacia is caused by vitamin D deficiency, which results in bone losing calcium and becoming soft. The disease is uncommon in the United States. It is the same disorder as rickets in children, except that the epiphyseal growth plates are closed in adults.
- Vitamin D is required for absorption of calcium from the intestine. Insufficient vitamin D intake can interfere with the normal bone mineralization; with little or no calcification, bones become soft.
- Causes include limited sun exposure (ultraviolet rays needed for vitamin D synthesis), gastrointestinal (GI) malabsorption (post–weight loss surgery, Celiac disease), chronic diarrhea, and pregnancy.

Common manifestations are bone pain and muscle weakness. The pain is often worse at night and affects the lower back, pelvis, hips, legs, and ribs.
- Muscle weakness and progressive deformity of weight-bearing bones (e.g., spine, extremities) can lead to problems walking and a waddling gait. Fractures are common and slow to heal.

Laboratory findings include decreased serum calcium or phosphorus levels, decreased serum 25-hydroxyvitamin D, and increased serum alkaline phosphatase. X-rays may demonstrate generalized bone demineralization, especially a loss of calcium in the bones of the pelvis, and the presence of associated bone deformity.
- *Looser's transformation zones* (ribbons of decalcification in bone found on X-ray) are diagnostic of osteomalacia. Significant osteomalacia may exist without X-ray changes.

Treament is directed toward correcting vitamin D deficiency. When vitamin D_3 (cholecalciferol) and vitamin D_2 (ergocalciferol) are used as supplements, the patient often shows a dramatic response. Calcium or phosphorus supplements may also be prescribed.
- Exposure to sunlight and weight-bearing exercise are valuable.
- Encourage a diet rich in eggs, meat, oily fish, and milk and breakfast cereals fortified with calcium and vitamin D.

OSTEOMYELITIS

Description

Osteomyelitis is a severe infection of the bone, bone marrow, and surrounding soft tissue. Although *Staphylococcus aureus* is the most common cause, a variety of pathogens can cause osteomyelitis (Table 63).

Pathophysiology

Infecting microorganisms can invade by indirect or direct entry.

Indirect entry (hematogenous) is usually from infection with one microorganism. Indirect injury accounts for only 20% of cases. It most often affects children younger than 17 years of age.

- Risk factors in adults are older age, debilitation, hemodialysis, sickle cell disease, and IV drug use. The vertebrae are the most common site of infection in adults.

Direct entry (contiguous) osteomyelitis accounts for 80% of cases. It most often affects adults. It can occur when an open wound (e.g., penetrating wounds, fractures, surgery) allows microorganisms to enter the body.

- Osteomyelitis may also be related to a foreign body, such as an implant or an orthopedic prosthetic device (e.g., plate, total

TABLE 63 Organisms Causing Osteomyelitis	
Organism	**Predisposing problem**
Escherichia coli	Urinary tract infection
Fungi, mycobacteria	Immunocompromised host
Mycobacterium tuberculosis	Tuberculosis
Neisseria gonorrhoeae	Gonorrhea
Pseudomonas	Puncture wounds, IV drug use
Salmonella	Sickle cell disease
Staphylococcus aureus	Pressure injury, penetrating wound, open fracture, orthopedic surgery, vascular insufficiency (e.g., diabetes, atherosclerosis)
Staphylococcus epidermidis	Indwelling prosthetic devices (e.g., joint replacements, fracture fixation devices)
Streptococcus viridans	Abscessed tooth, gingival disease

joint prosthesis). It may occur in the feet of patients with diabetes or vascular disease–related ulcers or in the hips or sacrum near a pressure injury. More than one microorganism is usually involved.

After entering the blood, the microorganisms grow. The increased pressure leads to ischemia and vascular compromise of the periosteum.

- The infection spreads through the bone cortex and marrow cavity, ultimately resulting in cortical devascularization and necrosis. Bone death occurs resulting from ischemia.
- The area of dead bone eventually separates from the surrounding living bone, forming *sequestra*. It is difficult for blood-borne antibiotics or white blood cells (WBCs) to reach the sequestra. A sequestrum may become a reservoir for microorganisms that spread to other sites, including the lungs and brain. If the sequestrum does not resolve on its own or is not debrided surgically, a sinus tract may develop with chronic, purulent drainage.

Acute osteomyelitis refers to the initial infection or an infection of <1 month in duration.

Chronic osteomyelitis refers to a bone infection that persists for more than 1 month or did not respond to an initial course of therapy. Chronic osteomyelitis may be a continuous, persistent, or recurrent problem.

Clinical Manifestations
Acute Osteomyelitis
Local manifestations include constant bone pain that is unrelieved by rest and worsens with activity; swelling, tenderness, and warmth at the infection site; and restricted movement of the affected part.

- Systemic manifestations include fever, night sweats, restlessness, nausea, and malaise.
- Later signs include drainage from the sinus tracts to the skin and/or fracture site.

Chronic Osteomyelitis
Local signs of infection include constant bone pain and swelling and warmth at the infection site. Systemic signs may be less severe than those seen with the acute form.

Diagnostic Studies
- Bone or soft tissue biopsy is definitive for determining the microorganism.
- Blood and/or wound cultures are frequently positive.
- Elevated WBC and erythrocyte sedimentation rate (ESR) may be found.

- MRI and CT scan may be used to help identify the extent of the infection.
- Radionuclide bone scans (gallium and indium) show abnormalities earlier than X-ray.
- X-ray signs of osteomyelitis usually do not appear until 2–4 weeks after symptoms appear.

Interprofessional Management

Aggressive and prolonged IV antibiotic therapy is the treatment of choice for acute osteomyelitis if bone ischemia has not occurred. Any related soft tissue abscess or ulceration often needs surgical debridement or drainage.

- Most patients start on IV antibiotics and then switch to oral therapy. Some though may only receive oral agents. IV antibiotic therapy may be started in the hospital and then continued at home for 4–6 weeks. A few persons need therapy for 3–6 months.
- Patients are often discharged to home care with IV antibiotics delivered through a central venous access device (CVAD). A variety of antibiotics are used, depending on the culture results. Common antibiotics used include oxacillin, nafcillin, clindamycin, vancomycin, ceftriaxone, ciprofloxacin, and linezolid.

Treatment of chronic osteomyelitis includes extended use of antibiotics and surgical removal of the poorly perfused tissue and dead bone. Antibiotic-impregnated acrylic bead chains may be implanted during surgery. Intermittent or constant irrigation of the affected bone with antibiotics may be used.

- In adults, oral therapy with a fluoroquinolone (ciprofloxacin [Cipro]) for 6–8 weeks may be prescribed instead of IV antibiotics.
- Oral antibiotic therapy may also be given for 4–8 weeks after IV therapy.
- Patient response is monitored through bone scans and ESR tests.
- Hyperbaric oxygen therapy using 100% oxygen may be given as an adjunct therapy.

If an orthopedic prosthetic device is a source of chronic infection, it must be removed. Muscle flaps or skin grafting provides wound coverage over the dead space (cavity) in the bone. Bone grafts may help restore blood flow. However, flaps or grafts should never be placed in the presence of infection. Amputation may be needed (see Amputation).

- Rare complications of osteomyelitis include septicemia, septic arthritis, pathologic fractures, and amyloidosis.

Nursing Management

Goals

The patient with osteomyelitis will have satisfactory pain and fever management, be free from complications, and adhere to the treatment plan.

Interventions

Control of other infections (e.g., urinary and respiratory tract, deep pressure injuries) is important in preventing osteomyelitis. Those at risk for osteomyelitis are immunocompromised or have diabetes, orthopedic implants, or vascular insufficiency.

- Teach patients at risk signs of osteomyelitis to immediately report to the health care provider (HCP): bone pain, fever, swelling, and restricted limb movement.

Some immobilization of the affected limb (e.g., splint, traction) may be needed to decrease pain. Carefully handle the involved limb to avoid undue manipulation, which increases pain and may cause a pathologic fracture.

- Assess the patient's pain. Muscle spasms may cause minor to severe pain. Nonsteroidal antiinflammatory drugs (NSAIDs), opioid analgesics, and muscle relaxants may be given.

Dressings are used to absorb wound drainage and to debride devitalized tissue. Sterile technique is essential for dressing changes.

The patient is often placed on bed rest in the early stages of acute infection. Good body alignment and position changes prevent complications associated with immobility and promote comfort.

Monitor peak and trough blood levels of most antibiotics to avoid adverse drug effects.

▼ Patient and Caregiver Teaching

- Teach the patient the possible adverse and toxic reactions associated with prolonged high-dose antibiotic therapy. These reactions include hearing deficit, impaired renal function, and neurotoxicity (e.g., limb weakness or numbness, cognitive changes, vision changes, headache, behavioral problems).
- Long-term antibiotic therapy can result in an overgrowth of *Candida albicans* and *Clostridium difficile* in the mouth or genitourinary tract. Teach the patient to report any whitish yellow, curd-like lesions or itching and discharge to the HCP.
- If at home, teach patient and family about managing the venous access device, administering the antibiotic when scheduled and follow-up laboratory testing. Stress the importance of continuing to take antibiotics after the symptoms have improved.
- Instruct the patient and caregiver in the technique for wound dressing changes and assist them to obtain supplies.

- The patient and caregivers may be anxious and discouraged because of the serious nature of the disease, uncertainty of the outcome, and the long, costly treatment. Provide continued emotional support.

OSTEOPOROSIS

Description

Osteoporosis, or porous bone (fragile bone disease), is a chronic, progressive metabolic bone disease marked by low bone mass and deterioration of bone tissue, leading to bone fragility.

Risk factors for osteoporosis are female gender, advancing age (older than 65 years), white or Asian ethnicity, family history, low body weight, surgical or age-related menopause, sedentary lifestyle, smoking, excess alcohol use, a diet low in calcium, or vitamin D deficiency. Low testosterone levels are a major risk factor in men.

- Current guidelines recommend an initial bone density test in all women over age 65 years. Women who are younger than 65 years and at high risk (e.g., low body weight, smoker, prior fractures) should have a bone density test earlier. Testing should start earlier and be done more frequently if a person is at high risk for fractures.

Pathophysiology

Peak bone mass (maximum bone tissue) is typically achieved before age 20 years. It is largely determined by four factors: heredity, nutrition, exercise, and hormone function. Heredity may be responsible for up to 70% of peak bone mass.

- Bone loss from midlife (age 35–40 years) onward is inevitable, but the rate of loss varies. Women have rapid bone loss when estrogen production declines at menopause. This rate of loss then slows and eventually matches the rate of bone lost by men aged 65–70 years.

Bone is continually deposited by osteoblasts and resorbed by osteoclasts, a process called *remodeling.* Normally, the rates of bone deposition and resorption are equal, and total bone mass remains constant. In osteoporosis, bone resorption exceeds bone deposition.

- Diseases associated with osteoporosis include inflammatory bowel disease, intestinal malabsorption, kidney disease, rheumatoid arthritis, hyperthyroidism, alcohol use disorder, cirrhosis, hypogonadism, and diabetes.

- Many drugs can interfere with bone metabolism. These include corticosteroids, antiseizure drugs (e.g., divalproex sodium, phenytoin), aluminum-containing antacids, heparin, some chemotherapy drugs, and excess thyroid hormones. Long-term corticosteroid use is a major contributor to osteoporosis.

Clinical Manifestations

Bone loss occurs without symptoms. People may not know they have osteoporosis until a sudden strain, bump, or fall causes a hip, wrist, or vertebral fracture.

- A person who has a spinal vertebral fracture because of osteoporosis has an increased risk for a second vertebral fracture within a year.
- Over time, wedging and fractures of the vertebrae produce loss of height and a humped back known as "dowager's hump" or *kyphosis.*

Diagnostic Studies

Osteoporosis cannot be detected by conventional X-ray until 25%–40% of the calcium in the bone is lost.

- Serum calcium, phosphorus, and alkaline phosphatase levels remain normal, although alkaline phosphatase may be increased after a fracture.
- Bone mineral density (BMD) measurements are used to measure bone density.
- Quantitative ultrasound (QUS) measures bone density with sound waves in the heel, kneecap, or shin.

  Dual-energy X-ray absorptiometry (DEXA) measures bone density in the spine, hips, and forearm (the most common sites of fractures with osteoporosis). DEXA studies are useful to evaluate changes in bone density and the effectiveness of treatment.

- DEXA results are reported as T-scores: A T-score of 0 means the BMD is equal to the norm for a healthy young adult. The greater the negative number, the more severe the osteoporosis.
- Sometimes the health care provider (HCP) asks for a Z-score instead of a T-score. For this score, a person is compared with someone their own age, gender, and/or ethnic group instead of a healthy 30-year-old. Among older adults, Z-scores can be misleading because decreased bone density is common.

Interprofessional and Nursing Management

Care focuses on proper nutrition, calcium and Vitamin D supplementation, exercise, prevention of falls and fractures, and drugs. Treatment is recommended for postmenopausal women who have:

(1) a T-score of <-2.5, (2) a T-score between -1 and -2.5 with additional risk factors, or (3) a prior history of a hip or vertebral fracture.

- A patient's risk of fracture caused by osteoporosis can be calculated using the Fracture Risk Assessment (FRAX) tool.

The recommended calcium intake is 1000 mg/day for women aged 19–50 years and men aged 19–70 years and 1200 mg/day in women 51 years or older and men 71 years or older.

- If diet intake of calcium is inadequate, supplements may be needed. Teach the patient to take calcium supplements as divided doses to increase absorption.
- Vitamin D is important in calcium absorption and function. Being in the sun for 20 minutes a day is generally enough. However, supplemental vitamin D (800–1000 IU) is recommended for postmenopausal women, older adults, people who are homebound or in long-term care settings, and those with decreased sun exposure.

Regular physical activity is important to build up and maintain bone mass. The best exercises are those that are weight bearing and force a person to work against gravity, such as walking, hiking, weight training, tennis, stair climbing, and dancing.

- Walking is preferred to high-impact aerobics or running, which may stress the bones and result in fractures.

Vertebroplasty and kyphoplasty are minimally invasive procedures to treat osteoporotic vertebral fractures. In *vertebroplasty,* bone cement is injected to stabilize the collapsed vertebra, but it does not correct the deformity. In *kyphoplasty,* an air bladder is inserted into the collapsed vertebra and inflated to restore vertebral body height, and then bone cement is injected.

Drug Therapy

The recommended drug therapies for preventing and treating osteoporosis are the bisphosphonates alendronate and risedronate. Bisphosphonates inhibit osteoclast-mediated bone resorption and slow the cycle of bone remodeling. Although a modest increase in BMD is common, bone remodeling may be suppressed to the extent that normal bone formation is impaired and fracture risk increases. Treatment should continue for 5 years.

- Ensure an adequate intake of calcium and vitamin D, including supplements, when osteoporosis drugs are prescribed.
- A rare, but serious, side effect of bisphosphonates is osteonecrosis (bone death) of the jaw. Its cause is unknown. Those with dental disease, cancer, Paget's disease, or renal disease are most at risk for this complication.

Women no longer routinely use estrogen replacement therapy or estrogen with progesterone after menopause to prevent osteoporosis because of the increased risk for heart disease and breast and uterine cancer.

- A woman who takes short-term estrogen therapy to treat menopausal symptoms, such as hot flashes, may receive some protection against bone loss and hip and vertebrae fractures. Estrogen may inhibit osteoclast activity, leading to decreased bone resorption.

Patients receiving corticosteroids should receive the lowest effective dose for the shortest possible time.

OVARIAN CANCER

Description

Ovarian cancer is a malignant tumor of the ovaries. The cause is unknown. It is the fifth leading cause of cancer deaths in women in the United States. Most women with ovarian cancer have advanced disease at diagnosis.

- Risk factors include a personal or family history of cancer, genetic predisposition, family history of Lynch syndrome (hereditary nonpolyposis colorectal cancer [HNPCC]), endometriosis, nulliparity (never having given birth), and infertility.
- Women who have given birth, breastfed, or used hormonal contraceptive pills for 5 or more years have a reduced risk of ovarian cancer. These factors may have a protective effect because they reduce the number of ovulatory cycles over the lifetime.

Intraperitoneal dissemination is a common characteristic of ovarian cancer. It metastasizes to the uterus, bladder, bowel, and omentum. In advanced disease, ovarian cancer may spread to the stomach, colon, and liver.

Clinical Manifestations

Early ovarian cancer usually has no obvious symptoms. There may be nonspecific symptoms such as pelvic or abdominal pain, bloating, urinary urgency or frequency, and difficulty eating or feeling full quickly.

- In later stages, abdominal enlargement with ascites (fluid in the abdominal cavity), unexplained weight loss or gain, nausea, and abnormal vaginal discharge or bleeding may occur. Adnexal mass or lymphadenopathy may be present on physical exam.

Diagnostic Studies

No accurate screening test exists for early detection of ovarian cancer.

- Bimanual pelvic examinations may identify an ovarian mass.
- Abdominal or vaginal ultrasound or MRI can be used to detect ovarian masses.
- CA-125 is also used to monitor the course of the disease and response to treatment. The problem is that CA-125 levels can be high with other cancers (e.g., pancreatic cancer) or with benign gynecologic problems, including fibroids and endometriosis.

Interprofessional Management

Options for women at high risk include prophylactic removal of the ovaries and fallopian tubes and the use of oral contraceptives. While salpingo-oophorectomy significantly reduces the risk for ovarian cancer, it does not completely eliminate the risk for cancer in the peritoneum.

- The initial treatment for all stages of ovarian cancer is a total abdominal hysterectomy and bilateral salpingo-oophorectomy (TAH-BSO) with removal of the omentum and as much of the tumor as possible (tumor debulking).

Depending on the grade and stage of cancer, treatment options include intraperitoneal and systemic chemotherapy, intraperitoneal instillation of radioisotopes, and external abdominal and pelvic radiation therapy. Combination chemotherapy and radiation therapy should be considered before a single-modality treatment.

- The chemotherapy agents most commonly used are taxanes (paclitaxel, or docetaxel) and platinum agents (carboplatin, or cisplatin).
- Targeted therapy used to treat advanced ovarian cancer includes bevacizumab (Avastin), rucaparib (Rubraca), and olaparib (Lynparza). Rucaparib and olaparib are poly ADP-ribose polymerase (PARP) inhibitors. They block enzymes involved in repairing damaged DNA. They are used for women with ovarian cancer that is associated with defective BRCA genes.

Nursing Management

See Cervical Cancer.

PAGET'S DISEASE

Description

Paget's disease (osteitis deformans) is a chronic skeletal bone disorder in which excessive bone resorption is followed by replacement of normal marrow by vascular, fibrous connective tissue. The new bone is larger, disorganized, and weaker. Areas often affected include the pelvis, long bones, spine, ribs, sternum, and skull. Up to 5% of adults in the United States have Paget's disease. Men are affected twice as often.

- We do not know what causes Paget's disease. The cause may be viral or genetic. Up to 40% of all patients with the disease have a relative with the disorder.

Clinical Manifestations

In mild forms of Paget's disease, patients may not have any symptoms. The disease may be discovered incidentally on X-ray or serum chemistry findings indicating a high alkaline phosphatase (ALP) level.

- Bone pain may gradually progress to severe intractable pain. Other early manifestations include fatigue and progressive development of a waddling gait.
- Headaches, dementia, vision deficits, and loss of hearing can result with an enlarged, thickened skull. Increased bone volume in the spine can cause spinal cord or nerve root compression.

Pathologic fracture may be the first sign of the disease. Other complications include osteosarcoma, osteoclastoma (giant cell tumor), and fibrosarcoma.

Diagnostic Studies

- Serum ALP levels are markedly increased (indicating rapid bone turnover) in advanced disease.
- X-rays may show curvature of an affected bone and thickened bone cortex, especially in weight-bearing bones and the cranium.
- Bone scans using a radiolabeled bisphosphate show increased uptake in the affected skeletal areas.

Interprofessional and Nursing Management

Treatment is usually limited to symptomatic and supportive care, with correction of secondary deformities by either surgical intervention or braces.

- Bisphosphonate drugs are used to slow bone resorption. Zoledronic acid may also be given as a bone-building drug. Calcium and vitamin D are often given to decrease hypocalcemia, a common side effect with these drugs. Monitor drug effectiveness by regular assessment of serum ALP.
- Calcitonin is an option for patients who cannot tolerate bisphosphonates.
- Pain is usually managed with nonsteroidal antiinflammatory drugs (NSAIDs).

- Orthopedic surgery for fractures, hip and knee replacements, and knee realignment may be necessary.

A firm mattress can provide back support and relieve pain. The patient may need to wear a corset or light brace to relieve back pain and to provide support. Teach the patient to correctly apply the device and examine the skin for friction damage.

- Good body mechanics are essential. Discourage lifting and twisting. Physical therapy may increase muscle strength.
- A healthy diet with vitamin D, calcium, and protein is important for bone formation.
- Teach the patient to use an assistive device and make environmental changes (e.g., do not use throw rugs) to decrease risk for falls and related fractures.

PANCREATIC CANCER

Description

Pancreatic cancer is most often an adenocarcinoma. More than half of the tumors occur in the head of the pancreas. As the tumor grows, the common bile duct becomes obstructed and obstructive jaundice develops. Tumors starting in the body or the tail of the pancreas often remain silent until their growth is advanced.

The median age at diagnosis is around 68 years of age. The majority of cancers have metastasized at the time of diagnosis, with a poor prognosis. Most patients die within 5–12 months of the initial diagnosis, and the 5-year survival rate is only 9%.

Pathophysiology

The cause is unknown. Smokers are 2–3 times more likely to develop pancreatic cancer than nonsmokers. Other risk factors include chronic pancreatitis, diabetes, age, family history of pancreatic cancer, high-fat diet, and exposure to chemicals, such as benzidine. Blacks have the highest incidence of pancreatic cancer.

Clinical Manifestations

Signs and symptoms of pancreatic cancer are similar to those of chronic pancreatitis. Manifestations include abdominal pain (dull or aching), anorexia, rapid and progressive weight loss, nausea, and jaundice.

- Cancer in the head of the pancreas commonly causes pain, jaundice, and weight loss. Weight loss is due to poor digestion and absorption caused by lack of digestive enzymes from the pancreas.

- Pain is related to the location of the cancer. The pain is often in the upper abdomen or left hypochondrium and often radiates to the back. Pain is often related to eating and occurs at night. Extreme, unrelenting pain occurs with extension of the cancer into the retroperitoneal tissues and nerve plexuses.
- Pruritus may accompany obstructive jaundice.

Diagnostic Studies

- Abdominal ultrasound or endoscopic ultrasound (EUS), spiral CT scan, MRI, and MR cholangiopancreatography (MRCP) are used for diagnosing and staging pancreatic cancer.
- Endoscopic retrograde cholangiography (ERCP) allows for visualization and collection of secretions and tissues from the pancreatic duct and biliary system.
- Carbohydrate antigen (CA)19-9, which is increased in pancreatic cancer, is the most commonly used tumor marker.

Interprofessional Management

Surgery is the most effective treatment, but only 15%–20% of patients have resectable tumors at the time of diagnosis. The classic surgery is a *radical pancreaticoduodenectomy* or *Whipple procedure*. This procedure is a resection of the proximal pancreas (proximal pancreatectomy), the adjoining duodenum (duodenectomy), the distal part of the stomach (partial gastrectomy), and the distal segment of the common bile duct. An anastomosis of the pancreatic duct, common bile duct, and stomach to the jejunum is done. Pancreatic body and/or tail tumors require a distal pancreatectomy procedure.

- If the pancreatic tumor cannot be removed surgically, palliative measures include a cholecystojejunostomy to relieve biliary obstruction and/or endoscopic placement of biliary stents.
- Radiation therapy alters survival rates little but is effective for pain relief.
- The role of chemotherapy in pancreatic cancer is limited. Chemotherapy usually consists of fluorouracil (5-FU) and gemcitabine (Gemzar), either alone or in combination with agents such as capecitabine (Xeloda), paclitaxel (Abraxane), erlotinib (Tarceva), or irinotecan (Onivyde). Erlotinib is a targeted therapy agent.

Nursing Management

Because the patient with pancreatic cancer has many of the same problems as the patient with pancreatitis, nursing care includes the same measures (see Pancreatitis, Acute).

- Provide symptomatic and supportive nursing care, including comfort measures and medications to relieve pain.
- Psychologic support is essential, especially during times of anxiety or depression.
- Support nutrition with measures to manage anorexia, nausea, and vomiting. Offer frequent and supplemental feedings.
- Because bleeding can result from impaired vitamin K production, assess for bleeding from body orifices and mucous membranes.
- Helping the patient and caregivers through the grieving process is an important aspect of nursing care.

PANCREATITIS, ACUTE

Description

Acute pancreatitis is inflammation of the pancreas, varying from mild edema to severe hemorrhagic necrosis. Pancreatic enzymes spilling into the surrounding pancreatic tissue cause autodigestion and severe pain.

Acute pancreatitis is most common in middle-aged men and women, with the rate three times higher in blacks than in whites.

Pathophysiology

Many factors can cause injury to the pancreas. In the United States, the most common cause is gallbladder disease (gallstones), which is more common in women. The second most common cause is chronic alcohol intake, which is more common in men. Less common causes include drug reactions, pancreatic cancer, and hypertriglyceridemia.

Autodigestion of the pancreas follows injury to pancreatic cells or activation of pancreatic enzymes in the pancreas rather than in the intestine. The pathophysiologic involvement in acute pancreatitis is classified as either *mild pancreatitis* (also known as *edematous* or *interstitial*) or *severe pancreatitis* (also called *necrotizing pancreatitis*).

- Shock may occur from hemorrhage into the pancreas, toxemia from the activated pancreatic enzymes, or hypovolemia because of massive fluid shifts into the retroperitoneal space. Patients with severe pancreatitis are at high risk for developing pancreatic necrosis, organ failure, and sepsis.

Clinical Manifestations

Abdominal pain is the predominant symptom of acute pancreatitis. The pain is usually in the left upper quadrant but may be in the midepigastric area. It often radiates to the back.

- The pain has a sudden onset and is described as severe, deep, piercing, and continuous or steady. Eating worsens the pain, which is not relieved by vomiting. Pain often begins when the patient is lying down. Abdominal tenderness with muscle guarding is common. The pain may be accompanied by flushing, cyanosis, and dyspnea.
- Other manifestations include nausea and vomiting, low-grade fever, leukocytosis, hypotension, tachycardia, and jaundice. Bowel sounds may be decreased or absent. Paralytic ileus may occur and causes marked abdominal distention. The lungs are often involved, with crackles present.
- Intravascular damage from circulating trypsin may cause areas of cyanosis or greenish to yellow-brown discoloration of the abdominal wall. Other areas of ecchymoses are the flanks (*Gray Turner's spots* or *sign,* a bluish flank discoloration) and the periumbilical area (*Cullen's sign,* a bluish periumbilical discoloration).

Complications

The severity of the disease varies according to the extent of pancreatic destruction. Some patients recover completely, others have recurring attacks, and still others develop chronic pancreatitis. Acute pancreatitis can be life-threatening. Local complications of acute pancreatitis are pseudocyst and abscess.

- A *pancreatic pseudocyst* is an accumulation of fluid, pancreatic enzymes, tissue debris, and inflammatory exudates surrounded by a wall. Manifestations of pseudocyst are abdominal pain, palpable epigastric mass, nausea, vomiting, and anorexia. The serum amylase level is often high. CT, MRI, and endoscopic ultrasound (EUS) may be used in the diagnosis. The cysts usually resolve spontaneously within a few weeks but may perforate, causing peritonitis, or rupture into the stomach or the duodenum. Treatment options include surgical drainage, percutaneous catheter placement and drainage, and endoscopic drainage.
- A *pancreatic abscess* is a collection of pus resulting from extensive necrosis in the pancreas. It may perforate into adjacent organs. Manifestations include upper abdominal pain, abdominal mass, high fever, and leukocytosis. Pancreatic abscesses need prompt surgical drainage to prevent sepsis.

The main systemic complications are cardiovascular and pulmonary (pleural effusion, atelectasis, pneumonia, acute respiratory distress syndrome [ARDS]), and hypocalcemia leading to tetany.

Diagnostic Studies

- High serum amylase and lipase are primary diagnostic findings.
- Liver enzymes, triglycerides, glucose, and bilirubin are high with a decrease in calcium.
- Abdominal ultrasound, X-ray, or contrast-enhanced CT scan can identify pancreatic problems.
- Endoscopic retrograde cholangiopancreatography (ERCP) is used along with EUS, magnetic resonance cholangiopancreatography (MRCP), and angiography to diagnose pancreatic problems.

Interprofessional Management

Goals of management for acute pancreatitis include relief of pain, prevention or alleviation of shock, reduction of pancreatic secretions, correction of fluid and electrolyte imbalances, prevention or treatment of infections, and removal of the precipitating cause, if possible.

Treatment is focused on supportive care, including aggressive hydration, pain management, management of metabolic complications, and minimization of pancreatic stimulation. If shock is present, blood volume replacements, volume expanders, and fluids may be given. Treatment and control of pain are very important. Pain medications may be combined with spasmolytics.

It is important to reduce or suppress pancreatic enzymes to decrease stimulation of the pancreas.

- Usually the patient is NPO with nasogastric (NG) suction to reduce vomiting and prevent gastric digestive juices from entering the duodenum.
- Drugs such as antacids, histamine H_2-receptor antagonists, and proton pump inhibitors may help suppress gastric acid secretion.
- As pancreatitis resolves, the patient resumes oral intake. Enteral nutrition support may be needed.
- Other drugs used to prevent and treat problems associated with pancreatitis include antacids, antispasmodics, opioids, proton pump inhibitors, antibiotics, insulin, and pancreatic enzyme products.

When the acute pancreatitis is related to gallstones, an urgent ERCP with endoscopic sphincterotomy may be performed. This may be followed by laparoscopic cholecystectomy to reduce the potential for recurrence. Patients with severe acute pancreatitis may need drainage of a percutaneous pseudocyst or necrotic fluid collection performed surgically, under CT guidance, or endoscopically.

Nursing Management

Goals

The patient with acute pancreatitis will have relief of pain, normal fluid and electrolyte balance, minimal to no complications, and no recurrent attacks.

Interventions

During the acute phase, it is important to monitor vital signs. Hypotension, fever, and tachypnea may compromise hemodynamic stability. Monitor the response to IV fluids. Closely monitor fluid and electrolyte balance. Frequent vomiting, along with gastric suction, may result in decreased chloride, sodium, and potassium levels.

- Because hypocalcemia can occur, observe for symptoms of tetany, including jerking, irritability, and muscular twitching. Numbness or tingling around the lips and in the fingers is an early sign of hypocalcemia. Assess the patient for a positive Chvostek's sign or Trousseau's sign. Give calcium gluconate as ordered to treat symptomatic hypocalcemia. Monitor serum magnesium levels since hypomagnesemia may develop.

Respiratory tract infections are common because the retroperitoneal fluid raises the diaphragm, which causes the patient to take shallow, guarded abdominal breaths. Measures to prevent respiratory tract infections include turning, coughing, deep breathing, and assuming a semi-Fowler's position.

- Respiratory failure may develop in the patient with severe acute pancreatitis. Assess respiratory function (e.g., lung sounds, O_2 saturation levels). If acute respiratory distress syndrome (ARDS) develops, the patient may need intubation and mechanical ventilation support. See ARDS.

A major focus of your care is pain relief. Pain and restlessness can increase the metabolic rate and stimulate pancreatic enzymes. Measures such as comfortable positioning, frequent changes in position, and relief of nausea and vomiting assist in reducing the restlessness that usually accompanies the pain.

- A side-lying position with the head elevated 45 degrees decreases tension on the abdomen and may help ease the pain.
- For the patient who is on NPO status or has an NG tube, provide frequent oral and nasal care to relieve dryness.

Patients may require follow-up home care. Physical therapy may be needed because of loss of muscle strength.

▼ Patient and Caregiver Teaching

- Counseling about abstinence from alcohol is important to prevent future attacks of acute pancreatitis and development of chronic pancreatitis.

- Because nicotine can stimulate the pancreas, smoking should be avoided.
- Encourage carbohydrates, which are less stimulating to the pancreas. Dietary teaching should include fat restriction because fats stimulate the secretion of cholecystokinin, which then stimulates the pancreas. Teach the patient to avoid crash and binge dieting, which can precipitate attacks.
- Teach the patient and caregiver to recognize symptoms of infection, diabetes, or *steatorrhea* (foul-smelling, frothy stools). These changes indicate ongoing destruction of pancreatic tissue and a possible need for exogenous enzyme supplementation.

PANCREATITIS, CHRONIC

Description

Chronic pancreatitis is a continuous, prolonged, inflammatory, and fibrosing process involving the pancreas. The pancreas is progressively destroyed as it is replaced by fibrotic tissue with strictures and calcifications. Chronic pancreatitis may follow acute pancreatitis or occur in the absence of any history of an acute condition.

Pathophysiology

The most common cause of *obstructive* pancreatitis is inflammation of the sphincter of Oddi associated with gallstones. Cancer of the ampulla of Vater, duodenum, or pancreas can also cause this type of chronic pancreatitis.

The most common cause of *nonobstructive* pancreatitis (the most common type of chronic pancreatitis) is chronic alcohol use. In nonobstructive pancreatitis, there is inflammation and sclerosis, mainly in the head of the pancreas and around the pancreatic duct.

Chronic pancreatitis may occur with systemic diseases (e.g., systemic lupus erythematosus), autoimmune pancreatitis, and cystic fibrosis. Some patients may not have an identifiable risk factor (idiopathic pancreatitis).

Clinical Manifestations

As with acute pancreatitis, a major manifestation of chronic pancreatitis is abdominal pain. The patient may have episodes of acute pain, but it usually is chronic (recurrent attacks at intervals of months or years). The attacks may become more frequent until the pain is almost constant. Sometimes they decrease as pancreatic fibrosis develops. The pain is in the same areas as in acute pancreatitis but is usually described as a heavy, gnawing feeling, or sometimes as burning and cramp-like. Food or antacids do not relieve the pain.

- Signs and symptoms of pancreatic insufficiency include weight loss, constipation, mild jaundice with dark frothy urine, steatorrhea, and diabetes. The steatorrhea may become severe, with voluminous, foul, fatty stools. Abdominal tenderness may be present.

Complications of chronic pancreatitis may include pseudocyst formation, bile duct or duodenal obstruction, pancreatic ascites or pleural effusion, or pancreatic cancer.

Diagnostic Studies

Confirming the diagnosis of chronic pancreatitis can be challenging and is based on the patient's signs and symptoms, laboratory studies, and imaging.

- Serum amylase and lipase levels may be slightly increased.
- Serum bilirubin and alkaline phosphatase levels may be high.
- Mild leukocytosis and elevated sedimentation rate may be found.
- Endoscopic retrograde cholangiopancreatography (ERCP) is used to visualize the pancreatic and biliary ductal system.
- CT, MRI, MR cholangiopancreatography (MRCP), abdominal ultrasound, and endoscopic ultrasound may be used in the diagnostic workup.
- A secretin test can assess the degree of pancreatic dysfunction.

Interprofessional and Nursing Management

When the patient with chronic pancreatitis has an acute attack, the therapy is identical to that for acute pancreatitis. At other times the focus is on the prevention of further attacks, relief of pain, and control of pancreatic exocrine and endocrine insufficiency. Sometimes large, frequent doses of opioid analgesics are needed to relieve the pain.

- A bland diet low in fat and high in carbohydrates, pancreatic enzyme replacement such as pancrelipase (Pancrease, Zenpep, Creon, Viokace), and management of diabetes are measures used to control the pancreatic insufficiency. Pancreatic enzyme products, such as pancrelipase, contain amylase, lipase, and trypsin. They are taken with meals and snacks to replace the deficient pancreatic enzymes.
- Bile salts may be given to help with fat-soluble vitamin (A, D, E, and K) absorption and prevent further fat loss.
- Treatment of chronic pancreatitis sometimes requires endoscopic therapy or surgery. When biliary disease is present or

obstruction or pseudocyst develops, surgery may divert bile flow or relieve ductal obstruction.

▼ **Patient and Caregiver Teaching**

- Instruct the patient to take measures to prevent further attacks. Explain dietary control and consistency in taking pancreatic enzymes with meals and snacks.

- Teach the patient and caregiver to observe the stools for steatorrhea to help determine the effectiveness of the enzyme replacement.

- Teach the patient not to consume alcohol and caffeinated beverages. If the patient is dependent on alcohol, refer to other agencies or resources as needed.

- If diabetes develops, teach the patient regarding blood glucose testing and drug therapy (see Diabetes Mellitus).

PARKINSON DISEASE

Description

Parkinson disease (PD) is a chronic, progressive neurodegenerative disorder characterized by slowness in the initiation and execution of movement (*bradykinesia*), increased muscle tone (*rigidity*), tremor at rest, and gait disturbance. It is the most common form of *parkinsonism,* a syndrome of several disorders with similar symptoms.

Almost 1 million Americans are living with PD in the United States. Around 60,000 persons are diagnosed each year. Occurrence of PD increases with age, with average age of onset around 70 years. Men are 1.5 times more likely to have PD than women.

Pathophysiology

The exact cause of PD is unknown. We think it is an interplay of genetic and environment risk factors. Traumatic brain injury has been shown to increase the risk of PD. Exposure to industrial manganese, pesticides, herbicides (paraquat), industrial solvents, and chemicals (polychlorinated biphenyl) may increase risk.

- Parkinsonism is a syndrome made up of disorders that mimic PD. Many forms of secondary (atypical) parkinsonism exist. Because of the similarity, PD and parkinsonism can be confused.

- Symptoms of parkinsonism have occurred after exposure to a variety of chemicals and metals. Drug-induced parkinsonism can follow therapy with metoclopramide, methyldopa, lithium, haloperidol, or chlorpromazine. It can be seen after the use of illicit drugs such as methamphetamine. After removing the cause, symptoms of parkinsonism often disappear.

- Other causes include hydrocephalus, neurodegenerative disorders, hypoparathyroidism, infections, stroke, tumor, and trauma.
- Around 20%–25% of patients with PD have a family history of PD. Several gene mutations have been linked to various forms of PD.

The pathology of PD involves the degeneration of the dopamine (DA)-producing neurons in the substantia nigra of the midbrain. This disrupts the balance between dopamine (DA) and acetylcholine (ACh) in the basal ganglia.

- DA is essential for normal functioning of the extrapyramidal motor system, including control of posture, support, and voluntary motion. Initial symptoms of PD do not occur until 60%–80% of DA-producing neurons are lost.
- *Lewy bodies,* unusual clumps of protein, are found in the brains of patients with PD. Their presence indicates abnormal brain functioning.

Clinical Manifestations

The onset of PD is gradual, with ongoing progression. One limb or side of the body may be involved at first. Common manifestations are tremors, rigidity, bradykinesia, and postural instability. Early in the disease, only a mild tremor, a flattened affect, slowing of ADLs (dressing, feeding), or decreased arm swing may be seen. Shoulder rigidity may be mistaken for arthritis. Later, the patient may have a shuffling gait and appear unable to stop. There may be speech problems (hypokinetic dysarthria) that affect communication.

- *Tremor*, often the first sign, is more prominent at rest and is aggravated by emotional stress or increased concentration. The hand tremor is described as "pill rolling" because the thumb and forefinger appear to move in a rotary fashion as if rolling a pill, coin, or other small object. Tremor can involve the diaphragm, tongue, lips, and jaw.
- *Rigidity* is increased resistance to passive motion when the limbs are moved through their range of motion. Parkinsonian rigidity is typified by jerky (cogwheel) rigidity, as if there were intermittent catches when the joint is passively moved. Sustained muscle contraction causes the patient to feel stiff with muscle soreness, feeling tired and achy.
- *Bradykinesia* (slow movement) is present in both spontaneous and automatic actions. Tasks that were once easy are now frustratingly slow because of the absence or loss of control

P

of voluntary muscle movements. Bradykinesia is particularly evident in the loss of automatic movements, secondary to the physical and chemical alteration of the basal ganglia. A lack of spontaneous activity (blinking of the eyelids, swinging of the arms while walking, swallowing of saliva, self-expression with facial and hand movements, and minor movement of postural adjustment) in PD accounts for the stooped, bent forward posture, masked face (deadpan expression), drooling of saliva, and shuffling gait.

- *Postural instability* is common, and patients may report being unable to stop themselves from going forward (propulsion) or backward (retropulsion). This increases the risk of falling.

Other signs and symptoms include depression, anxiety, apathy, fatigue, inability to plan, poor attention, pain, urinary incontinence, constipation, erectile dysfunction, and memory changes. Problems with eating include early satiety and loss of taste. Patients have trouble communicating due to a lack of expressive voice and low volume (hypophonia). Sleep problems include difficulty staying asleep at night, restless sleep, nightmares, and excessive daytime sleepiness.

Complications

- As PD progresses, complications increase. Swallowing becomes more difficult (dysphagia) and malnutrition or aspiration may result. Increasing weakness may lead to immobility problems.
- Orthostatic hypotension is common. Along with loss of postural reflexes, it can cause falls or other injury. The increased fall risk means caregivers must be aware of environment conditions that may contribute to falls.
- Other complications include dyskinesias (spontaneous, involuntary movements), weakness, and neuropsychiatric problems (e.g., depression, hallucinations). Dementia often results and is associated with increased mortality.

Diagnostic Studies

Diagnosis is based on the history and clinical features. Confirmation is a positive response to antiparkinsonian drugs (levodopa or DA agonist).

Interprofessional Management

Management is aimed at relieving symptoms.

Drug Therapy

Drug therapy for PD is aimed at correcting the imbalance of central nervous system (CNS) neurotransmitters. Antiparkinsonian drugs either enhance the release or supply of DA (dopaminergic) or antagonize or block the effects of overactive cholinergic neurons in the striatum (anticholinergic). Levodopa with carbidopa (Sinemet) is the primary treatment for symptomatic patients. Levodopa is a precursor of DA and can cross the blood–brain barrier. It is converted to DA in the basal ganglia. Prolonged use of levodopa can result in dyskinesias and "off/on" periods when the medication will unpredictably start or stop working. See Table 64 for the actions of drugs commonly used to manage PD.

Surgical Therapy

Surgical procedures such as ablation (destruction) and deep brain stimulation (DBS) are aimed at relieving symptoms of PD for patients who are unresponsive to drug therapy or who have developed severe motor complications.

Nursing Management

Goals

The patient with PD will maximize neurologic function, maintain independence in activities of daily living for as long as possible, prevent injury, and optimize psychosocial well-being.

Interventions

Promotion of physical exercise and a well-balanced diet are major nursing concerns. Exercise can limit the consequences of decreased mobility, such as muscle atrophy, contractures, and constipation. Include exercises for overall muscle tone and to strengthen the muscles involved with speaking and swallowing.

- Patients who have dysphagia and bradykinesia need appetizing foods that are easily chewed and swallowed, with adequate fiber to avoid constipation. Provide ample time for eating to avoid frustration.
- Protein ingestion can impair the absorption of levodopa. Limiting protein intake to the evening meal can decrease this problem.

Because PD is a chronic degenerative disorder, focus on teaching and nursing care directed toward maintaining good health, encouraging independence, and avoiding complications such as contractures.

▼ Patient and Caregiver Teaching

- Teach the patient to facilitate getting out of a chair by using an upright chair with arms and placing the back legs on small (2-inch) blocks.
- An elevated toilet seat can facilitate getting on and off the toilet.
- Encourage environmental alterations for safety, such as removing rugs and excess furniture to avoid stumbling.

TABLE 64 Drug Therapy: Parkinson's Disease

Drug	Mechanism of Action	Side Effects	Considerations
Dopaminergics			
Dopamine Precursors			
Levodopa (L-dopa) Levodopa/carbidopa (Sinemet)	Converted to dopamine (DA) in basal ganglia	Dry mouth GI distress	Do not take with meals. Limit Vitamin B6 intake. Teach about ways to decrease dry mouth.
Dopamine Receptor Agonists			
Pramipexole (Mirapex) Ropinirole (Requip, requip XL) Rotigotine (Neupro [transdermal patch])	Stimulate DA receptors	Dizziness GI distress Hallucinations Insomnia Orthostatic BP	Monitor orthostatic BP. Change positions slowly. Use safety measures if CNS effects occur. Rotate patch sites.
Dopamine Agonists			
Amantadine	Blocks NMDA-type glutamate receptors, increases DA release, and blocks DA reuptake	Dizziness Insomnia	Do not stop abruptly. Use safety measures if CNS effects occur.
Apomorphine (Apokyn)	Stimulates postsynaptic DA receptors	Chest pain Drowsiness GI distress Liver toxicity Sweating	Monitor liver function tests. Rotate injection sites. Give in abdomen, thigh, upper arm.

TABLE 64 Parkinson's Disease—cont'd

Drug	Mechanism of Action	Side Effects	Considerations
Anticholinergics			
Benztropine (Cogentin) Trihexyphenidyl	Block cholinergic receptors, thus helping to balance cholinergic and dopaminergic activity	Dizziness Dry mouth Urinary retention Vision changes	Stop if swallowing problems occur. Avoid alcohol, hot weather. Use safety measures if CNS effects occur.
Antihistamine			
Diphenhydramine	Has anticholinergic effect	Drowsiness Dry mouth Urinary retention Vision changes	Avoid alcohol. Use safety measures if CNS effects occur. Do not take with MAO inhibitors.
Monoamine Oxidase Type B Inhibitors			
Rasagiline (Azilect) Safinamide (Xadago) Selegiline	Block breakdown of DA	Dizziness Dry mouth Headache Orthostatic BP	Use safety measures if CNS effects occur. Avoid tyramine-containing foods. Many drug interactions. Avoid direct sunlight. Change positions slowly.

Continued

P

TABLE 64	Parkinson's Disease—cont'd		
Drug	Mechanism of Action	Side Effects	Considerations
Catechol *O*-Methyltransferase (COMT) Inhibitors			
Entacapone (Comtan) Opicapone (Ongentys)	Block COMT and slow the breakdown of levodopa, thus prolonging the action of levodopa	Confusion Dizziness GI distress Hypotension	Only give with levodopa. Avoid pregnancy. Use safety measures if CNS effects occur.

*NMDA, N-*Methyl-*D*-aspartic acid.

- Clothing can be simplified by the use of slip-on shoes and hook-and-loop (Velcro) fasteners or zippers on clothing instead of buttons and hooks. Allow extra time for dressing.
- As the disease progresses, the impact on the psychologic well-being of the patient increases. Assist the patient through listening, providing education, encouraging social interactions, and referral to the American Parkinson Disease Association (www.apdaparkinson.org).

Family members provide care for most patients with PD. Their burden increases as the disease progresses. Help them find appropriate resources.

PELVIC INFLAMMATORY DISEASE

Description
Pelvic inflammatory disease (PID) is a clinical syndrome, which includes a spectrum of infectious and inflammatory diseases of the upper genital tract. Ascending organisms cause inflammation in the endometrium, fallopian tubes, ovaries, and pelvic peritoneum.

Pathophysiology
PID is caused by an infectious organism ascending from the vagina or upper urogenital tract. Untreated sexually transmitted Neisseria gonorrhoeae and *Chlamydia trachomatis* are common causes of PID, as are microbes associated with bacterial vaginosis. Organisms can ascend past the endocervical barrier through normal physiologic processes such as menstruation or with gynecologic procedures (e.g., IUD insertion). Other risk factors include high-risk sexual behaviors, young age, vaginal douching, recent cervical manipulation, and prior history of PID.

Clinical Manifestations
The classic presentation of acute PID is pelvic or lower abdominal pain with tenderness in the cervix, uterus, or adnexa.
- Pain varies from mild to severe. The pain often occurs with intercourse and urination. Movement, such as walking, can increase the pain.
- Spotting after intercourse and purulent cervical or vaginal discharge may occur.
- Fever and chills may be present.

Complications
PID can cause serious complications including infertility, ectopic pregnancy, chronic pelvic pain, or tubo-ovarian abscess

(TOA). These result from scarring, adhesions, or obstruction of the fallopian tubes. TOA or perihepatitis (Fitz-Hugh–Curtis syndrome) are potential immediate and serious risks of untreated PID.

Diagnostic Studies

A health and sexual history and physical assessment are important to explore the presenting symptoms and rule out other causes of abdominal or pelvic pain.

Physical assessment will include abdominal, pelvic, and speculum examinations.

- Diagnostic testing includes examination for *N. gonorrhoeae* and *C. trachomatis.* Testing for other STIs such as HIV is recommended.
- A pregnancy test is done to rule out ectopic pregnancy.
- Ultrasound, endometrial biopsy, or laparoscopy may be useful to rule out other potential complications.

Interprofessional and Nursing Management

PID is usually treated on an outpatient basis with a combination of broad-spectrum antibiotics. Symptoms should improve within 72 hours of starting treatment. Hospitalization may be needed for patients with suspected PID who do not respond within 48–72 hours.

- Patients who are pregnant or present with severe symptoms such as high fever or nausea and vomiting may be hospitalized. In those instances, IV antibiotics, further tests, or surgery may be needed. Analgesics to relieve pain and IV fluids to prevent dehydration are also used.
- Recent sexual partners should be treated presumptively for gonorrhea and chlamydia.

Prevention, early recognition, and prompt treatment of vaginal and cervical infections can help prevent PID and its serious complications. Provide teaching about sexual practices and health screening to reduce transmission of STIs in the future.

- Urge women to seek medical attention for any unusual vaginal discharge or possible infection of the reproductive organs.
- Advise patients to abstain from sexual intercourse until treatment is completed and sexual partners have been treated.
- The patient may feel guilty about having PID, especially if it was associated with a sexually transmitted infection, and concerned about possible infertility or ectopic pregnancy. Discuss her feelings and concerns to assist her to cope.

PEPTIC ULCER DISEASE

Description

Peptic ulcer disease (PUD) is an erosion of the mucosa resulting from the digestive action of hydrochloric acid (HCl) and pepsin. Any part of the gastrointestinal (GI) tract that comes into contact with gastric secretions is susceptible to ulcer development. This includes the lower esophagus, stomach, duodenum, and margin of a gastrojejunal anastomosis after surgical procedures. PUD affects about 4.6 million people in the United States each year.

Peptic ulcers are acute or chronic, depending on the degree and duration of mucosal involvement, and gastric or duodenal, according to the location.

- An *acute ulcer* is associated with superficial erosion and minimal inflammation. It is of short duration and resolves quickly when the cause is identified and removed.
- A *chronic ulcer* is of long duration, eroding through the muscular wall with the formation of fibrous tissue. It is continuously present for many months or recurs intermittently. Chronic ulcers are more common than acute erosions.
- *Gastric* and *duodenal* ulcers are distinctly different in etiology and incidence (Table 65). Generally, the treatment of all ulcer types is similar.

Pathophysiology

Peptic ulcers develop in the presence of an acid environment. The back-diffusion of HCl into the gastric mucosa causes cellular destruction and inflammation. Histamine is released from the damaged mucosa. This results in vasodilation and increased capillary permeability and further secretion of acid and pepsin. Several factors may damage the mucosal barrier.

- *Helicobacter pylori* is associated with chronic gastritis and peptic ulcer development. Eighty percent of gastric and 90% of duodenal ulcers are related to *H. pylori*. In the United States, *H. pylori* affects 20% of persons younger than 30 years and 50% of those older than 60 years. The rate is highest in Hispanics.
- Nonsteroidal antiinflammatory drug (NSAID) use is responsible for most non–*H. pylori* peptic ulcers. NSAIDs inhibit prostaglandin synthesis, increase gastric acid secretion, and reduce the integrity of the mucosal barrier. NSAID use in the presence of *H. pylori* further increases the risk of PUD.

TABLE 65 Comparison of Gastric and Duodenal Ulcers

Gastric Ulcers	Duodenal Ulcers
Lesion	
Superficial, smooth margins. Round, oval, or cone shaped	Penetrating (deformity of duodenal bulb from healing of recurrent ulcers)
Location of Lesion	
Predominantly antrum, also in body and fundus of stomach	First 1–2 cm of duodenum
Gastric Secretion	
Normal to decreased	Increased
Incidence	
Greater in women	Greater in men, but increasing in women (especially postmenopausal)
Peak age 50–60 yr	Peak age 35–45 yr
Increased cancer risk	No increase in cancer risk
H. pylori infection in 80%	*H. pylori* infection in 90%
↑ With incompetent pyloric sphincter and bile reflux	Associated with other diseases (e.g., chronic obstructive pulmonary disease, pancreatic disease, hyperparathyroidism, Zollinger-Ellison syndrome, chronic renal failure)
Clinical Manifestations	
Burning or gaseous pressure in epigastrium	Burning, cramping, pressure-like pain across midepigastrium and upper abdomen. Back pain with posterior ulcers.
Pain 1–2 hr after meals. If penetrating ulcer, aggravation of discomfort with food	Pain 2–5 hr after meals and midmorning, midafternoon, middle of night. Periodic and episodic. Pain relief with antacids and food.
Recurrence Rate	
High	High

Clinical Manifestations

Discomfort associated with gastric ulcer is generally high in the epigastrium and occurs about 1–2 hours after meals. The pain is described as burning or gaseous. If the ulcer has eroded through the gastric mucosa, food tends to worsen the pain.

Duodenal ulcer symptoms occur when gastric acid comes in contact with the ulcer, generally 2–5 hours after a meal. The pain is described as "burning" or "cramp-like." It is most often located in the midepigastric region beneath the xiphoid process. Duodenal ulcers can also produce back pain. Duodenal ulcers tend to occur continuously for a few weeks or months and then disappear for a time, only to recur some months later.

- Not all patients with gastric or duodenal ulcers have discomfort. Silent peptic ulcers are more likely to occur in older adults and those taking NSAIDs. The presence or absence of symptoms is not directly related to the size of the ulcer or the degree of healing.

Diagnostic Studies

- Endoscopy is used to obtain tissue for biopsy, confirm the absence of cancer, obtain specimens to test for *H. pylori,* and determine the degree of ulcer healing after treatment.
- Biopsy of the antral mucosa and testing for urease (rapid urease testing) confirm a diagnosis of *H. pylori* infection. A noninvasive urea breath test can identify active infection.
- Complete blood count (CBC), urinalysis, liver enzyme studies, serum amylase determination, and stool examination may provide further diagnostic information.

Interprofessional Management

Conservative Therapy

The aim of treatment is to decrease gastric acidity and enhance mucosal defense mechanisms. The regimen consists of rest, drug therapy, smoking cessation, and long-term follow-up care. Strict adherence to the prescribed drug regimen is important because ulcers frequently recur. Pain disappears after 3–6 days, but complete healing may take 3–9 weeks of therapy.

- *Drug therapy* includes the use of histamine H_2-receptor antagonists, proton pump inhibitors (PPIs), antisecretory agents, cytoprotective agents, antacids, and anticholinergics. Aspirin and NSAIDs are stopped for 4–6 weeks. When aspirin must be continued, coadministration with a PPI, H_2-receptor blocker, or misoprostol may be prescribed.

- The patient is given antibiotics and a PPI for 10–14 days to eradicate *H. pylori* infection. Because of the development of antibiotic-resistant organisms, patients may need more than one round of therapy.

An acute exacerbation is frequently accompanied by bleeding, increased pain and discomfort, and nausea and vomiting.

- Management of hemorrhage is similar to that described for upper GI bleeding (see Gastrointestinal Beedling, Upper). Blood volume is replaced with IV solutions, and packed red blood cells (RBCs) may be necessary.
- With perforation, the immediate focus is to stop the spillage of gastric or duodenal contents into the peritoneal cavity and restore blood volume. A nasogastric (NG) tube can provide continuous aspiration and gastric decompression. Broad-spectrum antibiotic therapy is started immediately to treat bacterial peritonitis. Pain medication is also given.
- With gastric outlet obstruction, the aim of therapy is to decompress the stomach using an NG tube. Pain relief results from the decompression. IV fluids and electrolytes may be given for dehydration, vomiting, and electrolyte imbalances.

Nutritional Therapy
There is no specific diet to treat PUD. Patients should eat and drink foods and fluids that do not cause distressing symptoms. Foods that may cause gastric irritation include pepper, carbonated beverages, broth (meat extract), and hot, spicy foods. Caffeinated beverages and foods can increase symptoms in some patients. Teach the patient to avoid alcohol use because it can delay healing.

Surgical Therapy
Surgery is done for complications unresponsive to medical management. Surgical procedures include partial gastrectomy, vagotomy, or pyloroplasty. Partial gastrectomy with removal of the distal two-thirds of the stomach and anastomosis of the gastric stump to the duodenum is a *gastroduodenostomy* or *Billroth I* operation; removal of the distal two-thirds of the stomach with anastomosis of the gastric stump to the jejunum is a *gastrojejunostomy* or *Billroth II* operation. *Vagotomy* (severing of the vagal nerve) decreases gastric acid secretion. *Pyloroplasty* is the surgical enlargement of the pyloric sphincter to facilitate the passage of contents from the stomach.

Postoperative complications from surgery are dumping syndrome, postprandial hypoglycemia, and bile reflux gastritis.

- *Dumping syndrome* occurs when surgery drastically reduces the capacity of the stomach. A large bolus of hypertonic fluid enters the intestine, drawing fluid into the bowel lumen. This creates a decrease in plasma volume, distention of the bowel lumen, and rapid intestinal transit. Symptoms begin within 15–30 minutes after eating and last about an hour. The patient reports generalized weakness, sweating, palpitations, and dizziness. The patient may have abdominal cramps, borborygmi, and the urge to defecate.

- *Postprandial hypoglycemia* is a variant of dumping syndrome. It is the result of uncontrolled gastric emptying of a bolus of fluid high in carbohydrates into the small intestine. This causes initial hyperglycemia and the release of excess amounts of insulin into the circulation followed by reflex hypoglycemia. Symptoms are like those of any hypoglycemic reaction. They include sweating, weakness, mental confusion, palpitations, tachycardia, and anxiety. Symptoms generally occur 2 hours after eating.

- Gastric surgery that involves the pylorus can result in reflux of bile into the stomach. The major symptom of *bile reflux gastritis* is continuous epigastric distress that increases after meals. Vomiting relieves distress temporarily. Cholestyramine before or with meals has been used to treat this problem. It binds with the bile salts that are the source of gastric irritation.

Because of surgical changes, the stomach's reservoir is diminished, and meal size must be reduced accordingly. Advise the patient to limit fluids with meals. Dry foods with a low carbohydrate content and moderate protein and fat content are better tolerated initially. Dietary changes and a short rest period after each meal reduce the risk of dumping syndrome.

Nursing Management

Goals

The overall goals are that the patient with PUD will adhere to the therapeutic regimen, achieve pain relief, be free from complications, have complete healing of the peptic ulcer, and make appropriate lifestyle changes to prevent recurrence.

Interventions

During an acute phase, the patient may be NPO, have an NG tube connected to intermittent suction, and have IV fluid replacement. Explain the rationale for this therapy to the patient and caregiver. When the stomach is kept empty of gastric secretions, pain decreases and ulcer healing begins. The patient's immediate environment should be quiet and restful.

Major complications of peptic ulcers such as hemorrhage, perforation, and gastric outlet obstruction are emergencies and may require surgical intervention. Manifestations of perforation are sudden and dramatic. They include severe upper abdominal pain that quickly spreads throughout the abdomen. Bowel sounds are usually absent.

If the patient has surgery, postoperative care is similar to that after abdominal laparotomy (see Abdominal Pain, Acute). Additional considerations for a patient with a partial gastrectomy include:

- It is essential that the NG suction be working and that the tube remain patent so that accumulated secretions do not put a strain on the anastomosis. If the tube must be replaced or repositioned, call the health care provider (HCP) to perform this task because of the danger of perforating the gastric mucosa or disrupting the suture line.
- Observe the gastric aspirate for color, amount, and odor
- While the NG tube is connected to suction, maintain IV therapy. Add potassium and vitamin supplements (as ordered) to the infusion until oral feedings are resumed.
- Observe the patient for signs of decreased peristalsis and lower abdominal discomfort that may indicate impending intestinal obstruction.
- Observe the dressing for signs of bleeding or odor and drainage indicative of an infection.
- Keep the patient comfortable and free of pain by administering prescribed drugs and by frequent changes in position.
- Encourage early ambulation.
- The patient may require cobalamin therapy.

▼ **Patient and Caregiver Teaching**
General instructions should cover aspects of the disease process, drugs, possible changes in lifestyle, and regular follow-up evaluation (Table 66). Stress the need for long-term follow-up care. Encourage the patient to seek immediate intervention if symptoms return.

TABLE 66   **Patient and Caregiver Teaching: Peptic Ulcer Disease (PUD)**

1. Avoid foods that cause epigastric distress, such as acidic foods.
2. Avoid cigarettes. Smoking promotes ulcer development and delays ulcer healing.
3. Reduce or eliminate alcohol intake.
4. Avoid over-the-counter (OTC) drugs unless approved by the HCP. Many preparations contain ingredients, such as aspirin, which should not be taken unless approved by the HCP. Check with the HCP about the use of nonsteroidal antiinflammatory drugs.
5. Do not interchange brands of PPIs, antacids, or H_2-receptor blockers that can be bought OTC without checking with the HCP. This can lead to harmful side effects.
6. Take all medications as prescribed. This includes both antisecretory and antibiotic drugs. Failing to take medications as prescribed can result in relapse.
7. It is important to report any of the following:
   • increased nausea or vomiting
   • increased epigastric pain
   • bloody emesis or tarry stools
8. Stress can be related to signs and symptoms of PUD. Learn and use stress management strategies.
9. Share concerns about lifestyle changes and living with a chronic illness.

P

PERICARDITIS, ACUTE

Description

Pericarditis is a condition caused by inflammation of the pericardium, often with fluid accumulation. The pericardium is composed of the inner serous membrane (visceral pericardium) and the outer fibrous (parietal) layer. The pericardial space between these two layers normally holds 10–15 mL of serous fluid. The pericardium anchors the heart, provides lubrication to decrease friction between heart contractions, and helps prevent excess dilation of the heart during diastole.

Pathophysiology

Acute pericarditis is most often idiopathic (unknown) or viral. Viral pericarditis is often seen after respiratory or GI illness. Other causes include uremia, bacterial infection, acute myocardial infarction (MI), neoplasm, and trauma.

- *Acute pericarditis* develops rapidly, causing the pericardial sac to become inflamed and leak fluid (pericardial effusion). *Subacute pericarditis* occurs weeks to months after an event. We refer to pericarditis lasting more than 6 months as *chronic.*
- About 20% of cases are due to cardiac injury. Post-MI syndrome (Dressler syndrome) pericarditis can occur 4–6 weeks after transmural MI. This syndrome is more common after a large anterior infarct.

An inflammatory response is the characteristic pathologic finding in acute pericarditis. There is an influx of neutrophils, increased pericardial vascularity, and eventual fibrin deposition on the pericardium.

Clinical Manifestations

Clinical symptoms include progressive, severe sharp chest pain. The pain generally worsens with deep inspiration and when lying flat. Sitting up and leaning forward relieve the pain.

- The pain may radiate to the neck, arms, or left shoulder, making it hard to distinguish from angina. One distinction is that pericarditis pain can be referred to the trapezius muscle (shoulder, upper back).
- Dyspnea that accompanies acute pericarditis is related to the patient's breathing in rapid, shallow breaths to avoid chest pain. Pain may be aggravated by fever and anxiety.
- The hallmark finding is a *pericardial friction rub,* which is a scratching, grating, high-pitched sound believed to arise from friction between the roughened pericardial and epicardial surfaces. It is best heard with the stethoscope diaphragm firmly placed at the lower left sternal border of the chest with the patient leaning forward. Because it is hard to tell a pericardial friction rub from a pleural friction rub, ask the patient to hold their breath. If you still hear the rub, then it is cardiac. Pericardial friction rubs may be intermittent.

Complications

Pericardial effusion is buildup of fluid in the pericardium. Heart sounds are distant and muffled. BP is usually maintained. Large effusions compress nearby structures. Pulmonary tissue compression can cause cough, dyspnea, and tachypnea. Phrenic nerve compression can induce hiccups. Compression of the recurrent laryngeal nerve may cause hoarseness.

Cardiac tamponade develops as the pericardial effusion volume increases and compresses the heart. The speed of fluid accumulation affects the severity of clinical signs. Cardiac tamponade can occur acutely (e.g., rupture of heart, trauma) or subacutely (e.g., from renal failure, cancer). The patient may report chest pain and is often confused, anxious, and restless. Heart sounds become muffled, pulse pressure is narrowed, and the patient develops tachypnea, tachycardia, and decreased cardiac output. Increased jugular venous pressure causes neck vein distention. *Pulsus paradoxus* is a decrease in systolic BP with inspiration.

Diagnostic Studies

- Electrocardiogram (ECG) changes (e.g., diffuse ST-segment elevation) are noted in approximately 90% of the cases.
- Echocardiography is used to determine the presence of pericardial effusion or cardiac tamponade.
- Doppler and color M-mode imaging assess diastolic function and help diagnose constrictive pericarditis.
- Laboratory findings include leukocytosis and increased erythrocyte sedimentation rate (ESR) and C-reactive protein (CRP). Troponin levels may be increased in patients with ST-segment elevation and acute pericarditis, indicating myocardial damage.
- CT scan and MRI permit visualization of the pericardium and pericardial space.

Interprofessional Management

Management is aimed at identifying and treating the underlying problem and symptoms. Antibiotics treat bacterial pericarditis, and nonsteroidal antiinflammatory drugs (NSAIDs) (e.g., salicylates [aspirin], ibuprofen) control the pain and inflammation. Corticosteroids are reserved for patients with pericarditis secondary to systemic lupus erythematosus, those already taking corticosteroids for a rheumatologic or other immune system condition, or those who do not respond to NSAIDs. Colchicine, an antiinflammatory drug used to treat gout, can be used in recurrent pericarditis.

- Pericardiocentesis is usually done for pericardial effusion with acute cardiac tamponade, purulent pericarditis, or suspected cancer.
- Hemodynamic support before pericardiocentesis may include administering volume expanders and inotropic agents (e.g., dopamine) and discontinuing anticoagulants.
- A *pericardial window* is a surgical procedure that allows the excess pericardial fluid to drain continuously into the peritoneum or chest.

Nursing Management

Assess to distinguish the pain of myocardial ischemia (angina) from the pain of pericarditis. Pericarditis pain is in the precordium or over the left trapezius ridge and has a sharp quality that increases with inspiration. Relief is often obtained by sitting or leaning forward and pain is worse when the patient is lying flat.

- Position the patient on bed rest with the head of the bed elevated to 45 degrees and an overbed table for arm support.
- Antiinflammatory agents help alleviate the patient's pain. Give these drugs with food. Tell the patient to avoid alcohol because of the risk of gastrointestinal (GI) bleeding. Other drugs, such as a proton pump inhibitor (e.g., pantoprazole, omeprazole), can reduce stomach acid.
- Monitor for the signs and symptoms of tamponade and prepare for possible pericardiocentesis.
- Provide simple, complete explanations of procedures and possible causes of the pain to help reduce anxiety.

PERIPHERAL ARTERY DISEASE

Description

Peripheral artery disease (PAD) involves thickening of artery walls and progressive narrowing of the arteries in the arms and legs. PAD is strongly related to other types of cardiovascular disease (CVD) and their risk factors. In the United States, about 8.5 million people over age 40 years have PAD, with a higher prevalence in blacks.

Pathophysiology

The leading cause of PAD is atherosclerosis, which is a gradual thickening of the *intima* (the innermost layer of the arterial wall) and *media* (middle layer of the arterial wall). This results from cholesterol and lipids deposited within the vessel walls and leads to narrowing of the artery. Although the exact causes of atherosclerosis are unknown, inflammation and endothelial injury play a major role.

- Risk factors for PAD are tobacco use (most important), diabetes, hypertension, high cholesterol, and age over 60 years.
- Symptoms occur when vessels are 60%–75% blocked.

Peripheral Artery Disease: Lower Extremities

Lower extremity PAD may affect the iliac, femoral, popliteal, tibial, or peroneal arteries (see Fig. 22.) The femoral-popliteal area is the most common site in nondiabetic patients. Those with diabetes tend to develop PAD in arteries below the knee.

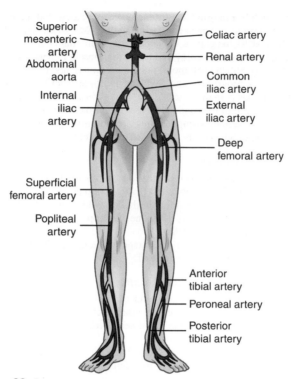

Fig. 22 Common anatomic locations of atherosclerotic lesions (shown in yellow) of the abdominal aorta and lower extremities.

Clinical Manifestations

Severity of the symptoms depends on the site and extent of the obstruction and the amount of collateral circulation.

- The classic symptom of PAD is *intermittent claudication,* which is ischemic muscle pain that is caused by exercise, resolves within 10 minutes or less with resting, and is reproducible.
- Some persons with PAD either have no symptoms or atypical leg symptoms (e.g., burning, hardness, heaviness, knotting, pressure, soreness, tightness, weakness) in atypical locations (e.g., ankle, foot, hamstring, hip, knee, shin).
- *Paresthesia* (numbness or tingling) in the toes or feet may result from nerve tissue ischemia. Reduced blood flow to neurons causes loss of pressure and deep pain sensation.

- Pallor (blanching) of the foot is noted in response to leg elevation. *Reactive hyperemia* (redness) develops when the limb is allowed to hang in a dependent position *(dependent rubor)*. The skin becomes shiny and taut. The lower legs lose their hair. Pedal, popliteal, or femoral pulses are diminished or absent.
- As PAD progresses and involves multiple arterial segments, continuous pain develops at rest. Rest pain most often occurs in the forefoot or toes and is worse with limb elevation.

The most serious complications are nonhealing arterial ulcers and gangrene, which may require lower extremity amputation.

Diagnostic Studies

- Doppler ultrasound and duplex imaging assess blood flow.
- Segmental BPs are obtained (using Doppler ultrasound and a sphygmomanometer) at the thigh, below the knee, and at ankle level while the patient is supine. A drop in segmental BP of >30 mm Hg suggests PAD.
- Angiography or magnetic resonance angiography (MRA) delineates location and extent of PAD.

Interprofessional Management

The first treatment goal is to reduce cardiovascular risk factors. Tobacco cessation and aggressive management of diabetes, hypertension, and hyperlipidemia are essential. Lifestyle interventions and drug therapy are needed.

- Statins (e.g., simvastatin [Zocor]) and a fibric acid derivative (gemfibrozil [Lopid]) lower low-density lipoprotein (LDL) and triglyceride levels.
- Antiplatelet agents are critical for reducing the risk of CVD events and death. Oral antiplatelet therapy should include low-dose aspirin therapy. Aspirin-intolerant patients may take clopidogrel (Plavix) daily.
- Two drugs are available to treat intermittent claudication: cilostazol and pentoxifylline. Pentoxifylline, a xanthine derivative, improves the flexibility of red blood cells (RBCs) and white blood cells (WBCs) and decreases fibrinogen concentration, platelet adhesiveness, and blood viscosity.

A supervised exercise program is recommended for all patients with intermittent claudication. The patient should exercise for 30–45 minutes/day, at least three times per week, for a minimum of 3 months. Although walking is most commonly prescribed exercise, other modes of exercise (e.g., cycling) also improve walking ability and quality of life.

- Teach patients to adjust caloric intake to achieve and maintain a body mass index (BMI) less than $25\,kg/m^2$. Recommend a diet high in fruits, vegetables, and whole grains and low in cholesterol, saturated fat, and salt.

Critical limb ischemia is characterized by chronic ischemic rest pain lasting more than 2 weeks, nonhealing arterial leg ulcers, or gangrene of the leg from PAD. Conservative management goals for critical limb ischemia include protecting the patient's extremity from trauma, decreasing ischemic pain, preventing and controlling infection, and maximizing perfusion. Carefully inspect, cleanse, and lubricate both feet to prevent skin cracking and infection.

Various surgical approaches can be used to improve arterial blood flow beyond a blocked artery.

- The most common is a peripheral arterial bypass operation with autogenous (native) vein or synthetic graft material to bypass or carry blood around the lesion.
- Other surgical options include endarterectomy (opening the artery and removing the obstructing plaque) and patch graft angioplasty (opening the artery, removing the plaque, and sewing a patch to the opening to widen the lumen).

Interventional radiology catheter-based procedures are alternatives to open surgery for treatment of lower extremity PAD.

- *Percutaneous transluminal angioplasty* uses a catheter with a balloon at the tip. The end of the catheter is advanced to the stenotic area of the artery. The balloon is inflated, compressing the atherosclerotic intimal lining.
- *Stents,* expandable metallic devices, are positioned to hold the artery open immediately after balloon angioplasty. The stents may be covered with Dacron or a drug-eluting agent (e.g., paclitaxel) to reduce restenosis by limiting the new tissue growth into the stent.
- *Atherectomy* removes the obstructing plaque. A directional atherectomy device uses a high-speed cutting disk that cuts long strips of the atheroma. Laser atherectomy uses ultraviolet energy to break apart the atheroma.

Amputation may be needed if tissue necrosis is extensive, gangrene or osteomyelitis develops, or all major arteries are blocked.

Nursing Management
Goals
The patient with lower extremity PAD will have adequate tissue perfusion, relief of pain, increased exercise tolerance, and intact, healthy skin on extremities. Additional information on care for the

patient with PAD of the lower extremities is presented in eNursing Care Plan 41-1 on the website.

Interventions

After surgical or radiologic intervention, check the operative extremity every 15 minutes initially and then hourly for color, temperature, capillary refill, presence of peripheral pulses, and movement and sensation. Immediately notify the health care provider (HCP) of any loss of palpable pulses or a change in the Doppler sound over a pulse.

After the patient leaves the recovery area, continue to monitor extremity perfusion and assess for complications such as bleeding, hematoma, thrombosis, embolization, and compartment syndrome. A dramatic increase in pain, loss of previously palpable pulses, extremity pallor or cyanosis, numbness or tingling, or a cold extremity suggests blockage of the graft or stent. Report these findings to the HCP immediately.

- Do not place the patient in a knee-flexed position except for exercise. Turn the patient frequently and position with pillows to support the incision. On postoperative day 1, assist the patient out of bed several times. Walking even short distances is desirable.
- Discourage prolonged sitting with legs lowered since it may cause pain and edema, increase the risk of venous thrombosis, and place stress on the suture lines. Graduated compression stockings may help control leg edema. If edema develops, position the patient supine and elevate the leg above the heart level.

▼ Patient and Caregiver Teaching

- Encourage supervised exercise training after revascularization. Explain that exercise decreases CVD risk factors including hypertension, hyperlipidemia, obesity, and glucose levels.
- Teach foot care to all patients with PAD. Meticulous foot care is especially important for the diabetic patient with PAD. Thick or overgrown toenails and calluses need regular attention by an HCP (e.g., podiatrist).
- Tell patients to inspect their legs and feet daily for changes in skin color or texture. Show patients how to check skin temperature and capillary refill and to palpate pulses. Stress reporting any changes in these findings or the development of ulceration or inflammation to the HCP.
- Encourage patients to wear clean, all-cotton or all-wool socks and comfortable shoes with rounded (not pointed) toes and soft insoles. Tell patients to lace shoes loosely and to break in new shoes gradually.

PERITONITIS

Description

Peritonitis, inflammation of the peritoneum, may result from contamination of the peritoneal cavity with bacteria, irritating chemicals, or both. Causes are listed in Table 67. Primary peritonitis occurs when blood-borne organisms enter the peritoneal cavity. For example, the ascites that occurs with cirrhosis of the liver provides an excellent liquid environment for bacteria to flourish. Secondary peritonitis is more common and occurs when abdominal organs perforate or rupture and release their contents (bile, enzymes, bacteria) into the peritoneal cavity.

Pathophysiology

Intestinal contents irritate the normally sterile peritoneum, producing an initial chemical peritonitis that is followed a few hours later by bacterial peritonitis. The resulting inflammatory response leads to massive fluid shifts (peritoneal edema) and formation of adhesions as the body tries to wall off the infection.

Clinical Manifestations and Complications

- Severe, continuous abdominal pain is the most common symptom.
- A universal sign of peritonitis is tenderness over the involved area. Rebound tenderness, rigidity, and spasm are other major signs of peritoneal irritation.
- Abdominal distention or ascites, fever, tachycardia, tachypnea, nausea, vomiting, and altered bowel habits may also be present.

Complications include hypovolemic shock, sepsis, intraabdominal abscess, paralytic ileus, and acute respiratory distress syndrome. If treatment is delayed, peritonitis may be fatal.

Diagnostic Studies

- Complete blood count (CBC) will determine elevations in WBC count and hemoconcentration from fluid shifts.
- Peritoneal aspiration and analysis for blood, bile, pus, bacteria, fungi, and amylase content.
- Abdominal X-ray may show dilated loops of bowel consistent with paralytic ileus, free air if perforation has occurred, or air-fluid levels if an obstruction is present.
- CT scan and ultrasound may be useful in identifying ascites or abscesses.
- Peritoneoscopy may be helpful in patients without ascites.

TABLE 67	Causes of Peritonitis

Primary
- Blood-borne organisms
- Cirrhosis with ascites

Secondary
- Appendicitis with rupture
- Blunt or penetrating trauma to abdominal organs
- Diverticulitis with rupture
- Intestinal cancer
- Ischemic bowel disorders
- Pancreatitis
- Perforated intestine, uterus, urinary bladder, stomach
- Perforated peptic ulcer
- Peritoneal dialysis
- Postoperative (breakage of anastomosis)

Interprofessional Management

Patients with milder cases of peritonitis or who are poor surgical candidates may be managed conservatively with antibiotics, nasogastric (NG) suction, analgesics, and IV fluid administration. Surgery is indicated to locate the cause, drain purulent fluid, and repair damage such as perforated organs.

Nursing Management

Goals

The patient with peritonitis will have resolution of inflammation, relief of abdominal pain, freedom from complications (hypovolemic shock, sepsis), and normal nutritional status.

Interventions

The patient with peritonitis is extremely ill and needs skilled supportive care. Establish IV access to replace lost fluids and deliver antibiotic therapy. Monitor the patient for pain and response to analgesics. The patient may be positioned with knees flexed to increase comfort. Sedatives may be given to promote rest.

- Monitor vital signs frequently.
- Accurately monitor fluid intake and output and electrolyte status to determine replacement therapy.
- Antiemetics may be given to decrease nausea and vomiting and prevent further fluid and electrolyte losses. The patient is NPO and may have an NG tube in place to decrease gastric distention and further leakage of bowel contents into the peritoneum.

- If the patient has an open surgical procedure, drains may be in place to remove purulent drainage and excess fluid. Postoperative care is similar to that for the patient after a laparotomy (see Abdominal Pain, Acute).

PNEUMONIA

Description

Pneumonia is an infection of the lung parenchyma. Despite progress in antibiotic therapy, pneumonia still has significant morbidity and mortality. Pneumonia and lower respiratory tract infections were the fourth leading cause of death worldwide in 2019. Pneumonia can be caused by bacteria, viruses, *Mycoplasma* organisms, fungi, and parasites.

Pneumonia is classified as *community-acquired pneumonia* (CAP) or *hospital-acquired pneumonia* (HAP). Classifying pneumonia helps the HCP identify the most likely cause (Table 68) and the choice of antimicrobial therapy.

- *CAP* is an acute infection of the lung occurring in patients who have not been hospitalized or lived in a long-term care facility within 14 days of the onset of symptoms.
- *HAP* is pneumonia in a nonintubated patient that begins 48 hours or longer after admission to a hospital and was not present at the time of admission.
- *Ventilator-associated pneumonia (VAP)*, a type of HAP, refers to pneumonia that develops more than 48 hours after endotracheal intubation.

Pathophysiology

Normally, various defense mechanisms protect the airway distal to the larynx from infection. Pneumonia is more likely when defense mechanisms are incompetent or overwhelmed by infectious agents because of:

- a weak cough or epiglottal reflexes;
- tracheal intubation interfering with the normal cough reflex and the mucociliary escalator mechanism;
- impaired mucociliary mechanism caused by air pollution, smoking, viral upper respiratory tract infections, and normal aging changes;
- chronic diseases, which suppress the immune system.

Organisms that cause pneumonia reach the lungs by aspiration from the nasopharynx or oropharynx, inhalation of microbes

P

TABLE 68 Organisms Causing Pneumonia

Community-Acquired Pneumonia (CAP)	Hospital-Acquired Pneumonia (HAP)
Typical • *Escherichia coli* • *Haemophilus influenzae*[a] • *Klebsiella pneumoniae*[a] • *Methicillin resistant staphylococcus aureus (MRSA)* • *Moraxella catarrhalis* • *Pseudomonas* • *Staphylococcus aureus*[a] • *Streptococcus pneumoniae*[a] Atypical • *Chlamydophila pneumoniae* • *Coxiella burnettii* • *Influenza A and B* • *Legionella pneumophilia* • *Mycoplasma pneumoniae* • *Mycobacterium tuberculosis* Respiratory viruses • *Emerging infections such as SARS-CoV-2* • *Parainfluenza virus* • *Respiratory syncytial virus* • *Rhinovirus* Other causes of CAP • Fungi • Oral anaerobes	• *Escherichia coli*[b] • *Haemophilus influenzae* • *Klebsiella pneumoniae*[b] • *Microaspiration of bacteria that colonize the mouth, oropharynx* • *Pseudomonas aeruginosa*[b] • *Proteus species* • *Serratia marcescens* • *Staphylococcus aureus* • *Streptococcus pneumoniae*[a]

[a]Most common causes of CAP.
[b]Most common causes of HAP.

present in the air, or hematogenous spread from a primary infection elsewhere in the body. Most organisms trigger an inflammatory response in the lung. Inflammation, characterized by an increase in blood flow and vascular permeability, activates neutrophils to engulf and kill the offending organisms. The inflammatory process attracts more neutrophils, edema of the airways occurs, and fluid leaks from the capillaries and tissues into alveoli. Normal O_2 transport is impaired, leading to signs of hypoxia (e.g., tachypnea, dyspnea, tachycardia).

Consolidation occurs in bacterial pneumonia when normally air-filled alveoli are filled with fluid and debris. Macrophages lyse and process the debris, normal lung tissue is restored, and gas exchange returns to normal if there are no complications.

Clinical Manifestations and Complications

The most common presenting symptoms of pneumonia are cough, fever, shaking chills, dyspnea, tachypnea, and pleuritic chest pain.

- Cough may or may not be productive. Sputum may be green, yellow, or rust-colored (bloody).
- Viral pneumonia may initially seem to be influenza, with respiratory symptoms appearing and/or worsening 12–36 hours after onset.
- In older adults or debilitated patients, confusion or stupor (possibly related to hypoxia) may be the only finding.

Fine or coarse crackles may be auscultated over the affected area. If consolidation is present, bronchial breath sounds, egophony, and increased fremitus may be noted.

- Complications include atelectasis (collapsed, airless alveoli), pleurisy (inflammation of the pleura), pleural effusion, bacteremia, pneumothorax, lung abscess, sepsis, and acute respiratory failure.

The COVID-19 pandemic (caused by SARS-CoV-2) has forever impacted communities worldwide. Human-to-human spread occurs mainly through respiratory droplets, causing upper and/or lower respiratory infection. Since this viral infection was first recognized toward the end of 2019, it has caused significant morbidity and mortality globally.

- In the most severe cases of COVID-19 pneumonia and respiratory failure, a significant inflammatory cascade is triggered, leading to acute respiratory distress syndrome (ARDS) and multiorgan dysfunction (MODS). See Fig. 23 for the range of body systems affected in COVID-19. (See ARDS and SIRS/MODS.)

Diagnostic Studies

- History, physical examination, and chest X-ray provide information for early treatment decisions. Chest X-ray often shows a pattern characteristic of the infecting organism.
- Sputum culture with gram stain and blood cultures are used to identify the causative organism.
- Arterial blood gases (ABGs) are used to assess for hypoxemia, hypercapnia, and acidosis.
- White blood cell (WBC) count often reveals leukocytosis.

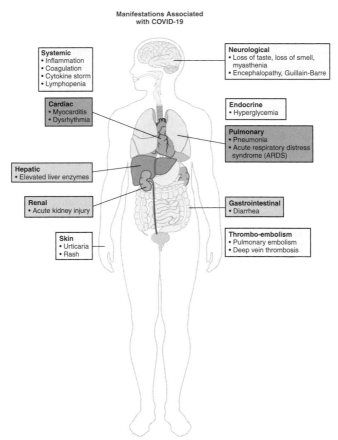

Fig. 23 Manifestations of COVID-19 (infection with SARS-CoV-2).

Interprofessional Management

Pneumococcal vaccine is used to prevent *Streptococcus pneumoniae* (pneumococcus) pneumonia.

- Vaccination is recommended for those 65 years of age or older and younger patients who are at high risk. A one-time repeat vaccination in 5 years is recommended for those who received their initial vaccination before the age of 65 years.

Vaccines immunizing against influenza or SARS-CoV-2 also are used to prevent pneumonia, but are effective for a shorter period of time.

Prompt treatment with appropriate antibiotics almost always cures bacterial pneumonia, including *Mycoplasma* pneumonia. In uncomplicated cases, the patient responds to drug therapy within 48–72 hours. A major problem today is pneumonia caused by multidrug-resistant (MDR) pathogens. Common culprits include methicillin-resistant *Staphylococcus aureus* and Gram-negative bacilli.

- Risk factors for MDR pneumonia include advanced age, immunosuppression, history of antibiotic use, and prolonged mechanical ventilation. Antibiotic susceptibility tests can identify MDR organisms.

Care is generally supportive for a majority of viral pneumonias.

- Helpful measures include oxygen therapy, analgesics to relieve chest pain, and antipyretics, such as aspirin or acetaminophen. Individualize rest and activity to the patient's tolerance.
- Hydration is important. IV administration of fluids and electrolytes may be needed. If the patient has heart failure, monitor fluid intake carefully.
- Small, frequent meals are easier for patients with dyspnea to tolerate. Offer foods high in calories and nutrients.

Nursing Management

Goals
The patient with pneumonia will have no signs of hypoxemia, normal breathing patterns, clear breath sounds, normal chest X-ray, normal WBC count, and no complications.

Interventions
To reduce the risk of pneumonia, teach patients to practice good health habits such as frequent hand washing, proper nutrition, adequate rest, regular exercise, and coughing or sneezing into the elbow rather than hands.

- Avoiding cigarette smoke is an important health-promoting behavior.
- Encourage those at increased risk for pneumonia to obtain both influenza and pneumococcal vaccines.
- If possible, avoid exposure to people with upper respiratory infections (URIs). If a URI occurs, it should be treated promptly with supportive measures (e.g., rest, fluids). If symptoms persist for more than 7 days, the person should seek medical care.

The eNursing Care Plan 30-1 (on the website) for a patient with pneumonia applies to people both at home and in the hospital. We provide supportive measures according to the patient's needs. These may include O_2 therapy to treat hypoxemia, antipyretics (e.g., acetaminophen) for fever, and analgesics to relieve chest pain.

- Place the patient with altered consciousness in positions (e.g., side-lying, upright) that will prevent or minimize aspiration. Reposition the patient at least every 2 hours to promote lung expansion and mobilization of secretions. Prone position may be useful for some patients.
- The patient who has a feeding tube requires attention to prevent aspiration.
- In the intensive care unit (ICU), strict adherence to "ventilator bundle" interventions reduces the incidence of VAP. These interventions are elevation of the head of the bed 30–45 degrees, daily "sedation holidays," assessment of readiness to extubate, prophylaxis for peptic ulcer disease and venous thromboembolism, and daily oral care with chlorhexidine.
- The patient who has difficulty swallowing (e.g., after a stroke) needs assistance in eating, drinking, and taking medication to prevent aspiration. After a patient has had local anesthesia to the throat, assess for a gag reflex before giving food or fluids.
- Patients with impaired mobility from any cause need assistance with turning and moving, as well as frequent encouragement to breathe deeply.
- Practice strict medical asepsis and adherence to infection control guidelines, including hand hygiene, to reduce the incidence of HAP.

▼ **Patient and Caregiver Teaching**
- Provide information about available vaccines.
- Teach the patient about the importance of taking every dose of the prescribed antibiotic, any drug–drug and food–drug interactions for the prescribed antibiotic, and the need for adequate rest to promote recovery.
- Tell the patient to drink plenty of liquids (at least 6–10 glasses/day, unless contraindicated) and to avoid alcohol and smoking.
- A cool mist humidifier or warm bath may help the patient breathe easier.

PNEUMOTHORAX

Description

A *pneumothorax* is a complete or partial collapse of a lung caused by accumulation of air in the pleural space. Pneumothorax can be described as *open* (air entering through an opening in the chest wall) or *closed* (no external wound).

Pathophysiology

Normally, negative (subatmospheric) pressure exists between the visceral pleura (surrounding the lung) and parietal pleura (lining

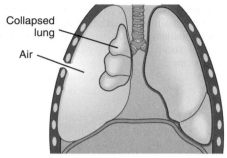

Fig. 24 Open pneumothorax resulting from collapse of lung following disruption of chest wall and outside air entering.

the chest cavity), known as the pleural space. The pleural space has a few milliliters of lubricating fluid to reduce friction when the tissues move. When air enters this normally subatmospheric space, lung volume decreases. The change to positive pressure causes a partial or complete lung collapse.

Types of Pneumothorax

Spontaneous pneumothorax occurs as a result of the rupture of small blebs (air-filled sacs) on the surface of the lung. These blebs occur in healthy, young people or from lung disease such as chronic obstructive pulmonary disease (COPD), asthma, cystic fibrosis, and pneumonia.

- Smoking increases the risk of bleb formation. Other risk factors include being tall and thin, male gender, family history, and previous spontaneous pneumothorax.

Traumatic pneumothorax can occur from either penetrating (open) or nonpenetrating (closed) chest trauma.

- A penetrating chest wound may be referred to as a "sucking chest wound," because air enters the pleural space through the chest wall during each inspiration (Fig. 24).

Iatrogenic pneumothorax can occur because of laceration or puncture of the lung during medical procedures such as transthoracic needle aspiration, subclavian catheter insertion, pleural biopsy, and transbronchial lung biopsy. Esophageal procedures may result in a pneumothorax from tearing of the esophageal wall.

- Barotrauma from excessive pressure during manual or mechanical ventilation can rupture alveoli, creating a pneumothorax.

Tension pneumothorax occurs when air enters the pleural space from either an open or a closed pneumothorax. The accumulation of air in the pleural space causes increasingly elevated intrapleural pressures. This results in compression of the lung on the affected side and pressure on the heart and great vessels, pushing them away from the affected side.

- The mediastinum shifts toward the unaffected side, compressing the "good" lung, which further compromises oxygenation. As pressure increases, venous return is decreased and cardiac output falls.

Hemothorax is an accumulation of blood in the pleural space from injury to the chest wall, diaphragm, lung, blood vessels, or mediastinum.

- The patient with a traumatic hemothorax needs immediate insertion of a chest tube for evacuation of the blood, which can be recovered and reinfused for a short time after the injury.

Clinical Manifestations

If the pneumothorax is small, only mild tachycardia and dyspnea may be present. If it is a large pneumothorax, shallow, rapid respirations, dyspnea, air hunger, and oxygen desaturation may occur.

- Chest pain and a cough with or without hemoptysis may be present.
- No breath sounds are auscultated over the affected area.
- Chest X-ray shows air or fluid in the pleural space with reduced lung volume.

Interprofessional Management

The most common treatment for a pneumothorax and hemothorax is to insert a chest tube and connect it to water-seal drainage (see Chest Tubes and Pleural Drainage). If the patient with a small pneumothorax is stable, the condition may resolve spontaneously, or the pleural space can be aspirated with a large-bore needle (thoracentesis). Repeated spontaneous pneumothoraces can be treated surgically by a partial pleurectomy, stapling, or pleurodesis to promote the adherence of pleurae to one another.

- Tension pneumothorax is a medical emergency, requiring urgent needle compression followed by chest tube insertion with water-seal drainage.
- Emergency treatment of an open pneumothorax consists of covering the wound with an occlusive dressing secured on three sides (vent dressing). During inspiration, as negative pressure is created in the chest, the dressing pulls against the wound, preventing air from entering the pleural space. During expiration, as the pressure rises in the pleural space, the

dressing is pushed out and air escapes through the wound and from under the dressing. If the object that caused the open chest wound is still in place, do not remove it. Stabilize the impaled object with a bulky dressing, and wait until a health care provider is present, or arrange transport to the nearest medical facility.

POLYCYSTIC KIDNEY DISEASE

Polycystic kidney disease (PKD) is a common genetic disorder. PKD is the fourth leading cause of end-stage renal disease (ESRD), affecting 5% of those with ESRD. A nongenetic PKD (acquired cystic kidney disease [ACKD]) can occur in those with severe kidney scarring and damage who receive dialysis. After 8 years on dialysis, 90% of patients will have ACKD.

- The *childhood form* of PKD is a rare autosomal recessive disorder that is often rapidly progressive. The *adult form* of PKD is an autosomal dominant disorder, which is usually manifested between 30 and 50 years of age. It involves both kidneys. The cortex and medulla are filled with large, thin-walled cysts up to several centimeters in diameter. The cysts enlarge and destroy surrounding tissue by compression.

Many people have no symptoms until the cysts begin to enlarge. Often the first manifestations are hypertension, hematuria (from rupture of cysts), or pain or a sensation of heaviness in the back, side, or abdomen. However, the first manifestation can be a urinary tract infection (UTI) or urinary stones. Bilateral, enlarged kidneys are often palpable on physical examination.

- Both acute and chronic pain are common. Chronic pain can be constant and severe.
- The disease progresses to ESRD by age 60 years in 50% of patients.
- PKD can also affect the liver (liver cysts, pancreas, heart [abnormal heart valves]), blood vessels (aneurysms), and intestines (diverticulosis). The most serious complication is a cerebral aneurysm, which can rupture.

Diagnosis is based on manifestations, family history, ultrasound, and CT scan.

There is no specific treatment for PKD. A major aim is to prevent or treat UTIs with appropriate antibiotics. Nephrectomy may be necessary for chronic pain, bleeding, or infection. When the patient experiences progressive renal failure, interventions depend on the remaining renal function.

- Dialysis and kidney transplantation may be needed to treat ESRD. Nursing measures are those used for management of ESRD (see Kidney Disease, Chronic). They include diet modification, fluid restriction, drugs (e.g., antihypertensives), and assisting the patient and family in coping with the chronic disease process and financial concerns.
- The patient with the adult form of PKD often has children by the time the disease is diagnosed. Refer the patient and any adult children for genetic counseling.

POLYCYTHEMIA

Description

Polycythemia is the production and presence of increased number of red blood cells (RBCs). The increase in RBCs can be so great that blood circulation is impaired due to the increased blood viscosity and volume.

Pathophysiology

The two types of polycythemia are *primary polycythemia (polycythemia vera)* and *secondary polycythemia* (Fig. 25). Their causes and pathogenesis differ, although their complications and manifestations are similar.

Polycythemia vera is a chronic myeloproliferative disorder. It involves increased production of not only RBCs but also white blood cells (WBCs) and platelets. This leads to enhanced blood viscosity and blood volume and congestion of organs and tissues with blood. Splenomegaly and hepatomegaly are common. Patients have hypercoagulopathies that predispose them to clotting. The disease develops insidiously and follows a chronic, vacillating course. The median age at diagnosis is 60 years, with a slight male predominance.

- Polycythemia vera begins with 1 or more DNA mutations of a single hematopoietic stem cell. Most cases are not inherited but a familial predisposition may exist.

Secondary polycythemia can be either hypoxia-driven or hypoxia-independent. In *hypoxia-driven polycythemia*, hypoxia stimulates erythropoietin (EPO) production in the kidney, which in turn stimulates RBC production. The need for O_2 may result from high altitude, lung or heart disease, defective O_2 transport, or tissue hypoxia. In *hypoxia-independent polycythemia*, cancer or benign tumor tissue makes extra EPO.

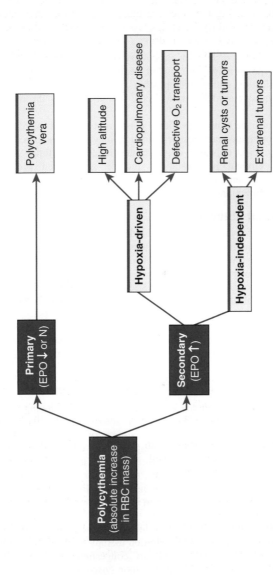

Fig. 25 Differentiating between primary and secondary polycythemia. *EPO*, Erythropoietin; *N*, normal; *RBC*, red blood cell.

Clinical Manifestations

Initial manifestations from hypertension caused by hypervolemia and hyperviscosity include headache, vertigo, dizziness, tinnitus, and visual changes.

- Blood vessel distention, circulatory stasis, thrombosis, and tissue hypoxia may cause angina, heart failure (HF), intermittent claudication, and thrombophlebitis.
- The most common serious acute complication is thrombotic stroke.
- Hemorrhage caused by either vessel rupture from overdistention or inadequate platelet function may result in petechiae, ecchymoses, epistaxis, or gastrointestinal (GI) bleeding.

Other clinical manifestations include generalized pruritus, hepatomegaly and splenomegaly, pain from peptic ulcer, *plethora* (ruddy complexion), hyperuricemia, and gout.

Diagnostic Studies

Diagnostic study abnormalities include:

- High hemoglobin (Hgb), hematocrit, and RBC mass;
- Bone marrow examination shows hypercellularity of RBCs, WBCs, and platelets;
- Presence of JAK2V617F or JAK2exon 12 mutation;
- Low to normal EPO level in polycythemia vera, high EPO level in secondary polycythemia;
- High WBC count with basophilia and neutrophilia;
- High platelets (thrombocytosis) and platelet dysfunction;
- Normal or high leukocyte alkaline phosphatase, uric acid, and cobalamin levels.

Interprofessional and Nursing Management

Treatment of polycythemia vera is directed toward reducing blood volume and viscosity and bone marrow activity. Phlebotomy is the mainstay of treatment to reduce the hematocrit and keep it < 45%. Initially, 300–500 mL of blood may be removed every few days until the hematocrit is reduced to acceptable levels. Phlebotomy may be needed every 2–3 months, reducing the blood volume by about 500 mL each time. A person managed with repeated phlebotomies eventually becomes deficient in iron, although the individual is rarely symptomatic.

- Hydration therapy can reduce the blood viscosity. Assess fluid intake and output during hydration therapy to avoid fluid overload (which worsens circulatory congestion) or fluid deficit (which can make the blood even more viscous).

- Myelosuppressive agents, such as hydroxyurea or busulfan (Myleran) may be given. Ruxolitinib (Jakafi), which inhibits the expression of the JAK2 mutation, is given to patients who have not responded to hydroxyurea.
- α-Interferon (α-IFN) and pegylated interferon are given to women of childbearing age or those with intractable pruritus. Teach the patient about the side effects of the drugs.
- Begin activities and/or medications to decrease thrombus formation. Start active or passive leg exercises and ambulation when possible. Low-dose aspirin can prevent clotting.
- Assess the patient's nutritional status, since inadequate food intake can result from GI symptoms of fullness, pain, and dyspepsia.

Because of its chronic nature, polycythemia vera requires ongoing evaluation. Assess the patient for complications.

PRESSURE INJURY

Description

A *pressure injury* is localized damage to the skin or underlying tissue. It usually occurs over a bony prominence or is related to a medical or other device. The injury occurs because of intense and/or prolonged pressure or pressure in combination with shear. The most common sites for pressure injuries are the sacrum and heels.

Factors influencing pressure injury development include amount of pressure (intensity), length of time pressure is exerted on skin (duration), and ability of patient's tissue to tolerate externally applied pressure. *Shear* (pressure exerted on skin when the surface layer of skin adheres to bedding while deeper skin layers slide in the direction of body movement) and excessive moisture also contribute to pressure injury. The tolerance of soft tissue for pressure and shear is affected by microclimate, nutrition, perfusion, comorbidities, and condition of the soft tissue.

- Patients at risk for the development of pressure injuries are those who are older, incontinent, unable to reposition or unable to feel the need to reposition (e.g., spinal cord injury), and bed- or wheelchair-bound.
- A medical device–related pressure injury results from the use of devices designed and applied for diagnostic or therapeutic purposes. The resulting injury generally conforms to the pattern

or shape of the device. The most implicated devices include splints, braces, indwelling lines, and respiratory devices. The most common site is the ears, from O_2 tubings and masks.

Clinical Manifestations

Pressure injuries are staged on the basis of the visible or palpable tissue in the injury bed. Table 69 shows the pressure injury stages. If the pressure injury becomes infected, the patient may show systemic signs of infection (e.g., leukocytosis, fever).

Interprofessional Management

Pressure injury management requires local wound care as well as support measures such as adequate nutrition, pain management, and pressure relief. Both conservative and surgical strategies are used in the treatment of pressure injuries, depending on the wound's stage and condition.

Nursing Management

Goals

The overall goals are that the patient with a pressure injury will have no deterioration of the wound, not develop an infection in the pressure injury, have healing of pressure injuries, and have no recurrence.

Interventions

Assess patients for pressure injury risk on admission and at periodic intervals, using a validated assessment tool, such as the Braden Scale (available at www.bradenscale.com). Implement prevention strategies for those identified as being at risk for a pressure injury. Table 70 lists guidelines for preventing pressure injuries.

- Reposition patients frequently to prevent pressure injuries. Although the past "standard" was every 2 hours, the frequency of turning and repositioning patients should be individualized on the basis of risk factors and the type of support surface. For example, some high-risk patients may need to be turned and repositioned every hour.

If a pressure injury has developed, document its size, depth, and appearance. Initiate interventions based on the injury's characteristics (e.g., size, stage, location, presence of infection or pain) and the patient's general clinical status. Pressure injuries generally heal by secondary intention. Local injury care may involve debridement, wound cleaning, relief of pressure, and the application of a dressing.

- Necrotic tissue or eschar (except for dry, stable necrotic heels) must be removed by surgical, mechanical, enzymatic, or

TABLE 69 Staging of Pressure Injuries

Definition and Description	Clinical Presentation
Stage 1 Pressure Injury: Nonblanchable Erythema of Intact Skin Intact skin with a localized area of nonblanchable erythema, which may appear differently in dark skin. Blanchable erythema or changes in sensation, temperature, or firmness may precede visual changes. May be hard to detect in persons with dark skin tones.	
Stage 2 Pressure Injury: Partial-Thickness Skin Loss with Exposed Dermis Blister or partial thickness loss of skin with exposed dermis. The wound bed is viable, pink or red, and moist. There is no slough, eschar, or granulation tissue.	

Continued

P

TABLE 69 Staging of Pressure Injuries—cont'd

Definition and Description	Clinical Presentation

Stage 3 pressure Injury: Full-Thickness Skin Loss

Full-thickness tissue loss, in which subcutaneous fat may be visible. Granulation tissue and rolled wound edges are often present. Slough and/or eschar may be visible. Depth of tissue damage varies by anatomical location. Areas of significant adiposity can develop deep wounds. Undermining and tunneling may occur.

Stage 4 Pressure Injury: Full-Thickness Skin and Tissue Loss

Full-thickness skin and tissue loss with involvement of muscle, tendon, ligament, cartilage, or bone. Slough and/or eschar may be visible. Often includes undermining and/or tunneling. Depth varies by anatomical location.

TABLE 69   Staging of Pressure Injuries—cont'd

Definition and Description	Clinical Presentation

Unstageable Pressure Injury: Obscured Full-Thickness Skin and Tissue Loss

Full-thickness skin and tissue loss in which the extent of the injury cannot be determined because the base of the injury is covered by slough or eschar. A stage 3 or stage 4 pressure injury is present after removing slough or eschar. Stable eschar (i.e., dry, adherent, intact without erythema redness or fluctuance) on the heel or ischemic limb should not be softened or removed.

Deep Tissue Pressure Injury (DTPI): Persistent Nonblanchable Deep Red, Maroon, or Purple Discoloration

Intact or nonintact skin with localized area of persistent nonblanchable deep red, maroon, purple discoloration, or epidermal separation revealing a dark wound bed or blood-filled blister. Pain and temperature changes often precede skin color changes. May evolve rapidly to detect in persons with dark skin. May evolve rapidly to reveal the actual extent of tissue injury or may resolve without tissue loss. Visible necrotic tissue, subcutaneous tissue, granulation tissue, fascia, muscle, or other underlying structures indicates a full-thickness pressure injury (Unstageable, stage 3 or stage 4).

Source: European Pressure Ulcer Advisory Panel, National Pressure Injury Advisory Panel and Pan Pacific Pressure Injury Alliance. Prevention and Treatment of Pressure Ulcers/Injuries: Quick reference guide.

P

autolytic debridement methods. Once the pressure injury has been successfully debrided and has a clean granulating base, the goal is to provide an appropriate wound environment that supports moist wound healing and prevents disruption of newly formed granulation tissue.

- Reconstruction of the pressure injury site by operative repair, using skin grafts, skin flaps, musculocutaneous flaps, or free flaps, may be necessary.
- Pressure injuries should be cleaned with noncytotoxic solutions, such as normal saline, which do not kill or damage cells.
- After cleansing the pressure injury, cover it with a proper dressing. (Dressings are discussed in Table 12.14, Harding et al., Lewis' *Medical-Surgical Nursing,* ed 12.)
- Choose appropriate pressure-redistributing techniques (e.g., mattress replacement, mattress overlay, integrated bed system, seat cushion, seat cushion overlay) to move pressure off of areas of pressure injury. Whenever possible, do not turn the patient onto a body surface that has blanchable erythema. Massage is contraindicated in the presence of acute inflammation and where there is the possibility of damaged blood vessels or fragile skin.
- Sliding down in bed causes shear. Encourage patients to reposition themselves by lifting rather than sliding and to use a trapeze if needed. Lift sheets may be used to move patients up in bed or to transfer them.
- Maintaining adequate nutrition is an important nursing responsibility when caring for a patient with a pressure injury. Oral feedings must be adequate in calories, protein, fluids, vitamins, and minerals to meet the patient's nutrition requirements. Enteral feedings or parenteral nutrition can supplement oral feedings.

The patient with a pressure injury often requires extensive care for other health problems, so the patient and caregiver may need your psychosocial support.

▼ **Patient and Caregiver Teaching**

Because recurrence of pressure injuries is common, it is extremely important to teach the patient and caregiver about prevention techniques (see Table 70).

TABLE 70 **Patient and Caregiver Teaching: Pressure Injury**

When teaching the patient or caregiver to prevent and care for pressure injuries, do the following:

1. Identify and explain risk factors and cause of pressure injuries to patient and caregiver.
2. Teach the caregiver techniques for incontinence. If incontinence occurs, cleanse skin at time of soiling and use absorbent pads or briefs.
3. Demonstrate correct positioning to decrease risk of skin breakdown. NEVER position the patient directly on the pressure injury if possible.
4. Teach caregiver to reposition a bed-bound patient at least every 2 hours, a chair-bound patient every hour.
5. Review the available resources (i.e., caregiver's availability and skill, finances, equipment) of patients who need pressure injury care at home.
6. Teach patient and/or caregiver to place clean dressings over sterile dressings using "no touch" technique when changing dressings. Review the disposal of contaminated dressings.
7. Teach patient and caregiver to inspect skin daily. Tell them to report any significant changes to the health care provider.
8. Teach patient and caregiver the importance of good nutrition to enhance injury healing.

PROSTATE CANCER

Description

Prostate cancer is a tumor of the prostate gland. It is the most common cancer among men, excluding skin cancer, and is the second leading cause of cancer death in men (exceeded only by lung cancer). A man has a 1 in 9 risk of developing prostate cancer in his lifetime. More than 3.1 million men in the United States are prostate cancer survivors.

- Black men have the highest rate of prostate cancer.

Pathophysiology

Prostate cancer is a slow-growing androgen-dependent cancer. It is most likely to develop in the outer part of the prostate, called the peripheral zone. Tumor spread is by three routes: direct extension, through the lymph system, or through the bloodstream. Spread by direct extension involves the seminal vesicles, urethral mucosa, bladder wall, and external sphincter. Later spread occurs through the lymphatic system. The bloodstream is the route for spread to the pelvic bones, head of the femur, lower lumbar spine, liver, and lungs.

- The incidence of prostate cancer increases markedly after age 50 years, with a median age at diagnosis of 66 years.
- Dietary factors and obesity may be related to prostate cancer. A diet high in red and processed meats and high-fat dairy products along with a low intake of vegetables and fruits may increase the risk of prostate cancer.
- There is an increased prevalence of prostate cancer among farmers and commercial pesticide applicators, possibly caused by exposure to chemicals.
- It is not clear if smoking is a risk factor.
- Persons with a family history of prostate cancer are at increased risk.

Clinical Manifestations

Prostate cancer usually has no early symptoms. Eventually the patient may have signs and symptoms similar to those of benign prostatic hyperplasia (BPH), including dysuria, hesitancy, dribbling, frequency, urgency, hematuria, nocturia, retention, interruption of urinary stream, and inability to urinate.

- Pain in the lumbosacral area that radiates down to the hips or legs, when coupled with urinary symptoms, may indicate metastasis. As the cancer spreads to the bones, spinal cord compression and bone destruction cause severe back and leg pain.

Diagnostic Studies

Most men in the United States with prostate cancer are diagnosed by prostate-specific antigen (PSA) screening. The discussion about screening should take place at: (1) age 50 years for men who are at average risk of prostate cancer and are expected to live at least 10 more years; (2) age 45 years for men at high risk for development of prostate cancer, including blacks and men who have a first-degree relative (father, brother, or son) diagnosed with prostate cancer at an early age (younger than age 65 years); and (3) age 40 years for men at even higher risk (those with more than 1 first-degree relative who had prostate cancer at an early age).

- Mild elevations in PSA may occur with aging, BPH, recent ejaculation, constipation, or prostatitis, or after long bike rides. Cystoscopy, indwelling urethral catheters, and prostate biopsies may cause transient increases in PSA levels. Decreases in the PSA level can occur with drugs such as finasteride (Proscar) and dutasteride (Avodart). When prostate cancer treatment is successful, PSA levels should fall to undetectable levels.

- On digital rectal examination (DRE), the prostate gland may feel hard, nodular, and asymmetric.
- Biopsy using transrectal ultrasound can confirm the diagnosis.
- CT scan, bone scan, or MRI can assess cancer spread.
- Elevated serum alkaline phosphatase may indicate bone metastasis.

Interprofessional Management
Staging
The most common classification system for determining the extent of the prostate cancer is the tumor-node-metastasis (TNM) system (see TNM Classification System).

Currently, the Gleason score and the Grade Group system (Table 71) are used together with the TNM system to determine the stage of the tumor.

- Most patients with prostate cancer are diagnosed when the cancer is in either a local or a regional stage. The 5-year survival rate with a diagnosis at these stages is 100%.

The decision of which treatment course to pursue should be made jointly by patients, their partners, and the interprofessional team.

- A conservative approach to slow-growing tumors is active surveillance or "watchful waiting." This strategy is appropriate for: (1) a life expectancy of <10 years (low risk of dying of the disease), (2) the presence of a low-grade, low-stage tumor, and (3) serious coexisting medical conditions. Patients are monitored with frequent PSA testing and DREs. Significant changes in PSA level, DRE findings, or symptoms warrant a reevaluation of treatment options.

Surgical Therapy
With radical prostatectomy, the entire prostate gland, seminal vesicles, and part of the bladder neck (ampulla) are removed. Retroperitoneal lymph node dissection is performed only on men with a high risk for metastatic disease. A pelvic lymph node dissection is typically done at the same time as prostatectomy to pathologically assess for nodal metastases in the local pelvic area. Typically, a higher number of lymph nodes are removed and dissected if the prostate cancer is higher grade/higher risk on biopsy. Surgery is not an option for advanced-stage disease, except to relieve symptoms associated with obstruction.

- Traditional approaches for radical prostatectomy are retropubic (low abdominal incision) and perineal (incision between the scrotum and anus).

TABLE 71 Staging of Prostate Cancer

Stage	Tumor Size	Lymph Node Involvement	Metastasis	PSA Level	Gleason Score
I	Not felt on DRE Not seen by visual imaging	No	No	<10	≤6
II	Felt on DRE Seen by imaging Tumor confined to prostate	No	No	10–20	6–7
III	Cancer outside prostate Possible spread to seminal vesicles	No	No	Any level	Any score
IV	Any size	Any nodal involvement	Yes	Any level	Any score

DRE, Digital rectal examination; *PSA,* prostate-specific antigen.
Adapted from American Cancer Society: How is prostate cancer staged? Retrieved from www.cancer.org/Cancer/ProstateCancer/DetailedGuide/prostate-cancer-staging.

- Robotic-assisted (e.g., da Vinci system) laparoscopic prostatectomy is associated with less bleeding, less pain, and a faster
  recovery.
- After surgery, the patient has a large indwelling catheter with
  a 20- or 30-mL balloon placed in the bladder via the urethra. A
  drain is left in the surgical site.

Two major adverse outcomes after a radical prostatectomy are
erectile dysfunction (ED) and urinary incontinence.

- The incidence of ED depends on the patient's age, preoperative
  sexual functioning, whether nerve-sparing surgery was done,
  and the expertise of the surgeon. A nerve-sparing technique is
  sometimes used to reduce the risk of ED.
- Problems with urinary control may occur for the first few
  months because the bladder must be reattached to the urethra
  after the prostate is removed. Kegel exercises strengthen the
  pelvic floor muscles and the urinary sphincter and may help
  improve continence.

Cryotherapy is a surgical technique that destroys cancer cells by
freezing. The treatment takes about 2 hours, with the patient under
general or spinal anesthesia.

A bilateral orchiectomy is the surgical removal of the testes
that may be done alone or in combination with prostatectomy for
advanced stages of prostate.

Radiation Therapy
Radiation therapy is a common option as the only treatment, or
in combination with surgery or hormonal therapy. (See Radiation
Therapy.) Salvage radiation therapy for cancer recurrence after a
radical prostatectomy may improve survival.

- External beam radiation is the most widely used method.
  Brachytherapy using radioactive seed implants placed in the
  prostate gland is best suited for patients with early-stage disease.

Drug Therapy
The types of drug therapy available for the treatment of advanced
or metastatic prostate cancer are androgen deprivation (hormone)
therapy, chemotherapy, or a combination.

Androgen deprivation therapy (ADT) is focused on reducing the
levels of circulating androgens to reduce the tumor growth. Almost
all tumors treated will become resistant to ADT therapy *(hormone-
refractory)* within a few years. Androgen deprivation can be produced
by inhibiting androgen production or blocking androgen receptors.

- Luteinizing hormone–releasing hormone (LHRH) agonists
  (e.g., goserelin [Zoladex], leuprolide [Lupron, Eligard], trip-
  torelin [Trelstar]) produce a chemical castration similar to the
  effects of an orchiectomy.

- Degarelix (Firmagon) is an LHRH antagonist. It lowers testosterone levels to castration levels.
- Androgen receptor blockers such as bicalutamide (Casodex), enzalutamide (Xtandi), apalutamide (Erleada), darolutamide (Nubeqa), and nilutamide (Nilandron) compete with circulating androgens at the receptor sites.
- Combining an androgen receptor blocker with an LHRH agonist results in combined androgen blockade.

Chemotherapy is generally reserved for patients with hormone-refractory prostate cancer (HRPC) in late-stage disease. The goal of chemotherapy is palliative (see Chemotherapy).

- Men with advanced prostate cancer who have HRPC may receive a vaccine (sipuleucel-T [Provenge]). The vaccine stimulates the patient's system against the cancer and may prolong survival.

Nursing Management

Goals

The patient with prostate cancer will be an active participant in the treatment plan, have acceptable pain control, follow the therapeutic plan, understand the effect of the therapeutic plan on sexual function, and find an acceptable way to manage the impact on bladder or bowel function.

Interventions

One of your most important roles is to encourage patients to have an annual prostate screening (PSA and DRE).

- Provide support for the patient and the family to help them cope with the cancer diagnosis.
- Care during the preoperative and postoperative phases of radical prostatectomy is similar to that with surgical procedures for BPH (see BPH).
- See Radiation Therapy, Chemotherapy for nursing interventions.
- Pain control is the primary nursing intervention for the terminally ill patient. It is managed through pain assessment, giving prescribed medications (both opioid and nonopioid agents), and nonpharmacologic methods of pain relief (e.g., relaxation breathing).
- In advanced prostate cancer, palliative and end-of-life care is often appropriate and beneficial.

▼ Patient and Caregiver Teaching

Teach appropriate catheter care for the patient discharged with an indwelling catheter in place.

- Teach the patient to clean the urethral meatus with soap and water once each day; maintain a high oral fluid intake; keep the collecting bag lower than the bladder at all times; keep the catheter securely anchored to the inner thigh or abdomen; and report any signs of bladder infection such as bladder spasms, fever, or hematuria.

If urinary incontinence is a problem, encourage the patient to practice pelvic floor muscle exercises (Kegel) with urination and throughout the day. Continuous practice during the 4–6-week healing process improves the success rate.

PSORIATIC ARTHRITIS

Psoriatic arthritis (PsA) is a progressive, inflammatory disease affecting about 30% of the people with psoriasis. *Psoriasis* is a common, benign, inflammatory skin disorder characterized by the presence of red, irritated, and scaly patches.

- Both PsA and psoriasis appear to have a genetic link with human leukocyte antigens (HLAs) in many patients. Although the exact cause of PsA is unknown, a combination of immune, genetic, and environmental factors is suspected.

PsA can occur in different forms. *Asymmetric oligoarthritis* involves different joints on each side of the body. *Symmetric polyarthritis* resembles RA. It affects joints on both sides of the body at the same time. These two forms are the most common types of PsA. *Distal interphalangeal predominant PsA* involves the ends of the fingers and toes. The patient often has pitting and color changes in the fingernails and toenails. *Spondylitis* is marked by pain and stiffness in the spine and neck. *Arthritis mutilans* affects less than 5% of people with PsA. It is the most severe form of the disease, causing complete destruction of small joints.

- On X-ray, cartilage loss and erosion are similar to those seen in RA. Advanced cases of PsA often reveal widened joint spaces.
- A "pencil in cup" deformity is common in the distal interphalangeal (DIP) joints as a result of thin, weakened bone. In this deformity, the narrowed end of the affected metacarpals or phalanges inserts into the expanded end of the other (adjacent) bone sharing the joint.
- Elevated erythrocyte sedimentation rate (ESR), elevated serum uric acid, and mild anemia are seen in some patients. Therefore, the diagnosis of gout must be excluded.

Treatment includes splinting, joint protection, and physical therapy. Nonsteroidal antiinflammatory drugs (NSAIDs) may help with inflammation early in the course of the disease. Drug therapy includes disease-modifying antirheumatic drugs (DMARDs), such as methotrexate. They are effective for both articular and skin manifestations. Sulfasalazine, cyclosporine, and BRMs (e.g., etanercept, golimumab, adalimumab, infliximab) may be used. Apremilast (Otezla), a phosphodiesterase-4 inhibitor, can treat adults with active PsA.

P

PULMONARY EMBOLISM

Description

Pulmonary embolism (PE) is the blockage of pulmonary arteries by a thrombus, fat, or air embolus or tumor tissue. An *embolus* is a mobile clot that travels with blood flow through ever-smaller blood vessels until it lodges and obstructs the pulmonary circulation. Most PEs arise from deep vein thrombosis (DVT) formed in the deep leg veins. Other sites of origin of PE include femoral or iliac veins, right side of the heart (atrial fibrillation), pelvic veins (especially after surgery or childbirth) or upper extremities. *Venous thromboembolism (VTE)* is the preferred term to describe the spectrum of pathologic conditions from DVT to PE.

■ Risk factors for PE include immobility or reduced mobility, surgery within the last 3 months (especially pelvic and lower extremity surgery), history of DVT, cancer, obesity, oral contraceptives, hormone therapy, cigarette smoking, prolonged air travel, heart failure, pregnancy, and clotting disorders.

Approximately 10% of patients with massive PE die within the first hour. Treatment with anticoagulants significantly reduces mortality.

Clinical Manifestations

Manifestations of PE are varied and nonspecific, making diagnosis hard.

■ Dyspnea occurs in 85% of patients with PE.
■ Other signs and symptoms are hypoxemia, tachypnea, cough, chest pain, hemoptysis, crackles, wheezing, fever, accentuation of the pulmonic heart sound, tachycardia, and syncope.
■ Massive PE may cause a sudden change in mental status, hypotension, feelings of impending doom, shock, and cardiorespiratory arrest.
■ Small emboli may go undetected or cause vague, transient symptoms. However, in the patient with underlying conditions, even small emboli may result in severe compromise.

Complications

Pulmonary infarction (death of lung tissue) is most likely when there is occlusion of a large or medium-sized pulmonary vessel (more than 2 mm in diameter), insufficient collateral blood flow from the bronchial circulation, or preexisting lung disease. Infarction results in alveolar necrosis and hemorrhage with pleural effusion.

Pulmonary hypertension results from hypoxemia or involvement of a large surface area of the pulmonary bed. A single embolus rarely causes pulmonary hypertension. Recurrent emboli may result in *chronic thromboembolic pulmonary hypertension*, leading to dilation and hypertrophy of the right ventricle. Outcomes can vary. Some patients die within months and others live for decades (see Pulmonary Hypertension).

Diagnostic Studies

- Spiral (or helical) CT scan is the most common test for diagnosis of PE. If the patient cannot have the contrast media used in a spiral CT, then a ventilation-perfusion (V/Q) scan is done.
- D-dimer testing assists in screening for a clotting condition such as an embolism.
- Arterial blood gases (ABGs) may show hypoxemia.

Interprofessional Management

Treatment is started as soon as PE is suspected. The goals are to facilitate optimal cardiorespiratory function, ensure adequate blood flow, prevent further growth or extension of thrombi, and prevent and avoid further recurrence and any complications. Supportive therapy varies according to the severity of the PE.

- O_2 needs are determined by ABG analysis. Mask, cannula, or endotracheal intubation and mechanical ventilation may be used to maintain oxygenation.
- Respiratory measures such as turning, coughing, deep breathing, and incentive spirometry help prevent or treat atelectasis.
- If shock is present, fluids and vasopressor agents are given as needed to support circulation. If heart failure is present, diuretics are used.

Immediate coagulation is required for patients with PE. Subcutaneous administration of low-molecular-weight heparin (LMWH) (e.g., enoxaparin, fragmin, fondaparinux) is the recommended treatment for patients with acute PE. LMWH is safer and more effective than unfractionated heparin. Warfarin (Coumadin), an oral anticoagulant, should be started at the time of diagnosis. Warfarin should be given for at least 3–6 months and then reevaluated. Alternatives to warfarin include apixaban (Eliquis), dabigitran (Pradaxa), and edoxaban (Savaysa). Anticoagulant therapy may be contraindicated if the patient has complicating factors related to clotting.

- Fibrinolytic agents, such as the tissue plasminogen activator alteplase (Activase), may be used to dissolve the PE lesion as well as the clots at the thrombus source.

Hemodynamically unstable patients with massive PE and contra-indications to fibrinolytic therapy may be candidates for pulmonary embolectomy. This can be done via a diagnostic imaging (vascular catheter) or surgical approach. Percutaneous interventional techniques, surgical embolectomy, ultrasound-guided catheter thrombolysis, and aspiration thrombectomy are newer, moderately invasive procedures for PE.

In patients who are at high risk and patients for whom anticoagulation is contraindicated, an inferior vena cava (IVC) filter may be the treatment of choice.

Nursing Management

Prevention of PE begins with prevention of DVT. Identification of the "at risk" patient is essential.

- Nursing measures aimed at prevention of PE are similar to those for prophylaxis of VTE (see Venous Thrombosis). These include the use of intermittent pneumatic compression devices, early ambulation, and anticoagulant medications.

The prognosis for a patient with acute PE is good if therapy is instituted promptly. Keep the patient in bed in a semi-Fowler's position to facilitate breathing. Maintain an IV line for drugs and fluid therapy. Administer O_2 therapy as ordered. Carefully monitor vital signs, ABGs, cardiac rhythm, pulse oximetry, and lung sounds to assess the patient's clinical status.

- The patient may be anxious because of pain, inability to breathe, and fear of death. Provide information emotional support and reassurance to help relieve the patient's anxiety.
- Monitor laboratory results to ensure therapeutic ranges of INR (for warfarin) and aPTT (for IV heparin). Monitor platelet counts for thrombocytopenia and the development of heparin-induced thrombocytopenia (see HIT).
- Observe the patient for complications of anticoagulant and fibri-nolytic therapy (e.g., bleeding, bruising). Implement fall pre-cautions once the patient can be out of bed.

▼ Patient and Caregiver Teaching

- Long-term management is similar to that for the patient with VTE (see Venous Thrombosis).
- Patient teaching regarding long-term anticoagulant therapy is critical. Patients with recurrent emboli are treated with antico-agulants indefinitely. INR levels are obtained at intervals, and warfarin dosage is adjusted accordingly.
- Discharge planning is aimed at preventing worsening of the current condition and avoiding complications and recurrence. Reinforce the need for the patient to return to the health care provider for regular follow-up care.

PULMONARY HYPERTENSION

Description

Pulmonary hypertension is elevated pulmonary artery pressure (greater than 20 mm Hg) from increased resistance to blood flow through the pulmonary circulation. Pulmonary hypertension can occur as a primary disease (idiopathic pulmonary arterial hypertension) or as a secondary complication of a respiratory, heart, autoimmune, hepatic, or connective tissue disorder (secondary pulmonary arterial hypertension).

Idiopathic pulmonary arterial hypertension (IPAH) is pulmonary hypertension that occurs without an apparent cause. It is associated with connective tissue diseases, cirrhosis, and human immunodeficiency virus (HIV) infection. Untreated IPAH can cause right-sided heart failure (HF) and death within a few years.

Pathophysiology

An insult (e.g., hormonal, mechanical) to the pulmonary endothelium may cause a cascade of events leading to vascular scarring, endothelial dysfunction, and smooth muscle proliferation. IPAH affects more females.

Clinical Manifestations

Classic symptoms are dyspnea on exertion and fatigue. Exertional chest pain, dizziness, and syncope may occur. As the disease progresses, dyspnea occurs at rest. Pulmonary hypertension increases the workload of the right ventricle and causes right ventricular hypertrophy (a condition called *cor pulmonale*) (see Cor Pulmonale) and eventually HF (see Heart Failure).

- Right-sided cardiac catheterization is the definitive test to diagnose pulmonary hypertension. By the time patients become symptomatic, the pulmonary artery pressure is 2–3 times normal value.
- Confirmation of IPAH requires excluding conditions that may cause secondary pulmonary arterial hypertension. Diagnostic evaluation includes electrocardiography (ECG), chest X-ray, pulmonary function testing, echocardiogram, and CT scan.

Interprofessional and Nursing Management

Treatment can relieve symptoms, improve quality of life, and prolong life. Drug therapy consists of agents that dilate the pulmonary blood vessels, reduce right ventricular overload, and reverse remodeling

P

- Diuretics are used to manage peripheral edema.
- Anticoagulants reduce the risk of thrombus formation.
- Because hypoxia is a potent pulmonary vasoconstrictor, low-flow O_2 gives symptomatic relief. The goal is to keep O_2 saturation 90% or greater.

Surgical interventions include pulmonary thromboendarterectomy (PTE), in which clots are removed from the pulmonary arteries. Atrial septostomy is a palliative procedure that involves creating an intraatrial right-to-left shunt to decompress the right ventricle. It is used for some patients awaiting lung transplantation. A lung transplant is indicated for patients who do not respond to drug therapy and progress to severe right-sided HF.

Secondary Pulmonary Arterial Hypertension

Secondary pulmonary arterial hypertension (SPAH) occurs when another disease causes anatomic or vascular changes with a chronic increase in pulmonary artery pressures. SPAH can develop because of parenchymal lung disease, left ventricular dysfunction, intracardiac shunts, chronic PE, or systemic connective tissue disease. Diagnosis of SPAH is similar to that of IPAH.

- Symptoms include dyspnea, fatigue, lethargy, and chest pain.
- Treatment of SPAH consists mainly of treating the underlying primary disorder. When irreversible pulmonary vascular damage has occurred, therapies used for IPAH are started.

PYELONEPHRITIS

Description

Pyelonephritis is an inflammation of the renal parenchyma and collecting system (including the renal pelvis). The most common cause is bacterial infection. *Urosepsis* is a systemic infection arising from a urologic source. If not treated promptly, it can lead to septic shock and death (see Shock).

Pathophysiology

Pyelonephritis usually begins with infection of the lower urinary tract via the urethra. Bacteria normally found in the intestinal tract, including *E. coli* or *Proteus, Klebsiella,* or *Enterobacter* species, often cause pyelonephritis. A preexisting factor can be present, such as *vesicoureteral reflux* (retrograde [backward] movement of urine from lower to upper urinary tract) or dysfunction of the lower urinary tract (e.g., obstruction from benign prostatic hyperplasia [BPH], stricture, stones).

- Pregnancy-induced changes in the urinary system are an important risk factor for acute pyelonephritis.
- For residents of long-term care facilities, catheter-associated urinary tract infections (CAUTIs) are common causes of pyelonephritis and urosepsis.
- *Acute pyelonephritis* often starts in the renal medulla and spreads to the adjacent cortex.
- In *chronic pyelonephritis*, the kidneys are continually infected. This leads to inflammation and fibrosis (scarring). There may be a loss of renal function and renal atrophy (shrinkage). Chronic pyelonephritis is usually the result of significant anatomic abnormalities, such as vesicoureteral reflux or recurring infections involving the upper urinary tract. It can rarely occur due to a substantial inflammatory response from an infection. It often progresses to end-stage renal disease (ESRD) when both the kidneys are involved, even if the underlying infection or problem is successfully eradicated (see Kidney Disease, Chronic).

Clinical Manifestations

The classic manifestations of acute pyelonephritis include fever, chills, nausea, vomiting, malaise, and flank pain with costovertebral angle (CVA) tenderness to percussion on the affected side. Lower urinary tract symptoms such as dysuria, urgency, and frequency may also be present.

Diagnostic Studies

- Urinalysis may show pyuria, bacteriuria, hematuria, and white blood cell (WBC) casts.
- Complete blood count (CBC) count with WBC differential identifies leukocytosis.
- Urine and blood cultures with sensitivities identify the infecting organism.
- Ultrasound helps identify anatomic abnormalities, hydronephrosis, renal abscesses, or stones.

Chronic pyelonephritis is diagnosed by radiologic imaging and biopsy rather than clinical features. A renal biopsy can show the loss of functioning nephrons, infiltration of the parenchyma with inflammatory cells, and fibrosis.

Interprofessional and Nursing Management

Goals for the patient with pyelonephritis include normal renal function, no complications, relief of pain, and no recurrence of symptoms. Patients with severe infections or complicating factors, such as nausea and vomiting with dehydration, require hospital admission.

- Parenteral antibiotics are often given initially in the hospital to rapidly establish high drug levels.

The patient with mild symptoms may be treated as an outpatient with antibiotics for 7–14 days. Symptoms and signs typically improve or resolve within 48–72 hours after starting therapy. Relapses may be treated with a 6-week course of antibiotics. Antibiotic prophylaxis may also be used for recurrent infections.

- Emphasize continuing medications as prescribed, having a follow-up urine culture, and recognizing manifestations of recurrence. Stress the need for regular health care.
- Encourage the patient to drink at least 8 glasses of fluid every day, even after the infection has been treated.

RAYNAUD'S PHENOMENON

Description

Raynaud's phenomenon is an episodic vasospastic disorder of the small cutaneous arteries, most often in the fingers and toes. It occurs more often in women 15–40 years of age. Abnormalities in the vascular, intravascular, and neuronal mechanisms cause an imbalance between vasodilation and vasoconstriction.

Primary Raynaud's phenomenon occurs in isolation while secondary Raynaud's phenomenon occurs with an underlying disease (e.g., thyroid conditions, rheumatoid arthritis, scleroderma, systemic lupus erythematosus). Other contributing factors include use of vibrating machinery or work in cold environments, exposure to heavy metals (e.g., lead), and high homocysteine levels.

Clinical Manifestations

Cold exposure, stress, tobacco use, and caffeine often trigger symptoms.

- The disorder is characterized by vasospasm-induced color changes (white, red, and blue) of fingers, toes, ears, and nose. Decreased perfusion results in pallor (white). The digits then become cyanotic (bluish purple). These changes are subsequently followed by rubor (red), caused by the hyperemic response when blood flow is restored.
- The patient usually describes cold and numbness in the vasoconstrictive phase, with throbbing and aching pain, tingling, and

swelling in the hyperemic phase. An episode usually lasts only minutes but may persist for several hours.

- The skin may become thickened and the nails brittle. Complications include punctate lesions (small holes) of the fingertips and superficial gangrenous ulcers in advanced stages.
- Diagnosis is based on persistent symptoms for at least 2 years.

Interprofessional and Nursing Management

Sustained-release calcium-channel blockers (e.g., nifedipine [Procardia]) relax smooth muscles of the arterioles by blocking the influx of calcium into the cells. This reduces the frequency and severity of vasospastic attacks.

- Other vasodilators (e.g., phosphodiesterase-5 inhibitors [sildenafil]) or topical nitroglycerin 2% ointment may be used.

Prompt intervention is needed for patients with digital ulceration or critical ischemia. Treatment options include prostacyclin infusion therapy (e.g., iloprost), antibiotics, analgesics, and surgical debridement of necrotic tissue. Botulinum toxin A and statins may lessen the severity of Raynaud's phenomenon. Sympathectomy is considered in advanced cases.

▼ Patient and Caregiver Teaching

Teaching should be directed toward preventing recurrent episodes.

- Loose, warm clothing should be worn for protection from cold, including gloves for working in a refrigerator or freezer or handling cold objects.
- Temperature extremes should be avoided. Immersing hands in warm water often decreases the spasm.
- Patients should stop using all tobacco products and avoid caffeine and other drugs with vasoconstrictive effects (e.g., pseudoephedrine).
- Provide patients with information about stress management techniques.

REACTIVE ARTHRITIS

Reactive arthritis (*Reiter's syndrome*) is associated with a symptom complex that includes urethritis (in men) or cervicitis (in women), conjunctivitis, and mucocutaneous lesions. It occurs more often in young men.

- Although the exact cause is unknown, reactive arthritis appears to be a reaction triggered in the body after exposure to specific genitourinary or gastrointestinal (GI) tract infections. *Chlamydia trachomatis* is spread through sexual contact.

- Reactive arthritis is also associated with GI infections from *Shigella, Salmonella, Campylobacter,* or *Yersinia* species and other microorganisms.

Those who are positive for human leukocyte antigen (HLA)-B27 are at increased risk for developing reactive arthritis after sexual contact or exposure to certain gastrointestinal pathogens.

- Urethritis or cervicitis develops within 1–2 weeks after sexual contact or GI infection. Low-grade fever, conjunctivitis, and arthritis may occur over the next several weeks.
- This arthritis tends to be asymmetric, often involving the toes and the large joints of the lower extremities. Lower back pain may occur with severe disease.
- Lesions commonly occur as small, painless, superficial ulcerations on the tongue, oral mucosa, and glans penis. Soft tissue manifestations include Achilles tendinitis or plantar fasciitis.
- The erythrocyte sedimentation rate (ESR) may be elevated.

Most patients recover within a few months. Because *C. trachomatis* can cause reactive arthritis, treatment with doxycycline is recommended for patients and their sexual partners. Antibiotics have no effect on arthritis or other symptoms. Conjunctivitis and skin lesions generally do not need treatment. Topical ophthalmic corticosteroids are helpful for uveitis. Drug therapy may also include nonsteroidal antiinflammatory drugs (NSAIDs) and disease-modifying antirheumatic drugs (DMARDs). Physical therapy may be helpful during recovery.

REFRACTIVE ERRORS

Refractive errors are the most common visual problem. Irregularities in corneal curvature, lens-focusing power, or eye length prevent light rays from converging to a point on the retina. Types of refractive errors include:

- *Myopia* (nearsightedness), the most common refractive error, is an inability to accommodate for objects at a distance. It causes light rays to be focused in front of the retina. The person can see near objects but distant objects are blurred.
- *Hyperopia* (farsightedness) is an inability to accommodate for near objects. It causes the light rays to focus behind the retina. The person with hyperopia can see distant objects clearly but near objects are blurred.
- *Presbyopia* is an age-related loss of accommodation with an inability to focus on near objects. The lens becomes larger,

firmer, and less elastic. The condition generally becomes noticeable in the early to mid-40s.

- *Astigmatism* is an uneven or irregular curvature of the cornea.
Incoming light rays are bent unequally, causing visual distortion. Astigmatism can occur with any of the other refractive
errors.

Refractive errors cause blurred vision. Patients may report ocular discomfort, eye strain, or headaches. Vision correction options
include eyeglasses, contact lenses, refractive surgery, or surgical
implantation of an artificial lens.

RESPIRATORY FAILURE, ACUTE

Description

Acute respiratory failure (ARF) occurs when oxygenation, ventilation, or both are inadequate. ARF is not a disease, but a condition
that reflects insufficient lung function. In ARF, not enough O_2 is
transferred to the blood or an inadequate amount of CO_2 is removed
from the lungs. ARF occurs with problems involving the lungs or
other body systems (Table 72).

Conditions that interfere with O_2 diffusion result in *hypoxemia,*
a decrease in arterial O_2 (PaO_2), and saturation (SaO_2) to less than
normal values. Insufficient CO_2 removal results in hypercapnia.
This is an increase in arterial CO_2 ($PaCO_2$). Arterial blood gases
(ABGs) are used to assess changes in pH, PaO_2, $PaCO_2$, bicarbonate, and SaO_2. We use pulse oximetry (SpO_2) to assess arterial O_2
saturation noninvasively.

ARF is classified as hypoxemic or hypercapnic.

- *Hypoxemic respiratory failure* (also called *oxygenation failure*),
is defined as a $PaO_2 < 60$ mm Hg when the patient is receiving an
inspired O_2 concentration of 60% or more. The main problem
is inadequate exchange of O_2 between the alveoli and pulmonary capillaries. The SaO_2 level shows low O_2 saturation in the
patient despite receiving supplemental O_2.
- *Hypercapnic respiratory failure* (or *ventilatory failure*)
is defined as a $PaCO_2 > 50$ mm Hg with acidemia (arterial
pH < 7.35). The main problem is insufficient CO_2 removal. This
causes the $PaCO_2$ to be higher than normal and acidemia occurs.

Major changes in PaO_2 and $PaCO_2$ with ARF may develop over
minutes to hours. The patient may have hemodynamic instability
(e.g., tachycardia, hypotension), increased respiratory effort, and
decreased level of consciousness. Urgent intervention is needed.

R

TABLE 72 Common Causes of Respiratory Failure	
Hypoxemic Respiratory Failure	**Hypercapnic Respiratory Failure**
ARDS	
Asthma	
Chronic Bronchitis	
Emphysema	
Pulmonary Edema	
Respiratory System	**Respiratory System**
• Bronchiectasis	• COPD
• Hepatopulmonary syndrome (e.g., low-resistance flow state, V/Q mismatch)	• Cystic fibrosis
	• Hypoventilation syndrome (causes include CNS, obesity, chest wall, and neuromuscular)
• Pneumonia	• Upper airway obstruction
• Pneumothorax	**Chest wall**
• Pulmonary embolism (e.g., thrombus emboli, fat emboli)	• Kyphoscoliosis
• Pulmonary fibrosis	• Pain
• Toxic inhalation (e.g., smoke inhalation)	• Severe obesity
	• Thoracic trauma (e.g., flail chest)
Cardiac	**CNS**
• Anatomic shunt (e.g., ventricular septal defect)	• Brainstem injury or infarction
• Cardiogenic pulmonary edema	• Sedative and opioid overdose
	• Severe head injury
• Cardiogenic shock (decreasing blood flow through pulmonary vasculature)	• Spinal cord injury
	Neuromuscular
• High CO states: diffusion limitation	• Amyotrophic lateral sclerosis
	• Critical illness polyneuropathy
	• Guillain-Barré syndrome
	• Muscular dystrophy
	• Multiple sclerosis
	• Myasthenia gravis
	• Phrenic nerve injury
	• Poliomyelitis
	• Toxin exposure or ingestion

Chronic respiratory failure develops more slowly, over several days to weeks. The patient is usually more stable as the body had time to compensate for the small, but subtle, changes that have occurred.

■ Patients may have acute and chronic respiratory failure at the same time. This happens when a patient with a chronic respiratory problem develops a new acute problem. For example, a patient with chronic obstructive pulmonary disease (COPD) who has pneumonia could have "acute-on-chronic" respiratory failure.

Pathophysiology

Hypoxemic Respiratory Failure

Four physiologic mechanisms may cause respiratory failure: (1) mismatch between ventilation (V) and perfusion (Q), referred to as *V/Q mismatch*; (2) shunt; (3) diffusion limitation; and (4) hypoventilation. The most common causes are V/Q mismatch and shunt.

- Many diseases and conditions cause V/Q mismatch. The most common ones involve increased secretions in the airways (e.g., COPD) or alveoli (e.g., pneumonia) or bronchospasms (e.g., asthma). V/Q mismatch may result from pain, alveolar collapse (atelectasis), or pulmonary emboli.

- *Shunt* occurs when blood exits the heart without having taken part in gas exchange. A shunt is an extreme V/Q mismatch. O_2 therapy alone is not effective in increasing the PaO_2 if hypoxemia is caused by shunt.

- *Diffusion limitation* occurs when gas exchange across the alveolar-capillary membrane is compromised by a process that damages the alveolar membrane or affects blood flow through the pulmonary capillaries. Conditions that cause the alveolar-capillary membrane to become thicker (fibrotic) slow gas transport. These include pulmonary fibrosis, interstitial lung disease, and acute respiratory distress syndrome (ARDS). An accumulation of fluid, white blood cells, or protein in the alveoli can decrease gas exchange between the alveolus and the capillary bed. This occurs in pulmonary edema. The classic sign of diffusion limitation is hypoxemia that worsens with exercise.

- *Alveolar hypoventilation* is a decrease in ventilation that results in an increase in the $PaCO_2$. Alveolar hypoventilation may be caused by central nervous system (CNS) conditions, chest wall dysfunction, acute asthma, or restrictive lung diseases. Although alveolar hypoventilation is mainly a mechanism of hypercapnic respiratory failure, it contributes to hypoxemia.

Frequently, hypoxemic respiratory failure is caused by a combination of V/Q mismatch, shunt, diffusion limitation, and alveolar hypoventilation.

Hypercapnic Respiratory Failure

In acute hypercapnic respiratory failure (*ventilatory failure*), the respiratory system cannot maintain the CO_2 level within normal limits. This occurs from increased CO_2 production or decreased alveolar ventilation. Hypercapnic respiratory failure can be acute or chronic.

R

- Conditions that cause impaired ventilation are CNS problems, neuromuscular problems, chest wall problems, or conditions affecting the airways and/or alveoli (see Table 72).

Clinical Manifestations

Signs of respiratory failure are related to the extent of change in PaO_2 or $PaCO_2$, the speed of change (acute or chronic), and the patient's ability to compensate. A lack of O_2 or excess of CO_2 affects all body systems (see Table 73).

One of the first signs of hypoxemic ARF is a change in mental status (restlessness, confusion, agitation) because the brain is extremely sensitive to inadequate O_2 and acid–base balance. Permanent brain damage can result if hypoxia is severe and prolonged. On the other hand, a morning headache and slow respiratory rate with decreased level of consciousness may indicate problems with CO_2 removal.

- Tachycardia, tachypnea, slight diaphoresis, and mild hypertension are early signs of ARF. These changes indicate attempts by the heart and lungs to compensate for decreased O_2 and rising CO_2 levels.
- Cyanosis is an unreliable indicator of hypoxemia. It is a late sign in ARF that often does not occur until hypoxemia is severe (PaO_2 45 mm Hg or less).

Observing the patient's position helps assess the *work of breathing* (WOB), the effort needed by the respiratory muscles to move air into the lungs. In moderate distress, patients may prefer to sit. With severe distress, they may be unable to breathe unless sitting upright.

- The tripod position helps decrease the WOB in patients with moderate to severe COPD and ARF. The patient sits with the arms propped on the overbed table or on the knees. Propping the arms increases the anteroposterior diameter of the chest and changes pressure in the thorax.

The patient in ARF may have a rapid, shallow breathing pattern (hypoxemia) or a slower respiratory rate (hypercapnia). Increased respiratory rates require a substantial amount of work and can lead to respiratory muscle fatigue. A change from a rapid rate to a slower rate in a patient in respiratory distress, such as with acute asthma, suggests severe respiratory muscle fatigue and increased chance of respiratory arrest.

- The dyspneic patient may be able to speak only a few words at a time between breaths.
- Dyspneic patients may be using pursed-lip breathing. This technique increases PaO_2 by slowing respirations, increasing

TABLE 73 Common Manifestations of Hypoxemia and Hypercapnia

Specific	Nonspecific
Hypoxemia	
Respiratory	*Cardiovascular*
Accessory muscle use	↑ BP (early), ↓BP (late)
Dyspnea	Dysrhythmias (late)
Intercostal muscle	↑ HR
retraction	Skin cool, clammy, and diaphoretic
Nasal flaring	*CNS*
Paradoxical chest or	Agitation
abdominal wall	Confusion
movement with	Disorientation
respiratory cycle (late)	↓ Level of consciousness
Prolonged expiration	Restless, combative behavior
↓ SpO$_2$ (<90%)	Coma (late)
Tachypnea	*Other*
Cyanosis (late)	Fatigue
	Inability to speak in complete sentences
	without pausing to breathe
Hypercapnia	
Respiratory	*Cardiovascular*
Dyspnea	↑ BP
Limited chest wall	Dysrhythmias
movement	↑ HR
Pursed-lip breathing	*CNS*
Tripod position	Agitation
↓ Respiratory rate or	Confusion, disorientation
rapid rate with shallow	Morning headache
respirations	Progressive somnolence
↓ Tidal volume	↑ ICP
↓ Minute ventilation	Coma (late)
	Neuromuscular
	↓ Deep tendon reflexes
	Muscle weakness
	Tremors, seizures (late)

R

time for expiration, and preventing small bronchioles from collapsing.

- You may see *retraction* (inward movement) of the intercostal spaces or supraclavicular area and accessory muscles use (e.g., sternocleidomastoid) with a moderate degree of respiratory distress.

- *Paradoxical breathing* occurs with severe respiratory distress. With paradoxical breathing, the abdomen and chest move in the opposite manner—outward during exhalation and inward during inspiration.

Fine crackles may occur with pulmonary edema. Coarse crackles heard on expiration indicate fluid in the airways. This may be a sign of pneumonia or heart failure (HF). Absent or decreased breath sounds occur with atelectasis, pleural effusion, or hypoventilation. Bronchial breath sounds over the lung periphery occur with lung consolidation from pneumonia. You may hear a pleural friction rub if pneumonia involves the pleura.

Diagnostic Studies

- ABGs determine the levels of $PaCO_2$, PaO_2, bicarbonate, and pH.
- Chest X-ray helps identify possible causes of respiratory failure.
- A peripheral arterial catheter may be inserted for monitoring BP and obtaining ABGs.
- Pulse oximetry monitors oxygenation status indirectly but reveals little about lung ventilation.
- Other studies may include complete blood count (CBC), serum electrolytes, urinalysis, and electrocardiography (ECG).
- Sputum and blood cultures determine sources of possible infection.
- If pulmonary embolus is suspected, a V/Q lung scan or CT scan may be done.

For the patient in severe ARF who needs mechanical ventilation, end-tidal CO_2 ($EtCO_2$) can measure trends in ventilation.

Interprofessional and Nursing Management

Preventing atelectasis, pneumonia, and complications of immobility while optimizing hydration and nutrition can decrease the risk of ARF in acutely ill patients. The interprofessional team collaborates to tailor management strategies for ARF to the patient's unique needs. In severe ARF, the patient is cared for in an intensive care unit (ICU).

- Additional information on care for the patient with acute respiratory failure is presented in eNursing Care Plan 32.1: Patient with Acute Respiratory Failure (available on the website).

Respiratory Therapy

The goals of respiratory care include maintaining adequate oxygenation and ventilation and correcting acid–base imbalance. Interventions include O_2 therapy, mobilization of secretions, and positive pressure ventilation (PPV).

Oxygen Therapy

The primary goal of O_2 therapy is to correct hypoxemia (see Oxygen Therapy). Always administer O_2 at the lowest possible FiO_2 (O_2 concentration) needed to keep SpO_2 and PaO_2 within patient-specific goals. Never withhold O_2 from a patient. Closely monitor patients' response to O_2 therapy and changes in mental status, respiratory rate, and ABGs until their PaO_2 level has reached their baseline normal value. The selected O_2 delivery device should maintain PaO_2 at 60 mm Hg or higher and SaO_2 at 90% or higher.

- Hypoxemia secondary to an intrapulmonary shunt is usually not responsive to high O_2 concentrations. The patient usually requires PPV (see Mechanical Ventilation).
- Chronic hypercapnia blunts the response of chemoreceptors to high CO_2 levels as a respiratory stimulant. Initial O_2 therapy may be provided to patients with chronic hypercapnia through a low-flow device, such as a nasal cannula at 1–2 L/minute or a Venturi mask at 24%–28%. Those who do not respond to O_2 therapy or other interventions may need mechanically ventilation with higher FiO_2.

Mobilization of Secretions

Retained pulmonary secretions may cause or worsen ARF. This occurs because the movement of O_2 into the alveoli and removal of CO_2 is severely limited or blocked. Secretions can be mobilized by proper positioning, effective coughing, chest physiotherapy, suctioning, humidification, hydration, and when possible, early ambulation.

Effective Coughing and Positioning

When secretions are present, encourage the patient to cough. Unfortunately, not all patients will have enough strength or force to produce a cough that will clear the airway of secretions.

- Augmented coughing (quad coughing) may help some patients. To aid with augmented coughing, place one or both hands at the anterolateral base of the patient's lungs. As you observe deep inspiration end and expiration begin, move your hands forcefully upward. This increases abdominal pressure and helps the patient cough. It increases expiratory flow and promotes secretion clearance.
- Position the patient upright. Elevate the head of the bed at least 30 degrees or use a reclining chair or chair bed. This helps maximize respiratory expansion, decrease dyspnea, and mobilize secretions. Lateral or side-lying positioning may be used in patients with disease involving only one lung, such as right-sided pneumonia. This position, termed *good lung down,* allows for improved V/Q matching in the affected lung.

R

Hydration and Humidification

Thick and viscous secretions are difficult to expel. Adequate fluid intake (2–3 L/day) keeps secretions thin and easier to remove. A patient who is unable to take sufficient fluids orally needs IV hydration.

- Assess for signs of fluid overload by clinical evaluation (e.g., crackles, dyspnea) and invasive monitoring (e.g., increased central venous pressure) at regular intervals.
- Humidification helps with secretion management. Thin secretions with aerosols of sterile normal saline or mucolytic drugs (e.g., acetylcysteine mixed with a bronchodilator) given by nebulizer.

Airway Suctioning

Suctioning through an artificial airway (e.g., endotracheal tube, tracheostomy) may be needed if the patient cannot expectorate secretions (see Artificial Airways). Perform suctioning with caution, while monitoring the patient for complications. These include hypoxia, increased intracranial pressure (ICP), dysrhythmias, hypotension (from sudden increase in intrathoracic pressure), hypertension and tachycardia (from noxious stimulation), and bradycardia (possible vasovagal response).

Positive Pressure Ventilation

If the patient continues to show signs of acute respiratory failure despite intensive measures, ventilatory assistance may be needed (see Mechanical Ventilation). PPV may be provided invasively using orotracheal or nasotracheal intubation or noninvasively by a nasal or face mask.

Drug Therapy

Drug therapy depends on the cause of ARF, the patient's preexisting health condition, and whether infection is present. Goals of drug therapy include: (1) reduce airway inflammation and bronchospasm; (2) relieve pulmonary congestion; (3) treat infection; and (4) reduce anxiety, pain, and restlessness.

Reduce Airway Inflammation and Bronchospasm

Corticosteroids (e.g., IV methylprednisolone) are often used in combination with other drugs to relieve inflammation and bronchospasm. It may take several hours to see their effects. Inhaled corticosteroids require 4–5 days for optimum therapeutic effects.

Relief of bronchospasm increases alveolar ventilation. In acute bronchospasm, short-acting bronchodilators (e.g., albuterol) may be given at 15–30-minute intervals until a response occurs. Give these drugs using a handheld nebulizer or a metered-dose inhaler with a spacer. Side effects include tachycardia and hypertension. Prolonged use can increase the risk of dysrhythmias and cardiac ischemia. Monitor the patient's vital signs and ECG for changes.

Relieve Pulmonary Congestion

Interstitial fluid can accumulate in the lungs because of injury to the alveolar capillary membrane, HF, or fluid overload. Use of IV diuretics (e.g., furosemide), morphine, or nitroglycerin can decrease pulmonary congestion caused by HF. Use caution when giving these drugs. Changes in heart rate and rhythm and significant decreases in BP are common.

Treat Infections

Lung infections (e.g., pneumonia, acute bronchitis) can result in excessive mucus production, fever, increased O_2 consumption, and inflamed, fluid-filled, and/or collapsed alveoli. Alveoli that are fluid-filled or collapsed cannot take part in gas exchange. Infections can cause or worsen ARF. IV antibiotics are often given to treat infection.

Reduce Anxiety, Pain, and Restlessness

Assess for treatable causes of restlessness (e.g., hypoxemia, pain, delirium) and manage as needed. Anxiety, pain, and restlessness may result from hypoxia. They increase O_2 consumption and CO_2 production (from an increased metabolic rate) and increase WOB. For the nonintubated patient, this may cause tachypnea and ineffective ventilation. For the intubated patient, this may cause ventilator dyssynchrony and increase the risk of unplanned extubation. Sedation and analgesia are used to decrease anxiety, agitation, and pain. Follow an evidence-based protocol to meet patient-specific goals.

Nutritional Therapy

Maintaining protein and energy stores is important in patients with ARF. The hypermetabolic state increases the caloric requirements needed to maintain body weight and muscle mass. Nutritional depletion causes a loss of muscle mass, including the respiratory muscles, which may delay recovery. Nutritional support should start early and focus on a diet that addresses the person's caloric, protein and nutrient requirements needs. Ideally, enteral nutrition (EN) should begin within 24–48 hours (see Enteral Nutrition).

R

RESTLESS LEGS SYNDROME

Description and Pathophysiology

Restless legs syndrome (RLS), also known as *Willis–Ekbom disease* (WED), is a relatively common sleep problem with unpleasant sensory (paresthesia) and motor abnormalities of the legs. RLS is more common in older adults. It is also more common in women than men.

There are two types of RLS: primary (idiopathic) and secondary. Most people have primary RLS. Secondary RLS can occur with metabolic problems from iron deficiency, renal disease and hemodialysis, or neuropathy as in multiple sclerosis. RLS has a genetic link. Many pregnant women develop RLS.

- Symptoms may be worsened by sleep deprivation, sleep apnea, stress, sedentary lifestyle, obesity, alcohol, nicotine, caffeine use, diabetes, peripheral neuropathy, and some medications (antihistamines, antiemetics, lithium, and some antipsychotics.

RLS is believed to be related to a dysfunction in the brain's basal ganglia circuits that use the neurotransmitter dopamine (DA). Disruption in these pathways can cause involuntary movement.

Clinical Manifestations

The severity of RLS sensory symptoms ranges from infrequent minor discomfort (numbness, tingling, "pins and needles" sensation) to severe pain. Symptoms may disappear for a while, but they eventually reappear. Sensory symptoms often appear first.

- Some persons compare the sensations to bugs crawling on the skin.
- A tingling, itching, "creepy-crawling," or throbbing feeling in the calf muscle is accompanied by an irresistible urge to move. Symptoms most often begin when the patient is inactive or lying still, commonly at night. Some patients have pain in the arms.
- Pain at night can disrupt sleep. Physical activity, such as walking, stretching, rocking, or kicking, often relieves the pain.

Diagnostic Studies

RLS is a clinical diagnosis based on the patient's history or the report of the bed partner related to nighttime activities.

- Polysomnography studies during sleep distinguish RLS from other clinical conditions that disturb sleep.
- Complete blood count, serum ferritin, and renal function tests (e.g., serum creatinine) may help exclude secondary causes of RLS. A patient with diabetes may have paresthesia caused by peripheral neuropathy.

Interprofessional and Nursing Management

RLS is lifelong and has no cure. The goal is to reduce discomfort and distress and improve sleep quality. When RLS is secondary to renal failure or iron deficiency, treatment of these conditions will decrease symptoms.

- Lifestyle changes may help with mild-to-moderate RLS. For example, decreasing the use of caffeine, alcohol, or tobacco, maintaining regular sleep habits, exercising, relaxation techniques, and massaging and stretching the legs may be helpful.

- The patient should avoid antihistamine medications (e.g., diphenhydramine).
- A vibratory counterstimulation device can compete with and diminish RLS sensations.
- Some health care providers recommend foot wraps or pneumatic compression devices.

If nondrug measures fail to provide symptom relief, drug therapy is an option.

- The antiseizure drugs gabapentin, enacarbil (Horizant), or pregabalin are first-line drugs for RLS. They may decrease the sensory sensations and nerve pain.
- DA agonists (e.g., ropinirole [Requip], pramipexole [Mirapex], rotigotine [Neupro]) can treat pain and provide more restful sleep. These drugs can cause impulse disorders (gambling, shopping).
- The patient with iron-deficiency anemia may need iron supplements. Other supplements that may help RLS include magnesium, zinc, and vitamin D.

RETINAL DETACHMENT

Description

Retinal detachment is a separation of the sensory retina and underlying pigment epithelium with fluid accumulation between the two layers. A retinal detachment is an ocular emergency. If it is not treated quickly, more of the retina can detach. This increases the risk of permanent vision loss or blindness.

Pathophysiology

Risk factors include age, age-related macular degeneration (AMD), diabetic retinopathy, eye surgery, eye trauma, family or personal history of retinal detachment, severe myopia, and thinning of the peripheral retina.

The most common cause is a retinal break, a full-thickness interruption in the retinal tissue. Retinal holes are spontaneous atrophic breaks. Retinal tears occur when the vitreous shrinks with aging and pulls on the retina. Once there is a retinal break, liquid vitreous may leak between the layers, causing detachment.

Clinical Manifestations

Symptoms of a detaching retina flashes of light, floaters, and a "cobweb" or ring in the vision field. Once the retina is detached, a

R

gradual and painless loss of peripheral or central vision occurs "like a curtain" across the field of vision.

Diagnostic Studies

- Direct and indirect ophthalmoscopy or slit lamp microscopy
- Ultrasound to help identify a detachment

Interprofessional Management

For those retinal breaks less likely to progress to detachment, the ophthalmologist monitors the patient and instructs the patient to seek immediate evaluation for any symptoms of impending detachment.

Surgical treatment to seal retinal breaks may include laser photocoagulation and cryopexy. Inward retinal traction can involve a scleral buckling procedure, pneumatic retinopexy, and vitrectomy.

- Visual prognosis depends on the extent, length, and area of detachment.

Nursing Management

In most cases, retinal detachment is an urgent situation requiring an unexpected surgery. Provide the patient with emotional support, especially during the immediate preoperative period.

- Give prescribed drugs for postoperative pain, and teach the patient to take these drugs as necessary when discharged.
- Begin discharge planning as early as possible because the patient may be discharged a few hours after surgery.

▼ **Patient and Caregiver Teaching**

- Teach the patient with an increased risk of retinal detachment about the signs and symptoms of detachment and to seek immediate evaluation if any of these occur.
- Promote the use of protective eyewear to help avoid traumatic retinal detachment.
- Review the signs and symptoms of retinal detachment with the patient because the risk of detachment in the other eye is increased.

Patient and caregiver teaching after eye surgery is described in Table 22.

RHEUMATIC FEVER AND HEART DISEASE

Description

Rheumatic fever (RF) is an acute inflammatory disease, which can involve all the heart layers. *Rheumatic heart disease* (RHD) is a chronic scarring and deformity of the heart valves resulting from RF. Over 15 million people worldwide have evidence of RHD.

Pathophysiology

RF occurs as a complication 2–3 weeks after a group A streptococcal pharyngitis. RF affects the heart, skin, joints, and central nervous system (CNS).

About 50% of RF episodes are *rheumatic pancarditis*, involving all layers of the heart (endocardium, myocardium, pericardium).

- Rheumatic endocarditis is found mainly in the valves, with swelling and erosion of the valve leaflets. Vegetations form and initially create a fibrous thickening of the valve leaflets, fusion of commissures and chordae tendineae, and fibrosis of the papillary muscle. Stenosis and regurgitation may occur in valve leaflets. The mitral and aortic valves are most commonly affected.
- Nodules, called Aschoff's bodies, are formed by a reaction to inflammation, with swelling and fragmentation of collagen fibers. As the Aschoff's bodies age, they become more fibrous, and scar tissue forms in the myocardium.
- Rheumatic pericarditis affects both layers of the pericardium, which becomes thickened and covered with a fibrinous exudate.

Systemic lesions of RF involve the skin, joints, and CNS. Painless subcutaneous nodules, arthralgias or arthritis, and chorea may develop.

Clinical Manifestations

The presence of two major criteria or one major and two minor criteria, plus evidence of a preceding group A streptococcal infection, indicates a high probability of acute RF.

Major Criteria

- *Carditis* is the most important manifestation of RF. It results in three signs: (1) an organic heart murmur or murmurs of mitral or aortic regurgitation or mitral stenosis; (2) heart enlargement and heart failure (HF) occurring from myocarditis; and (3) pericarditis resulting in distant heart sounds, chest pain, a pericardial friction rub, or signs of effusion.
- *Monoarthritis or polyarthritis* is the most common finding in RF, occurring in up to 75% of patients. The larger joints (particularly the knees, ankles, elbows, and wrists) are most severely affected by swelling, warmth, redness, tenderness, and limitation of motion.
- *Sydenham's chorea* is the major CNS manifestation. It is characterized by involuntary movements (especially of the face and limbs), muscle weakness, and speech and gait problems.
- *Erythema marginatum* lesions are a less common feature. The bright pink, nonpruritic, map-like macular lesions occur mainly

on the trunk and proximal extremities. The lesions intensify with heat (e.g., warm bath).

- *Subcutaneous nodules* are small, hard, painless swellings found over extensor surfaces of the joints, especially the knees, wrists, and elbows.

Minor Criteria

Minor clinical manifestations include fever, polyarthralgia, and certain laboratory tests (e.g., elevated C-reactive protein [CRP], elevated white blood cell [WBC] count).

Evidence of Infection

In addition to the major and minor criteria, there must also be evidence of a preceding group A streptococcal infection. Such evidence includes a positive result on a rapid antigen test for group A streptococci, an elevated antistreptolysin-O titer, or a positive throat culture.

Diagnostic Studies

- Chest X-ray may show an enlarged heart if HF is present.
- Echocardiogram may show valvular insufficiency and pericardial fluid or thickening.
- Electrocardiography (ECG) reveals a prolonged PR interval with delayed atrioventricular (AV) conduction.

Interprofessional Management

Treatment consists of drug therapy and supportive measures. Antibiotic therapy does not change the course of the acute disease or the development of carditis. It eliminates residual group A streptococci in the tonsils and pharynx and prevents the spread of organisms to close contacts. Salicylates, nonsteroidal antiinflammatory drugs (NSAIDs), and corticosteroids are the antiinflammatory agents most widely used to control the fever and joint manifestations.

Nursing Management

Goals

The goals for a patient with RF and rheumatic heart disease include: (1) normal or baseline heart function, (2) resumption of daily activities without joint pain, and (3) ability to manage the long-term antibiotic therapy.

Interventions

RF can be prevented by early detection and immediate treatment of group A streptococcal pharyngitis. Teach people in the community to seek medical attention for symptoms of streptococcal pharyngitis.

Administer antibiotics as ordered and teach the patient that oral antibiotics require adherence to the full course of therapy. Promote optimal rest to reduce cardiac workload and the body's metabolic needs. Position painful joints for proper alignment and apply heat for comfort. Give salicylates, NSAIDs, and corticosteroids as prescribed for joint pain.

- After acute symptoms have subsided, the patient without carditis can ambulate. If the patient has carditis with HF, promote strict bed rest.

▼ **Patient and Caregiver Teaching**

- Teach the patient that completing the full course of antibiotics is vital to successful treatment.
- Teach the patient with a history of previous RF about the disease process, possible sequelae, and the need for continuous prophylactic antibiotics. Patients with RF without carditis need prophylaxis until age 20 and for a minimum of 5 years. Patients with rheumatic carditis and residual heart disease (e.g., persistent valve disease) need lifelong prophylaxis.
- Encourage good nutrition, hygiene practices, and adequate rest.
- Caution the patient about the possible development of heart valve disease. Teach the patient to seek medical attention for excessive fatigue, dizziness, palpitations, or exertional dyspnea.

RHEUMATOID ARTHRITIS

Description

Rheumatoid arthritis (RA) is a chronic, systemic autoimmune disease characterized by inflammation of connective tissue in the diarthrodial (synovial) joints. RA is typically marked by periods of remission and exacerbation and often has extraarticular manifestations.

RA occurs globally, affecting all ethnic groups. RA most often begins in women between ages 30 and 60 years. Almost three times as many women have the disease as men.

Pathophysiology

The exact cause of rheumatoid arthritis is unknown. However, it likely results from an autoimmune response to genetic and environmental triggers. RA is marked by the presence of autoantibodies against abnormal immunoglobulin G (IgG). The autoantibodies, known as *rheumatoid factor* (RF), combine with IgG to form

R

TABLE 74	Stages of Rheumatoid Arthritis
Stage	**Characteristics**
I	• No destructive change on X-ray • X-ray evidence of osteoporosis possible
II	• X-ray evidence of osteoporosis at joint, with or without slight subchondral bone destruction • Slight cartilage destruction possible • Joint mobility may be limited, but no joint deformities noted • Muscle atrophy near joints • Soft tissue lesions (nodules, tenosynovitis) possible near joints
III	• X-ray evidence of cartilage and bone destruction, osteoporosis at joint • Joint deformity without joint fusion • Extensive muscle atrophy near joints • Soft tissue lesions possible near joints
IV	• Criteria from stage III, plus • Fibrous or bony joint fusion

WBC, White blood cell.
Modified from Medscape Drugs & Diseases (https://emedicine.medscape.com/), Rheumatoid Arthritis (RA), 2022, available at: https://emedicine.medscape.com/article/331715-overview.

immune complexes that deposit on synovial membranes or superficial articular cartilage in the joints.

■ Immune complex formation leads to complement activation and an inflammatory response. Neutrophils attracted to the site release proteolytic enzymes that damage articular cartilage and thicken the synovial lining.

■ Other inflammatory cells include T helper ($CD4^+$) cells and pro-inflammatory cytokines, such as interleukin-1 (IL-1), interleukin-6 (IL-6), and tumor necrosis factor (TNF).

■ Genetic predisposition is important in the development of RA.

Symptoms and outcomes of RA can vary greatly. See Table 74 for the stages of disease progression. Joint damage can be slowed or stopped with aggressive, early treatment.

Clinical Manifestations

The onset of RA is typically subtle. Fatigue, anorexia, weight loss, and generalized stiffness may precede the onset of joint symptoms. The stiffness becomes more localized after weeks to months.

Joint Manifestations

Specific joint involvement is marked by pain, stiffness, limitation of motion, and signs of inflammation (heat, swelling, tenderness). Joint symptoms are symmetrical and often affect the small joints of the hands and feet, as well as the larger peripheral joints, including wrists, elbows, shoulders, knees, hips, ankles, and jaw.

- The patient typically has joint stiffness after periods of inactivity. (See Table 60 for a comparison of RA and osteoarthritis [OA].)
- As RA progresses, inflammation and fibrosis of the joint capsule and supporting structures may cause deformity and disability. Muscle atrophy and tendon destruction around the joint can cause one articular surface to slip past the other *(subluxation)*. Typical hand distortions include "ulnar drift," "swan neck," and boutonniere deformities.

Extraarticular Manifestations

RA can affect nearly every system in the body.

Atherosclerosis can result from chronic inflammation that damages endothelial cells within blood vessels. More cholesterol plaques may be formed. When plaques break loose, they can lead to heart attack or stroke. Risk of heart attack in people with RA is 60% higher than in persons without RA.

Rheumatoid nodules appear as firm, nontender, granuloma-type masses under the skin on bony areas such as the fingers and elbows.

Sjögren syndrome can occur by itself or in conjunction with other arthritic disorders, such as RA and systemic lupus erythematosus (SLE). The inflammation of RA can damage the tear-producing (lacrimal) glands, making the eyes feel dry and gritty (see Sjögren syndrome).

Felty syndrome is rare but can occur in patients with long-standing RA. It is characterized by an enlarged spleen and low white blood cell (WBC) count. Patients with Felty syndrome are at increased risk for infection and lymphoma.

Flexion contractures and hand deformities cause diminished grasp strength, affecting the patient's ability to perform self-care tasks. Depression may also occur.

Diagnostic Studies

A diagnosis is often made based on history and physical findings. Some laboratory tests are useful to confirm the diagnosis and to monitor disease progression.

- Erythrocyte sedimentation rate (ESR) and C-reactive protein (CRP) are elevated as general indicators of active inflammation.

- Antinuclear antibody (ANA) titers may increase.
- High levels of antibodies to citrullinated peptide (anti-CCP) are more specific than RF for RA. Testing may allow an early, accurate diagnosis.
- Synovial fluid analysis in early disease often shows a straw-colored fluid with many fibrin flecks. The WBC count of synovial fluid is elevated (up to 25,000/μL).
- Tissue biopsy can confirm inflammatory changes in the synovium.
- X-rays alone are not diagnostic of RA. They may show only soft tissue swelling and bone demineralization in early disease. A narrowed joint space, articular cartilage destruction, erosion, subluxation, and deformity are seen in later disease. Poor alignment and fusion (ankyloses) may be noted in advanced disease.

Interprofessional Management

Care of the patient with RA begins with a thorough program of education and drug therapy. The physical therapist helps the patient maintain joint motion and muscle strength. An occupational therapist helps the patient maintain upper extremity function and encourages use of splints or other assistive devices for joint protection. A balance of rest and activity is encouraged.

Drug Therapy

Drugs are the cornerstone of RA treatment. Because irreversible joint changes can occur as early as the first year of RA, health care providers (HCPs) aggressively prescribe disease-modifying antirheumatic drugs (DMARDs). These drugs may slow disease progression and lessen risk of joint erosion and deformity. The choice of drug is based on disease activity, the patient's functional level, and lifestyle considerations, such as the desire to become pregnant.

- Methotrexate is preferred for early treatment because it has a lower toxicity than other drugs. Rare but serious side effects include bone marrow suppression and liver toxicity. Methotrexate therapy requires frequent laboratory monitoring.
- Sulfasalazine (Azulfidine) and the antimalarial drug hydroxychloroquine (Plaquenil) may be effective DMARDs for mild to moderate disease.
- Leflunomide (Arava) is a synthetic DMARD that blocks immune cell overproduction and has efficacy similar to that of methotrexate and sulfasalazine.

Biologic response modifiers (BRMs) (also called *biologics* or *immunotherapy agents*) are also used to slow disease progression in RA. They can be used alone or in combination therapy with a

DMARD, such as methotrexate. These drugs all inhibit the inflammatory response.

- Tumor necrosis factor inhibitors include etanercept (Enbrel), infliximab (Remicade), adalimumab (Humira), certolizumab (Cimzia), and golimumab (Simponi).

Other biologic and targeted inhibitors that may be used include anakinra (Kineret), tocilizumab (Actemra), sarilumab (Kevzara), abatacept (Orencia), and rituximab (Rituxan). Nonsteroidal antiinflammatory drugs (NSAIDs) and salicylates treat pain and inflammation. All nonaspirin NSAIDs increase the risk of blood clots, heart attack, and stroke. Corticosteroid therapy can be used to manage symptoms during disease flares. Intraarticular injections may temporarily reduce acute pain and inflammation.

Nursing Management
Goals
The patient with RA will have satisfactory pain relief and minimal loss of joint function, participate in planning and implementing the therapeutic regimen, maintain a positive self-image, and perform self-care to the maximum amount possible.

Interventions
Prevention of RA is not possible at this time. Smoking cessation can reduce the risk of developing RA. Teach symptom recognition to promote early diagnosis and treatment.

Interventions begin with a careful physical assessment (joint pain, swelling, range of motion, general health status), psychosocial assessment (family support, sexual satisfaction, emotional stress, financial constraints, vocation and career limitations), and environmental assessment (transportation, home, and work modifications).

- Inflammation may be managed with NSAIDs, DMARDs, and biologic/targeted therapy agents. Discuss the action and side effects of each drug and any needed laboratory monitoring. Make the drug regimen as understandable as possible.
- Lightweight splints can rest an inflamed joint and prevent deformity. Remove splints regularly to assess, give skin care, and perform range-of-motion (ROM) exercises. Reapply splints as prescribed.
- Plan care around the patient's morning stiffness. Sitting or standing in a warm shower, sitting in a tub with warm towels around the shoulders, or soaking the hands in a basin of warm water may relieve joint stiffness and allow the patient to perform activities of daily living comfortably. Application of ice may help during periods of exacerbation.

- Alternating rest periods with activity helps relieve fatigue and pain. Help the patient identify activity changes to avoid overexertion.
- Relaxation techniques, joint protection, biofeedback, transcutaneous electrical nerve stimulation (TENS), and hypnosis may be helpful.
- Good body alignment while resting can be maintained with a firm mattress or bed board. Encourage positions of extension and teach the patient to avoid positions of flexion. Avoid pillows under the knees. A small, flat pillow may be used under the head and shoulders.
- Assistive devices such as built-up utensils, button hooks, and raised toilet seats simplify tasks. A cane or a walker offers support and pain relief when walking.
- Gentle ROM exercises are usually done daily to keep the joints functional. Reinforce correct performance of exercises.
- Balanced nutrition is important. Fatigue, pain, and depression may cause a loss of appetite. Limited endurance and mobility may make it hard to shop for and prepare food. The occupational therapist can help the patient modify the home environment and use assistive devices for easier food preparation.

▼ Patient and Caregiver Teaching
- Self-management requires that the patient understand the nature and course of RA and the goals of therapy. Consider the patient's value system and perception of the disease.
- Help the patient recognize fears and concerns of living with a chronic illness.
- Evaluate the family support system. Financial planning may be needed. Community resources such as home care nurse visits, homemaker services, vocational rehabilitation, and self-help groups may provide support.

SCLERODERMA

Description

Scleroderma (systemic sclerosis) is a disorder of the connective tissue characterized by fibrotic, degenerative, and sometimes inflammatory changes in the skin, blood vessels, synovium, skeletal muscle, and internal organs. *Localized scleroderma* mainly affects the skin. It is more common in children. Skin changes of localized disease are usually limited to a few places on the skin or muscle. The prognosis of patients with limited disease is better than for those with systemic disease. *Systemic scleroderma* (or *systemic sclerosis*) is more common in adults. Skin and connective tissue changes progress rapidly during the first months of systemic scleroderma. It is associated with internal organ involvement.

Pathophysiology

We think immunologic and vascular abnormalities play a role in the development of systemic scleroderma. Risk factors include environmental or occupational exposure to coal, plastics, and silica dust. In scleroderma, the body makes too much collagen (protein that gives normal skin its strength and elasticity). This leads to progressive tissue fibrosis and occlusion of blood vessels. Collagen overproduction disrupts normal function of internal organs, such as the lungs, kidney, heart, and GI tract. Vascular problems, which involve the small arteries and arterioles, are almost always present.

Clinical Manifestations

Manifestations range from benign limited skin disease to diffuse skin thickening with rapidly progressive and widespread organ involvement. Diffuse scleroderma involves widespread thickening of the skin. This especially occurs in the hands, arms, thighs, chest, abdomen, and face. Blood vessels, heart and lungs, joints and muscles, esophagus, and intestines may be damaged. Limited scleroderma affects the face, fingers, hands, and lower arms and legs.

Some patients with limited scleroderma have *CREST syndrome*:

Calcinosis: painful deposits of calcium in the skin of fingers, forearms, pressure points

Raynaud phenomenon: intermittent vasospasm of fingertips in response to cold or stress

Esophageal dysfunction: difficulty swallowing because of internal scarring

Sclerodactyly: tightening of skin on fingers and toes

Telangiectasia: red spots on hands, forearms, palms, face, and lips from capillary dilation

Raynaud phenomenon (sudden vasospasm of the digits) is the most common first symptom in localized scleroderma. Patients have decreased blood flow to the fingers and toes when exposed to cold (blanching or white phase). This is followed by cyanosis as hemoglobin releases O_2 to the tissues (blue phase), then erythema during rewarming (red phase). Numbness and tingling often occur (see Raynaud Phenomenon).

- About 20% of people with scleroderma develop secondary Sjögren syndrome, a condition associated with dry eyes and dry mouth (see Sjögren Syndrome). Dysphagia, gum disease, and dental decay can result.

- Reflux of gastric acid can occur due to esophageal fibrosis. If swallowing is difficult, the patient may decrease food intake and lose weight. GI effects include constipation from colonic hypomotility and diarrhea caused by malabsorption from bacterial overgrowth.
- Lung involvement includes pleural thickening, pulmonary fibrosis, pulmonary artery hypertension, and abnormal pulmonary function.
- Heart disease consists of pericarditis, pericardial effusion, and dysrhythmias. Heart failure from myocardial fibrosis occurs most often with systemic disease.
- Recent improvements in dialysis, bilateral nephrectomy in patients with uncontrollable hypertension, and kidney transplant have offered hope to patients with renal failure. Angiotensin-converting enzyme (ACE) inhibitors (e.g., lisinopril [Prinivil]) have a marked effect on renal disease.

Diagnostic Studies

- Blood studies may reveal mild hemolytic anemia.
- Anticentromere antibodies occur in people with CREST syndrome. Antibodies to topoisomerase-1 are present in about 30% of people with diffuse disease.
- If renal involvement is present, urinalysis may show proteinuria, microscopic hematuria, and casts.
- X-rays may show subcutaneous calcification, distal esophageal hypomotility, or bibasilar pulmonary fibrosis.
- Pulmonary function studies reveal decreased vital capacity and lung compliance.
- Thermography can detect temperature differences between affected and normal tissue.
- Soft tissue can be assessed with ultrasound and MRI.

Interprofessional Management

There is no specific treatment. Supportive care is directed to preventing or treating the complications. Physical therapy helps maintain joint mobility and preserve muscle strength. Occupational therapy assists the patient in maintaining functional abilities.

Drug Therapy

Vasoactive agents are often prescribed in early disease. Calcium-channel blockers (nifedipine [Procardia], diltiazem [Cardizem]) and the angiotensin II blocker losartan are common treatments for Raynaud's phenomenon. Reserpine, an α-adrenergic blocking agent, increases blood flow to the fingers. Bosentan (Tracleer), an endothelin-receptor antagonist, and the vasodilator epoprostenol (Flolan) may improve blood flow to the lung.

- Nonsteroidal antiinflammatory drugs (NSAIDs) and topical agents may give some relief from joint pain. Capsaicin cream may be useful not only as a local analgesic but also as a vasodilator.

Other therapies prescribed to treat specific systemic problems include: (1) tetracycline for diarrhea caused by bacterial overgrowth, (2) histamine (H2) receptor blockers (e.g., cimetidine) and proton pump inhibitors (e.g., omeprazole) for esophageal symptoms, and (3) antihypertensive agent (e.g., captopril, propranolol, methyldopa) for hypertension with renal involvement.

- Immunosuppressive drugs (e.g., cyclophosphamide, mycophenolate mofetil) are used in severe cases.

Nursing Management

Emotional stress and cold ambient temperatures may aggravate Raynaud's phenomenon. Teach the patient to protect the hands and feet from cold exposure and possible burns or cuts that might heal slowly.

- Encourage the patient to avoid smoking because of its vasoconstricting effect. Alcohol-free lotions may help alleviate skin dryness and cracking but must be rubbed in for a long time because of skin thickness.

A consultation with a dietitian is beneficial. Dysphagia may be reduced by eating small, frequent meals, chewing carefully and slowly, and drinking fluids. Decrease risk for heartburn by using antacids 45–60 minutes after each meal and sitting upright for at least 2 hours after eating. Using extra pillows or raising the head of the bed on blocks may reduce gastroesophageal reflux during the night.

- Emphasize daily oral hygiene to avoid to tooth and gum disease.

Teach the patient to actively carry out therapeutic exercises. Encourage the use of moist heat applications or paraffin baths to promote skin flexibility in the hands and feet. Teach the patient to use assistive devices as needed and organize activities to preserve strength and reduce disability.

- Job modifications are often needed because of problems with stair climbing, typing, writing, and cold exposure.

Provide sensitive counseling about sexual dysfunction from body changes, pain, muscular weakness, limited mobility, decreased self-esteem, erectile dysfunction, and decreased vaginal secretions.

S

SEIZURE DISORDER

Description

A *seizure* is a sudden abnormal, excessive, electrical discharge of neurons in the brain. During a seizure, multiple neurons fire at a rate much faster than normal, causing involuntary movements, sensory phenomena, emotional expression, and unusual behaviors. Seizures may accompany a variety of disorders, or they may occur without any apparent cause.

Seizure disorder, or *epilepsy*, is a group of neurologic diseases marked by recurring seizures. If a person has two or more seizures more than 24 hours apart without an underlying problem that caused the seizure, they may have seizure disorder. Seizures from systemic and metabolic problems are not seizure disorder if they stop when the underlying problem is corrected. About 3.4 million or 1.2% of Americans have seizure disorder.

Etiology and Pathophysiology

One or more genetic abnormalities are known to affect up to 70% of people with seizure disorder. For most persons, the cause of seizure disorder is unknown. These cases are known as idiopathic generalized epilepsy (IGE). Known causes include stroke, brain tumors, cerebral infection, traumatic brain injury, hypoxic birth injury, neurodevelopmental disorders (e.g., autism spectrum disorders), or neurodegenerative disease (e.g., Alzheimer disease). Other common causes include low or very high glucose levels, abnormal serum electrolytes (sodium, magnesium, calcium), eclampsia with pregnancy, lack of sleep, and alcohol withdrawal. Children may have seizures with high fever. Medical problems that may cause seizures include hypertension, sepsis, and heart, lung, liver, or kidney diseases. Patients with autoimmune disease, such as systemic lupus erythematosus and multiple sclerosis, have inflammatory changes in the brain, increasing seizure risk.

Seizure disorder is characterized by a group of abnormal neurons that seem to fire without a clear cause. This may happen due to the release of excitatory neurotransmitters or by an absence of neuroinhibitory activity. Both allow abnormal excitement of neurons, leading to excessive discharge of electrical activity. Any stimulus that causes the neuron's cell membrane to depolarize can cause this firing, which spreads by physiologic pathways. Localizing the seizure focus (the place where the seizure originates) is critical to the success of any surgical treatment.

Clinical Manifestations

Seizures are classified based on where the seizure activity begins: generalized onset, focal onset, and unknown onset; 60% of patients have focal seizures. Motor, nonmotor, and level of awareness descriptors address what occurs during the seizure. It may not be easy to figure out what type of seizure a patient is having. Seizures may begin with a single focus and then become generalized throughout the brain.

Depending on the type, a seizure may progress through several phases: (1) *prodromal phase,* with sensations or behavior changes that precede a seizure by hours or days; (2) *aural phase,* with a sensory warning that is similar each time a seizure occurs; (3) *ictal phase,* from first symptoms to the end of seizure activity; and (4) *postictal phase,* the recovery period after the seizure. Not all patients have every phase.

Generalized-Onset Seizures

Generalized-onset seizures involve both sides of the brain and are characterized by bilateral synchronous neural discharges. In most cases, the patient has impaired consciousness for a few seconds to several minutes. Generalized seizures are either motor or nonmotor. Motor movements are bilateral.

- *Tonic–clonic* (formerly known as "grand mal") seizures are the most common generalized seizures. During a tonic–clonic seizure, the patient loses consciousness and if upright, falls to the ground. The body stiffens (tonic phase) for 10–20 seconds and the extremities jerk (clonic phase) for 30–40 seconds, up to several minutes. Cyanosis, excessive salivation, tongue or cheek biting, and incontinence may occur. In the postictal phase, the patient usually has muscle soreness, feels tired, and may sleep for several hours. Some patients may not feel normal for several hours or days after a seizure. The patient has no memory of the seizure.
- Other types of generalized-onset motor seizures include tonic and clonic. A *tonic* seizure involves a sudden onset of increased tone in the extensor muscles, contributing to sudden stiff movements. Tonic seizures most often occur in sleep and affect both sides of the body. Patients will fall if they are standing when the seizure occurs. Tonic seizures usually last <20 seconds. The patient usually remains aware. *Clonic* seizures begin with loss of awareness and sudden loss of muscle tone, followed by rhythmic limb jerking that may or may not be symmetric. Clonic seizures are rare.
- A generalized *atonic seizure* (or *drop attack*) involves a brief, sudden loss of tone. It may affect just the head and neck or result

S

in the person falling to the ground. Seizures typically last a few seconds. There is a brief loss of consciousness and a brief post-ictal confusion. Patients with atonic seizure are at great risk for head injury and often need protective helmets.

- *Absence* ("petit mal") seizures most often occur in children. A typical absence seizure is marked by a sudden onset brief star-ing spell that resembles daydreaming and sudden recovery. It often goes unnoticed because it lasts less than 10–20 seconds. Usually, the patient is unresponsive when spoken to during the seizure.

- In *atypical absence seizure,* the staring spell is accompanied by other signs and symptoms, such as eye blinking or jerk-ing movements of the lips and repetitive finger movements (automatisms).

Focal-Onset Seizures

Focal-onset seizures (formerly called *partial seizures*) begin in one hemisphere of the brain in a localized region of the cortex. Focal seizures are motor or nonmotor. Motor activities include atonic (loss of tone, relaxed muscles), tonic (sustained stiffening), clonic (rhythmic jerking), or myoclonic (very rapid, irregular, brief jerk-ing). Some people show strange behavior, such as lip smacking, picking at clothes, or other repetitive, purposeless actions (automa-tisms). With a focal nonmotor seizure, the patient can have emo-tional manifestations or autonomic symptoms.

Complications

Status epilepticus (SE) is a state of continuous seizure activity, any seizure lasting longer than 5 minutes or seizures occurring so close together the patient cannot recover between them. The patient does not return to consciousness between seizures. The longer a seizure lasts, the less likely it is to stop without drug therapy.

SE is a neurologic emergency.

- During repeated seizures, the brain uses more energy than can be supplied. As neurons become exhausted and cease to func-tion, permanent brain damage may result.

- *Convulsive status epilepticus* can cause potentially fatal respira-tory insufficiency, hypoxemia, dysrhythmias, hyperthermia, and systemic acidosis.

- Severe injury and death can result from physical trauma during a seizure. Patients who lose consciousness during a seizure are at greatest risk.

Perhaps the most common complication of seizure disorder is the effect it has on the patient's lifestyle. Antiseizure medications and the continued need to manage a chronic disease can contribute to depression. Patients may experience discrimination in employment and educational opportunities. Transportation may be difficult if state law does not allow the person to drive.

Diagnostic Studies

- Accurate and comprehensive descriptions of the seizures and the patient's health history are important.
- EEG is useful only if it shows abnormalities. Some patients who do not have seizure disorder have abnormal EEG patterns, while many patients with seizure disorder have normal EEGs between seizures.
- Complete blood count (CBC), serum chemistry panel, studies of liver and kidney function, and urinalysis can rule out metabolic disorders.
- CT scan and MRI can rule out a structural lesion.
- Cerebral angiography, single-photon emission computed tomography (SPECT), magnetic resonance spectroscopy (MRS), magnetic resonance angiography (MRA), and positron emission tomography (PET) may be used.

Interprofessional Management

Most seizures are self-limiting. However, medical care should be sought immediately in cases of status epilepticus, injury, or first-time seizure. Table 75 summarizes the emergency care of the patient with a generalized tonic–clonic seizure.

Drug Therapy

Seizure disorder is treated primarily with medications that stabilize the nerve cell membranes and prevent the spread of the epileptic discharge.

The principle of drug therapy is to begin with a single drug based on the patient's age and weight with consideration of the type, frequency, and cause of seizure. Then the dosage is increased until the seizures are controlled or toxic side effects occur. If seizure control is not achieved with a single drug, the drug dosage and timing or administration may be changed or a second drug may be added.

- The main drugs to treat tonic–clonic and focal-onset seizures are phenytoin, carbamazepine (Tegretol), and divalproex (Depakote).
- The drugs used most often to treat generalized onset nonmotor and myoclonic seizures include ethosuximide (Zarontin), divalproex, and clonazepam (Klonopin).

S

TABLE 75 Emergency Management of Tonic–Clonic Seizures

Assessment Findings	Interventions
Aural Phase	**Initial**
• Bowel and bladder incontinence	• Ensure patent airway.
• Diaphoresis	• Protect patient from injury during seizure. *Do not restrain.* Pad side rails.
• Loss of consciousness	
• Pallor, flushing, or cyanosis	
• Peculiar sensations that precede seizure	• Remove sharp objects and glasses.
• Tachycardia	• Never force anything between patient's clenched teeth.
• Warm skin	
Tonic Phase	
• Continuous muscle contractions	• Remove or loosen tight clothing.
Hypertonic Phase	
• Extreme muscular rigidity lasting 5–15 sec	• Establish IV access.
	• Stay with patient until seizure has passed.
Clonic Phase	
• Rigidity and relaxation alternating in rapid succession	• Anticipate giving phenytoin, benzodiazepines (e.g., diazepam, midazolam, lorazepam) to try to stop seizures.
Postictal Phase	
• Altered level of consciousness, lethargy	
• Confusion and headache	• Suction as needed.
• Repeated tonic-clonic seizures for several minutes	• Assist ventilations if patient does not breathe spontaneously after seizure.
	• Anticipate need for intubation.
	Ongoing Monitoring
	• Monitor vital signs, level of consciousness, O_2 saturation, Glasgow Coma Scale results, pupil size and reactivity.
	• Reassure and orient patient after seizure.
	• Give IV dextrose for hypoglycemia.
	• Maintain NPO until awake with gag reflex.

- Treatments for focal seizures are carbamazepine, lamotrigine (Lamictal), or levetiracetam (Keppra). Pregabalin (Lyrica) is an added treatment for focal aware or impaired awareness seizures not controlled with one medication.

Treatment of SE requires a rapid-acting antiseizure drug. The drugs most often used are benzodiazepines. Options include midazolam IM autoinjector (Seizalam) and buccal or intranasal midazolam (Nayzilam). If a patient has an IV, then IV lorazepam is preferred. Because these are short-acting drugs, we follow their administration with long-acting drugs, such as fosphenytoin. Ongoing administration of IV antiseizure and anesthetic drugs is needed if the seizures are not. People with a defined site of seizure origin (epileptogenic zone) can benefit from surgical resection of that focal area, laser ablation, or radiosurgery over continued use of antiseizure drugs. For severe cases, hemispherectomy can be done.

Goals

The patient with seizures will be free from injury during a seizure, have optimal mental and physical functioning while taking antiseizure drugs, and have satisfactory psychosocial functioning.

Interventions

The patient with seizure disorder should practice good general health habits (e.g., maintaining a proper diet, getting adequate rest, exercising). Help the patient identify events or situations that cause seizures and provide suggestions for handling them better. Teach the patient to avoid excess alcohol intake, fatigue, and loss of sleep. Help the patient handle stress constructively.

Nursing care for a hospitalized patient with seizures should focus on maintaining safety, observation and treatment of the seizure, teaching, and psychosocial support.

- Carefully observe and record details of the seizure event because the diagnosis and subsequent treatment often rest on the seizure description. What events preceded the seizure? When did the seizure occur? How long did each phase (aural [if any], ictal, postictal) last? What occurred during each phase?
- The description should include the exact onset of the seizure (which body part was affected first and how); the course and nature of the seizure activity (loss of consciousness, tongue biting, automatisms, stiffening, jerking, total lack of muscle tone); the body parts involved and their sequence of involvement; and the presence of autonomic signs (dilated pupils, excessive salivation, altered breathing, cyanosis, flushing, diaphoresis, or incontinence).
- Assessment of the postictal period should include a detailed description of the level of consciousness (LOC), vital signs,

memory loss, muscle soreness, speech disorders (aphasia, dysarthria), weakness or paralysis, sleep period, and the duration of each sign or symptom.

- During the seizure, maintain a patent airway for the patient, protect the patient's head, turn the patient to the side, loosen constrictive clothing, and ease the patient to the floor if seated. Do not restrain the patient or place any objects in the patient's mouth.
- After the seizure, the patient may require suctioning and oxygen.
- A seizure can be a frightening experience for the patient and others who witnessed it. Assess the level of their understanding and provide information about how and why the event occurred.

▼ Patient and Caregiver Teaching
Prevention of recurring seizures is the major goal in the treatment of epilepsy. Drugs must be taken regularly and continually, often for a lifetime. You have an important role in teaching the patient and caregivers. Guidelines for teaching are shown in Table 76.

TABLE 76 Patient and Caregiver Teaching: Seizure Disorder

Include the following information in the teaching plan for the patient with seizure disorder.

1. Take antiseizure medications as prescribed. Report all drug side effects to the HCP.
2. When needed, blood is drawn to ensure therapeutic drug levels. Schedule regular visits with the HCP to discuss treatment options.
3. Do not add any supplements without HCP approval.
4. Use nondrug techniques, such as relaxation therapy and diet modification, to try to reduce the number of seizures.
5. Be aware of community and online resources for education and help with tracking and explaining seizure activity.
6. Wear a medical alert bracelet or necklace and carry an identification card.
7. Avoid excess alcohol use, fatigue, and loss of sleep.
8. Eat regular meals and snacks in between if feeling shaky, faint, or hungry.
9. Be knowledgeable as a woman of childbearing age about antiseizure medications and contraceptive use.

TABLE 76   Patient and Caregiver Teaching: Seizure Disorder—cont'd

Caregivers should receive the following information.

Focal-Onset Seizures

1. Stay calm. Guide patient to safety to prevent injury but do not restrain.
2. Observe for asymmetry of activity and focus on specific actions, such as lip smacking and abnormal movements.
3. Assess patient's level of consciousness and ability to converse and respond appropriately.
4. Note the time the seizure started and stopped. Take note of the time of return to baseline.
5. Provide respect and explanation of occurrence.

Generalized-Onset Tonic-Clonic Seizures

1. When seizure occurs outside the hospital setting, activate EMS if the duration is greater than 5 minutes; events recur without the patient recovering to baseline; the patient is unable to establish a normal breathing pattern, is injured or pregnant; or you do not know if this is a first-time seizure event.
2. Maintain patient safety. Lower the patient to the floor or bed, remove glasses if worn, and loosen restrictive clothing.
3. Do not place anything in the patient's mouth. Patient's teeth/dentures may be damaged.
4. Position patient on side (if possible) to improve the patient's ability to drain oral secretions.
5. Note the time the seizure started and stopped. Take note of the time of return to baseline.
6. Assess for any injury and lingering motor weakness.

SEXUALLY TRANSMITTED INFECTIONS

Sexually transmitted infections (STIs) are diseases that spread through sexual contact with the penis, vagina, anus, mouth, or body fluids of an infected person. Mucosal tissues in the genitals (urethra in men, vagina in women), rectum, and mouth are especially susceptible to the bacteria and viruses that cause STIs.

- Infections that are associated with sexual transmission can also be contracted by other routes, such as through blood or blood products or by autoinoculation (spread of infection by touching or scratching an infected area and transferring it to another part of the body).

Common infections that are transmitted sexually are listed in Table 77.

An estimated 26 million new STIs are diagnosed in the United States each year. Many risk factors contribute to the high rates of STIs (Table 78). In the United States, nurses and other health care

S

TABLE 77   Causes of Sexually Transmitted Infections (STIs)

Sexually Transmitted Infection	Cause
Bacteria	
Chlamydia	*Chlamydia trachomatis*
Gonorrhea	*Neisseria gonorrhoeae*
Syphilis	*Treponema pallidum*
Viruses	
Genital herpes	Herpes simplex virus (HSV 1 or 2)
Genital warts (condylomata acuminata)	Human papillomavirus (HPV)
Human immunodeficiency virus (HIV) infection/acquired immunodeficiency syndrome (AIDS)	HIV
Hepatitis B and C	Hepatitis B and C viruses
Molluscum contagiosum	Poxvirus (molluscum contagiosum virus)
Parasites/Protozoa	
Trichomoniasis	*Trichomonas vaginalis*

providers (HCPs) are mandated to report all cases of gonorrhea, chlamydia, and syphilis to public health authorities for surveillance and partner notification. See Gonorrhea, Syphilis, Herpes, Genital, Warts, Genital and Chlamydial Infection.

Interprofessional and Nursing Management

The overall goals are that the patient with an STI will understand the mode of transmission of STIs and the risks related to STIs, complete treatment and return for appropriate follow-up, notify or assist in notifying sexual contacts about their need for testing and treatment, abstain from sexual contact until the infection is resolved and all partners have been treated, and show knowledge of safer sex practices.

The diagnosis of an STI may be met with a variety of emotions such as embarrassment, shame, guilt, anger, and even a desire for vengeance.

- Provide counseling and encourage the patient to voice feelings. A referral for professional counseling to explore the impact of an STI on a relationship may be indicated.

TABLE 78 Risk Factors for Sexually Transmitted Infections (STIs)

High-Risk Behaviors

- Alcohol or substance use (inhibits judgment)
- Having new sexual partners
- Having more than one sexual partner
- Having sexual partners who have/have had multiple partners
- Inconsistent or incorrect use of condoms or other barrier methods
- Exchanging sex for money, shelter, or other needs

High-Risk Medical History

- Having one STI is a risk factor for getting another
- Not being vaccinated for STIs or other infections that may be transmitted through some forms sexual activity (HPV, hepatitis A and B)
- Receiving multiple courses of nonoccupational postexposure prophylaxis to prevent HIV infection

High-Risk Populations

- Adolescents and young adults (under age 25)
- Ethnicity/Race (e.g., Black, American Indian/Alaskan Native, Native Hawaiian/Other Pacific Islander, Hispanic)
- Men who have sex with men
- Persons in correctional facilities
- Transgender women
- Victims of sexual assault
- Women

Single-dose treatment for gonorrhea, chlamydia, and syphilis helps prevent problems from nonadherence with drug therapy. Stress the need for the patient receiving multiple-dose therapy to complete the prescribed treatment. Patients should return to the treatment center for a repeat culture from infected sites or serologic testing at designated times to determine effectiveness of treatment.

- Advise the patient to inform sexual partners of the need for treatment, regardless of whether they are free of or have symptoms.
- Emphasize hygiene measures such as frequent hand washing.
- Bathing and cleaning of involved areas can provide local comfort and prevent secondary infection.
- Teach patients not to douche after sex. It can push bacteria higher into the reproductive tract.
- Sexual abstinence is needed during the communicable phase of the infection. After the patient has completed treatment, condoms or other barrier methods may prevent spread of infection and reinfection.

S

- Be prepared to discuss decreasing exposure to STIs with all patients.

  See Table 79 for a patient teaching guide regarding STIs.

TABLE 79   Patient Teaching: Sexually Transmitted Infections (STIs)

When teaching the patient with an STI:

1. Explain precautions to take, such as
   - Using condoms and other barrier methods with every sexual encounter
   - When being monogamous, defining what monogamy means with your partner
   - Limiting the number of sexual partners
   - Asking potential partners about their sexual history
   - Asking potential partners if they have been tested for STIs
   - Avoiding sex with partners who have visible oral, inguinal, genital, perineal, or anal lesions, or those who use IV drugs
   - Voiding and washing genitalia and surrounding area after sex to flush out/wash away organisms to reduce potential for transmitting infection
2. Explain the importance of taking all antibiotics or antiviral agents as prescribed. Symptoms will improve after 1–2 days of treatment, but organisms may still be present.
3. Teach patients diagnosed with gonorrhea, chlamydia, syphilis, or trichomoniasis that all sexual partners need to be treated to prevent transmission and reinfection.
4. Teach patients to abstain from sexual contact during and for 7 days after treatment. Review the use of condoms or other barrier methods when sexual activity is resumed to prevent spread of infection and reinfection.
5. Explain the importance of follow-up examination and retesting at least once after treatment (if appropriate) to confirm complete cure and prevent relapse.
6. Allow patients and partners to voice their concerns and clarify areas that need explanation.
7. Teach patients about the signs and symptoms of complications and need to report problems to their HCP to ensure proper follow-up and early treatment of reinfection.
8. Tell patients of the infectious nature of these infections to avoid a false sense of security, which may result in careless sexual practices or poor personal hygiene.
9. Tell patients about health department requirements for anonymously reporting certain STIs.

SHOCK

Description

Shock is a life-threatening syndrome of decreased tissue perfusion and impaired cellular metabolism. The four main categories of shock are cardiogenic, hypovolemic, distributive, and obstructive.

- While the cause, initial presentation, and management strategies vary for each type, the physiologic responses of cells to hypoperfusion are similar.

Cardiogenic Shock

Cardiogenic shock occurs when either systolic or diastolic dysfunction of the heart's pumping action results in reduced cardiac output (CO). The patient has impaired tissue perfusion and cellular metabolism because of cardiogenic shock, which is most often caused by acute myocardial infarction (MI).

- The patient presents with tachycardia, hypotension, and a narrowed pulse pressure. A low CO (<4 L/min) and *cardiac index* (<2.5 L/min/m^2) result from systolic dysfunction.
- Tachypnea and crackles are evidence of pulmonary congestion. The pulmonary artery wedge pressure (PAWP) and pulmonary vascular resistance are increased.
- Signs of peripheral hypoperfusion (e.g., cyanosis, pallor, diaphoresis, diminished pulses, delayed capillary refill) are apparent.
- Decreased renal blood flow results in sodium and water retention and decreased urine output.
- Anxiety, confusion, and agitation develop as cerebral perfusion is impaired.

Studies helpful in diagnosing cardiogenic shock include laboratory studies (e.g., cardiac biomarkers, b-type natriuretic peptide [BNP]), electrocardiogram (ECG), chest X-ray, and echocardiogram.

Hypovolemic Shock

Hypovolemic shock occurs when there is inadequate fluid volume in the intravascular space to support perfusion. The volume loss may be either absolute or relative.

- *Absolute hypovolemia* results when fluid is lost through hemorrhage, gastrointestinal (GI) loss (e.g., vomiting, diarrhea), fistula drainage, diabetes insipidus, or diuresis.
- In *relative hypovolemia,* fluid volume moves out of the vascular space into the extravascular space (e.g., intracavity space). This fluid shift is called *third spacing.* One example of relative

S

volume loss is fluid leakage from the vascular space to the inter-stitial space because of increased capillary permeability, as seen in burns.

Reduced intravascular volume results in decreased venous return to the heart, decreased preload, decreased stroke volume, and decreased CO. A cascade of events results in decreased tissue per-fusion and impaired cellular metabolism, the hallmarks of shock (Fig. 26).

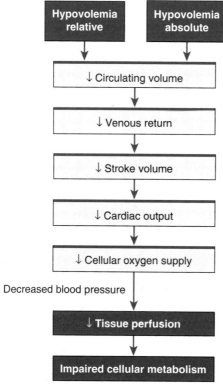

Fig. 26 The pathophysiology of hypovolemic shock. (Modified from Urden L.D., Stacy K.M., Lough M.E. *Critical care nursing: diagnosis and management,* ed 6, St Louis, 2010, Mosby.)

- A total blood loss of 15%–30% results in a sympathetic nervous system (SNS)–mediated response that increases heart rate, CO, and respiratory rate and depth. If hypovolemia is corrected at this time, tissue dysfunction is generally reversible.
- If volume loss is >30%, it must be immediately replaced with blood products.
- A loss of more than 40% of the total blood volume results in irreversible tissue destruction.

Laboratory studies include serial measurements of hemoglobin and hematocrit levels, electrolytes, lactate, blood gases, and central venous oxygenation ($ScvO_2$), as well as hourly urine outputs.

Distributive Shock (Neurogenic, Anaphylactic, Septic)

Neurogenic Shock

Neurogenic shock is a hemodynamic phenomenon that can occur within 30 minutes of a spinal cord injury and last up to 6 weeks. The injury results in massive vasodilation without compensation because of the loss of SNS vasoconstrictor tone. This leads to a pooling of blood in the blood vessels, tissue hypoperfusion, and impaired cellular metabolism.

Spinal anesthesia can also temporarily block transmission of impulses from the SNS. Depression of the vasomotor center of the medulla from drugs (e.g., opioids, benzodiazepines) may result in decreased vasoconstrictor tone of the peripheral blood vessels and neurogenic shock.

- Manifestations are hypotension (from massive vasodilation) and bradycardia (from unopposed parasympathetic stimulation).

The patient in neurogenic shock may not be able to regulate body temperature. Initially, the skin is warm because of the vasodilation. As the heat disperses, the patient is at risk for hypothermia.

Anaphylactic Shock

Anaphylactic shock is an acute and life-threatening hypersensitivity (allergic) reaction to a substance such as a drug, chemical, vaccine, food, or insect venom. The reaction quickly causes massive vasodilation, release of vasoactive mediators, and an increase in capillary permeability.

- As capillary permeability increases, fluid leaks from the vascular space into the interstitial space. Anaphylactic shock can lead to respiratory distress as a result of laryngeal edema or severe bronchospasm and to circulatory failure because of massive vasodilation.

S

- Patients present with a sudden onset of dizziness, chest pain, incontinence, swollen lips and tongue, wheezing, and stridor. Skin changes include flushing, pruritus, urticaria, and angioedema.
- A patient can develop a severe allergic reaction leading to anaphylactic shock after contact with, inhalation or ingestion of, or injection with an antigen (allergen) to which the person has previously been sensitized.

Septic Shock

Septic shock occurs with *sepsis* (systemic inflammatory response to infection). Septic shock is characterized by persistent hypotension, despite adequate fluid resuscitation, and inadequate tissue perfusion that results in tissue hypoxia. The main organisms that cause sepsis are Gram-negative and Gram-positive bacteria. Parasites, fungi, and viruses can also lead to the development of sepsis.

- Microorganisms entering the body trigger normal immune and inflammatory responses. However, in sepsis and septic shock, the body's response is exaggerated. Both proinflammatory and antiinflammatory responses are activated. Inflammation and coagulation increase along with a decrease in fibrinolysis. Endotoxins from the microorganism cell wall stimulate the release of cytokines and other proinflammatory mediators. The combined effects of the mediators result in endothelial damage, vasodilation, increased capillary permeability, and neutrophil and platelet aggregation and adhesion to the endothelium. Septic shock has three major pathophysiologic effects: vasodilation, maldistribution of blood flow, and myocardial depression.
- Persistent high CO and low systemic vascular resistance (SVR) beyond 24 hours is an ominous finding associated with severe hypotension and multiple organ dysfunction syndrome (MODS) (see Systemic Inflammatory Response Syndrome [SIRS] and MODS).
- Respiratory failure is common. The patient initially hyperventilates, resulting in respiratory alkalosis. Once the patient can no longer compensate, respiratory acidosis develops.
- Other clinical signs include decreased urine output, alteration in neurologic status, and GI problems such as GI bleeding and paralytic ileus.

Obstructive Shock

Obstructive shock develops when a physical obstruction to blood flow occurs with a decreased CO. This can be caused from a restriction to diastolic filling of the right ventricle caused by compression (e.g., cardiac tamponade, tension pneumothorax, pulmonary embolism, superior vena cava syndrome).

- Patients have decreased CO, increased afterload, and variable left ventricular filling pressures, depending on the obstruction. Other signs include jugular venous distention and pulsus paradoxus. Rapid assessment and immediate treatment are important to prevent further hemodynamic compromise and possible cardiac arrest.

Stages of Shock

Shock is categorized into four overlapping stages: (1) initial stage, (2) compensatory stage, (3) progressive stage, and (4) refractory stage.

Initial Stage

The *initial stage* of shock at the cellular level is usually not clinically apparent. Metabolism changes at the cellular level from aerobic to anaerobic, causing lactic acid buildup. Lactic acid is a waste product that is removed by the liver. However, this removal process requires oxygen, which is unavailable because of the decrease in tissue perfusion.

Compensatory Stage

In the *compensatory stage,* the body activates neural, hormonal, and biochemical mechanisms to try to overcome the consequences of anaerobic metabolism and maintain homeostasis.

- A classic sign of shock is a drop in BP. The SNS stimulates vasoconstriction and the release of the potent vasoconstrictors epinephrine and norepinephrine. Blood flow to the heart and brain is maintained. Blood flow to the kidneys, GI tract, and lungs is diverted.
- The myocardium responds to SNS stimulation and the increase in oxygen demand by increasing heart rate and contractility, which also increases myocardial O_2 consumption.
- Some areas of the lungs that are being ventilated will not be perfused because of the decreased blood flow to the lungs. Arterial O_2 levels will decrease, and the patient will have a compensatory increase in the rate and depth of respirations.
- Decreased blood flow to the kidneys activates the renin-angiotensin-aldosterone system, resulting in vasoconstriction and sodium and water reabsorption.

If the cause of shock is corrected at this stage, the patient recovers with few or no residual effects. If the cause of shock is not corrected and the body is unable to compensate, the patient goes on to the progressive stage of shock.

S

Progressive Stage

The *progressive stage* of shock begins as compensatory mechanisms fail. Continued decreased cellular perfusion and altered capillary permeability are distinguishing features of this stage, causing profound edema *(anasarca)*. Aggressive interventions are needed to prevent the development of MODS.

- CO begins to fall, causing a decrease in BP and coronary artery, cerebral, and peripheral perfusion. Decreased perfusion results in dysrhythmias, myocardial ischemia, and possibly MI.
- The combined effects of pulmonary vasoconstriction and bronchoconstriction are impaired gas exchange, decreased compliance, and worsening ventilation–perfusion mismatch. The patient presents with tachypnea, crackles, and an overall increased work of breathing.
- As the blood supply to the GI tract is decreased, the normally protective mucosal barrier becomes ischemic, which predisposes the patient to ulcers and GI bleeding.
- Prolonged hypoperfusion to the kidneys causes renal tubular ischemia and may lead to acute kidney injury (AKI). The patient has a decreased urine output and an elevated blood urea nitrogen (BUN) and serum creatinine. Metabolic acidosis occurs from an inability to excrete acids and reabsorb bicarbonate.
- Loss of liver function leads to a failure to metabolize drugs and waste products such as ammonia and lactate. Jaundice results from accumulated bilirubin.
- The patient is at risk for the development of disseminated intravascular coagulation (DIC) with hemorrhage (see Disseminated Intravascular Coagulation).

Refractory Stage

In the *refractory stage,* decreased perfusion from peripheral vasoconstriction and decreased CO worsen anaerobic metabolism. The loss of intravascular volume worsens hypotension and tachycardia and decreases coronary and cerebral blood flow.

- The patient has profound hypotension and hypoxemia. Recovery from this stage is unlikely. The organs are failing, and the body's compensatory mechanisms are overwhelmed.

Diagnostic Studies

- A thorough medical and surgical history and a history of recent events (e.g., surgery, chest pain, trauma) provide valuable data.

- Blood studies may include complete blood count (CBC), DIC screen, cardiac enzymes, BUN, glucose, electrolytes, arterial blood gases (ABGs), blood cultures, and liver enzymes.
- Decreased tissue perfusion leads to an increased lactate level with a base deficit (the amount needed to bring the pH back to normal). These changes reflect increased anaerobic metabolism.
- Twelve-lead ECG, continuous cardiac monitoring, and chest X-ray.
- Continuous pulse oximetry, invasive and noninvasive hemodynamic monitoring.

Interprofessional Management

Early recognition and treatment are critical factors in shock management. Prompt intervention in the early stages may prevent the decline to the progressive or irreversible stage. Successful management of the patient in shock includes: (1) identifying patients at risk for developing shock; (2) integrating the patient's history, physical assessment, and clinical findings to establish a diagnosis; (3) interventions to control or eliminate the cause; (4) protecting target and distal organs from dysfunction; and (5) providing multisystem supportive care. Emergency care of the patient in shock is presented in Table 80. General management strategies begin with ensuring that the patient is responsive and has a patent airway. Once the airway is established with either a natural airway or an endotracheal tube, O_2 delivery must be optimized.

- Supplemental O_2 and mechanical ventilation may be needed to maintain an arterial oxygen saturation of at least 90% (arterial partial pressure of O_2 [PaO_2] > 60 mm Hg) and avoid hypoxemia (see Artificial Airways: Endotracheal Tubes, Oxygen Therapy, and Mechanical Ventilation).

In addition to general management of shock, there are specific interventions for different types of shock (Table 81). The mean arterial pressure and circulating blood volume are optimized with fluid replacement and drug therapy (Table 82).

Nursing Management
Goals
The overall goals for a patient in shock include adequate tissue perfusion, restoration of normal or baseline BP, recovery of organ function, avoiding complications from prolonged states of hypoperfusion, and preventing health care–associated complications.

S

TABLE 80 Emergency Management: Shock

Common Causes	Assessment Findings	Interventions
Medical • Addisonian crisis • Dehydration • Diabetes • Diabetes insipidus • MI • Pulmonary embolus • Sepsis **Surgical** • Aortic dissection • GI bleeding • Postoperative bleeding • Ruptured ectopic pregnancy or ovarian cyst • Ruptured organ or vessel • Vaginal bleeding **Trauma** • Fractures, spinal injury • Multiorgan injury • Ruptured or lacerated vessel or organ (e.g., spleen)	• Anxiety • Chills • Confusion • Cool, clammy skin (warm skin in early onset of septic and neurogenic shock) • Cyanosis • Dysrhythmias • Extreme thirst • Feeling of impending doom • Hypotension • ↓ Level of consciousness • Narrowed pulse pressure • Nausea and vomiting • Obvious hemorrhage or injury • ↓ O$_2$ saturation • Pallor • Rapid, weak, thready pulses • Restlessness • Tachypnea, dyspnea, or shallow, irregular respirations • Temperature dysregulation • Weakness	**Initial** • If unresponsive, assess circulation, airway, and breathing (CAB). • If responsive, monitor airway, breathing, and circulation (ABC). • Stabilize cervical spine as appropriate. • Control any external bleeding with direct pressure or pressure dressing. • Give high-flow O$_2$ (100%) by nonrebreather mask or bag-valve-mask. • Anticipate need for intubation and mechanical ventilation. • Establish IV access with 2 large-bore catheters (14- to 16-gauge) or an intraosseous access device; aid with central line insertion. • Begin fluid resuscitation with crystalloids (e.g., 30 mL/kg repeated until hemodynamic improvement is seen). • Draw blood for laboratory studies (e.g., blood cultures, lactate, WBC). • Assess for life-threatening injuries (e.g., cardiac tamponade, liver laceration, tension pneumothorax). • Consider vasopressor therapy if hypotension persists after fluid resuscitation. • Insert an indwelling urinary catheter and nasogastric tube. • Start antibiotic therapy after blood cultures if sepsis is suspected. • Obtain 12-lead ECG and treat dysrhythmias. **Ongoing Monitoring** • ABCs • Level of consciousness • Vital signs, including pulse oximetry; peripheral pulses, capillary refill, skin color and temperature • Respiratory status • Heart rate and rhythm • Urine output

ECG, Electrocardiogram; *GI,* gastrointestinal; *WBC,* white blood cell.

TABLE 81 Interprofessional Care: Shock

Oxygenation	Circulation	Drug Therapies	Supportive Therapies
Cardiogenic Shock			
• Provide supplemental O_2 (e.g., nasal cannula, nonrebreather mask) • Intubation and mechanical ventilation, if needed • Monitor $ScvO_2$ or SvO_2	• Restore blood flow with angioplasty with stenting, emergent coronary revascularization • Reduce workload of heart with circulatory assist devices: IABP, VAD	• Nitrates (e.g., nitroglycerin) • Inotropes (e.g., dobutamine) • Diuretics (e.g., furosemide) • β-Adrenergic blockers (contraindicated with ↓ ejection fraction)	• Treat dysrhythmias
Hypovolemic Shock			

• Provide supplemental O_2
 • Monitor $ScvO_2$ or SvO_2
	• Rapid fluid replacement using two large-bore (14–16 gauge) peripheral IV lines, an intraosseous access device, or central venous catheter
	 • Restore fluid volume (e.g., blood or blood products, crystalloids)
	 • End points of fluid resuscitation:
	   • CVP 15 mm Hg
	   • PAWP 10–12 mm Hg
		• No specific drug therapy	• Correct the cause (e.g., stop bleeding, GI losses)
			 • Use warmed IV fluids, including blood products (if appropriate)

Continued

S

TABLE 81 Interprofessional Care: Shock—cont'd

Oxygenation	Circulation	Drug Therapies	Supportive Therapies
Septic Shock			
• Provide supplemental O_2 • Intubation and mechanical ventilation, if needed • Monitor $ScvO_2$ or SvO_2	• Aggressive fluid resuscitation (e.g., 30 mL/kg of crystalloids repeated if hemodynamic improvement is noted) • End points of fluid resuscitation are based on: Focused physical assessment including vital signs, cardiopulmonary assessment, capillary refill, peripheral pulses, and skin or any two of the following: • $ScvO_2$ >70 or SvO_2 >65 • CVP 8–12 mm Hg • Cardiovascular ultrasound • Fluid responsiveness with passive leg raise or fluid challenge	• Antibiotics as ordered • Vasopressors (e.g., norepinephrine) • Inotropes (e.g., dobutamine) • Anticoagulants (e.g., low-molecular-weight heparin)	• Obtain cultures (e.g., blood, wound) before beginning antibiotics • Monitor temperature • Control blood glucose • Stress ulcer prophylaxis

TABLE 81 Interprofessional Care: Shock—cont'd

Oxygenation	Circulation	Drug Therapies	Supportive Therapies
Neurogenic Shock			
• Maintain patent airway • Provide supplemental O_2 • Intubation and mechanical ventilation (if needed)	• Cautious administration of fluids	• Vasopressors (e.g., phenylephrine) • Atropine (for bradycardia)	• Minimize spinal cord trauma with stabilization • Monitor temperature
Anaphylactic Shock			
• Maintain patent airway • Optimize oxygenation with supplemental O_2 • Intubation and mechanical ventilation, if needed	• Aggressive fluid resuscitation with colloids	• Epinephrine (IM or IV) • Antihistamines (e.g., diphenhydramine) • Histamine (H_2)-receptor blockers • Bronchodilators: nebulized (e.g., albuterol) • Corticosteroids (if hypotension persists)	• Identify and remove offending cause • Prevent via avoidance of known allergens • Premedicate with history of prior sensitivity (e.g., contrast media)

Continued

S

TABLE 81 Interprofessional Care: Shock—cont'd

Oxygenation	Circulation	Drug Therapies	Supportive Therapies
Obstructive Shock			
• Maintain patent airway • Provide supplemental O₂ • Intubation and mechanical ventilation, if needed	• Restore circulation by treating cause of obstruction • Fluid resuscitation may provide temporary improvement in CO and BP	• No specific drug therapy	• Treat cause of obstruction (e.g., pericardiocentesis for cardiac tamponade, needle decompression or chest tube insertion for tension pneumothorax, embolectomy for pulmonary embolism)

CO, Cardiac output; *CVP,* central venous pressure; *GI,* gastrointestinal; *IABP,* intraaortic balloon pump; *MAP,* mean arterial pressure; *PAWP,* pulmonary artery wedge pressure; *ScvO₂/SvO₂,* central venous oxygenation/mixed venous oxygenation; *VAD,* ventricular assist device.

TABLE 82 Drug Therapy for Shock

Drug[a]	Mechanism of Action	Type of Shock	Nursing Implications
Angiotensin II (Giapreza)	↑ BP, ↑ MAP ↑SVR	Septic and other distributive shock	Give via central line. Monitor for thromboembolic events. Provide VTE prophylaxis.
Dobutamine	↑ Myocardial contractility ↓ Ventricular filling pressures ↓ SVR, PAWP ↑ CO, SV, CVP ↑/↓ HR	Used in cardiogenic shock with severe systolic dysfunction Used in septic shock to increase O_2 delivery and raise $ScvO_2$ or SvO_2 to 70% if Hgb >7 g/dL or Hct ≥30%	Give via central line (infiltration leads to tissue sloughing). Do not give in same line with $NaHCO_3$. Monitor HR, BP (hypotension may worsen, requiring addition of a vasopressor). Stop infusion if tachydysrhythmias develop.

Continued

S

TABLE 82   Drug Therapy for Shock—cont'd

Drug[a]	Mechanism of Action	Type of Shock	Nursing Implications
Dopamine	Positive inotropic effects: ↑ Myocardial contractility ↑ Automaticity ↑ Atrioventricular conduction ↑ HR, CO ↑ BP, ↑ MAP ↑ MVO₂ Can cause progressive vasoconstriction at high doses	Cardiogenic shock	Give via central line (infiltration leads to tissue sloughing). Do not give in same line with NaHCO₃. Monitor for tachydysrhythmias. Monitor for peripheral vasoconstriction (e.g., paresthesias, coldness in extremities) at moderate to high doses.
Epinephrine (Adrenalin)	*Low doses:* β-Adrenergic agonist (cardiac stimulation, bronchodilation, peripheral vasodilation) ↑ HR, contractility, CO ↓ SVR *High doses:* α-Adrenergic agonist (peripheral vasoconstriction) ↑ SV, SVR ↑ Systolic/↓ diastolic BP, widened pulse pressure ↑ CVP, PAWP	Cardiogenic shock Anaphylactic shock Septic shock, if 2nd agent needed after norepinephrine Cardiac arrest, pulseless ventricular tachycardia, ventricular fibrillation, asystole	Monitor for HR >110 beats/min. Monitor for dyspnea, pulmonary edema. Monitor for chest pain, dysrhythmias from ↑ MVO₂. Monitor for renal failure due to ischemia.

S

Continued

TABLE 82 Drug Therapy for Shock—cont'd

Drug[a]	Mechanism of Action	Type of Shock	Nursing Implications
Hydrocortisone (Solu-Cortef)	↓ Inflammation, reverses ↑ capillary permeability ↑ BP, HR	Septic shock requiring vasopressor therapy (despite fluid resuscitation) to maintain adequate BP Anaphylactic shock if hypotension persists after initial therapy	Monitor for hypokalemia, hyperglycemia. Consider use as continuous infusion.
nitroglycerin	Venous dilation Dilates coronary arteries ↓ Preload, MVO_2, SVR, BP	Cardiogenic shock	Continuously monitor BP and HR, since reflex tachycardia may occur. Glass bottle recommended for infusion.
norepinephrine (Levophed)	β_1-Adrenergic agonist (cardiac stimulation) α-Adrenergic agonist (peripheral vasoconstriction) Renal and splanchnic vasoconstriction ↑ BP, MAP, CVP, ?AWP, SVR ↑/↓ CO	Cardiogenic shock after MI Septic shock—first drug of choice for BP unresponsive to adequate fluid resuscitation	Give via central line (infiltration leads to tissue sloughing). Monitor for dysrhythmias due to ↑ MVO_2 requirements.

TABLE 82	Drug Therapy for Shock—cont'd		
Drug[a]	Mechanism of Action	Type of Shock	Nursing Implications
Phenylephrine	α-Adrenergic agonist (peripheral vasoconstriction) Renal, mesenteric, splanchnic, cutaneous, and pulmonary blood vessel constriction ↑ HR, BP, SVR ↑/↓ CO	Neurogenic shock	Monitor for reflex bradycardia, headache, restlessness. Monitor for renal failure from ↓ renal blood flow. Give via central line (infiltration leads to tissue sloughing).
Sodium nitroprusside	Arterial and venous vasodilation ↓ Preload, afterload ↓ CVP, PAWP ↑/↓ CO ↓ BP	Cardiogenic shock with ↑ SVR	Continuously monitor BP. Protect solution from light. Wrap infusion bottle with opaque covering. Give with D_5W only. Monitor serum cyanide levels and for signs of cyanide toxicity (e.g., metabolic acidosis, tachycardia, altered level of consciousness, seizures, coma, almond smell on breath).

TABLE 82 Drug Therapy for Shock—cont'd

Drug[a]	Mechanism of Action	Type of Shock	Nursing Implications
Vasopressin	Antidiuretic hormone Nonadrenergic vasoconstrictor ↑MAP ↑Urine output	Shock states (most often septic shock) refractory to other vasopressors	Given with norepinephrine and in low doses. Infusions are not titrated. Monitor hemodynamic pressures and urine output.

CVP, Central venous pressure; *MVO₂,* myocardial O$_2$ consumption; *PAWP,* pulmonary artery wedge pressure; *SVR,* systemic vascular resistance.
[a]Consult agency guidelines, pharmacist, pharmacology references, and drug manufacturer's materials for more information and dosing recommendations.

S

Interventions

Your important role in the prevention of shock begins with identifying patients at risk. Patients who are older, immunocompromised, or have chronic illnesses are at an increased risk. A person who has surgery or trauma is at risk for shock from conditions such as hemorrhage, spinal cord injury, and sepsis.

Do not underestimate the effects of fear and anxiety on the patient and caregiver faced with a life-threatening situation. Fear, anxiety, and pain may worsen respiratory distress and increase the release of catecholamines. Encourage caregivers to perform simple comfort measures if desired. Provide privacy and assure the patient and caregivers that assistance is readily available.

- Monitor the patient's mental state and level of pain using valid assessment tools. Give drugs to decrease anxiety and pain as needed.
- Talk to the patient and encourage the caregiver to talk to the patient, even if the patient is intubated, sedated, or appears comatose. Patients who cannot respond may still be able to hear. If the intubated patient is capable of writing, provide a "magic slate" or a pencil and paper.
- Reduce noise and light levels to control sensory input. Keep a day–night cycle of activity and rest as much as possible. Sensory overload and disruption of the patient's diurnal cycle may contribute to delirium.
- Do not overlook the patient's spiritual needs. Offer to call a member of the clergy.

Rehabilitation of the patient after critical illness requires correction of the precipitating cause, prevention or early treatment of complications, and education on disease management and/or prevention of recurrence.

- Continue to monitor the patient for complications, including decreased range of motion, decreased physical endurance, renal failure after acute tubular necrosis, and fibrotic lung disease because of acute respiratory distress syndrome (ARDS).
- Patients recovering from shock may require diverse services after discharge. These can include admission to transitional care units (e.g., for mechanical ventilation weaning) or rehabilitation centers (inpatient or outpatient), or management by home health care agencies. Start planning a safe transition from the hospital to home as soon as the patient is admitted to the hospital.
- See also eNursing Care Plan 66-1: Patient in Shock, on the website.

SICKLE CELL DISEASE

Description

Sickle cell disease (SCD) is a group of inherited, autosomal recessive disorders characterized by an abnormal form of hemoglobin (Hgb) in the red blood cell (RBC). This abnormal Hgb, *hemoglobin S* (Hgb S), causes the erythrocyte to stiffen and elongate, taking on a sickle shape in response to low O_2 levels.

Because this is a genetic disorder, SCD is usually identified during routine neonatal screening. Although median survival now exceeds 50 years of age, the disease often results in irreversible damage of the lungs, kidneys, brain, retina, or bones and significantly affects patients' quality of life.

Pathophysiology

Types of SCD include sickle cell anemia, sickle cell thalassemia, sickle cell Hgb C disease, and sickle cell trait.

Sickle cell anemia is the most severe of the SCD syndromes. It occurs when a person inherits Hgb S from both parents.

Sickle cell thalassemia and *sickle cell Hgb C* occur when a person inherits Hgb S from one parent and another type of abnormal Hgb (e.g., thalassemia or Hgb C) from the other parent. These forms of SCD are less common and less severe than sickle cell anemia.

Sickle cell trait occurs when a person is heterozygous for Hgb S (Hgb AS). The person has inherited Hgb S from one parent and normal Hgb (Hgb A) from the other parent. Sickle cell trait is typically a mild to asymptomatic condition.

The main trigger of sickling episodes is low O_2 tension in the blood. Infection is the most common cause of hypoxia or deoxygenation of the RBCs. Other causes include high altitude, emotional or physical stress, surgery, and blood loss. Other triggering events include dehydration, increased hydrogen ion concentration (acidosis), increased plasma osmolality, decreased plasma volume, and low body temperature. A sickling episode can also occur without an obvious cause.

- Sickled RBCs become rigid and take on an elongated, crescent shape. Sickled cells cannot easily pass through capillaries or other small vessels and can cause vascular occlusion, leading to acute or chronic tissue injury. The resulting hemostasis promotes a cycle of local hypoxia, deoxygenation of more erythrocytes, and more sickling.
- Circulating sickled cells are hemolyzed by the spleen, leading to anemia.

S

- Initially the sickling of cells is reversible with reoxygenation, but eventually the condition becomes irreversible because of cell membrane damage from recurrent sickling.

Sickle cell crisis is a severe, painful, acute exacerbation of RBC sickling causing a vasoocclusive crisis. As sickled cells impair blood flow, vasospasm occurs, further restricting blood flow. Tissue ischemia, infarction, and necrosis eventually occur from lack of oxygen. Shock is a possible life-threatening consequence because of severe tissue hypoxia and decreased circulating fluid volume. Sickle cell crisis can begin suddenly and persist for weeks.

- The frequency, extent, and severity of sickling episodes are unpredictable but largely depend on the percentage of Hgb S present. People with sickle cell anemia have the most severe form because the RBCs contain a high percentage of Hgb S.

Clinical Manifestations

Many people with sickle cell anemia are in reasonably good health most of the time. However, they may have chronic health problems and pain because of organ hypoxia and damage (e.g., involving the kidneys or liver). The typical patient is anemic but asymptomatic except during sickling episodes.

- Because most persons with sickle cell anemia have dark skin, pallor is easier to detect by examining the mucous membranes. The skin may have a grayish cast. Because of the hemolysis, jaundice is common. Patients are prone to gallstones (cholelithiasis).
- During sickle cell crisis, the pain of tissue ischemia is severe. The back, chest, extremities, and abdomen are most often affected. Pain is accompanied by fever, tachypnea, hypertension, and nausea and vomiting.

Complications

With repeated episodes of sickling, there is gradual involvement of all body systems, especially the spleen, lungs, kidneys, and brain.

- Infection is a major contributor to morbidity and mortality in patients with sickle cell disease. Pneumonia is the most common infection.
- The spleen becomes infarcted and dysfunctional because of repeated scarring.
- *Acute chest syndrome* is a pulmonary complication that includes pneumonia, tissue infarction, and fat embolism, resulting in

pulmonary hypertension, myocardial infarction (MI), and ultimately cor pulmonale.
- The kidneys may be injured from the lack of oxygen, resulting in renal failure.
- Stroke can result from thrombosis and infarction of cerebral blood vessels.
- The heart may become ischemic and enlarged, leading to heart failure.
- Retinal vessel obstruction may result in hemorrhage, scarring, retinal detachment, and blindness.
- Bone changes may include osteoporosis and osteosclerosis after infarction. Chronic leg ulcers can result from hypoxia.

Diagnostic Studies
- Peripheral blood smear may reveal sickled cells and abnormal reticulocytes.
- Hgb electrophoresis may determine the amount of Hgb S and SCD from other variants.
- Findings of hemolysis (jaundice, elevated serum bilirubin levels) and abnormal laboratory test results (see Table 8, p. XX) may be present.
- Skeletal X-rays, MRI, and Doppler studies may be used to assess for bone and joint deformities, stroke, and deep vein thromboses, respectively.

Interprofessional and Nursing Management
Care is directed toward preventing and alleviating symptoms from complications of SCD, minimizing end-organ damage, and promptly treating serious sequelae such as acute chest syndrome. Review steps to avoid dehydration and hypoxia. Teach patients with SCD to avoid high altitudes, maintain adequate fluid intake, and treat infections promptly.
- Sickle cell crises may require hospitalization. O_2 treats hypoxia and controls sickling. Rest may reduce metabolic needs. Fluids and electrolytes are administered to reduce blood viscosity and maintain renal function.
- During an acute crisis, optimal pain control usually includes large doses of continuous opioid analgesics along with breakthrough analgesia, often in the form of patient-controlled analgesia (PCA).
- Acute chest syndrome is treated with broad-spectrum antibiotics, O_2 therapy, and fluid therapy.
- Priapism is managed with pain medication and fluids.

S

- Chronic leg ulcers may be treated with bed rest, antibiotics, warm saline soaks, mechanical or enzyme debridement, and grafting if necessary.
- Transfusion therapy is indicated when an aplastic crisis occurs. Chelation therapy may be needed to reduce transfusion-produced iron overload.
- Encourage routine immunizations such as pneumococcal, influenza, and hepatitis.
- Hematopoietic stem cell transplantation (HSCT) is the only available treatment that can cure some patients with SCD, but is not widely available.

Various drugs can reduce sickling episodes. Hydroxyurea (Hydrea) increases the production of hemoglobin F (fetal hemoglobin) and alters the adhesion of sickled RBCs to the endothelium. The increase in Hgb F is accompanied by a reduction in hemolysis, an increase in hemoglobin concentration, and a decrease in sickled cells and painful crises. Adakveo (crizanlizumab–tmca) reduces sickle cell and blood vessel adhesion. Voxelotor (Oxbryta) stabilizes an oxygenated hemoglobin cell, reducing sickling. Oral glutamine, an amino acid, decreases endothelial adhesion and can reduce the number and frequency of pain crises and hospitalizations.

SJÖGREN SYNDROME

Sjögren syndrome is an autoimmune disease that targets the moisture-producing exocrine glands. This leads to *xerostomia* (dry mouth) and *keratoconjunctivitis sicca* (dry eyes). The nose, throat, airways, and skin can become dry. It may affect other glands, including those in the stomach, pancreas, and intestines, increasing the risk for non-Hodgkin's lymphoma. The disease is usually diagnosed in people over age 40 years. Most people with Sjögren syndrome are women.

Sjögren syndrome appears to be caused by genetic and environmental factors. The trigger may be a viral or bacterial infection that stimulates the immune system. In Sjögren syndrome, lymphocytes attack and damage the lacrimal and salivary glands.

- Decreased tearing causes dry eyes, which leads to a gritty sensation in the eyes, burning, blurred vision, and photosensitivity.
- Dry mouth causes buccal membrane fissures, changes in taste, dysphagia, and increased mouth infection or dental decay.

- Dry skin and rashes, joint and muscle pain, and thyroid problems may be present. Other exocrine glands can be affected. For example, vaginal dryness may lead to painful intercourse (dyspareunia).

Ophthalmologic examination (Schirmer test for tear production), measures of salivary gland function, and lower lip biopsy of minor salivary glands aid in diagnosis.

Treatment is symptomatic, including preservative-free artificial tears or ophthalmic antiinflammatory drops (e.g., cyclosporine [Restasis]). Some patients have surgical punctal occlusion.

Increased fluids with meals and dental hygiene are important. Pilocarpine (Salagen) and cevimeline (Evoxac) can treat dry mouth and decrease risk of dental caries.

Increased humidity at home may reduce respiratory tract infections. Vaginal lubrication with a water-soluble product, such as K-Y jelly, may increase comfort during intercourse.

SPINAL CORD INJURY

Description

Spinal cord injury (SCI) can result in temporary or permanent alteration in spinal cord function. SCIs are usually caused by trauma, including motor vehicle collisions, falls, violence, and sports injuries.

Pathophysiology

The extent of the neurologic damage caused by an SCI results from both *primary injury* (initial disruption of axons) and *secondary injury* (processes such as ischemia, hypoxia, hemorrhage, and edema).

Primary SCI can be caused by cord compression by bone displacement, interruption of blood supply, or distraction from pulling on the cord. Penetrating trauma, such as gunshot and stab wounds, causes tearing and transection.

Secondary injury refers to ongoing, progressive damage after the primary injury. Possible causes include vascular changes resulting from hemorrhage, vasospasm, thrombosis, loss of autoregulation, breakdown of the blood–brain barrier, and infiltration of inflammatory cells that cause ischemia, edema, and cellular necrosis.

- *Apoptosis* (programmed cell death) may continue for weeks after injury and may contribute to postinjury demyelination.

These processes lead to scar tissue formation, irreversible nerve damage, and permanent neurologic deficit. This ongoing destructive process makes it critical to initiate care and management of the patient with an SCI as soon as possible, to limit the damage.

- The extent of injury and prognosis for recovery are most accurately determined at 72 hours or more after injury. Fig. 27 shows the cascade of events causing secondary injury after traumatic SCI.

PATHOPHYSIOLOGY MAP

Fig. 27 Cascade of metabolic and cellular events that leads to spinal cord ischemia and hypoxia of secondary injury. *RBCs,* Red blood cells; *SCBF,* spinal cord blood flow.

Spinal and Neurogenic Shock

Spinal shock may occur after acute SCI. It is characterized by loss of deep tendon and sphincter reflexes, loss of sensation, absent thermoregulation, and flaccid paralysis below the level of injury. This syndrome lasts days to weeks and may mask postinjury neurologic function.

Neurogenic shock results from the loss of vasomotor tone caused by injury and is characterized by hypotension and bradycardia. Loss of sympathetic innervation causes peripheral vasodilation, venous pooling, and decreased cardiac output. These effects are generally associated with a cervical or high thoracic injury. Neurogenic shock may persist for as long as 5 weeks after injury.

Classification

SCIs are classified by the mechanism of injury, level of injury, and degree of injury. The major mechanisms of injury are flexion, flexion-rotation, hyperextension, vertical compression, extension-rotation, and lateral flexion. The level of injury may be cervical, thoracic, lumbar, or sacral. Cervical and lumbar injuries are the most common because these areas are associated with the greatest flexibility and movement. The degree of spinal cord involvement may be either complete or incomplete (partial).

- *Complete cord involvement* results in total loss of sensory and motor function below the level of the injury.
- *Incomplete cord involvement* (partial transection) results in a mixed loss of voluntary motor activity and sensation and leaves some tracts intact. The degree of sensory and motor loss varies depending on the level of the injury and reflects the specific nerve tracts damaged.
- If the cervical cord is involved, paralysis of all four extremities results in *tetraplegia* (formerly termed *quadriplegia*). The lower the level of injury, the more function is retained in the arms.
- If the thoracic, lumbar, or sacral spinal cord is damaged, the result is *paraplegia* (paralysis and loss of sensation in the legs).

Clinical Manifestations

Manifestations of SCI are related to the level and degree of injury. The patient with an incomplete lesion may demonstrate a mixture of symptoms—the higher the injury, the more serious the effects because of the proximity of the cervical cord to the medulla and brainstem.

Movement and rehabilitation potential related to specific locations of the SCI are described in Table 65.2, Harding et al., *Lewis' Medical-Surgical Nursing,* ed 12. In general, sensory function closely parallels motor function at all levels.

Complications

Respiratory System

Cervical injuries above the level of C3 vertebra cause a total loss of respiratory muscle function. Injury or fracture at levels C3–C5 can result in diaphragmatic breathing with respiratory insufficiency and hypoventilation.

Cardiovascular System

Cord injury above the level of T6 leads to dysfunction of the sympathetic nervous system. The result is bradycardia, peripheral vasodilation, and hypotension (neurogenic shock).

Urinary System

Urinary retention is common in acute SCI and spinal shock. While the patient is in spinal shock, the bladder is atonic and fails to empty (urinary retention). In the postacute phase, the bladder may become hyperirritable, with reflex emptying (urinary incontinence).

Gastrointestinal System

Decreased gastrointestinal (GI) motor activity contributes to gastric distention and development of paralytic ileus. Excessive release of hydrochloric acid (HCl) in the stomach may cause stress ulcers. Loss of voluntary control of the bowel after SCI results in neurogenic bowel.

- SCI above the level of the conus medullaris causes the anal sphincter to remain tight, and the ability to sense a full rectum is lost. Bowel movement occurs on a reflex basis when the rectum is full (incontinence).
- SCI at or below the conus medullaris causes the bowel to be areflexic. Peristalsis is impaired and stool propulsion is slow. The defecation reflex may be damaged and anal sphincter tone relaxed (retention). This leads to constipation, increased risk of incontinence, and possible impaction, ileus, or megacolon.

Integumentary System

Lack of movement and sensation increases the potential for skin breakdown over bony prominences. Pressure injuries can occur quickly, leading to major infection or sepsis.

Thermoregulation

Poikilothermia is the inability to maintain a constant core temperature, with the patient assuming the temperature of the environment. It occurs because the interruption of the sympathetic nervous system prevents peripheral temperature sensations from reaching the hypothalamus. With SCI, there is decreased ability to sweat or shiver below the level of injury, which also affects body temperature regulation.

Peripheral Vascular Problems

Venous thromboembolism (VTE) is a common problem in the first 3 months (see Venous Thrombosis). Pulmonary embolism is a leading cause of death in patients with SCI.

Pain

Pain after SCI can be nociceptive or neuropathic.

- *Nociceptive pain* in SCI can result from musculoskeletal, visceral, and/or other types of injury (e.g., skin ulceration, headache). Patients often describe musculoskeletal pain as dull or aching. It starts or worsens with movement. Visceral pain is located in the thorax, abdomen, and/or pelvis and may be dull, tender, or cramping.
- *Neuropathic pain* in SCI occurs from damage to the spinal cord or nerve roots. The pain can be located at or below the level of injury. Patients often identify neuropathic pain as hot, burning, tingling, "pins and needles," cold, and/or shooting. Even light touch can cause significant pain.

Autonomic Dysreflexia

Autonomic dysreflexia (also known as *hyperreflexia*) is a massive uncompensated cardiovascular reaction mediated by the sympathetic nervous system. It involves stimulation of sensory receptors below the level of the SCI. The intact sympathetic nervous system below the SCI responds to the stimulation by increasing BP, but the parasympathetic nervous system is unable to directly counteract these responses via the injured spinal cord. Baroreceptors in the carotid sinus and aorta sense the hypertension and stimulate the parasympathetic system. This results in a decreased heart rate, but visceral and peripheral vessels do not dilate because efferent impulses cannot pass through the injured spinal cord.

- *Autonomic hyperreflexia* is a life-threatening situation requiring immediate resolution to prevent status epilepticus, myocardial infarction, stroke, and even death.
- The most common precipitating cause is a distended bladder or rectum.
- Manifestations include hypertension, blurred vision, throbbing headache, marked flushing and diaphoresis above the level of the lesion, bradycardia (30–40 beats/minute), piloerection, nasal congestion, nausea, and anxiety. Measure BP when the patient with an SCI reports a headache. Suspect AD in adults with SBP elevation of 20–40 mm Hg above baseline.

S

- Elevate the head of the bed 45 degrees or sit the patient upright, determine the cause, and notify the health care provider (HCP). If symptoms persist after the source has been relieved, a rapid-onset and short-duration agent, such as nitroglycerin, nitroprusside, or hydralazine, is administered. Continue careful monitoring until vital signs stabilize.
- Teach the patient and caregivers the causes and symptoms of autonomic hyperreflexia (throbbing headache, marked flushing and sweating above the level of injury, piloerection [goosebumps], blurred vision or seeing spots, nasal congestion, anxiety, and nausea). They must understand the life-threatening nature of this dysfunction, know how to relieve the cause, and be prepared to call for emergency care.

Diagnostic Studies

- CT scan is the preferred imaging study to diagnose the location and degree of injury and degree of spinal canal compromise. Cervical X-rays are obtained when CT scan is not readily available.
- MRI is used to assess soft tissue and neurologic changes and for neurologic deficits or worsening of neurologic status.
- Comprehensive neurologic examination is done along with assessment of the head, chest, and abdomen for additional injuries or trauma.
- Patients with cervical injuries who demonstrate altered mental status may need vertebral angiography to rule out vertebral artery damage.

Interprofessional Management

After stabilization at the injury scene, the person is transferred to a health care facility. A thorough assessment is done to evaluate the specific degree of deficit and establish the level and degree of injury. The patient may go directly to surgery after initial immobilization and assessment or to the intensive care unit (ICU) for monitoring and management.

Stabilization

Nonoperative treatments are focused on stabilization of the injured spinal segment and decompression, through either traction or realignment, to prevent secondary spinal cord damage caused by repeated contusion or compression.

When cord compression is certain or the neurologic disorder progresses, immediate surgery may stabilize the spinal column and reduce secondary injury.

- A fixation procedure involves attaching metal screws, plates, or other devices to align the bones of the spine. This is usually done when two or more vertebrae have been injured. Small pieces of bone may be attached to the injured area to help the bones fuse into one solid piece.

Drug Therapy

The American Association of Neurological Surgeons and Congress of Neurological Surgeons does not recommend methylprednisolone for treatment in acute SCI.

- Low-molecular-weight heparin (LMWH) (e.g., enoxaparin [Lovenox]) is used to prevent VTE unless contraindicated.
- Vasopressor agents, such as phenylephrine or norepinephrine, may be used in the acute phase to maintain mean arterial pressure and the perfusion to the spinal cord.

Nursing Management

Goals

The patient with an SCI will maintain an optimal level of neurologic functioning, have minimal or no complications of immobility, be able to care for self or direct others to do so, and return to home at an optimal level of functioning.

Interventions

Nursing interventions for the prevention of SCI include identifying high-risk persons and providing teaching.

- Support measures to combat distracted and impaired driving.
- Teach people to use child safety seats and helmets for motorcyclists and bicyclists.
- Promote programs for older adults aimed at preventing falls and injury.

High cervical injury resulting from flexion-rotation is the most complex SCI and is discussed in this section. Interventions for this type of injury can be modified for patients with less severe problems.

Immobilization

- Proper immobilization of the neck involves maintaining a neutral position. Closed reduction with skeletal traction is used for early realignment of cervical injuries. Crutchfield or Gardner–Wells tongs or halo (halo ring) can provide this type of traction. A rope extends from the center of the device over a pulley to weights attached at the end. Traction must be maintained at all times. Possible displacement of the skull pins is a disadvantage of tongs. If pin displacement occurs, hold the patient's head in a neutral position and get help. Immobilize the head while the HCP reinserts the tongs.
- Infection at the sites of tong insertion is a potential problem. A common protocol involves cleansing the sites twice a day with chlorhexidine and applying an antibiotic ointment as a mechanical barrier to the entrance of bacteria.

S

After cervical fusion or other stabilization surgery, a hard cervical collar or sternal-occipital-mandibular immobilizer brace can be worn. A patient with a stable injury may have a halo fixation apparatus applied. Patients with stable thoracic or lumbar spine injuries may be immobilized with a custom thoracolumbar sacral orthosis (TLSO, body jacket).

Respiratory Problems

Respiratory complications are the leading cause of morbidity and mortality in SCI. The possibility of respiratory arrest requires careful monitoring and readiness for prompt action. If the patient is exhausted from labored breathing or if arterial blood gases indicate inadequate oxygenation or ventilation, endotracheal intubation or tracheostomy and mechanical ventilation are needed (see Artificial Airways: Endotracheal Tubes, Tracheostomy and Mechanical Ventilation). Pneumonia and atelectasis may occur because of reduced vital capacity and the loss of intercostal and abdominal muscle function, resulting in diaphragmatic breathing, pooled secretions, and an ineffective cough.

- Regularly assess breath sounds, arterial blood gases (ABGs), tidal volume, vital capacity, skin color, breathing patterns (especially the use of accessory muscles), subjective comments about the effort to breathe, and the amount and color of sputum.
- Support gas exchange and ventilation by the administration of O_2, chest physiotherapy and assisted coughing, incentive spirometry, and tracheal suctioning.

Cardiovascular Instability

If bradycardia is symptomatic, give an anticholinergic medication such as atropine. A pacemaker may be inserted (see Pacemakers). Hypotension is managed with fluid replacement and a vasopressor agent such as phenylephrine or norepinephrine. Monitor the patient for indications of hypovolemic shock secondary to hemorrhage, which may require blood transfusion.

- Use LMWH or low-dose heparin in combination with intermittent pneumatic compression devices (IPCs) or graduated compression stockings to promote venous return and reduce the risk of VTE.
- Perform range-of-motion (ROM) exercises and stretching regularly. Assess the thighs and calves of the legs for the signs of deep vein thrombosis (DVT) every shift (e.g., deep reddish color, edema).

Fluid and Nutritional Maintenance

During the first 48–72 hours after the injury, the GI tract stops functioning (paralytic ileus). A nasogastric (NG) tube can be inserted to suction.

- Once bowel sounds are present or flatus is passed, and the patient is not receiving mechanical ventilation, a formal swallow evaluation should be done. If no risk of aspiration is identified, gradually introduce oral food and fluids.
- If the patient fails the swallow evaluation or is unable to eat because of an endotracheal tube or tracheostomy, a more secure feeding tube may be placed in the stomach or jejunum.

Bowel and Bladder Management

An indwelling catheter is inserted soon after the injury. Strict aseptic technique for catheter care is essential.

- *Catheter-acquired urinary tract infection* (CAUTI) is a common problem. After the patient is stabilized, assess the best means of managing long-term urinary function. Clean intermittent catheterization (CIC) is the preferred method for emptying the bladder.

To combat constipation from neurogenic bowel, start a bowel program.

- A rectal stimulant (suppository or mini-enema) is inserted daily, followed by gentle digital stimulation or manual evacuation. Include adequate fluid intake, a diet high in fiber and vegetables, and increased activity as able.

Temperature Control

Monitor the environment closely to maintain an appropriate temperature. Regularly assess the patient's temperature. Do not use excess covers or unduly expose the patient.

Skin Care

The most common long-term complication in SCI is pressure injury (PI). Healthy skin requires adequate blood circulation. Constant pressure can compress blood vessels and limit blood supply, causing cell death and PI. Factors that increase risk for PI include duration of SCI, higher level of injury, smoking, being underweight, and comorbid medical conditions.

- Preventing PI requires diligent nursing care. Perform a risk assessment with a daily skin assessment. Areas most vulnerable to breakdown include the sacrum, ischia, trochanters, and heels. Assess surgical incisions for healing and skin integrity under collars and braces.
- Regularly assess nutrition status. Both weight loss and gain can contribute to skin breakdown. Teach the patient and caregiver about the causes and risk factors for PI development.

Stress Ulcers

Stress ulcers can occur because of the physiologic response to severe trauma and psychologic stress. Peak incidence is 6–14

S

days after injury. Monitor hematocrit for a slow drop. Histamine (H_2)-receptor blockers or proton pump inhibitors (e.g., pantoprazole, omeprazole) may be given prophylactically to decrease HCl secretion.

Pain Management

Antiinflammatory drugs, such as ibuprofen (Motrin), or opioids may help with musculoskeletal nociceptive pain. Visceral nociceptive pain is a dull, tender, or cramping pain in the thorax, abdomen, or pelvis. It may originate in the bladder or bowel. Assess the patient's bowel and bladder function to avoid bladder distention or constipation. Other causes of nociceptive pain include urinary tract infection (UTI) and renal stones.

- Notify the HCP if the patient has persistent pain despite treatment. Diagnostic imaging may be needed to determine the cause.

Neuropathic pain in the initial phase is usually at the level of SCI. It may occur on one or both sides of the body within the affected dermatome, and up to three levels below. The patient will describe hot, burning, tingling, shooting, electric pain. Pregabalin (Lyrica) is used to reduce pain.

Sensory Deprivation

To prevent sensory deprivation, compensate for the patient's absence of sensations by stimulating the patient above the level of injury. Conversation, music, and interesting foods can be a part of the nursing care plan. If the head of the bed must remain flat, provide prism glasses to help the patient read and watch television. Make every effort to prevent the patient from withdrawing from the environment.

Reflexes

Once spinal shock is resolved, reflexes often return with hyperactive and exaggerated responses. Penile erections can occur from a variety of stimuli, causing embarrassment and discomfort. Spasms ranging from mild twitches to convulsive movements below the level of the lesion may also occur. Reflex activity may be interpreted by the patient or caregiver as a return of function. Tactfully explain the reason for the activity. Spasms may be controlled with antispasmodic medications such as baclofen, dantrolene (Dantrium), or tizanidine (Zanaflex).

Rehabilitation

Physiologic and psychologic rehabilitation is complex. Many of the problems identified in the acute period may continue throughout life. Rehabilitation focuses on refined retraining of physiologic processes and extensive patient, caregiver, and family teaching about how to manage the changes resulting from injury.

SPINAL CORD TUMORS

Description

Spinal cord tumors are classified as *primary* (arising from some component of cord, dura, nerves, or vessels) or *secondary* (from primary growths that have metastasized to the spinal cord).

Spinal cord tumor locations are as *extradural* (outside the dura), *intradural-extramedullary* (between the spinal cord and dura), or *intramedullary* (within the substance of spinal cord itself). The most common lesions are astrocytes and ependymomas.

Symptoms are caused by the mechanical effects of slow compression and irritation of nerve roots, displacement of the spinal cord, or gradual obstruction of the vascular supply. The slow growth does not cause a secondary injury as in traumatic spinal cord injury (SCI). Complete function may be possible after the tumor is removed.

Clinical Manifestations

A common early symptom of a spinal cord tumor is back pain, with the location depending on the level of compression. The pain worsens with activity, coughing, straining, and lying down.

- Slowly increasing clumsiness, weakness, spasticity, and paralysis can develop.
- Sensory disruption occurs as coldness, numbness, and tingling in one or more extremities.
- Bladder problems are marked by urgency, with difficulty in starting the flow and progressing to retention with overflow incontinence.

Diagnostic Studies

Extradural tumors can be seen on routine spinal X-rays. Intradural and intramedullary tumors require MRI or CT scans or CT myelogram for detection. Cerebrospinal fluid (CSF) analysis may reveal tumor cells.

Interprofessional and Nursing Care

Spinal cord compression is an emergency. Relief of the ischemia related to the compression is the goal of therapy.

- Corticosteroids (e.g., dexamethasone) are given immediately to relieve tumor-related edema.

Emergency surgery may be needed to decompress the spinal cord, obtain tissue for pathology, and determine appropriate adjunctive treatment. Primary spinal tumors may be removed with the goal of cure. In patients with metastatic tumors, treatment is primarily palliative, with the goal of restoring or preserving neurologic function, stabilizing the spine, and alleviating pain. Radiation therapy and/or chemotherapy may be used to treat the tumor.

- Ensure that the patient receives pain medication as needed.
- Assess the patient's neurologic status before and after treatment. Depending on the neurologic dysfunction, the patient may require care similar to that of a patient recovering from an SCI. Depending on the amount of neurologic dysfunction, care of the patient may be similar to that of a patient recovering from SCI (see Spinal Cord Injury).

SPLEEN DISORDERS

Many illnesses can affect the spleen. Most can cause some degree of *splenomegaly* (enlarged spleen). However, an enlarged spleen may be present in some people without any evidence of disease. When the spleen enlarges, its normal blood cell filtering and storage capacity increase, reducing the number of circulating blood cells.

- The degree of splenic enlargement varies with the disease. Massive splenic enlargement occurs with mononucleosis, chronic myelogenous leukemia, and thalassemia major. Mild splenic enlargement occurs with heart failure and systemic lupus erythematosus.

A slight to moderate enlargement of the spleen is usually asymptomatic and found during routine examination of the abdomen. Massive splenomegaly may be tolerated. Patients report abdominal discomfort and early satiety. Other ways we assess the size of the spleen include ultrasound, CT or PET scan, MRI, and liver/spleen nuclear scan.

Sometimes splenectomy is part of treatment of splenomegaly. Another reason for splenectomy is splenic rupture from trauma and diseases such as mononucleosis, malaria, and cancers. After a splenectomy, peripheral red blood cell (RBC), white blood cell (WBC), and platelet counts can increase dramatically.

Nursing responsibilities for patients with spleen disorders vary. Splenomegaly may be painful and require analgesics.

- Take care in moving, turning, and positioning.
- Assess lung expansion because spleen enlargement may impair diaphragmatic excursion.

- If anemia, thrombocytopenia, or leukopenia develops from splenic enlargement, institute nursing measures to support the patient and prevent life-threatening complications.

  If splenectomy was performed, observe the patient for hemorrhage and shock.

- After a splenectomy, patients may develop immunologic deficiencies and be at lifelong risk for infection from encapsulated organisms, such as pneumococcus. This risk is reduced by pneumococcal vaccination.

STOMACH CANCER

Description

Stomach (gastric) cancer is an adenocarcinoma of the stomach wall. The average age at diagnosis is 68 years. The overall 5-year survival rate of all people with stomach cancer is about 32%.

Pathophysiology

Stomach cancer likely begins with a nonspecific mucosal injury because of infection (with *Helicobacter pylori*), autoimmune-related inflammation, repeated exposure to irritants such as bile or nonsteroidal antiinflammatory drugs (NSAIDs), or tobacco use.

- Increased risk is related to smoking, obesity, and diets high in smoked foods, salted fish and meat, and pickled vegetables. Whole grains and fresh fruits and vegetables reduce stomach cancer risk.

- Other risk factors include atrophic gastritis, pernicious anemia, adenomatous polyps, hyperplastic polyps, and achlorhydria (absent or low production of gastric HCl). People with lymphoma of the stomach (mucosa-associated lymphoid tissue [MALT]) have a higher risk. Although first-degree relatives of patients with stomach cancer are at increased risk, only about 10% of stomach cancers have an inherited component.

  Stomach cancer spreads by direct extension and infiltrates rapidly to the surrounding tissue and liver. Seeding of tumor cells into the peritoneal cavity occurs late in the disease.

Clinical Manifestations

Stomach cancers often spread to adjacent organs before any distressing symptoms occur. Manifestations include unexplained weight loss, early satiety, indigestion, abdominal discomfort or pain, and signs and symptoms of anemia.

S

- Anemia occurs with chronic blood loss as the lesion erodes the stomach mucosa. The patient appears pale and weak with fatigue, dizziness, weakness, and positive occult stools.
- Hard and enlarged supraclavicular lymph nodes suggest metastasis via the thoracic duct. Ascites is a poor prognostic sign.

Diagnostic Studies

- Upper gastrointestinal (GI) endoscopy is the best diagnostic tool.
- Endoscopic ultrasound and CT and positron emission tomography (PET) scans can be used to stage the disease.
- Laparoscopy can be done to determine peritoneal spread.
- Blood studies detect anemia and also liver and pancreatic involvement.
- Stool examination provides evidence of occult or gross bleeding.

Interprofessional Management

Treatment of choice is surgical removal of the tumor. Surgical procedures used are similar to those used for peptic ulcer disease (see Peptic Ulcer Disease). Patients with lesions in the antrum or pyloric region generally have either a Billroth I or II procedure. When the lesion is in the fundus, a total gastrectomy with esophagojejunostomy is done. When metastasis has occurred to adjacent organs, such as the spleen, ovaries, or bowel, the surgical procedure is extended as needed. If the tumor extends into the transverse colon, partial colon resection is done.

- Therapy for localized stomach cancer is surgical resection followed by chemotherapy agents used in combination. These include fluorouracil, capecitabine, carboplatin, cisplatin, docetaxel, epirubicin, irinotecan, oxaliplatin, and paclitaxel. Intraperitoneal administration of chemotherapy agents may also be used to treat metastatic disease (see Chemotherapy).
- Trastuzumab (Herceptin) and ramucirumab (Cyramza) are targeted therapy agents used to treat stomach cancer. Ramucirumab binds to the receptor for vascular endothelial growth factor (VEGF) and prevents VEGF from binding to the receptor, thus preventing the growth and spread of cancer.
- Combined radiation therapy and chemotherapy can reduce recurrence or be given as a palliative measure to decrease tumor mass and provide temporary relief of obstruction (see Radiation Therapy).

Nursing Management
Goals
The overall goals are that the patient with stomach cancer will experience minimal discomfort, achieve optimal nutritional status, and maintain a degree of spiritual and psychologic well-being appropriate to the disease stage.

Interventions
Your role in the early detection of stomach cancer focuses on identifying patients at risk, such as those with *H. pylori* infection, pernicious anemia, or achlorhydria. Encourage patients with a positive family history of stomach cancer to undergo diagnostic evaluation if manifestations of anemia, peptic ulcer disease, or vague epigastric distress are present.

When diagnostic tests confirm cancer, offer emotional and physical support, provide information, and clarify test results. Patient teaching is similar to that for peptic ulcer disease surgery (see Peptic Ulcer Disease).

- Preoperative management focuses on correcting nutrition deficits and treating anemia. Gastric decompression may be needed if gastric outlet obstruction is present.

Postoperative care is also similar to that after a Billroth I or II procedure for peptic ulcer disease.

- After a total gastrectomy, closely observe the patient for signs of fluid leakage at the site of anastomosis, as evidenced by an elevation in temperature and increasing dyspnea. Dumping syndrome may also occur with this procedure (see Peptic Ulcer Disease).
- Postoperative wound healing may be impaired because of poor nutritional intake. IV or oral replacement of vitamins C, D, and K; the B complex vitamins; and cobalamin may be needed because they are normally absorbed in the duodenum.

▼ Patient and Caregiver Teaching
Before discharge, teach the patient and caregivers about comfort measures and the use of analgesics. Additional considerations include:

- Recurrence of cancer is common. Patients need regular follow-up examinations and imaging assessments.
- Teach wound care, if needed, to the primary caregiver in the home setting.
- Dressings, special equipment, or special services may be required for the patient's care at home.
- Provide a list of community resources and referral to Home Health services, if needed.

S

STROKE

Description

Stroke occurs when there is *ischemia* (inadequate blood flow) to a part of the brain or *hemorrhage* (bleeding) into the brain that results in death of brain cells. In a stroke, functions such as movement, sensation, thinking, talking, or emotions that were controlled by the affected area of the brain are lost or impaired. The severity of the loss of function varies based on the location and extent of the brain damage. Stroke is the fifth most common cause of death in the United States. An estimated 800,000 people have a stroke annually, and 15%–30% will live with permanent disability.

- The terms *brain attack* and *cerebrovascular accident* (CVA) are also used to describe stroke. The term *brain attack* communicates the urgency of recognizing the warning signs of a stroke and treating it as a medical emergency, as would be done with a heart attack (Table 83).

Risk factors associated with stroke can be divided into non-modifiable and modifiable. Stroke risk increases with multiple risk factors.

Nonmodifiable risk factors include age, gender, ethnicity or race, and family history or heredity. Two-thirds of all strokes occur in persons older than 65 years, but stroke can occur at any age. Strokes are more common in men, but more women die from stroke than men.

- Blacks have twice the incidence of stroke and a higher death rate from stroke compared to any other ethnic groups. This may be related in part to an increased incidence of hypertension, obesity, and diabetes.
- People with a family history of stroke are at higher risk for stroke.

Modifiable risk factors include hypertension, heart disease, diabetes, smoking, obesity, sleep apnea, metabolic syndrome, lack of physical exercise, poor diet, and drug or alcohol use. Hypertension is the most important modifiable risk factor. Treating hypertension reduces stroke risk by up to 50%.

Transient Ischemic Attack

A *transient ischemic attack* (TIA) is an episode of neurologic dysfunction caused by focal brain, spinal cord, or retinal ischemia, but without acute brain infarction. TIAs may be caused by microemboli that temporarily block the blood flow. Clinical symptoms

TABLE 83 Patient and Caregiver Teaching: FAST for Warning Signs of Stroke

FAST is an easy way to remember the signs of stroke. Include the following information in the teaching plan for a patient at risk for stroke and the patient's caregiver.

F	Face drooping	Does one side of the face droop or is it numb? Ask the person to smile. Is the smile uneven?
A	Arm weakness	Is one arm weak or numb? Ask the person to raise both arms. Does one arm drift downward?
S	Speech difficulties	Is speech slurred? Is the person unable to speak or hard to understand? Ask the person to repeat a simple sentence like "The sky is blue." Is the sentence repeated correctly?
T	Time	Time is CRITICAL! If someone shows any of these signs (even if they go away), call 911 and get the person to the hospital. Note the time when the signs first appeared.

In addition, report the sudden onset of the following:
- confusion
- numbness or weakness, especially in one side of the body
- severe headache with no known cause
- trouble seeing in one or both eyes
- trouble walking, dizziness, loss of balance or coordination

American Stroke Association: FAST. Retrieved from www.strokeassociation.org/STROKEORG/WarningSigns/Stroke-Warning-Signs-and-Symptoms_UCM_308528_SubHomePage.jsp.

typically last <1 hour. TIAs are a warning sign of progressive cerebrovascular disease.

Most TIAs resolve. However, it is important to teach the patient to seek treatment for any stroke symptoms because there is no way to predict if a TIA will resolve. One-third of those who have a TIA do not have another one, one-third have more TIAs, and one-third progress to stroke. TIA signs and symptoms depend on the blood vessel involved and the brain area that is ischemic.

- If the carotid system is involved, patients may have a temporary loss of vision in one eye, transient hemiparesis, numbness or loss of sensation, or a sudden inability to speak.

- Signs and symptoms of a TIA involving the vertebrobasilar system may include tinnitus, vertigo, darkened or blurred vision, ptosis, dysphagia, ataxia, and unilateral or bilateral numbness or weakness.

A TIA is a medical emergency. Teach people at risk for TIA to seek medical attention at once with any stroke-like symptom and to identify the time of symptom onset.

Pathophysiology

Unlike a TIA, in which ischemia occurs without infarction, a stroke results in infarction (cell death). Strokes are classified as ischemic or hemorrhagic, based on the cause and underlying pathophysiology (Fig. 28 and Table 84).

Ischemic Stroke

An *ischemic stroke* results from inadequate blood flow to the brain from partial or complete occlusion of an artery. Ischemic strokes may be either thrombotic or embolic.

Thrombotic Stroke

A *thrombotic stroke* occurs from injury to a blood vessel wall and formation of a blood clot. The lumen of the blood vessel becomes narrowed, and if it becomes occluded, infarction occurs. It is the most common cause of stroke.

- Thrombotic strokes are more common in older adults. Most thrombotic strokes are associated with hypertension or diabetes. The extent of the stroke depends on speed of onset, size of the

A **Thrombotic stroke.**
The process of clot formation (thrombosis) results in a narrowing of the lumen, which blocks the passage of the blood through the artery.

B **Embolic stroke.**
An embolus is a blood clot or other debris circulating in the blood. When it reaches an artery in the brain that is too narrow to pass through, it lodges there and blocks the flow of blood.

C **Hemorrhagic stroke.**
A burst blood vessel may allow blood to seep into and damage brain tissues until clotting shuts off the leak.

Fig. 28 Major causes of stroke. A-Thrombotic stroke. B-Embolic stroke. C-Hemorrhagic stroke.

TABLE 84 Types of Stroke

Gender and Age	Warning and Onset	Prognosis
Ischemic		
Incidence: accounts for 87% of strokes		
Embolic		
Men more than women	*Warning:* TIA (uncommon) *Onset:* sudden onset, most likely to occur during activity	Single event, signs and symptoms develop quickly, usually some improvement, recurrence common without aggressive treatment of underlying disease.
Thrombotic		
Men more than women Oldest median age	*Warning:* TIA (30%–50% of cases) *Onset:* often during or after sleep	Stepwise progression, signs and symptoms develop slowly, usually some improvement, recurrence in 20%–25% of survivors.
Hemorrhagic		
Incidence: accounts for 13% of strokes		
Intracerebral		
Slightly higher in women	*Warning:* Headache (25% of cases) *Onset:* activity (often)	Progression over 24 h. Poor prognosis, fatality more likely with presence of coma.
Subarachnoid		
Slightly higher in women Youngest median age	*Warning:* Headache (common) *Onset:* activity (often), sudden onset, most often related to head trauma	Usually single sudden event, fatality more likely with presence of coma.

TIA, Transient ischemic attack.

S

lesion, and presence of collateral circulation. Many times, a TIA precedes a thrombotic stroke.

- Most patients do not have a decreased level of consciousness in the first 24 hours unless it is caused by a brainstem stroke or a condition such as seizures, increased intracranial pressure (ICP), or hemorrhage.
- Ischemic stroke symptoms may progress in the first 72 hours as infarction and cerebral edema increase.

Embolic Stroke

Embolic stroke occurs when an embolus lodges in and occludes a cerebral artery, resulting in infarction and edema of the area supplied by the involved vessel. Embolism is the second most common cause of stroke.

Most emboli originate in the heart. The embolus travels to the cerebral circulation and lodges where a vessel narrows. Heart conditions associated with emboli are atrial fibrillation, myocardial infarction (MI), infective endocarditis, valvular heart prostheses, patent foramen ovale, and atrial septal defects. Less common causes of emboli include air and fat from long bone (e.g., femur) fractures.

- The embolic stroke often occurs rapidly. The patient usually remains conscious, and may have a headache.
- Recurrence is common unless the underlying cause is aggressively treated.

Hemorrhagic Stroke

A *hemorrhagic stroke* results from bleeding into the brain tissue (intracerebral or intraparenchymal hemorrhage) or into the subarachnoid space or ventricles (subarachnoid hemorrhage [SAH]).

Intracerebral Hemorrhage

Intracerebral hemorrhage is bleeding within the brain caused by a rupture of a blood vessel. Hypertension is the most common cause of intracerebral hemorrhage. Other causes include vascular malformations, coagulation disorders, anticoagulant and thrombolytic drugs, trauma, brain tumors, and ruptured aneurysm.

- Hemorrhage often occurs during periods of activity. Most often there is a sudden onset of symptoms, progressing over minutes to hours caused by ongoing bleeding.
- Manifestations include neurologic deficits, headache, nausea, vomiting, decreased level of consciousness, and hypertension. Extent of the symptoms varies depending on the amount, location, and duration of bleeding.

- Prognosis of patients with intracerebral hemorrhage is poor, with 40%–80% of patients dying within 30 days, and 50% of the deaths occurring within the first 48 hours.

Subarachnoid Hemorrhage

SAH occurs when there is intracranial bleeding into the cerebrospinal fluid (CSF)–filled space between the arachnoid and pia mater membranes on the surface of the brain. SAH is often caused by rupture of a cerebral aneurysm (congenital or acquired weakness with ballooning of vessels). Other causes of SAH include trauma and cocaine use.

- The patient may have warning symptoms if the ballooning artery applies pressure to brain tissue. Minor warning symptoms may result from leaking of an aneurysm before major rupture. Sudden onset of the "worst headache of one's life" is a characteristic symptom of a ruptured aneurysm.
- The patient's level of consciousness may range from alert to comatose, depending on the severity of the bleeding.
- Other manifestations include focal neurologic deficits (including cranial nerve deficits), nausea, vomiting, seizures, and stiff neck.
- Despite improvements in surgical techniques and management, many patients with SAH die. Survivors can have significant deficits, including cognitive problems.

Clinical Manifestations

Neurologic manifestations do not significantly differ between ischemic and hemorrhagic stroke, because destruction of neural tissue is the basis of manifestations for both types of stroke. Manifestations are related to the location of the stroke. Manifestations seen with specific cerebral artery involvement are listed in Table 85. Fig. 29 illustrates manifestations of right- and left-sided stroke.

Motor Function

Motor deficits are the most obvious effect of stroke. Motor deficits include impairment of mobility, respiratory function, swallowing and speech, gag reflex, and self-care abilities. Because the pyramidal pathway crosses at the level of the medulla, a lesion on one side of the brain affects motor function on the opposite side of the brain (contralateral). Impaired spatial-perceptual orientation may further affect mobility.

- The initial *hyporeflexia* (depressed reflexes) usually progresses to *hyperreflexia* (hyperactive reflexes).

TABLE 85   Stroke Manifestations Related to Artery Involvement

Artery	Manifestations
Anterior cerebral	Motor and/or sensory deficit (contralateral), sucking or rooting reflex, rigidity, gait problems, loss of proprioception and fine touch
Middle cerebral	*Dominant side:* aphasia, motor and sensory deficit, hemianopsia *Nondominant side:* neglect, motor and sensory deficit, hemianopsia
Posterior cerebral	Hemianopsia, visual hallucination, spontaneous pain, motor deficit
Vertebral	Cranial nerve deficits, diplopia, dizziness, nausea, vomiting, dysarthria, dysphagia, and/or coma

Communication

The left hemisphere is dominant for language skills in all right-handed people and most left-handed people.

- Language disorders involve the expression and comprehension of written or spoken words. *Aphasia* (loss of comprehension and use of language) occurs when a stroke damages the dominant hemisphere of the brain. Types of aphasia include *receptive aphasia* (loss of comprehension), *expressive aphasia* (inability to produce language), or *global aphasia* (total inability to communicate).
- Many stroke patients have *dysarthria,* a disturbance in the muscular control of speech.

Affect

Patients who have had a stroke may have a hard time expressing emotions. Emotional responses may be exaggerated, unpredictable, and unrelated to the situation. Depression and feelings associated with changes in body image and loss of function can make this worse. Patients may be frustrated by mobility and communication problems.

Intellectual Function

Patients who have had a stroke may show impaired memory and judgment.

- A left-brain stroke is more likely to result in memory problems related to language. Patients with a left-brain stroke often are cautious in making judgments.

Right-brain damage (stroke on right side of the brain)	**Left-brain damage** (stroke on left side of the brain)
• Paralyzed left side: hemiplegia	• Paralyzed right side: hemiplegia
• Left-sided neglect	• Impaired speech/language aphasias
• Spatial-perceptual deficits	• Impaired right/left discrimination
• Tends to deny or minimize problems	• Slow performance, cautious
• Rapid performance, short attention span	• Aware of deficits: depression, anxiety
• Impulsive, safety problems	• Impaired comprehension related to language, math
• Impaired judgment	
• Impaired time concepts	

Fig. 29 Manifestations of right- and left-brain stroke.

- The patient with a right-brain stroke tends to be impulsive and move quickly.

Spatial-Perceptual Ability

Those who had a stroke on the right side of the brain are more likely to have problems with spatial-perceptual orientation. Spatial-perceptual problems fall within four categories:

- Patients may deny their illnesses or not recognize their own body parts. This results from parietal lobe damage.
- Spatial neglect, when the patient neglects all input from the affected side (erroneous perception of self in space). This may be worsened by *homonymous hemianopsia*, in which blindness

occurs in the same half of the visual fields of both eyes. The patient has trouble with spatial orientation, such as judging distances.

- *Agnosia.* This is the inability to recognize an object by sight, touch, or hearing.
- *Apraxia.* This is the inability to carry out learned sequential movements on command.

Diagnostic Studies

Diagnostic study results confirm manifestations of a stroke, identify likely causes, and guide decisions about therapy.

- MRI is more effective in identifying ischemic stroke than CT scans. However, CT scan is a rapid tool to rule out hemorrhage.
- CT angiography (CTA) provides visualization of cerebral blood vessels and an estimate of perfusion. CTA also detects filling defects in the cerebral arteries.
- Magnetic resonance angiography (MRA) can detect vascular lesions and blockages similar to CTA.
- Angiography can identify cervical and cerebrovascular occlusion, atherosclerotic plaques, and malformation of vessels.
- Intraarterial digital subtraction angiography (DSA) involves injection of a contrast agent to visualize vessels in the neck and circle of Willis.
- Transcranial Doppler (TCD) ultrasonography has been effective in detecting microemboli and vasospasm in the major cerebral arteries.
- If the suspected cause of the stroke includes emboli from the heart, diagnostic cardiac tests should be done.

Interprofessional Management

Prevention

The goals of stroke prevention include management of modifiable risk factors to prevent a stroke. Health promotion focuses on healthy diet, weight control, regular exercise, not smoking, limiting alcohol use, and BP management. Patients with known risk factors (e.g., diabetes, hypertension, obesity, high serum lipids, cardiac disease) need close management.

- Measures to prevent the development of a thrombus or embolus are used in patients with TIAs because they are at high risk for stroke. Antiplatelet drugs are usually the chosen treatment to prevent stroke in patients who have had a TIA. Aspirin at a dose of 81 mg/day is the most often used antiplatelet agent.
- Other drugs include ticlopidine, clopidogrel (Plavix), dipyridamole (Persantine), and combined dipyridamole and aspirin (Aggrenox).

- For patients who have atrial fibrillation, oral anticoagulation can include warfarin (Coumadin) and the direct factor Xa inhibitors: rivaroxaban (Xarelto), dabigatran (Pradaxa), and apixaban (Eliquis).
- Statins (simvastatin [Zocor], lovastatin) have been shown to be effective in the prevention of stroke for people who have had a TIA in the past.
- Surgical therapy for the patient with TIA from carotid disease includes carotid endarterectomy, transluminal angioplasty, and stenting.

Acute Care: Ischemic Stroke

- The goals of acute care are preserving life, preventing further brain damage, and reducing disability. In the unresponsive person, acute care begins with managing the airway, breathing, and circulation. O_2 administration, artificial airway insertion, intubation, and mechanical ventilation may be required. Determine the time of symptom onset. This is important for all types of stroke, especially ischemic strokes, since the time can affect treatment decisions.
- It is important for the patient to rapidly undergo either a noncontrast head CT or MRI.
- After baseline neurologic assessment, patients are monitored closely for increasing neurologic deficits.
- Elevated BP is common right after a stroke and may be a protective response to maintain cerebral perfusion. After ischemic stroke in those patients who do not receive fibrinolytic therapy, the use of drugs to lower BP is recommended only if BP is markedly increased (systolic BP > 220 mm Hg or diastolic BP > 120 mm Hg). In a patient who is going to have fibrinolytic therapy, the BP must be less than 185/110 mm Hg and then maintained at or below 180/105 mm Hg for at least 24 hours after fibrinolytic therapy.
- Fluid and electrolyte balance must be controlled carefully. Adequate fluid intake is a priority but overhydration may increase cerebral edema.
- Managing increased intracranial pressure (ICP) includes practices that improve venous drainage, such as elevating the head of the bed, maintaining head and neck in alignment, and avoiding hip flexion. For additional measures that reduce ICP, see Increased Intracranial Pressure.

Drug Therapy

Recombinant tissue plasminogen activator (tPA) is given IV to reestablish blood flow and prevent cell death for patients with acute ischemic stroke. This drug must be given within 3–4.5 hours of the onset of clinical signs. Patients are screened carefully before tPA is given, including a CT or MRI scan to rule out hemorrhagic stroke, blood tests for coagulation disorders, and recent history of gastrointestinal (GI) bleeding, head trauma, or major surgery.

- During tPA infusion, closely monitor the patient's vital signs to assess for improvement or deterioration related to intracerebral hemorrhage.
- Control of BP is critical during and for 24 hours after treatment.
- Aspirin may be started at a dose of 325 mg within 24–48 hours of an ischemic stroke.
- For patients who have atrial fibrillation, oral anticoagulants include warfarin and the direct factor Xa inhibitors: rivaroxaban (Xarelto), dabigatran (Pradaxa), and apixaban (Eliquis). Platelet inhibitors include aspirin, ticlopidine, clopidogrel, and dipyridamole.
- Statins are effective after an ischemic stroke.

Surgical Therapy

Stent retrievers are a way to open blocked arteries in the brain using a removable stent system. Stent retrievers are becoming the most effective way of managing ischemic stroke.

Acute Care: Hemorrhagic Stroke

Drug Therapy

Anticoagulants and platelet inhibitors are contraindicated in patients with hemorrhagic stroke. The main drug therapy for patients with hemorrhagic stroke is for managing hypertension. Oral and IV agents may be used to maintain systolic BP < 160 mm Hg.

- Seizure prophylaxis is situation-specific.

Surgical Therapy

Surgical interventions for hemorrhagic stroke include immediate evacuation of aneurysm-induced hematomas or cerebellar hematomas larger than 3 cm.

- Treatment of arteriovenous malformation (AVM) is surgical resection and/or radiosurgery (i.e., gamma knife). Both may be preceded by interventional neuroradiology procedures to embolize the blood vessels that supply the AVM.

Subarachnoid hemorrhage is usually caused by a ruptured aneurysm. Patients may have multiple aneurysms. Treatment of an aneurysm involves clipping or coiling the aneurysm to prevent rebleeding.

- After aneurysmal occlusion via clipping or coiling, hyperdynamic therapy (hemodilution-induced hypertension achieved using vasoconstricting agents such as phenylephrine or dopamine and hypervolemia) may be used to increase the mean

arterial pressure and cerebral perfusion. Volume expansion is achieved with crystalloid or colloid solution.
- Patients with SAH may receive nimodipine, a calcium-channel blocker, to treat cerebral vasospasms and minimize cerebral damage.
- Bleeding into the ventricles of the brain can block CSF circulation, thus increasing pressure on the brain. Insertion of a ventriculostomy can dramatically improve CSF drainage and decrease ICP.

Rehabilitation Care

After the patient with a stroke has stabilized for 12–24 hours, care shifts from preserving life to lessening disability and reaching optimal function. Many of the interventions from the acute phase are maintained during this phase.

Nursing Management

Goals

Establish the goals of nursing care together with the patient, caregiver, and family. Typical goals are that the patient will: (1) maintain a stable or improved level of consciousness, (2) achieve maximum physical functioning, (3) attain maximum self-care abilities and skills, (4) maintain stable body functions (e.g., bladder control), (5) maximize communication abilities, (6) maintain adequate nutrition, (7) avoid complications of stroke, and (8) maintain effective personal and family coping. See eNursing Care Plan 62-1 for the patient with stroke on the website.

Interventions

Respiratory System

During the acute phase after a stroke, management of respiratory function is a nursing priority. An oropharyngeal airway may be used in comatose patients to prevent the tongue from falling back and obstructing the airway and to provide access for suctioning. Alternatively, a nasopharyngeal airway may be used to provide airway protection and access. Interventions include frequently assessing airway patency and function, providing oxygenation, suctioning, promoting patient mobility, positioning the patient to prevent aspiration, and encouraging deep breathing.

Neurologic System

The primary tool to evaluate and document neurologic status in acute stroke patients is the National Institutes of Health (NIH) Stroke Scale (NIHSS), which measures stroke severity (see NIHSS in Table 62.12, Harding et al., *Lewis' Medical-Surgical Nursing,* ed 12). Other neurologic assessment includes mental status, pupillary responses, and extremity movement and strength. Closely

S

monitor vital signs. A decreasing level of consciousness may indicate increasing ICP.

Cardiovascular System

Nursing goals for the cardiovascular system are aimed at maintaining homeostasis. Interventions include monitoring vital signs frequently, monitoring cardiac rhythm, assessing intake and output, regulating IV infusions, adjusting fluid intake, monitoring lung sounds for crackles and rhonchi indicating pulmonary congestion, and monitoring heart sounds for murmurs or for S_3 or S_4 heart sounds.

- After a stroke, the patient is at risk for venous thromboembolism (VTE), especially in a weak or paralyzed lower extremity. The most effective prevention is to keep the patient moving. Teach active range-of-motion (ROM) exercises if the patient has voluntary movement in the affected extremity. For the patient with hemiplegia, perform passive ROM exercises several times each day.
- Other measures to prevent VTE include positioning to minimize the effects of dependent edema and the use of intermittent pneumatic compression devices. VTE prophylaxis may include low-molecular-weight heparin (e.g., enoxaparin [Lovenox]).

Musculoskeletal System

The goal for the musculoskeletal system is to maintain optimal function by preventing joint contractures and muscle atrophy.

- ROM exercises and positioning are important interventions. Muscle atrophy from lack of innervation and inactivity can develop after a stroke, so passive ROM exercise is begun on the first day of hospitalization.

Interventions to optimize musculoskeletal function include: (1) trochanter roll at the hip to prevent external rotation; (2) hand cones (not rolled washcloths) to prevent hand contractures; (3) arm supports with slings and lap boards to prevent shoulder displacement; (4) avoidance of pulling the patient by the arm to avoid shoulder displacement; (5) posterior leg splints or high-top tennis shoes to prevent footdrop.

Integumentary System

Interventions for preventing skin breakdown include: (1) pressure relief by position changes, special mattresses, or wheelchair cushions; (2) good skin hygiene; (3) emollients applied to dry skin; and (4) early mobility. An example of a position change schedule is side-back-side, with a maximum duration of 2 hours for any position.

- Position the patient on the weak or paralyzed side for no more than 30 minutes. Control of pressure is the single most important factor in both the prevention and treatment of skin breakdown (see Pressure Injury).

Gastrointestinal System

The most common bowel problem is constipation. Fluid and fiber intake goals are determined with the stroke team based on the patient's nutritional and fluid status. Physical activity also promotes bowel function. Laxatives, suppositories, or additional stool softeners may be needed if the patient does not respond to increased fluid and fiber. Bowel retraining may continue into the rehabilitation phase.

Urinary System

In the acute stage of stroke, the primary urinary problem is poor bladder control, resulting in incontinence.

- Take steps to promote normal bladder function and avoid the use of an indwelling catheter.
- Long-term use of an indwelling catheter is associated with urinary tract infections and delayed bladder retraining. An intermittent catheterization program may be used for patients with urinary retention.

Nutrition

The patient may initially receive IV infusions to maintain fluid and electrolyte balance. Patients should have their nutritional needs addressed in the first 72 hours of admission to the hospital, because nutrition is important for recovery and healing. Some patients may require enteral or parenteral nutrition support.

- Many patients have dysphagia after a stroke. Keep patients NPO until a speech therapist performs a swallowing evaluation within 24 hours after the stroke. The nurse or another member of the team may perform the screen if a speech therapist is not available.
- Before starting feeding, assess the gag reflex. If the gag reflex is absent, defer the feeding and begin exercises to stimulate swallowing.
- To assess swallowing ability, elevate the head of the bed to an upright position (unless contraindicated) and give the patient a small amount of crushed ice or ice water to swallow. If the gag reflex is present and the patient is able to swallow safely, you may proceed with feeding.
- Place food on the unaffected side of the mouth. Follow feedings with scrupulous oral hygiene because food may collect on the affected side of the mouth.

Communication

During the acute stage, your role in meeting the psychologic needs of the patient is primarily supportive.

- An alert patient is usually anxious because of a lack of understanding of what has happened and the inability to communicate.

S

Give the patient extra time to comprehend and respond to communication. If the patient cannot understand words, use gestures to support verbal cues.

Sensory-Perceptual Alterations

Homonymous hemianopsia (blindness in the same half of each visual field) is common after a stroke.

- Initially help the patient by arranging the environment within the patient's perceptual field, such as food is on the right side or the left side to accommodate for field of vision.
- Later the patient learns to compensate for the visual defect by checking weak or paralyzed extremities for adequacy of dressing, hygiene, and trauma.

Other visual problems may include diplopia, loss of the corneal reflex, and ptosis, especially if the stroke is in the vertebrobasilar arterial distribution. Diplopia is treated with an eye patch. If the corneal reflex is absent, prevent corneal abrasions with artificial tears or gel to keep the eyes moist and an eye shield (especially at night).

Coping

A stroke is usually a sudden, extremely stressful event for the patient, caregiver, and significant others. Reactions may involve fear, apprehension, denial of stroke severity, depression, anger, and sorrow.

- Provide information and emotional support. Explanations should be clear and understandable. Decision-making and upholding the patient's wishes are of utmost importance.

Home Care and Rehabilitation

The patient is usually discharged from the acute care setting to home, an intermediate or long-term care facility, or a rehabilitation facility. You can prepare the patient and family through teaching and evaluating the transition plan for any barriers.

Follow-up care is carefully planned for continuing nursing, physical, occupational, and speech therapy, as well as medical care. Patient and caregiver can benefit from the combined expertise of an interprofessional rehabilitation team. You can facilitate communication and coordination of care to achieve the patient's goals for successful rehabilitation.

▼ Patient and Caregiver Teaching

- Provide the caregiver with instruction and practice in home care while the patient is hospitalized.
- Provide guidance and referrals for adjustments in the home environment so that modifications (e.g., removal of a door to accommodate a wheelchair) can be made before discharge.

- Teach about exercise and ambulation techniques; dietary requirements; recognizing signs of another stroke (e.g., headache, vertigo, numbness, visual changes); understanding emotional lability and the possibility of depression; medication routine; and time, place, and frequency of follow-up activities such as occupational therapy and physical therapy.
- Support the caregiver to stay healthy. Stress the importance of planning for respite or rest from caregiving activities on a regular basis.

SYPHILIS

Description

Syphilis is a sexually transmitted bacterial infection that can have serious long-term complications if not identified and treated effectively. The population most affected by syphilis is men who have sex with men (MSM), with the highest rates among MSM of color.

Pathophysiology

Syphilis is caused by *Treponema pallidum,* a bacterial spirochete. It is transmitted by direct contact with a syphilitic ulcer called a *chancre* or through the mucosal membranes of an infected person. A chancre can occur externally on the genitals, anus, or lips or internally in the vagina, rectum, mouth, or tongue.

- The incubation period can range from 10 to 90 days (average, 21 days).
- Having the infection does not provide protection from reinfection, even after successful treatment.
- An infected pregnant woman can transmit syphilis to her fetus during her pregnancy. There is a high risk for stillbirth or for having babies that develop complications after birth including seizures and death.

Clinical Manifestations

Signs and symptoms of syphilis mimic those of other infections, so it is hard to recognize syphilis. Without treatment, the infection progresses.

- The *primary stage* is the development of a chancre at the site of transmission. This can appear days to months following infection. In most patients, it occurs by 3 weeks. Chancres can be found on the genitals but often go unnoticed when inside the mouth, vagina, or anus.

S

- In the *secondary stage,* syphilis is systemic. The classic maculopapular rash appears on the palms of the hands or soles of the feet. It may involve the trunk or extremities. Without treatment, the rash will resolve, but the patient still has syphilis and will remain infectious for some time.
- *Tertiary (late) syphilis* is the final stage. Patients will not have obvious symptoms. During this stage, the organism is silently causing organ damage over many years. The formation of gummas can lead to serious complications.

Complications

The *gummas* (destructive lesions) of late syphilis produce irreparable damage to bone, liver, or skin.

- In cardiovascular syphilis, the resulting aneurysm may press on structures, such as the intercostal nerves, causing pain. Scarring of the aortic valve results in aortic valve insufficiency and heart failure.
- Neurosyphilis causes mental deterioration. Visual impairment, tabes dorsalis (progressive locomotor ataxia), and dementia are rare, extreme manifestations.

Diagnostic Studies

- Detailed and accurate sexual history is important.
- Darkfield microscopy and direct fluorescent antibody tests of lesion exudate or tissue can confirm the diagnosis.
- To screen for syphilis, Venereal Disease Research Laboratory (VDRL) and rapid plasma reagin (RPR) testing can detect non-specific antitreponemal antibodies, which are usually positive 10–14 days after chancre appearance.
- To confirm a diagnosis of syphilis, the fluorescent treponemal antibody absorption (FTA-ABs) test, the *T. pallidum* particle agglutination (TP-PA) test, and the syphilis qualitative enzyme-linked immunoassay (EIA) can detect specific antitreponemal antibodies.

Interprofessional and Nursing Management

Management is aimed at starting treatment early. However, treatment cannot reverse damage that is already present in the late stage of the disease.

- Penicillin G benzathine (Bicillin L-A) is the recommended treatment for all stages of syphilis. If contraindicated, doxycycline or tetracycline may be used. Aqueous procaine penicillin G is the treatment of choice for neurosyphilis.

- It is important that all sexual contacts in the last 90 days be treated.
- Reexamination and follow-up testing are recommended every 6 months for up to 2 years.
- Repeat human immunodeficiency virus (HIV) testing should be done on all HIV-negative patients diagnosed with primary or secondary syphilis given the higher risk of HIV transmission during these stages.

See Nursing Management: Sexually Transmitted Infections.

SYSTEMIC EXERTION INTOLERANCE DISEASE

Description

Systemic exertion intolerance disease (SEID), formerly called *chronic fatigue syndrome* or *myalgic encephalomyelitis*, is a serious, complex, multisystem disease in which exertion of any sort (physical, emotional, cognitive) is impaired and accompanied by profound fatigue. People with SEID are not able to do their usual activities and may even be confined to bed. SEID is a poorly understood condition that can have a devastating impact on the lives of patients and their families.

The condition is three times more common in women than men. SEID is more common in minorities and socioeconomically disadvantaged groups. The true prevalence of SEID is unknown because many people with the disease have not been diagnosed.

Pathophysiology

The precise mechanisms of SEID remain unknown. However, many theories exist. Several microorganisms have been researched as causative agents, including herpes viruses (e.g., Epstein–Barr virus [EBV], cytomegalovirus [CMV]), retroviruses, enteroviruses, Candida albicans, and mycoplasma. The condition may be triggered by how a patient's immune system responds to stress or illness.

Clinical Manifestations and Diagnostic Studies

Severe fatigue is the most common symptom and the problem that causes the patient to seek health care. SEID is often hard to discern from fibromyalgia because many clinical features are similar (Table 86). In about half the cases, SEID develops slowly, or the patient may have periodic episodes that gradually become chronic. SEID

TABLE 86   Common Features of Fibromyalgia and Systemic Exertion Intolerance Disease (SEID)

Occurrence
Previously healthy, young and middle-aged women

Etiology (theories)
Infectious trigger, dysfunction in HPA axis, CNS problem

Clinical Manifestations
Generalized musculoskeletal pain, malaise and fatigue, cognitive problems, headaches, sleep problems, depression, anxiety, fever

Disease Course
Variable intensity of symptoms, fluctuates over time

Diagnosis
No definitive laboratory tests or joint and muscle assessments
Mainly a diagnosis of exclusion

Management
Symptomatic treatment may include antidepressant drugs, such as amitriptyline and fluoxetine (Prozac).
Nondrug measures include heat, massage, regular stretching, biofeedback, stress management, and relaxation training.

CNS, Central nervous system; *HPA,* hypothalamic-pituitary-adrenal.

can arise suddenly in a previously active, healthy person. Associated symptoms may vary in intensity over time.

- Physical assessment and diagnostic studies can be used to rule out other possible causes of the patient's symptoms. No laboratory test can diagnose SEID or measure its severity. SEID is a diagnosis of exclusion, based on symptoms. The patient may become angry and frustrated with health care providers who cannot diagnose a problem.

Interprofessional and Nursing Management

No definitive treatment exists for SEID. Supportive management is essential. Tell the patient what is known about the disease.

- Nonsteroidal antiinflammatory drugs (NSAIDs) can be used to treat headaches, muscle and joint aches, and fever. Antihistamines and decongestants can be used to treat allergic symptoms.

- Tricyclic antidepressants (e.g., doxepin, amitriptyline) and selective serotonin release inhibitors (SSRIs) (e.g., fluoxetine, paroxetine) can improve mood and sleep. Clonazepam (Klonopin) can be used to treat sleep problems and panic disorders.
- Use of low-dose hydrocortisone to decrease fatigue and disability is being studied.
- Urge the patient to plan a carefully graduated exercise program. Teach the patient to avoid total rest or strenuous exertion.
- Behavioral therapy may be used to promote a positive outlook and improve overall disability and fatigue.
- One of the major problems facing many patients with SEID is economic security. When the illness strikes, they cannot work or must decrease work time. Loss of a job often leads to loss of medical insurance.

SEID does not appear to progress. Although most patients recover or at least gradually improve over time, some do not show substantial improvement. Recovery is more common in persons with a sudden onset of SEID.

SYSTEMIC INFLAMMATORY RESPONSE SYNDROME (SIRS) AND MULTIPLE ORGAN DYSFUNCTION SYNDROME (MODS)

Description

Systemic inflammatory response syndrome (SIRS) is a generalized organ response to a variety of insults, including infection (referred to as "sepsis"), ischemia, infarction, and injury. Many different mechanisms can trigger SIRS, including:

- *mechanical tissue trauma*: burns, crush injuries, surgery
- *abscess formation*: intraabdominal, extremities
- *ischemic* or *necrotic tissue*: pancreatitis, vascular disease, myocardial infarction
- *microbial invasion*: bacteria, viruses, fungi, parasites
- *endotoxin release*: Gram-negative and Gram-positive bacteria
- *global perfusion deficits*: postcardiac resuscitation, shock states
- *regional perfusion deficits*: distal perfusion deficits

Multiple organ dysfunction syndrome (MODS) is failure of two or more organ systems in an acutely ill patient such that homeostasis cannot be maintained without intervention. MODS results from SIRS.

S

- Prognosis for the patient with MODS is poor, with mortality rates at 40%–60%.

Pathophysiology and Clinical Manifestations

When the inflammatory response is activated, consequences include the release of mediators, direct damage to the endothelium, and hypermetabolism.

- Increased vascular permeability allows mediators and protein to leak out of the endothelium and into the interstitial space.
- White blood cells (WBCs) begin to digest the foreign debris, and the coagulation cascade is activated.
- Hypotension, decreased perfusion, microemboli, and redistributed or shunted blood flow eventually compromise organ perfusion.

The respiratory system is often the first system to show signs of dysfunction in SIRS and MODS. Inflammatory mediators damage the pulmonary endothelium, causing increased capillary permeability.

- Type I pneumocytes (alveolar cells) are destroyed. Type II pneumocytes are damaged. Surfactant production is decreased. The alveoli collapse. This creates an increase in shunt (blood flow to the lungs that does not take part in gas exchange) and worsening ventilation-perfusion mismatch. The result is acute respiratory distress syndrome (ARDS) (see ARDS).

Cardiovascular changes include myocardial depression and massive vasodilation. To compensate for hypotension, heart rate and stroke volume increase, but increased capillary permeability decreases venous return and preload.

- Eventually, either perfusion of vital organs is insufficient or the cells are unable to use oxygen, and their function is further compromised.

Neurologic dysfunction manifests as mental status changes, an early sign of SIRS or MODS.

- The patient may be confused and agitated, combative, disoriented, lethargic, or comatose due to hypoxemia, the effect of inflammatory mediators, or impaired perfusion.

Hypoperfusion and the effects of the mediators can cause acute kidney injury (AKI, see Acute Kidney Injury). Many antibiotics used to treat Gram-negative bacteria (e.g., aminoglycosides) can be nephrotoxic, so careful monitoring of drug levels is needed.

Decreased perfusion of the gastrointestinal (GI) mucosa leads to a breakdown of the mucosal barrier and increases the risk for ulceration, GI bleeding, and bacterial movement from the GI tract into circulation.

Metabolic changes in SIRS and MODS trigger a hypermetabolic response, a catabolic state, and loss of lean body mass (muscle).

- The liver is unable to synthesize albumin needed to maintain plasma oncotic pressure. Intravascular fluid leaks to the interstitial space.
- The patient is unable to convert lactate to glucose, and lactate accumulates (lactic acidosis) while the patient becomes hypoglycemic.

Disseminated intravascular coagulation (DIC) may result from dysfunction of the coagulation system.

- DIC causes microvascular clotting and bleeding at the same time because of the depletion of clotting factors and excessive fibrinolysis (see Disseminated Intravascular Coagulation).

Electrolyte imbalances are common from hormonal and metabolic changes and fluid shifts. These changes worsen mental status changes, neuromuscular dysfunction, and dysrhythmias.

- Release of antidiuretic hormone and aldosterone cause sodium and water retention; aldosterone increases urinary potassium loss, and catecholamines cause potassium to move into the cells, resulting in hypokalemia.
- Metabolic acidosis results from hypoxia, impaired tissue perfusion, the shift to anaerobic metabolism, and progressive renal dysfunction.
- Hypocalcemia, hypomagnesemia, and hypophosphatemia are common.

Interprofessional and Nursing Management

The most important goal is to prevent SIRS from progressing to MODS. Your role is vigilant assessment and ongoing monitoring to detect early signs of deterioration or organ dysfunction.

Interprofessional care for patients with SIRS and MODS focuses on (1) preventing and treating infection, (2) maintaining tissue oxygenation, (3) nutrition and metabolic support, and (4) appropriate support of individual failing organs.

- Aggressive infection control is essential to decrease the risk for health care–associated infections (HAIs). Early, aggressive surgery is recommended to remove necrotic tissue (e.g., early debridement of burn tissue) that provides a culture medium for microorganisms. Aggressive pulmonary management, including early ambulation, can reduce the risk of respiratory infection. Strict asepsis can decrease infections related to intraarterial

S

lines, endotracheal tubes, urinary catheters, IV lines, and other invasive devices or procedures.

- Hypoxemia frequently occurs in patients with SIRS or MODS. Sedation, mechanical ventilation, analgesia, and rest may decrease O_2 demand and should be considered. Treating fever, chills, and pain decrease O_2 demand. O_2 delivery may be optimized by individualizing tidal volumes with positive end-expiratory pressure, increasing preload (e.g., fluids) or myocardial contractility to enhance CO, or reducing afterload to increase CO.
- Hypermetabolism in SIRS or MODS can result in profound weight loss, cachexia, and further organ failure. Providing early and adequate nutritional support decreases morbidity and mortality. The enteral route is preferred to parenteral nutrition.

Support of any failing organ is a primary goal of therapy. For example, the patient with ARDS requires aggressive oxygen therapy and mechanical ventilation. Renal failure may require dialysis or continuous renal replacement therapy. A final consideration may be that further interventions are futile.

- Maintain communication between the health care team and the patient's family and caregivers about realistic goals and likely outcomes for the patient with MODS. Withdrawal of life support and providing end-of-life care may be discussed.

SYSTEMIC LUPUS ERYTHEMATOSUS

Description

Systemic lupus erythematosus (SLE) is a multisystem inflammatory autoimmune disease. It typically affects the skin, joints, and serous membranes (pleura, pericardium). Renal, hematologic, and neurologic systems are often affected. SLE has a chronic unpredictable course, with alternating remissions and exacerbations.

- Most people with lupus develop the disease between ages 15 and 45 years; 90% of those with SLE are women.

Pathophysiology

The cause of the abnormal immune response in SLE is unknown. It is a complex disorder of interactions among genetic, hormonal, environmental, and immunologic factors.

- Hormones play a role in the development of SLE. Worsening of disease symptoms may occur after menarche, with the use of oral contraceptives, and during or after pregnancy.
- Exposure to silica dust in agricultural or industrial settings can be a factor. Drug triggers include those that make a person more sensitive to the sun (e.g., sulfa drugs, diuretics, tetracycline) and penicillin or similar antibiotics.
- Drug-induced SLE should not be confused with drug side effects, which typically occur within a few hours or days of short-term drug use. SLE generally occurs months to years after continuous therapy with a causative drug.

In SLE, the body makes various autoantibodies against nucleic acids (e.g., single- and double-stranded DNA), erythrocytes, coagulation proteins, lymphocytes, platelets, and many other self-proteins. Autoimmune reactions (antinuclear antibodies [ANA]) are directed against elements of the cell nucleus, especially DNA. Circulating immune complexes with antibodies against DNA are deposited in the basement membranes of capillaries in the kidneys, heart, skin, brain, and joints. These complexes trigger inflammation that causes tissue destruction. Overaggressive autoimmune responses are related to activation of B and T cells. Specific effects depend on the involved cell types or organs. SLE is a type III hypersensitivity response.

Clinical Manifestations and Complications

No characteristic pattern occurs in the progression of SLE. General complaints including fever, weight loss, joint pain (*arthralgia*), and fatigue may precede increased disease activity.

Dermatology

Vascular skin lesions are most likely to develop in sun-exposed areas. Severe skin reactions can occur in people who are photosensitive. The classic butterfly rash over the cheeks and bridge of the nose looks like a sunburn. People with chronic cutaneous lupus (CCLE) have discoid (round, coin-shaped) lesions, usually on the scalp and face. Subacute cutaneous lupus (SCLE) is marked by areas of red, ring-shaped lesions.

- Oral or nasopharyngeal membrane ulcers can occur.
- Alopecia is common. The scalp becomes dry, scaly, and atrophied.

Musculoskeletal

Polyarthralgia, pain in multiple joints, with morning stiffness is often the patient's first symptom. Arthritis occurs in many patients with SLE. Diffuse swelling is accompanied by joint and muscle pain and stiffness. Lupus-related arthritis is generally nonerosive, but it may cause deformities.

Cardiopulmonary

Tachypnea and cough in patients with SLE suggest lung disease. Cardiac involvement includes dysrhythmias from fibrosis of the sinoatrial (SA) and atrioventricular (AV) nodes in advanced disease. Hypertension and hypercholesterolemia from steroid use require aggressive treatment.

Renal

About 40% of persons with SLE have kidney damage. Renal problems vary from mild proteinuria to rapid, progressive glomerulonephritis. Treatments include corticosteroids and immunosuppressive agents (e.g., azathioprine, cyclosporine). Oral prednisone or pulsed IV methylprednisolone may be used, especially in the initial treatment period when cytotoxic agents have not yet taken effect. Belimumab (Benlysta), a human monoclonal antibody, reduces autoantibody levels and controls autoimmune disease activity. Voclosporin (Lupkynis) binds to the protein calcineurin, stopping T cells from triggering an autoimmune response.

Nervous System

Neuropsychiatric manifestations range from headache to cerebrovascular disease. Focal neuropsychiatric SLE (NPSLE) is caused by clots, especially in the presence of antiphospholipid antibodies. A stroke or aseptic meningitis may occur. Headaches are common and can become severe during a disease flare. The patient may have psychosis, anxiety, depression, acute confusion, or cognitive problems.

Hematology

Antibodies against blood cells may cause anemia, leukopenia, thrombocytopenia, and coagulation disorders (excessive bleeding or clotting). People with SLE are likely to be resistant to the blood-thinning effects of aspirin. Hydroxychloroquine may decrease risk of clots.

Infection

Patients with SLE have increased susceptibility to infections. This may be due to impaired ability to destroy invading bacteria, deficient antibody production, and immunosuppressive effects of many antiinflammatory drugs. Pneumonia is the most common infection.

Diagnostic Studies

- Diagnosis of SLE is based on distinct criteria. No specific test is diagnostic for SLE, but a variety of abnormalities may be present. Ninety-seven percent of persons with SLE have ANA.
- Testing for anti-DNA antibodies, anti-Smith (Sm) antibodies, and antiphospholipid antibodies is expected to identify immunologic disorders typical of SLE.
- Elevated erythrocyte sedimentation rate (ESR) and C-reactive protein (CRP) levels indicate inflammation but are not diagnostic of SLE. They may be used to monitor disease activity and treatment effectiveness.

Interprofessional Management

A major challenge in SLE treatment is to manage the active phase of the disease while preventing complications of treatment. The prognosis of SLE can be improved with early diagnosis, prompt recognition of organ involvement, and effective therapy.

Drug Therapy

Nonsteroidal antiinflammatory drugs (NSAIDs) are an important intervention for patients with joint pain. The patient may need to try several different NSAIDs to find the most effective one. Antimalarial agents such as hydroxychloroquine and chloroquine are often used to treat fatigue and skin and joint problems. Corticosteroid therapy should be limited to the lowest dose for the shortest possible time until a slower medication becomes effective. Immunosuppressive drugs such as azathioprine (Imuran) and cyclophosphamide may be prescribed to suppress the immune system and reduce end-organ damage.

- Topical immunomodulators are an alternative to corticosteroids for treating serious skin conditions. Tacrolimus (Protopic, Prograf) and pimecrolimus (Elidel) suppress immune activity in the skin, including the butterfly rash and possibly discoid (round, coin-shaped) lesions.

Because blood clots can be a life-threatening complication of SLE, anticoagulants, such as warfarin or low-dose heparin, may be prescribed.

Nursing Management

Goals

The patient with SLE will have acceptable pain management, show awareness of and avoid activities that worsen the disease, and maintain optimal role function and positive self-image.

S

Interventions

During an SLE flare, the patient may quickly become very ill. Nursing interventions include accurately documenting the severity of symptoms and response to therapy. Specifically assess fever pattern, joint inflammation, limitation of motion, location and degree of discomfort, and fatigue.

- Monitor the patient's weight and fluid intake and output. This is especially important if corticosteroids are prescribed because of related fluid retention and possible renal failure. Collect 24-hour urine for protein and creatinine clearance as ordered.
- Carefully assess the patient's neurologic status. Assess for visual changes, headaches, personality changes, and forgetfulness. Psychosis may indicate central nervous system disease or may be the effect of corticosteroid therapy. Nerve irritation of the extremities (peripheral neuropathy) may produce numbness, tingling, and weakness of the hands and feet.
- Monitor the patient on long-term NSAID therapy for GI and renal effects. Observe for signs of bleeding that result from drug therapy, such as pallor, skin bruising, petechiae, or tarry stools.

▼ **Patient and Caregiver Teaching**

Patient involvement is important for successful self-management. Help the patient understand that adherence to the treatment plan is no guarantee against flares in this unpredictable disease. Several factors may increase disease activity. Help the patient and caregiver eliminate or reduce exposure to fatigue, sun, emotional stress, infection, drugs, and surgery. Patient and caregiver teaching is outlined in Table 87.

- Teach patients taking corticosteroid bursts that the dose must be tapered down rather than stopped abruptly.
- Remind patients taking hydroxychloroquine to schedule eye examinations every 6–12 months to asses for development of retinopathy.
- Many couples require pregnancy and sexual counseling. For the best outcome, pregnancy should be planned when the disease activity is minimal.
- Pain and fatigue may interfere with quality of life. Pacing techniques and relaxation therapy can help the patient remain involved in daily activities.

> ## TABLE 87 Patient and Caregiver Teaching: Systemic Lupus Erythematosus
>
> *Include the following information in the teaching plan for a patient with systemic lupus erythematosus and the patient's caregiver.*
>
> - Disease process
> - Names of drugs, actions, side effects, dosage, administration
> - Pain management strategies
> - Energy conservation and pacing techniques
> - Therapeutic exercise, heat therapy for arthralgia
> - Relaxation therapy
> - Avoid physical and emotional stress
> - Avoid exposure to people with infection
> - Avoid drying soaps, powders, household chemicals
> - Use of sunscreen protection (at least SPF 15) and protective clothing, with minimal sun exposure from 11:00 A.M. to 3:00 P.M.
> - Need for regular medical and laboratory follow-up
> - Marital and pregnancy counseling as needed
> - Community resources and health care agencies

SPF, Sun protection factor.

TESTICULAR CANCER

Description

Testicular cancer is rare, but it is the most common type of cancer in men between 15 and 34 years of age. Testicular tumors are more common in males who have had undescended testes (cryptorchidism) or a family history of testicular cancer or anomalies. Other predisposing factors include orchitis, human immunodeficiency virus (HIV) infection, maternal exposure to exogenous estrogen, and testicular cancer in the other testis. Most testicular cancers develop from two types of embryonic germ cells: seminomas and nonseminomas.

Clinical Manifestations

Testicular cancer may have a slow or rapid onset.

- The patient may notice a painless lump in his scrotum and scrotal swelling. The scrotal mass is usually very firm and nontender.
- Some patients report a dull ache or heavy sensation in the lower abdomen, perianal area, or scrotum.
- With metastasis, there may be lower back and/or chest pain, cough, and dyspnea.

T

Diagnostic Studies
- Palpation of scrotal contents for masses and swelling.
- Ultrasound of the testes.
- Blood serum levels of α-fetoprotein (AFP), lactate dehydrogenase (LDH), and human chorionic gonadotropin (hCG).
- Chest X-ray and CT scan of the abdomen and pelvis are used to detect metastasis.

Interprofessional and Nursing Management
Testicular cancer is one of the most curable types of cancer. Management generally involves a radical inguinal orchiectomy (surgical removal of the affected testis, spermatic cord, and regional lymph nodes). Retroperitoneal lymph node dissection and removal may also be done.
- Testicular germ cell tumors are sensitive to systemic chemotherapy than any other adult solid tumor. Chemotherapy protocols use a combination of agents, including bleomycin, cisplatin. etoposide, and ifosfamide (Ifex).

Most patients (95%) obtain complete remission if the disease is detected early. All patients require meticulous follow-up monitoring and regular physical examinations, chest X-ray, CT scan, and assessment of serum tumor markers (hCG, LDH, and AFP). The goal is to detect relapse when tumor burden is minimal.
- There is high risk for infertility after chemotherapy and/or pelvic radiation. The option of cryopreservation of sperm in a sperm bank before treatment begins should be sensitively discussed.

THALASSEMIA

Description
Thalassemia is a group of diseases involving inadequate production of normal hemoglobin (Hgb), which decreases red blood cell (RBC) production. Hemolysis also occurs in thalassemia.
- Thalassemia is common in members of ethnic groups whose origins are near the Mediterranean Sea and equatorial or near-equatorial regions of Southeastern Asia, the Middle East, India, Pakistan, China, Southern Russia, and Africa.

Pathophysiology
Thalassemia has an autosomal recessive genetic basis. α-Globin chains are absent or reduced in α-thalassemia, and β-globin chains are absent or reduced in β-thalassemia. Hemolysis occurs as mononuclear phagocytes in the marrow destroy most erythroblasts. Those

released into the blood are rapidly destroyed by macrophages in the spleen. A person with thalassemia may have a homozygous or heterozygous form of the disease.

- In *thalassemia major,* the person is homozygous, with two thalassemic genes. Thalassemia major is a severe form of the disease.
- In *thalassemia minor (thalassemic trait),* the person is heterozygous, with one thalassemic gene and one normal gene. Thalassemia minor is a mild form of the disease.

Clinical Manifestations

The patient with thalassemia major has symptoms of anemia (see Anemia).

- Marked splenomegaly, hepatomegaly, and jaundice result from hemolysis of RBCs. Chronic bone marrow hyperplasia leads to expansion of the marrow space. This may cause thickening of the cranium and the maxillary cavity walls.
- Cardiac complications from iron overload, lung disease, and hypertension contribute to early death.
- Endocrine problems (diabetes, growth retardation, hypogonadism), osteoporosis, pulmonary hypertension, and thrombosis may be present.
- The patient with thalassemia minor may be asymptomatic, with mild to moderate anemia, microcytosis (small cells), and hypochromia (pale cells). Thalassemia minor requires no treatment because the body adapts to the reduction in normal Hgb.

Interprofessional and Nursing Management

The laboratory findings in thalassemia major are summarized in Table 8.

- Thalassemia major is managed with blood transfusions or exchange transfusions. Chelating agents reduce the iron overloading that occurs with chronic transfusion therapy. Drugs used include oral deferasirox (Exjade, JadeNu) or deferiprone (Ferriprox), or IV or subcutaneous deferoxamine (Desferal).
- Luspatercept-aamt (Reblozyl) may be given subcutaneously every 21 days to improve hemoglobin levels and reduce transfusion needs. It blocks inhibitors of late-stage RBC production.
- Because RBCs are sequestered in the enlarged spleen, thalassemia may be treated by splenectomy.
- Although hematopoietic stem cell transplantation remains the only cure for patients with thalassemia, the risks may outweigh its benefits.

T

THROMBOANGIITIS OBLITERANS

Thromboangiitis obliterans (*Buerger's disease*) is a nonathero-sclerotic, segmental, recurrent inflammatory vasoocclusive disorder of the small and medium-sized arteries and veins of the arms and legs. It occurs mostly in men under 45 years of age with a long history of tobacco or marijuana use, but without other cardiovascular disease (CVD) risk factors (e.g., hypertension, hyperlipidemia, diabetes).

In the acute phase of Buerger's disease, an inflammatory thrombus blocks the vessel. Over time, the thrombus becomes more organized, and the vessel wall inflammation subsides.

During the chronic phase, thrombosis and fibrosis in the vessel cause tissue ischemia. The symptoms of Buerger's disease are often confused with peripheral artery disease (PAD) and other autoimmune diseases (e.g., scleroderma).

- Patients may have intermittent claudication of the feet, hands, or arms. As the disease progresses, rest pain and ischemic ulcerations develop.
- Other signs and symptoms may include color and temperature changes of the limbs, paresthesia, superficial vein thrombosis, and cold sensitivity.

There are no laboratory or diagnostic tests specific to Buerger's disease. Diagnosis is based on the age at onset, history, symptoms, involvement of distal vessels, presence of ischemic ulcerations, and exclusion of other sources of emboli.

Treatment is the complete cessation of tobacco and marijuana use.

- The amputation rate in patients who continue tobacco use is much higher than in those who stop.

Conservative management includes avoiding limb exposure to cold temperatures, a supervised walking program, antibiotics to treat any infected ulcers, and analgesics to manage the ischemic pain. IV iloprost (Ventavis), a prostaglandin analog that promotes vasodilation, is used to manage rest pain, promote healing of ischemic ulcers, and decrease the need for amputation.

- Teach patients to avoid trauma to the extremities. Painful ulcerations may require finger or toe amputations.

THROMBOCYTOPENIA

Description

Thrombocytopenia is a reduction of platelets below 150,000/µL (150×10^9/L). Acute, severe, or prolonged decreases from this normal range can result in prolonged bleeding from minor trauma or spontaneous bleeding without injury. Platelet disorders occur from impaired production, increased destruction, or abnormal distribution. While they can be inherited (e.g., Wiskott–Aldrich syndrome), most are acquired. Drugs are a common cause of acquired disorders. Although some drugs are directly myelo-suppressive (e.g., chemotherapy, ganciclovir), the usual mechanism of drug-related thrombocytopenia is accelerated platelet destruction.

- Some drugs affect platelet aggregation. Aspirin doses as low as 81 mg can alter platelet aggregation. Normal function is restored when new platelets are made.

Immune Thrombocytopenia

Immune thrombocytopenia (ITP), the most common acquired thrombocytopenia, is an autoimmune destruction of circulating platelets. Antibody-coated platelets, mistakenly identified as foreign, are destroyed by macrophages in the spleen. ITP generally presents as an acute condition in children and a chronic condition in adults.

Thrombotic Thrombocytopenic Purpura

Thrombotic *thrombocytopenic purpura* (TTP) is an uncommon syndrome characterized by microangiopathic hemolytic anemia (MAHA), fever (in the absence of infection), thrombocytopenia, neurologic abnormalities, and renal abnormalities. TTP is almost always associated with hemolytic-uremic syndrome (HUS).

- TTP is a medical emergency because bleeding and clotting occur simultaneously.
- In most cases, the syndrome is caused by the deficiency of a plasma enzyme (ADAMTS13) that usually breaks down the von Willebrand (vWF) clotting factor into normal size.
- TTP is associated with enhanced agglutination of platelets, which form microthrombi in arterioles and capillaries.
- TTP is seen primarily in previously healthy adults.
- The syndrome may be idiopathic (autoimmune disorder with antibodies against ADAMTS13), caused by certain drug toxicities (e.g., chemotherapy, cyclosporine, quinine, oral contraceptives, valacyclovir, clopidogrel [Plavix]), pregnancy or

T

preeclampsia, infection, or known autoimmune disorder such as systemic lupus erythematosus or scleroderma.

Heparin-Induced Thrombocytopenia

Heparin-induced thrombocytopenia (HIT), also called *heparin-induced thrombocytopenia* and *thrombosis syndrome* (HITTS), may develop 5–10 days after heparin therapy is initiated. In HIT, an immune-mediated response to heparin causes platelet destruction and vascular endothelial injury.

- Antibodies are created against a heparin-platelet complex, and platelets are removed prematurely from circulation, leading to thrombocytopenia and formation of platelet-fibrin thrombi.
- HIT leads to venous or arterial thrombosis. Deep vein thromboses and pulmonary emboli are common. Other complications may include arterial vascular infarcts resulting in skin necrosis, stroke, and end-organ damage (e.g., kidneys).
- As many as 5% of patients on IV heparin therapy develop HIT. Suspect HIT if the platelet count drops by more than 50% from baseline or if a thrombus forms while the patient is on heparin therapy.
- Symptoms of bleeding are unusual because the platelet count rarely drops below 20,000/µL.

Clinical Manifestations

Many patients with thrombocytopenia are asymptomatic. The major complication of thrombocytopenia is hemorrhage in any area of the body, including the joints, retina, and brain. Cerebral hemorrhage may be fatal.

- The most common symptom is bleeding, usually mucosal or cutaneous. Mucosal bleeding may manifest as epistaxis and gingival bleeding. Large bullous hemorrhages may appear on the buccal mucosa. Bleeding into the skin is seen as petechiae, purpura, or superficial ecchymoses.
- Prolonged bleeding after venipuncture or IM injection may indicate thrombocytopenia. Be aware of manifestations that reflect internal blood loss, including weakness, fainting, dizziness, tachycardia, abdominal pain, and hypotension.

Diagnostic Studies

- Platelet count is decreased below 150,000/µL (150×10^9/L). Spontaneous life-threatening hemorrhages (e.g., intracranial bleeding) may occur with counts below 20,000/µL (20×10^9/L).
- Specific assays for antigens help differentiate ITP from other types of thrombocytopenia.

- Bone marrow analysis may show normal or increased mega-karyocytes (precursors of platelets). It is done to rule out leukemia, aplastic anemia, and other myeloproliferative disorders.
- Flow cytometry can be used to detect antiplatelet antibodies.

Interprofessional Management

Immune Thrombocytopenia

Multiple therapies are used to manage the patient with ITP. If the patient is asymptomatic, therapy may not be used unless the platelet count is below 30,000/μL. Platelet transfusions are not indicated until the count is $< 10,000/\mu L$ ($10 \times 10^9/L$) or for anticipated bleeding before a procedure.

- Corticosteroids (e.g., prednisone) are used initially to suppress the phagocytic response of splenic macrophages.
- Romiplostim (Nplate) and eltrombopag (Promacta) are used for patients with chronic ITP who have an insufficient response to the other treatments. These thrombopoietin receptor agonists drugs increase platelet production.

Splenectomy may be indicated if the patient is not responding to the conservative treatments. Approximately two-thirds of patients benefit from splenectomy, resulting in a sustained remission. High doses of IV immunoglobulin (IVIG) and a component of IVIG, anti-$Rh_o(D)$ (anti-D, WinRho), may be used in the patient who is unresponsive to corticosteroids or splenectomy, or for whom splenectomy is not an option.

Thrombotic Thrombocytopenic Purpura

TTP may be managed in a variety of ways. The first step is to treat the underlying disorder (e.g., infection) or remove an identified cause. Plasma exchange (plasmapheresis) may be needed to reverse the process. Treatment should be continued daily until the patient's platelet counts normalize and hemolysis has ceased. Administration of platelets is generally contraindicated because it may lead to new vWF-platelet complexes and increased clotting. Corticosteroids may be added. Rituximab has been used for patients who are refractory to plasma exchange. Caplacizumab, an anti-VWF antibody, blocks VWF binding to platelets. Other immunosuppressants, such as cyclosporine or cyclophosphamide, may also be used.

- Splenectomy is considered.

Heparin-Induced Thrombocytopenia

All forms of heparin must be stopped when HIT is first recognized. This includes heparin flushes for vascular catheters. Platelet transfusions are not given because they may enhance thromboembolic events.

T

- To maintain anticoagulation, the patient should receive a direct thrombin inhibitor, such as argatroban. Other options are fondaparinux (Arixtra), a factor Xa inhibitor (indirect thrombin inhibitor), or bivalirudin (a synthetic thrombin inhibitor). Warfarin should be started only when the platelet count reaches 150,000/µL.
- If clotting is severe, the most common treatments are plasmapheresis to clear the platelet-aggregating IgG from the blood, thrombolytic agents to treat the thromboembolic events, and surgery to remove clots.

Patients who have had HIT should never receive heparin or low-molecular-weight heparin (LMWH) again. This should be clearly marked in the patient's health record.

Nursing Management

The patient with thrombocytopenia will have no bleeding, maintain vascular integrity, and manage self-care to prevent complications related to bleeding. See eNursing Care Plan 34-2 for the patient with thrombocytopenia, available on the website for Harding et al, *Lewis' Medical-Surgical Nursing,* ed 12.

Discourage the use of over-the-counter (OTC) medications known to be causes of acquired thrombocytopenia and reduced platelet function. Some contain aspirin, which reduces platelet adhesiveness and contributes to bleeding.

The goal during acute episodes of thrombocytopenia is to prevent or control hemorrhage. In the patient with thrombocytopenia, bleeding is usually from superficial sites. Deep bleeding (into the muscles, joints, and abdomen) usually occurs only when clotting factors are diminished. Stress that a seemingly minor nosebleed or new petechiae may indicate potential hemorrhage and that the health care provider should be notified.

- In a woman with thrombocytopenia, menstrual blood loss may exceed the usual amount and duration. Counting sanitary napkins used during menses is an important intervention to detect excess blood loss. Suppressing menses with hormonal agents may be needed during predictable periods of thrombocytopenia (e.g., during chemotherapy) to reduce menstrual blood loss.
- Observe for early signs of thrombocytopenia in patients receiving cancer chemotherapy drugs.
- Proper administration of platelet transfusions is an important nursing responsibility.
- Monitor patients with ITP for response to therapy.

▼ **Patient and Caregiver Teaching**
- Teach the person with acquired thrombocytopenia to avoid causes when possible.
- Remind the patient to avoid injury or trauma and to observe for signs and symptoms of bleeding.
- Patients with either ITP or acquired thrombocytopenia should have planned periodic medical evaluations to assess and treat situations in which exacerbations and bleeding are likely to occur.
- Discuss the impact of the condition on the patient's quality of life.

THYROID CANCER

Description

Thyroid cancer is the most common cancer of the endocrine system. The incidence of thyroid cancer has risen significantly in the past 25 years. Thyroid cancer affects more women than men, and the incidence is higher in whites and Asian Americans. Adults at increased risk include those who had head and neck radiation therapy during childhood, were exposed to radioactive fallout, or have a personal or family history of goiter.

Four main types of thyroid cancer are papillary, follicular, medullary, and anaplastic.

- *Papillary thyroid cancer* accounts for about 70%–80% of all thyroid cancers. Papillary cancer grows slowly and initially spreads to lymph nodes in the neck.
- *Follicular thyroid cancer* makes up about 10%–15% of all thyroid cancers and tends to occur in older patients. Follicular cancer first grows into the cervical lymph nodes and then spreads to the lungs and bones.
- *Medullary thyroid cancer* accounts for up to 10% of all thyroid cancers. It is more likely to occur in families and to be associated with other endocrine problems. It is diagnosed by genetic testing for a *protooncogene* called *RET*. Medullary thyroid cancer is a type of multiple endocrine neoplasia. This type of cancer is associated with early metastasis.
- *Anaplastic thyroid cancer,* found in <2% of patients with thyroid cancer, is the most advanced and aggressive thyroid cancer. It is the least likely to respond to treatment and has a poor prognosis.

T

Clinical Manifestations

The primary sign of thyroid cancer is painless, palpable nodule or nodules in an enlarged thyroid gland. Most nodules are found during palpation of the neck. Some patients may have difficulty swallowing or breathing if tumor growth invades the trachea or esophagus. Hemoptysis and airway obstruction may occur if the trachea is involved.

Diagnostic Studies

Nodular thyroid gland enlargement or palpation of a mass requires further evaluation.

- Ultrasound is often the first diagnostic test used. CT, MRI, positron emission tomography (PET), and ultrasound-guided fine-needle aspiration (FNA) are other options.
- A thyroid scan may be done to evaluate for cancer. A nodule that does not take up radioactive iodine has a higher risk of being malignant.
- High serum calcitonin is associated with medullary thyroid cancer. In papillary and follicular cancers, serum thyroglobulin is high.

Interprofessional and Nursing Management

Surgical procedures may range from unilateral total lobectomy with removal of the isthmus to near-total thyroidectomy with bilateral lobectomy.

- Radioactive iodine (RAI) may be given to destroy remaining cancer cells after surgery. External beam radiation therapy may be given as palliative treatment for patients with metastatic thyroid cancer.

Many thyroid cancers are thyroid-stimulating hormone (TSH)–dependent, and thyroid hormone therapy in high doses is often prescribed to inhibit pituitary secretion of TSH.

- Chemotherapy, including doxorubicin, may be used for advanced disease. Vandetanib (Caprelsa), lenvatinib (Lenvima), sorafenib tosylate (Nexavar), and cabozantinib (Cometriq) are targeted therapy agents used for treatment of metastatic thyroid cancer. These drugs inhibit tyrosine kinases, enzymes that promote the growth of cancer cells.

Nursing care for the patient with thyroid cancer is similar to that for the patient undergoing thyroidectomy (see Surgical Therapy section in Hyperthyroidism). Because of the surgical site location and the potential for hypocalcemia, the patient requires frequent postoperative assessment.

- Assess the patient for airway obstruction, bleeding, and tetany, because a parathyroid gland may have been disturbed or removed during surgery.

TRIGEMINAL NEURALGIA

Description

Trigeminal neuralgia (TN) (tic douloureux) is characterized by sudden, usually unilateral, brief, recurrent episodes of severe stabbing pain in the distribution of the trigeminal nerve. It is seen more often in women than in men and more often in people over age 40 years.

Pathophysiology

The trigeminal nerve, the fifth cranial nerve (CN V), has both motor and sensory branches. The sensory branches, primarily the maxillary and mandibular branches, are involved in TN. Most TN cases result from vascular compression of the trigeminal nerve root by an abnormal loop of the superior cerebellar artery. Constant compression appears to lead to chronic injury, flattening and atrophy of the nerve, and damage to the myelin sheath. TN may be related to underlying pathology, such as multiple sclerosis, shingles, or masses in the cerebellum or brainstem.

Clinical Manifestations

TN is classified as classic (TN 1) or atypical (TN 2). Patients may have both types.

TN 1 manifests with an abrupt onset of paroxysms of excruciating pain. It is described as burning or knife-like, or a lightning-like shock, in the lips, upper or lower gums, cheek, forehead, or side of the nose.

- Intense pain, twitching, grimacing, and frequent blinking and tearing of the eye occur during the acute attack (giving rise to the term *tic*). Some patients may have facial sensory loss.
- The attacks are usually brief, lasting seconds to 2 or 3 minutes, and are generally unilateral. Frequency ranges from 1 to over 50 times a day.
- After the refractory (pain-free) period, a phenomenon known as "clustering" is characterized by a cycle of pain and refractoriness that continues for hours.
- Pain episodes are usually triggered by light touch at a specific point (trigger zones) along the distribution of the nerve branches.

T

- Precipitating stimuli include chewing, toothbrushing, feeling a hot or cold blast of air on the face, washing the face, yawning, or even talking.
- As a result, the patient may neglect eating and hygiene practices, wear a cloth over the face, and withdraw from interaction. The patient may sleep excessively to cope with the pain.

The atypical form, TN 2, is distinguished by constant aching, burning, crushing, or stabbing pain. The pain has a lower intensity and does not subside completely.

Diagnostic Studies

- The first episode of TN is sudden with a memorable onset. Diagnosis is based on history and examination.
- Neurologic assessment and CT scan or MRI of the brain are used to rule out any lesions, tumors, or vascular abnormalities.

Interprofessional Management

The goal of treatment is relief of pain. Antiseizure drug therapy may reduce pain by stabilizing the neuronal membrane and blocking nerve firing. These drugs are usually effective in treating TN 1 but less effective for TN 2. First-line drugs include carbamazepine (Tegretol) and oxcarbazepine (Trileptal). Topiramate (Topamax), clonazepam (Klonopin), phenytoin (Dilantin), lamotrigine (Lamictal), gabapentin, and valproic acid are other options. Tricyclic antidepressants, such as amitriptyline or nortriptyline, can be used to treat constant burning or aching pain. Analgesics or opioids are usually not effective in controlling pain in TN1 but may help with pain in TN2.

- Electrical stimulation of the nerves and nerve blocks with local anesthetics or botulinum toxin are treatment options.

If a conservative approach is ineffective or the patient is unable to tolerate drug therapy, surgical therapy is available. In percutaneous procedures, affected nerve fibers are damaged to eliminate pain. Although most patients are pain-free after any of these procedures, pain relief lasts longer with microvascular decompression.

Nursing Management

Monitor the patient's response to drug therapy and note any side effects. Discuss other pain management measures, such as acupuncture, biofeedback, and yoga.

Environmental management is essential during an acute period to decrease triggering stimuli. Keep the room at an even, moderate temperature and free of drafts.

Teach the patient about the importance of nutrition, hygiene, and oral care.

- Hygiene activities are best done when analgesia is at its peak. A small, soft-bristled toothbrush or a warm mouthwash assists in promoting oral care.
- Serve food high in protein and calories that is easily chewed and lukewarm. Encourage small, frequent meals. If the patient's nutritional status is compromised, a nasogastric (NG) tube can be inserted on the unaffected side for enteral feedings.

General postoperative nursing care for a craniotomy is appropriate if intracranial surgery has been performed. Compare the postoperative pain level with the preoperative level. Frequently evaluate the corneal reflex, extraocular muscle function, hearing, sensation, and facial nerve function.

- After a percutaneous radiofrequency procedure, apply an ice pack to the jaw on the operative side for 3–5 hours. To avoid injuring the mouth, the patient should not chew on the operative side until sensation has returned.

▼ **Patient and Caregiver Teaching**

Plan for regular follow-up care and teach the patient about the dosage and side effects of prescribed drugs. Encourage the patient to manage environmental stimuli and to use stress reduction methods.

Long-term management after surgical intervention depends on the residual effects of the procedure. If anesthesia is present or the corneal reflex is altered, teach the patient to: (1) chew on the unaffected side, (2) avoid hot foods or beverages that can burn the mucous membranes, (3) check the oral cavity after meals to remove food particles, (4) practice meticulous oral hygiene and continue with semiannual dental visits, (5) protect the face against extremes of temperature, (6) use an electric razor, (7) wear a protective eye shield and avoid rubbing the eyes, and (8) examine eye regularly for symptoms of infection or irritation.

TUBERCULOSIS

Description

Tuberculosis (TB) is an infectious disease caused by *Mycobacterium tuberculosis*. It usually involves the lungs, but can infect any organ, including the brain, kidneys, and bones.

About 25% of the world's population are infected with TB. Increasing rates of TB are attributed to human immunodeficiency (HIV) disease and the emergence of drug-resistant strains of *M. tuberculosis*. TB is the leading cause of mortality in patients with HIV infection.

T

TB occurs disproportionately in the poor, underserved, and minorities. People most at risk include the homeless, residents of inner-city neighborhoods, foreign-born people, those living or working in institutions (long-term care facilities, prisons, shelters, hospitals), IV drug users, those in overcrowded living conditions and with less than optimal sanitation, and those with poor access to health care. Immunosuppression from any cause (e.g., HIV infection, cancer, long-term corticosteroid use) increases the risk of active TB infection.

- Once a strain of *M. tuberculosis* develops resistance to the first-line drug therapy (isoniazid and rifampin), it is defined as *multidrug-resistant tuberculosis (MDR-TB)*. Extensively drug-resistant TB (XDR-TB) is a rare type of MDR-TB. XDR-TB is also resistant to any fluoroquinolone and at least one second-line drug. Resistance results from several problems, including incorrect prescribing, lack of case management, and nonadherence to the prescribed regimen.

Pathophysiology

M. tuberculosis is a Gram-positive, aerobic, acid-fast bacillus. It is usually spread from person to person by airborne droplets produced when speaking, breathing, sneezing, and coughing.

- TB transmission usually requires close contact and frequent or prolonged exposure. The disease cannot be spread by touching, sharing food utensils, kissing, or other physical contact.
- Once inhaled by another person, *M. tuberculosis* particles lodge in bronchioles and alveoli. The organisms can grow in the lungs, kidneys, epiphyses of bone, cerebral cortex, and adrenal glands.

Classification

The American Thoracic Society classifies TB based on development of the disease (Table 88). We classify TB by (1) its presentation—primary, latent, or reactivated—and (2) whether it is pulmonary or extrapulmonary.

Primary infection starts when the bacteria are inhaled, but there is an effective immune response and the bacteria become inactive. Most people have effective immune responses to encapsulate these organisms for the rest of their lives.

Latent TB infection (LTBI) occurs in a person who does not have active TB disease. People with LTBI have a positive skin test but are asymptomatic. They cannot transmit the TB bacteria to others but can develop active TB disease later. Immunosuppression, diabetes, poor nutrition, aging, pregnancy, stress, and chronic disease can reactivate the disease.

TABLE 88	Classification of Tuberculosis (TB)	
Class	Exposure or infection	Description
0	No TB exposure	No TB exposure, not infected (no history of exposure, negative tuberculin skin test)
1	TB exposure, no infection	TB exposure, no evidence of infection (history of exposure, negative tuberculin skin test)
2	Latent TB infection, no disease	TB infection without disease (positive reaction to tuberculin skin test, negative bacteriologic studies, no X-ray findings compatible with TB, no clinical evidence of TB)
3	TB, clinically active	TB infection with clinically active disease (positive bacteriologic studies, or both a significant reaction to tuberculin skin test and clinical or X-ray evidence of current disease)
4	TB, but not clinically active	No current disease (history of previous episode of TB or abnormal, stable X-ray findings in a person with a positive reaction to tuberculin skin test. Negative bacteriologic studies if done. No clinical or X-ray evidence of current disease)
5	TB suspect	TB suspect (diagnosis pending). Person should not be in this classification for >3 mo.

Source: American Thoracic Society.

Active TB disease results if the initial immune response is not adequate and the bacteria replicate. Active disease developing within the first 2 years of infection is termed *primary TB*. Postprimary TB,

T

or *reactivation TB,* is TB disease occurring 2 or more years after the initial infection.

Clinical Manifestations

- Active TB disease may initially present with fatigue, malaise, anorexia, unexplained weight loss, low-grade fevers, and night sweats. An initially dry cough becomes productive with mucoid or mucopurulent sputum.
- Sometimes TB has a more acute, sudden presentation. The patient may have a high fever, chills, generalized flu-like symptoms, pleuritic pain, a productive cough, and acute respiratory failure.
- In patients with HIV infection, signs of TB, such as fever, cough, and weight loss, may be wrongly attributed to pneumonia caused by *Pneumocystis jiroveci* or other HIV-associated diseases.
- Renal TB can cause dysuria and hematuria. Bone and joint TB may cause severe pain. Headaches, vomiting, and lymphadenopathy may be present with TB meningitis.

Complications

Miliary TB results from widespread dissemination of the mycobacterium to distant organs. The infection may be fatal if left untreated.

- Manifestations may slowly progress over days, weeks, or months. Symptoms vary depending on which organs are infected.
- Hepatomegaly, splenomegaly, and generalized lymphadenopathy may be present.

Pleural TB is an infected fluid collection in the pleural space. *Empyema* may occur with large numbers of tubercular organisms in the pleural space.

Diagnostic Studies

- Tuberculin skin test (TST): induration (not redness) at the injection site means that the person has been exposed to TB and has developed antibodies. See Chapter 30, Harding et al., *Lewis' Medical-Surgical Nursing,* ed 12, for guidelines in performing and interpreting TSTs.
- Interferon (INF)-gamma release assays (IGRAs).
- Blood test to detect response to mycobacterial antigens.
- Chest X-ray: diagnosis cannot be based solely on X-ray because other diseases may mimic TB.
- Bacteriologic studies: stained sputum smears for acid-fast bacilli (AFB test) can identify tubercle bacilli; cultures to grow

tubercle bacilli confirm diagnosis. We need three consecutive sputum specimens, each collected at 8–24-hour intervals, with at least one early morning specimen.

Interprofessional Management

Most patients with TB are treated on an outpatient basis and continue to work and maintain their lifestyles with few changes. Hospitalization may be needed for severely ill or debilitated patients. The mainstay of TB treatment is drug therapy.

Active Tuberculosis Disease

Because of the growing prevalence of MDR-TB, it is important to manage the patient with active TB aggressively. Drug therapy is divided into two phases: initial and continuation. The treatment for patients with previously untreated TB is a 2-month initial phase with four-drug therapy—isoniazid, rifampin, pyrazinamide, and ethambutol.

- Nonadherence is a major factor in the emergence of multidrug resistance and treatment failures. Many people do not adhere to the treatment program.
- Directly *observed therapy* (DOT) involves providing the antituberculous drugs directly to patients and watching as they swallow the medications.

Latent Tuberculosis Infection

In people with LTBI, drug therapy helps prevent a TB infection from developing into active TB disease. The standard treatment regimen for LTBI is 9 months of daily isoniazid.

Nursing Management

Goals

The patient with tuberculosis will have normal pulmonary function, adhere with the therapeutic regimen, take appropriate measures to prevent the spread of the disease, and have no recurrence of disease.

Interventions

Bacille Calmette-Guérin (BCG) vaccine is given to infants in parts of the world with a high prevalence of TB. The BCG vaccine should be considered for persons who meet specific criteria (e.g., health care workers who are continually exposed to MDR-TB and when infection control precautions are not successful).

- Screening programs in known high-risk groups are of value in detecting people with TB.
- Persons with a positive TST should have a chest X-ray to assess for active TB disease.
- Reducing prevalence of HIV infection, poverty, overcrowded living conditions, malnutrition, smoking, and drug and alcohol abuse can help minimize TB infection rates.

T

If hospitalization is needed for patients suspected of having TB, special measures should be taken.

- Airborne infection isolation is indicated for the patient with pulmonary or laryngeal TB until the patient is noninfectious (defined as effective drug therapy, clinical improvement, and three negative AFB smears).
- High-efficiency particulate air (HEPA) or N95 masks are worn by everyone entering the patient's room.

▼ **Patient and Caregiver Teaching**

- Teach hospitalized patients to cover the nose and mouth with paper tissues every time they cough, sneeze, or produce sputum.
- Teach the patient and caregivers about the prescribed regimen. Strategies to improve adherence include teaching and counseling, reminder systems, incentives or rewards, contracts, and DOT.
- Because about 5% of people have relapses, teach the patient to recognize and promptly report symptoms of TB recurrence to the health care provider.
- Teach the patient about factors that could reactivate TB, such as immunosuppression or cancer.

ULCERATIVE COLITIS

Ulcerative colitis is an autoimmune disorder that, along with Crohn's disease, is referred to as *inflammatory bowel disease* (IBD). See Inflammatory Bowel Disease for a discussion of the disorder.

URETHRITIS

Description

Urethritis is inflammation of the urethra. Causes of urethritis include a bacterial or viral infection, *Trichomonas* or monilial infection (especially in women), chlamydial infection, and gonorrhea (especially in men).

- In men, purulent discharge can indicate gonococcal urethritis. A clear discharge typically signifies a nongonococcal urethritis. Urethritis produces bothersome lower urinary tract symptoms (LUTS), including dysuria, urgency, and frequent urination, similar to those seen with cystitis.
- In women, urethritis is hard to diagnose. It should be considered when WBCs are present on urinalysis, but there are no bacteria.

It frequently produces bothersome LUTS, but urethral discharge may not be present.

Interprofessional and Nursing Management

Treatment is based on identifying and treating the cause and providing symptomatic relief. Women with negative urine cultures and no pyuria usually do not respond to antibiotics. Drugs used to treat bacterial infections include trimethoprim/sulfamethoxazole, doxycycline (Vibramycin), ceftriaxone, and nitrofurantoin.

- Metronidazole (Flagyl) and tinidazole (Tindamax) are options for treating *Trichomonas* infection.
- Nystatin, clotrimazole, or fluconazole may be used for monilial infections.
- In chlamydial infections, doxycycline and azithromycin are options.
  Warm sitz baths may temporarily relieve symptoms.
- Teach female patients to avoid using vaginal deodorant sprays and contraceptive gels and to cleanse the perineal area after bowel movement or voiding.
- Teach all patients to avoid sexual intercourse for at least 7 days. Teach patients with sexually transmitted urethritis to refer their sex partners for evaluation and testing if they had sexual contact in the 60 days before onset of the symptoms or diagnosis.

URINARY INCONTINENCE

Description

Urinary incontinence (UI) is involuntary leakage of urine. Although UI is more prevalent among older adults, it is not a natural consequence of aging. UI has a major effect on quality of life and contributes to emotional, social, and potential serious health problems, especially in older adults. Many cases of UI can be cured or significantly improved.

Pathophysiology

UI occurs when bladder pressure exceeds urethral closure pressure. Anything that interferes with internal and/or external urethral sphincter control can result in UI.

- Risk factors for UI include obesity, BPH, smoking, recurrent UTIs, GU surgeries, vaginal delivery, impaired functional status, certain drugs, certain neurological problems, and a family history of UI.

- UI disorders include stress, urge, overflow, and reflex incontinence. Patients may have more than one type of incontinence. The combination of stress and urge incontinence is referred to as mixed incontinence.

Diagnostic Studies

- A focused history, physical assessment, and a bladder log or voiding diary provide information about the onset of UI, factors that provoke urinary leakage, and associated conditions.
- Pelvic examination assesses for organ prolapse and evaluates pelvic floor muscle strength.
- Urinalysis can identify factors contributing to incontinence (e.g., urinary infection, diabetes).
- Measure postvoid residual (PVR) urine in the patient undergoing evaluation for UI. The PVR volume is obtained by asking the patient to void, followed by catheterization or use of bladder ultrasound within 10–20 minutes.
- Urodynamic testing may be indicated.
- Imaging studies of the upper urinary tract (e.g., ultrasound) are done when incontinence is associated with urinary tract infections or there is evidence of upper urinary tract involvement.

Interprofessional Management

Transient, reversible factors are corrected first, followed by management of the type of UI. In general, less-invasive treatments are tried before more invasive methods are used. Pelvic floor muscle training (Kegel exercises) is used to treat UI, especially stress UI. Biofeedback can help the patient identify, isolate, contract, and relax the pelvic muscles. Bladder training may help.

Drug Therapy

Drug therapy varies according to UI type.

- No drugs are approved to treat stress UI.
- In *urge* and *reflex UI,* drugs play a key management role. Anticholinergic drugs (muscarinic receptor blockers) block the action of acetylcholine at muscarinic receptors. They relax the bladder muscle and inhibit overactive detrusor contractions. These preparations include tolterodine (Detrol, Detrol LA), oxybutynin (Ditropan, Oxytrol Transdermal System), trospium, solifenacin (VESIcare), darifenacin (Enablex), and fesoterodine (Toviaz). Botox (onabotulinumtoxin A) injected into the bladder results in relaxation of the bladder, an increase in its storage capacity, and a decrease in UI.

Surgical Therapy

Surgical techniques also vary according to the type of UI.

- Surgical correction of stress UI may reposition the urethra and/ or create a backboard of support, or otherwise stabilize the urethra and bladder neck and make them better able to adapt to changes in intraabdominal pressure.
- Another technique for stress UI augments the urethral resistance of the intrinsic sphincter unit with a sling or periurethral injectable.
- Placement of a suburethral sling can correct stress UI in women.
- Bulking agents can be injected underneath the mucosa of the urethra to correct stress UI in women or men.
- An artificial urethral sphincter can be inserted in men with intrinsic sphincter deficiency and severe stress UI.

Nursing Management

Recognize both the physical and emotional problems associated with incontinence. Support the patient's dignity, privacy, and feelings of self-worth. Take a two-step approach involving devices to manage urinary leakage and a definitive plan to reduce or resolve the factors leading to incontinence.

- Emphasize consuming an adequate volume of fluids and reducing or eliminating bladder irritants (particularly caffeine and alcohol).
- Advise the patient to maintain a regular, flexible schedule of urination (usually every 3–4 hours while awake).
- Advise patients to quit smoking, because it increases the risk of stress UI.
- Teach patients to manage constipation with adequate fluid intake, increased dietary fiber, light exercise, and judicious use of stool softeners.
- Behavioral treatments include bladder retraining and pelvic floor muscle training (Kegel) exercises.
- Assess patient strategies and share information on products designed to contain urine.
- In inpatient or long-term care facilities, management of UI includes maximizing toilet access. Offer the urinal or bedpan, or assist the patient to the bathroom every 2–3 hours (or at scheduled times), and ensure privacy.

URINARY RETENTION

Description

Urinary retention is the inability to empty the bladder or the accumulation of urine in the bladder because of an inability to void. In some cases, it is associated with urinary leakage or postvoid dribbling, called *overflow urinary incontinence* (UI).

- *Acute urinary retention*, which is the total inability to pass urine via micturition, is a medical emergency.
- Chronic urinary retention is incomplete bladder emptying despite urination. The postvoid residual (PVR) volumes in patients with chronic urinary retention vary widely. Normal PVR is under 50 mL and for the elderly, 50–100 mL. A PVR over 200 mL is abnormal. A PVR between 100 and 200 mL can justify further evaluation when the patient has issues such as recurring UTIs or LUTS suggestive of UTI.

Pathophysiology and Diagnostic Studies

Urinary retention is caused by two different dysfunctions of the urinary system: bladder outlet obstruction and deficient detrusor (bladder wall muscle) contraction strength.

- *Bladder outlet obstruction* leads to urinary retention when the blockage prevents the bladder from emptying its contents despite detrusor contraction. A common cause in men is an enlarged prostate.
- Common causes of *deficient detrusor contraction strength* include neurologic impairment, diabetic neuropathy, overdistention, chronic alcohol use, and drugs (e.g., anticholinergic drugs).

The diagnostic studies for urinary retention are the same as those for UI (see Urinary Incontinence).

Interprofessional Management

Behavioral therapies for UI may be used in the management of urinary retention. Scheduled toileting and double voiding may be effective in chronic urinary retention associated with moderate PVR volumes.

- Double voiding is an attempt to maximize bladder evacuation by having the patient urinate, sit on the toilet for 3–4 minutes, and urinate again before exiting the bathroom.
- If catheterization is required for urinary retention, intermittent catheterization decreases the risk of catheter-associated urinary tract infections (CAUTIs).

Drug Therapy

For the patient with obstruction at the level of the bladder neck, an α-adrenergic blocker may be prescribed. These drugs relax the smooth muscle of the bladder neck and prostatic urethra and may decrease urethral resistance.

U

Surgical Therapy

Surgical interventions are used to manage urinary retention caused by obstruction. Transurethral or open surgical techniques are used to treat benign or cancerous prostatic enlargement, bladder neck contracture, urethral strictures, or dyssynergia of the bladder neck.

- Pelvic reconstruction using an abdominal or transvaginal approach can correct bladder outlet obstruction in women with severe pelvic organ prolapse.
- Sacral neuromodulation involves a stimulator device and placement of a lead wire into the S3 foramen.
- An intraurethral valve pump can be placed to empty the patient's bladder as needed.

Nursing Management

Acute urinary retention is a medical emergency that requires prompt bladder drainage. Insert a catheter as prescribed. See Urinary Catheterization.

- Teach the patient with or predisposed to acute urinary retention how to minimize risk, including avoiding rapid intake of large volumes of fluid.
- Advise the patient who is unable to urinate to attempt to urinate while in a tub of warm water or a warm shower.
- If these measures do not lead to successful urination, have the patient seek immediate care.

Patients may manage chronic urinary retention with behavioral methods, an indwelling catheter, intermittent catheterization, surgery, or drugs. Scheduled toileting and double voiding are the primary behavioral interventions used for chronic retention.

URINARY TRACT CALCULI

Description

Calculi, or stones, can be found in various locations in the urinary tract. In their lifetime, 11% of men and 7% of women in the United States will have *nephrolithiasis* (kidney stone disease). The term *calculus* refers to the stone, and *lithiasis* refers to stone formation. Except for struvite (magnesium ammonium phosphate) stones associated with urinary tract infection (UTI), stone disorders are more common in men than in women. Most patients are middle-aged adults. Stone formation is more frequent in whites than in Blacks, Hispanics, and Asians.

- The incidence is higher in people with a family history of stone formation. Stones can recur in up to 50% of patients.

- Stone formation occurs more often in the summer months, supporting the possible contributing factors of a hot climate and dehydration.

Pathophysiology

We think kidney stones form when certain crystal-forming substances are not diluted by the kidney and/or the kidney's ability to keep crystals from sticking together is reduced. Crystals in a supersaturated concentration can precipitate and unite to form a stone. Keeping urine dilute and free-flowing reduces the risk of recurrent stone formation.

- Urinary pH, solute load, and inhibitors in the urine affect the formation of stones. The higher the pH, the less soluble are calcium and phosphate. The lower the pH, the less soluble are uric acid and cystine. When a substance is not very soluble in fluid, it is more likely to precipitate out of solution.
- Other key factors in stone formation include obstruction with associated urinary stasis and UTI with urea-splitting bacteria (e.g., Proteus, Klebsiella, Pseudomonas, and some species of staphylococci). These bacteria cause the urine to become alkaline and contribute to the formation of struvite stones. Infected stones trapped in the kidney may assume a staghorn configuration as the stone branches to occupy a larger part of the collecting system. These stones can lead to a renal infection, hydronephrosis, and loss of kidney function.

Genetic factors may contribute to stone formation. Cystinuria, an autosomal recessive disorder, causes a large increase in the urinary excretion of cysteine. There are five major categories of stones: calcium oxalate, calcium phosphate, cystine, struvite, and uric acid. Stone composition may be mixed, although calcium stones are the most common.

Clinical Manifestations

The first symptom is usually sudden, excruciating pain in the flank area, back, or lower abdomen.

- *Renal colic* is the term used for the severe pain from the stretching, dilation, and spasm of the ureter in response to the obstructing stone. Nausea and vomiting may also occur.
- Urinary stones cause manifestations when they obstruct urinary flow. The type of pain is determined by the location of the stone. If the obstruction is in a calyx or the ureteropelvic junction (UPJ), the patient may have dull costovertebral flank pain or renal colic. Pain resulting from the passage of a stone calculus down the ureter is intense and colicky. The patient may be in mild shock, with cool, moist skin. As a stone nears the

ureterovesical junction (UVJ), pain will be felt in the lateral flank and sometimes down into the groin and testicles or labia.
- Manifestations may include dysuria, fever, and chills.

Diagnostic Studies

- Noncontrast helical (spiral) CT scan, ultrasound, and intravenous pyelogram (IVP) may be used.
- Urinalysis is used to assess for hematuria, crystalluria, and urine pH. Measuring urine pH is useful in the diagnosis of struvite stones (tendency to alkaline or high pH) and uric acid or cystine stones (tendency to acidic or low pH).
- Retrieval and analysis of the stones are important in diagnosing the underlying problem contributing to stone formation.
- Serum calcium, phosphorus, sodium, potassium, bicarbonate, uric acid, and creatinine levels and blood urea nitrogen (BUN) are measured.

Interprofessional Management

Care of a patient with stones involves two concurrent approaches. The *first approach* is managing the acute pain, infection, or obstruction. Give opioids to relieve renal colic pain. Nonsteroidal antiinflammatory drugs (NSAIDs) can be considered if there is normal renal function. Many stones are 4 mm or less in size, so will pass spontaneously. However, such a stone may take weeks to pass. Tamsulosin (Flomax) or terazosin, α-adrenergic blockers that relax the smooth muscle in the ureter, can facilitate stone passage.

The *second approach* is evaluating the cause of stone formation and preventing further stone development. Information obtained from the patient includes family history of stone formation, geographic location of residence, nutritional assessment (including fluid intake and intake of vitamins C and D), and activity pattern. Obtain a complete health and medication history.

Adequate hydration, dietary sodium restrictions, dietary changes, and drugs minimize urinary stone formation.

- Drugs are prescribed that prevent stone formation by altering urine pH, preventing excessive urinary excretion of a substance, or correcting a primary disease (e.g., hyperparathyroidism).

Treatment of struvite stones requires control of infection. Acetohydroxamic acid inhibits the chemical action caused by persistent bacteria and can slow struvite stone formation. The stone may have to be removed surgically if the infection cannot be controlled. Indications for open surgical, endourology, or lithotripsy stone removal include:

- stones too large for spontaneous passage (usually larger than 7 mm), associated with bacteriuria or symptomatic infection,

or causing impaired renal function, persistent pain, nausea, or paralytic ileus;
- medical treatment not successful;
- patient with only 1 kidney.

Endourologic procedures include the use of endoscopes to reach stones in the urinary tract. *Cystoscopy* can remove small stones in the bladder. *Cystolitholapaxy* is performed using a lithotrite to crush large stones. A *cystoscopic lithotripsy* uses ultrasonic waves to break up stones. Complications with these procedures include hemorrhage, retained stone fragments, and infection. Flexible *ureteroscopes* can be used to remove stones from the renal pelvis and upper urinary tract with ultrasonic, laser, or electrohydraulic lithotripsy. The same types of lithotripsy can be used during a percutaneous nephrolithotomy when a nephroscope is inserted through the skin into the kidney pelvis.

Lithotripsy is a procedure for eliminating calculi from the urinary tract. Specific lithotripsy techniques include percutaneous ultrasonic lithotripsy, electrohydraulic lithotripsy, laser lithotripsy, and extracorporeal shock wave lithotripsy. Extracorporeal shock wave lithotripsy and laser lithotripsy are the most common.
- Hematuria is common after lithotripsy procedures. A self-retaining ureteral stent is placed to prevent obstruction caused by sand buildup in the ureter, then removed 2 weeks later.
- If a stone is large or positioned in the mid or distal ureter, additional treatment may be needed.

Some patients need open surgical procedures because of pain, obstruction, or infection. The type of open surgery (e.g., *nephrolithotomy, pyelolithotomy, ureterolithotomy*) depends on location of the stone. For open surgery on the kidney or ureter, a flank incision directly below the diaphragm and across the side is usually preferred.

Nutritional Therapy

A high fluid intake (around 3 L/day) is recommended after an episode of urolithiasis to produce urine output of at least 2.5 L/day and prevent recurrent stones.
- Limit consumption of colas, coffee, and tea, because high intake of these beverages tends to increase the risk of recurring urinary stones.
- A low-sodium diet is recommended, because high sodium intake increases calcium excretion in the urine. Foods high in calcium, oxalate, and purines are listed in Table 50.12, Harding et al., *Lewis' Medical-Surgical Nursing*, ed 12.

Nursing Management

Goals

The overall goals are that the patient with urinary tract stones will have pain relief, no urinary tract obstruction, and knowledge of ways to prevent stone recurrence.

Interventions

Preventive measures related to the person who is on bed rest or is immobile for a prolonged period include maintaining an adequate fluid intake, turning the patient every 2 hours, and helping the patient sit or stand if possible to maximize urinary flow.

Pain management is a key nursing responsibility when a patient has an obstructing stone and renal colic.

- To retrieve passed stones, strain all urine voided by the patient, using gauze or a urine strainer.
- Encourage ambulation to promote movement of the stone to the lower urinary tract. To ensure safety, tell the patient who has acute renal colic to ask for help when ambulating, particularly if opioid analgesics are given.

▼ Patient and Caregiver Teaching

- Encourage adequate fluid intake to produce a urine output of approximately 2.5 L/day.
- Teach about dietary restriction of purines to lower risk for developing uric acid stones.
- Teach the patient the dosage, scheduling, and potential side effects of drugs used to reduce the risk of stone formation.
- Some patients may learn to self-monitor urinary pH or urinary output.

URINARY TRACT INFECTIONS

Description

Urinary tract infections (UTIs) are the most common outpatient infection. *Escherichia coli* (*E. coli*) is the most common pathogen causing a UTI. It causes 75% of cases without urinary tract structural abnormalities or stones and 65% of complicated UTIs.

- Bacterial counts in the urine of 10^5 colony-forming units per milliliter (CFU/mL) or higher typically indicate a UTI. However, bacterial counts as low as 10^2–10^3 CFU/mL in a person with symptoms are also indicative of UTI.
- Fungal and parasitic infections sometimes cause UTIs. These are more common in patients who are immunosuppressed, have

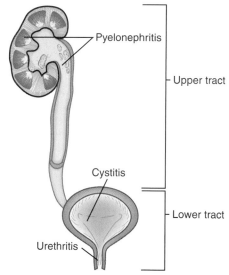

Fig. 30 Sites of infections in the upper and lower urinary tracts.

diabetes or kidney problems, or received multiple courses of antibiotic therapy.

Classification

A UTI can be described and classified as an upper or a lower UTI according to its location within the urinary system. Infection of the upper urinary tract (involving the renal parenchyma, pelvis, and ureters) typically causes fever, chills, and flank pain. A lower-urinary-tract infection does not usually have systemic manifestations.

Specific terms identify the UTI location. For example, *pyelonephritis* implies inflammation usually caused by infection of the renal parenchyma and collecting system. *Cystitis* indicates inflammation of the bladder wall, while *urethritis* is inflammation of the urethra. *Urosepsis* is a UTI that has spread systemically. It is a life-threatening condition requiring emergency treatment (Fig. 30).

- *Uncomplicated UTIs* occur in an otherwise normal urinary tract and usually involve only the bladder.
- *Complicated UTIs* are associated with an underlying disease or with a structural or functional problem in the urinary tract. Examples include obstruction, stones, catheters, abnormal genitourinary (GU) tract, acute kidney injury (AKI), chronic kidney disease (CKD), renal transplant, diabetes, or neurologic disease.

Pathophysiology

U

The urinary tract above the urethra is normally sterile. Organisms that cause UTIs are usually introduced from the urethra. Gram-negative aerobic bacilli normally found in the gastrointestinal (GI) tract cause most UTIs. However, Gram-positive organisms, such as streptococci, enterococci, and *Staphylococcus saprophyticus*, can also cause UTIs. Table 89 lists risk factors for UTIs.

- Urologic instrumentation (e.g., catheterization, cystoscopic examinations) allows bacteria normally present at the opening of the urethra to enter the urethra or bladder.
- Sexual intercourse promotes "milking" of bacteria from the vagina and perineum and may cause minor urethral trauma that predisposes women to UTIs.
- Blood-borne bacteria rarely invade the kidneys, ureters, or bladder unless there is a prior injury to the urinary tract,

UTIs are the most common health care–associated infection (HAI). They are mainly due to use of an indwelling catheter. *Catheter-associated urinary tract infections (CAUTIs)* often are caused by *E. coli* and, less often, *Pseudomonas* organisms. CAUTIs lead to extended hospital stays, increased health care costs, and increased mortality.

Clinical Manifestations

Manifestations of UTIs range from painful urination in uncomplicated urethritis or cystitis to severe systemic illness with abdominal or back pain, fever, and sepsis. Lower urinary tract symptoms (LUTSs) are seen in patients with UTIs of both the upper and lower urinary tracts.

- Symptoms include dysuria, frequent urination (more often than every 2 hours), urgency, and suprapubic discomfort or pressure. Older adults tend to experience generalized abdominal discomfort, rather than dysuria and suprapubic pain.
- The urine may contain visible blood (hematuria) or sediment, giving it a cloudy appearance.
- Flank pain, chills, and fever indicate an infection involving the upper urinary tract (pyelonephritis).

The common manifestations of a UTI are often absent in older adults, who tend to have general abdominal discomfort rather than dysuria and suprapubic pain. They may have impaired cognition or overall clinical deterioration.

Diagnostic Studies

- Dipstick urinalysis of a clean-catch specimen is done initially to identify presence of nitrites (indicating bacteriuria), white

TABLE 89   Risk Factors for Urinary Tract Infections

Anatomic Factors
- Congenital defects leading to obstruction or urinary stasis
- Fistula exposing urinary stream to skin, vagina, or fecal stream
- Obesity
- Shorter female urethra and colonization from normal vaginal flora

Foreign Bodies Factors Compromising Immune Response
- Aging
- Diabetes
- Human immunodeficiency virus infection

Factors Increasing Urinary Stasis
- Extrinsic obstruction (tumor, fibrosis compressing urinary tract)
- Intrinsic obstruction (stone, tumor of urinary tract, urethral stricture, benign prostatic hypertrophy)
- Renal impairment
- Urinary retention (e.g., neurogenic bladder)

Foreign Bodies
- Catheters (indwelling, external condom catheter, ureteral stent, nephrostomy tube, intermittent catheterization)
- Urinary tract instrumentation (cystoscopy)
- Urinary tract stones

Functional Disorders
- Constipation
- Voiding dysfunction with detrusor sphincter incoordination

Other Factors
- Habitual delay of urination ("nurse's bladder," "teacher's bladder")
- Pregnancy
- Menopause
- Sexual activity (women)
- Poor personal hygiene
- Use of spermicidal agents, contraceptive diaphragm (women), bubble baths, feminine sprays

blood cells (WBCs), and leukocyte esterase (an enzyme present in WBCs indicating pyuria).

- After confirmation of bacteriuria and pyuria, a urine culture with sensitivity may be obtained. A voided midstream technique (clean-catch urine sample) is best for obtaining a urine culture in most circumstances.
- A CT urogram or ultrasound may be obtained when obstruction of the urinary system is suspected.

Interprofessional Management

Drug Therapy

Uncomplicated UTIs are treated with a short-term course of antibiotics, typically for 3 days. In contrast, complicated UTIs need a longer period of treatment, lasting 7–14 days or more.

- First-choice drugs to treat uncomplicated or initial UTIs are trimethoprim/sulfamethoxazole (TMP-SMX), nitrofurantoin, cephalexin, and fosfomycin. TMP-SMX has the advantages of being inexpensive and taken twice daily. Nitrofurantoin is taken three or four times daily, but a twice-daily formulation is available.
- E. coli resistance to TMP-SMX, beta-lactams, and ciprofloxacin is an increasing problem in the United States.
- Other antibiotics used in the treatment of uncomplicated UTI include ampicillin, amoxicillin, and cephalosporins.
- Fluoroquinolones (e.g., levofloxacin, ciprofloxacin) are used to treat complicated UTIs.
- In patients with UTIs from fungi, fluconazole (Diflucan) is the preferred therapy.
- Prophylactic or suppressive antibiotics are sometimes given to patients who have repeated UTIs.
- A urinary analgesic, such as oral phenazopyridine, may relieve discomfort caused by severe dysuria.

Nursing Management

Goals

The goals for patient with a UTI are relief from bothersome symptoms, prevention of upper urinary tract involvement, and no recurrence. See eNursing Care Plan 50-1 for the patient with a UTI on the website.

Interventions

Health promotion activities, especially for persons who are at an increased risk for UTI, include teaching preventive measures, such as emptying the bladder regularly and completely, evacuating the bowel regularly, wiping the perineal area from front to back after urination and defecation, and drinking an adequate amount of liquid each day.

- All patients undergoing instrumentation of the urinary tract are at risk for developing CAUTI. Avoiding unnecessary catheterization and early removal of indwelling catheters are the most effective measures for reducing CAUTI. Always follow aseptic technique during these procedures.

- Wash your hands before and after contact with each patient. Wear gloves for care of urinary catheters. The American Nurses Association offers an evidence-based clinical tool for decreasing CAUTI.

- Promote adequate fluid intake. Fluid flushes out bacteria before they have a chance to colonize in the bladder. Caffeine, alcohol, citrus juice, chocolate, and highly spiced foods or beverages should be avoided because they may irritate the bladder.

- Application of local heat to the suprapubic area or lower back may relieve discomfort associated with a UTI. A warm shower or sitting in a tub of warm water filled to above the waist can provide temporary relief.

▼ **Patient and Caregiver Teaching**

Teach the patient about the prescribed drug therapy and side effects. Stress the importance of taking the full course of antibiotics.

- Teach patients to promptly report any of the following to their health care provider: (1) persistence of bothersome LUTS beyond the antibiotic treatment course, (2) onset of flank pain, or (3) fever. Recurrent symptoms associated with bacterial persistence or inadequate treatment typically occur within 1–2 weeks after completion of therapy.

- Teach the patient and caregiver about ongoing care, including taking antimicrobial drugs as ordered, maintaining adequate daily fluid intake, voiding regularly (approximately every 3–4 hours), urinating before and after intercourse, and temporarily discontinuing the use of a diaphragm.

- Teach patients prescribed phenazopyridine that the drug causes urine to turn orange or red.

VAGINAL, CERVICAL, AND VULVAR INFECTIONS

Lower genital tract infections include infections resulting from a disruption in the vaginal microbiome and sexually transmitted infections (STIs). The vaginal microbiome contains microorganisms such as yeast and healthy bacteria that protect against infection by maintaining an acidic environment. Inflammation of the vagina, known as vaginitis, can occur from a disruption of the vaginal flora.

TABLE 90 Vaginal Infections Associated with Vaginitis

Infection	Manifestations	Treatment Options
Bacterial vaginosis (bacterial infection)	"Fishy" odor Gray or white vaginal discharge	Oral or vaginal antibiotics • clindamycin (Cleocin) • metronidazole (Flagyl) • tinidazole (Tindamax)
Trichomonas vaginalis (protozoan infection)	Genital itching and inflammation Dysuria Frothy, thin, yellowish-greenish vaginal discharge Deep red or pink cervix and vagina ("strawberry cervix")	Antifungal agents • metronidazole (Flagyl) • tinidazole (Tindamax) Treatment of partner(s)
Vulvovaginal candidiasis (yeast infection)	Vaginal itching Red, swollen vulva Thick, white, curdy vaginal discharge	Oral or vaginal antifungals • butoconazole (Gynazole) • clotrimazole (Gyne-Lotrimin) • fluconazole (Diflucan) • miconazole (Monistat)

Pathophysiology and Clinical Manifestations

Organisms gain entrance to the lower genital tract through sexual intercourse, contact with contaminated hands or clothing, or douching. Table 90 presents the causes, manifestations and treatment of common infections of the female lower genital tract.

- Oral contraceptives, antibiotics, and corticosteroids may change the vaginal pH and trigger an overgrowth of the organisms present, such as *Candida albicans.*
- Vulvar infections, such as herpes and genital warts, can be sexually transmitted when no visible lesions are present (see Herpes, Genital, and Warts, Genital).

Abnormal vaginal discharge and a reddened vulva are common signs of infection.

Diagnostic Studies

Evaluation of genital problems begins with a history, including sexual history, and physical examination.

- Ulcerative lesions are cultured for herpesvirus.
- Vulvar dystrophies are examined by colposcope and biopsied.
- Vaginal discharge is examined and sent for culture.
- With cervicitis, endocervical cultures are obtained for chlamydia and gonorrhea.
- See Sexually transmitted infections.

Interprofessional and Nursing Management

Treatment options depend on the type of infection. A follow-up visit is often recommended to evaluate treatment effectiveness and provide teaching about sexual health and contraception.

- Discussing problems that concern the patient's genitalia or sexual intercourse is often hard. Use nonjudgmental communication to make women feel more comfortable while empowering them to ask questions. Review symptoms that indicate a problem, and help women seek care promptly.
- Teach patients about behavioral and lifestyle measures to reduce the risk for infection. This includes keeping the vulvar area dry and avoiding products such as harsh laundry detergents, scented menstrual products, or spermicides that can cause irritation. Discuss how to clean the vulva and vagina to reduce infections by using only gentle and unscented soaps to clean externally and avoiding douching.
- Review sexual practices to prevent infections such as inserting only clean objects (like washed hands or sex toys) into the vagina and using water- or silicone-based lubricants.
- Smoking cessation and nutrition teaching may help minimize risk of infection.
- Ensure that the patient fully understands the treatment. Provide information about comfort measures to improve symptoms. Vaginal creams should be inserted before going to bed so the medication will remain in the vagina for a long period. Teach where and how the applicator should be filled and inserted using visual aids or models.

VALVULAR HEART DISEASE

Description

Valvular heart disease is defined according to the affected valve or valves (mitral, aortic, tricuspid, pulmonary) and the type of dysfunction: *stenosis* or *regurgitation* (Fig. 31).

- The pressures on either side of an open valve normally are equal. In *stenosis,* the valve opening is smaller due to limited

Fig. 31 Valvular stenosis and regurgitation. (A) Normal position of the valve leaflets when the valve is open and closed. (B) Open position of a stenosed valve (left) and closed position of regurgitant valve (right). (C) Hemodynamic effect of mitral stenosis. The stenosed valve is unable to open sufficiently during left atrial systole, inhibiting left ventricular filling. (D) Hemodynamic effect of MR. The mitral valve does not close completely during left ventricular systole, letting blood reenter the left atrium. At the same time, blood is moving forward through the aortic valve. (From McCance K.L., Huether S.E. Pathophysiology: The biologic basis for disease in adults and children, ed 6, St Louis, 2010, Mosby.)

leaflet opening, impeding the forward flow of blood, and creating a pressure difference on the two sides of the open valve. The degree of stenosis (constriction or narrowing) is reflected in the pressure differences.

- In *regurgitation* (also called incompetence or *insufficiency*), incomplete closure of valve leaflets results in backward flow of blood.

Congenital heart conditions are the most common cause of valve disorders in children and adolescents. Aortic stenosis and mitral regurgitation are in older adults with heart disease. Other causes of valve disease in adults are related to endocarditis, rheumatic heart disease, hypertension, and autoimmune disorders.

Clinical manifestations of various types of valvular heart disease are presented in Table 91.

Mitral Valve Stenosis

Pathophysiology

Worldwide, the most common cause of mitral valve stenosis is rheumatic heart disease. Less common causes include congenital mitral stenosis, rheumatoid arthritis, radiation exposure, and systemic lupus erythematosus (SLE).

- Rheumatic endocarditis causes scarring of valve leaflets and chordae tendineae. Contractures and adhesions develop between the commissures (the junctional areas).
- The stenotic mitral valve takes on a "fish mouth" shape because of the thickening and shortening of mitral valve structures. Flow obstruction increases left atrial pressure and volume, resulting in higher pulmonary vasculature pressure and eventually involving the right ventricle.

Clinical Manifestations

The main symptom is exertional dyspnea caused by reduced lung compliance. Fatigue and palpitations from atrial fibrillation may also occur. Heart sounds include a loud first heart sound and a low-pitched, rumbling diastolic murmur (best heard at the apex with the stethoscope bell).

Other manifestations are identified in Table 91.

Mitral Valve Regurgitation

Pathophysiology

Mitral valve function depends on the integrity of mitral leaflets, chordae tendineae, papillary muscles, left atrium (LA), and left ventricle (LV). A defect in any of these structures can cause regurgitation. Myocardial infarction with left ventricular failure increases the risk for rupture of the chordae tendineae and acute mitral regurgitation (MR).

- Most cases of MR are caused by myocardial infarction, chronic rheumatic heart disease, mitral valve prolapse, ischemic papillary muscle dysfunction, and infective endocarditis (IE).
- MR allows blood to flow backward from the LV to the LA because of incomplete valve closure during systole. Both chambers of the left side of the heart must work harder to preserve an adequate cardiac output (CO).

TABLE 91 Manifestations of Valvular Heart Disease

Type	Manifestations
Mitral valve prolapse	Palpitations, dyspnea, chest pain, activity intolerance, syncope, holosystolic murmur
Mitral valve regurgitation	*Acute:* generally poorly tolerated. New systolic murmur with pulmonary edema. Cardiogenic shock develops rapidly *Chronic:* weakness, fatigue, exertional dyspnea, edema, palpitations, S_3 gallop, holosystolic murmur
Mitral valve stenosis	Dyspnea on exertion, hemoptysis, hoarseness, fatigue. Atrial fibrillation on ECG. Palpitations. Loud, accentuated S_1. Low-pitched, diastolic murmur
Aortic valve regurgitation	*Acute:* abrupt onset of profound dyspnea, chest pain, left ventricular failure and cardiogenic shock *Chronic:* fatigue, exertional dyspnea, orthopnea, PND. Water-hammer pulse, heaving precordial impulse, decreased or absent S_1, S_3, or S_4. Soft high-pitched diastolic murmur, Austin Flint murmur
Aortic valve stenosis	Angina, syncope, dyspnea on exertion, heart failure, normal or soft S_1, decreased or absent S_2, systolic murmur, prominent S_4
Tricuspid and pulmonic stenosis	*Tricuspid:* peripheral edema, ascites, hepatomegaly. Diastolic low-pitched murmur with increased intensity during inspiration *Pulmonic:* fatigue, loud midsystolic murmur

ECG, Electrocardiogram; *PND,* paroxysmal nocturnal dyspnea.

- In acute MR, the sudden increase in pressure and volume is transmitted to the pulmonary bed. This results in pulmonary edema and, if not treated, cardiogenic shock.
- In chronic MR, the added volume load results in left atrial enlargement and left ventricular dilation and hypertrophy and, finally, a decrease in CO.

Clinical Manifestations

Patients with acute MR have thready peripheral pulses and cool, clammy extremities. A low CO may mask a new systolic murmur.

Rapid assessment (e.g., cardiac catheterization) and intervention (e.g., valve repair or replacement) are critical for a positive outcome.

Patients with chronic MR may remain asymptomatic for years until the development of some degree of left ventricular failure. Manifestations are identified in Table 91.

Mitral Valve Prolapse

Pathophysiology

Mitral valve prolapse (MVP) is an abnormality of the mitral valve leaflets and papillary muscles or chordae that allows the leaflets to prolapse, or "buckle," back into the left atrium during systole. It is the most common form of valvular heart disease in the United States.

- MVP is usually benign, but serious complications can occur, including MR, IE, sudden cardiac death, and cerebral ischemia.
- There is an increased familial incidence in some patients resulting from a connective tissue defect affecting only the valve, or as part of Marfan's syndrome or other hereditary conditions that influence the structure of collagen in the body.

Clinical Manifestations

MVP covers a broad spectrum of severity. Most patients are asymptomatic for their entire lives. Clinical manifestations may include those identified in Table 91.

- If chest pain occurs, episodes tend to occur in clusters, especially during periods of emotional stress. Chest pain may occasionally be accompanied by dyspnea, palpitations, and syncope and does not respond to antianginal treatment (e.g., nitrates).

Patients with MVP generally have a benign course unless problems related to MR develop. Table 92 provides a teaching plan for patients with MVP.

Aortic Valve Stenosis

Pathophysiology

Congenital aortic stenosis is found in childhood, adolescence, or young adulthood. In older patients, *aortic stenosis* is a result of rheumatic fever or degeneration similar to that in coronary artery disease.

- In rheumatic valve disease, fusion and calcification cause the valve leaflets to stiffen and retract, resulting in stenosis.
- Aortic stenosis causes obstruction of flow from the LV to the aorta during systole. The result is left ventricular hypertrophy and increased myocardial oxygen consumption because of the increased myocardial mass.

TABLE 92   Patient and Caregiver Teaching: Mitral Valve Prolapse
Include the following information in the teaching plan for a patient with mitral valve prolapse (MVP) and the patient's caregiver.
• Take drugs as prescribed (e.g., β-adrenergic blockers to control palpitations, chest pain).
• Adopt healthy eating habits.
• Avoid caffeine because it is a stimulant and may worsen symptoms.
• If you use diet pills or other over-the-counter drugs, check for common ingredients that are stimulants (e.g., caffeine, ephedrine) because these can worsen symptoms.
• Begin or maintain an exercise program to achieve optimal health.
• Contact the health care provider (HCP) or emergency medical services if symptoms develop or worsen (e.g., palpitations, fatigue, shortness of breath, anxiety).

- As the disease progresses and compensation fails, reduced CO leads to pulmonary hypertension and heart failure.

Clinical Manifestations

Symptoms of aortic stenosis (AS) develop when the valve orifice becomes about one-third of its normal size. Symptoms include the classic triad of angina, syncope, and exertional dyspnea, reflecting left ventricular failure. Auscultation of AS often reveals a normal or soft S1, a decreased diminished or absent S2, a crescendo–decrescendo systolic murmur, with radiation to the carotids. Common manifestations are presented in Table 91.

Aortic Valve Regurgitation

Pathophysiology

Aortic regurgitation may be the result of primary disease of the aortic valve leaflets, the aortic root, or both.

- Acute aortic regurgitation is caused by IE, trauma, or aortic dissection and constitutes a life-threatening emergency.
- Chronic aortic regurgitation is generally the result of rheumatic heart disease, a congenital bicuspid aortic valve, syphilis, a connective tissue problem, or a postsurgical cause.
- Aortic regurgitation causes retrograde blood flow from the ascending aorta into the LV, resulting in volume overload.
- Myocardial contractility eventually declines, and blood volume increases in the LA and pulmonary bed. This leads to pulmonary hypertension and right ventricular failure.

Clinical Manifestations

Clinical manifestations of acute and chronic aortic valve regurgitation are presented in Table 91.

Tricuspid and Pulmonic Valve Disease

Diseases of the tricuspid and pulmonic valves are uncommon, with stenosis occurring more frequently than regurgitation. Tricuspid stenosis results in right atrial enlargement and elevated systemic venous pressures. Pulmonic stenosis results in right ventricular hypertension and hypertrophy. Table 91 presents clinical manifestations of these valve diseases.

Diagnostic Studies: Valvular Heart Disease

- Electrocardiogram (ECG) shows variations in heart rate (HR), rhythm, and possible ischemia or chamber enlargement.
- Echocardiogram reveals valve structure, function, and heart chamber size.
- Transesophageal echocardiography and Doppler color-flow imaging help diagnose and monitor valvular heart disease progression.
- Real-time three-dimensional echocardiography helps assess mitral valve and congenital heart disease.
- Chest X-ray reveals heart size, altered pulmonary circulation, and valve calcification.
- Cardiac catheterization detects chamber pressure changes and pressure gradients (differences) across the valves.

Interprofessional Care: Valvular Heart Disease

Overall treatment focuses on preventing exacerbations of heart failure, acute pulmonary edema, thromboembolism, and recurrent endocarditis. Heart failure is treated with vasodilators, positive inotropes, β-adrenergic blockers, diuretics, and a low-sodium diet.

- Anticoagulant therapy is used in patients with atrial fibrillation to prevent systemic or pulmonary emboli.
- Atrial dysrhythmias are common and treated with calcium-channel blockers, β-blockers, antidysrhythmic drugs, or electrical cardioversion.
- An alternative treatment for some patients with valvular stenosis is the *percutaneous transluminal balloon valvuloplasty* (PTBV) procedure in a heart catheterization laboratory. A balloon-tipped catheter is threaded from the femoral artery to the stenotic valve so that the balloon may be inflated to separate valve leaflets.

Transcatheter aortic valve replacement (TAVR) is an option for patients with severe, symptomatic AS. The insertion process is similar to the PTBV.

Surgical Therapy

The type of valve repair or replacement depends on the valves involved, disease pathology severity, and the patient's symptoms. Valve repair has a lower operative mortality rate than valve replacement, but may not restore total valve function.

- Open surgical valvuloplasty involves repairing the valve by suturing the torn leaflets, chordae tendineae, and papillary muscles. It is primarily used to treat mitral regurgitation or tricuspid regurgitation.

- For patients with mitral or tricuspid regurgitation, further valve repair or reconstruction using annuloplasty is an option. *Annuloplasty* involves reconstruction of the annulus, with or without the aid of prosthetic rings.

Valve replacement may be required for mitral, aortic, tricuspid, or pulmonic valve disease.

- *Mechanical valves* are made of combinations of metal alloys, pyrolytic carbon, and Dacron. Biologic valves are constructed from bovine, porcine, and human (cadaver) cardiac tissue.

- Mechanical prosthetic valves are more durable than biologic tissue valves, but they carry an increased risk of thromboembolism and patients need long-term anticoagulant therapy. Anticoagulation therapy is not needed with biologic valves. However, they are less durable and tend to develop early calcification, tissue degeneration, and stiffening of leaflets. Both valve types are subject to leaking and endocarditis.

- Long-term anticoagulation is needed for those patients with biologic valves who have atrial fibrillation. Some patients with biologic valves or annuloplasty with prosthetic rings may need anticoagulation the first few months after surgery, until the suture lines are covered by endothelial cells (endothelialized).

- The choice of valves depends on many factors. A mechanical valve may be best for a younger patient because it is more durable. If a patient cannot take an anticoagulant (e.g., women of childbearing age), a biologic valve is considered.

Nursing Management: Valvular Heart Disease

Goals

The overall goals for the patient with valve disease include: (1) normal heart function, (2) improved activity tolerance, and (3) an understanding of the disease process and health maintenance measures.

Interventions

Encouraging early treatment of streptococcal infection and providing prophylactic antibiotics for patients with a history of rheumatic fever are critical to prevent acquired rheumatic valve disease. Patients at risk for endocarditis and any patients with certain high-risk heart conditions must receive prophylactic antibiotics.

- Teach the person with a history of rheumatic fever, endocarditis, or congenital heart disease the symptoms of valvular heart disease to report.
- Design activities considering the patient's limitations. An appropriate exercise plan can increase cardiac tolerance. The patient should limit activities that cause fatigue and dyspnea.
- Emphasize conserving energy, setting priorities, and taking planned rest periods.
- Consider referral to a vocational counselor if the patient has a physically or emotionally demanding job.
- Perform ongoing cardiac assessments to monitor the effectiveness of medications. Teach the actions and side effects of drugs to increase adherence. Reinforce the importance of prophylactic antibiotic therapy to prevent IE.
- The patient on anticoagulants (e.g., warfarin) after surgery for valve replacement must have the international normalized ratio (INR) checked regularly to regulate therapy. INR values of 2.5–3.5 are therapeutic for patients with mechanical valves.

▼ Patient and Caregiver Teaching

- Teach the patient to notify the health care provider about any signs or symptoms of infection, heart failure, or bleeding.
- Encourage patients to wear a medical identification (Medic Alert) device.

VARICOSE VEINS

Description

Varicose veins (varicosities) are dilated (to 3 mm or larger in diameter), tortuous superficial veins, often found in the saphenous vein system. They may be small and innocuous or large and bulging.

- *Primary* varicose veins (idiopathic), caused by weakness of the vein walls, are more common in women.
- *Secondary* varicosities typically result from direct injury, a previous venous thromboembolism (VTE), or excessive vein distention. Secondary varicose veins may also occur in the esophagus (esophageal varices), vulva, spermatic cords (varicoceles), and

anorectal area (hemorrhoids), and as abnormal arteriovenous (AV) connections.

Pathophysiology

Risk factors include family history of chronic venous disease, weakness of the vein structure, female gender, tobacco use, increasing age, obesity, multiparity, history of VTE, venous obstruction resulting from extrinsic pressure by tumors, phlebitis, previous leg injury, and occupations that require prolonged standing or sitting.

- In primary varicose veins, weak vein walls allow the vein valve ring to enlarge so that the leaflets no longer fit together properly (incompetent). Incompetent vein valves allow backward blood flow, particularly when the patient is standing. This results in increased venous pressure and further venous distention.

Clinical Manifestations

Discomfort from varicose veins varies dramatically and tends to be worse after episodes of superficial thrombophlebitis. The most common varicose vein symptoms include a heavy, achy pain after prolonged standing or sitting, which is relieved by walking or limb elevation. Some patients feel pressure or a cramp-like, burning sensation. Swelling, restless or tired legs, fatigue, and nocturnal leg cramps may also occur.

Superficial venous thrombosis is the most frequent complication of varicose veins and may occur spontaneously or after trauma, surgical procedures, or pregnancy.

Diagnostic Studies

- Superficial varicose veins can be diagnosed by appearance.
- Duplex ultrasound detects obstruction and reflux in the venous system.

Interprofessional Management

Conservative treatment involves rest with limb elevation, graduated compression stockings, leg-strengthening exercise such as walking, and weight loss if indicated.

Venoactive drugs have been used to treat varicose veins and advanced chronic venous disease.

- These include micronized purified flavonoid fraction, rutosides (e.g., horse chestnut seed extract [*Aesculus hippocastanum*]), proanthocyanidins (from grapes and apples), and Ruscus (butcher's broom). Therapeutic benefits of venoactive drugs include pain relief, edema reduction, and decreased leg cramping and restless legs symptoms. These drugs have been widely used in Europe. They are not approved by the U.S. Food and Drug Administration (FDA); however, many are available over the counter as dietary or herbal supplements.

Sclerotherapy involves the injection of a substance that obliterates venous telangiectasias (i.e., spider veins) and small superficial varicose veins. Direct IV injection of a sclerosing agent, such as hypertonic saline, induces inflammation and causes thrombosis of the vein. After injection, a graduated compression stocking or bandage is worn. Patients should not travel long distances during the first week after sclerotherapy to minimize the risk of a VTE.

- Other noninvasive options include transcutaneous laser therapy for telangiectasias and high-intensity pulsed-light therapy for reticular veins.

Surgical intervention is needed for recurrent superficial vein thrombosis or when chronic venous insufficiency cannot be controlled. Traditional surgical intervention involves ligating the entire vein (usually the greater saphenous) and removing its incompetent branches. An alternative but time-consuming technique is ambulatory phlebectomy, which involves pulling the varicosity through a "stab" incision, followed by excision of the vein.

Nursing Management

Prevention is a key factor related to varicose veins. Teach the patient to avoid sitting or standing for long periods, maintain ideal body weight, avoid injury to the extremities, avoid wearing constrictive clothing, and walk daily.

After vein ligation surgery, check extremities regularly for color, movement, sensation, temperature, presence of edema, and pedal pulses. Some bruising and discoloration are considered normal.

- Elevate the patient's legs 15 degrees to decrease edema.
- Apply graduated compression stockings or bandages. Remove them every 8 hours for a short period and then reapply them.
- Encourage the patient to deep breathe, which promotes venous return.

Long-term management of varicose veins is directed toward improving circulation and appearance, relieving discomfort, and avoiding complications. Varicose veins can recur in other veins after surgery.

▼ Patient and Caregiver Teaching

- Teach the patient to apply custom-fitted graduated compression stockings in bed, before rising in the morning.
- Stress the importance of periodically elevating the legs above heart level.

- The overweight patient may need help with weight loss.
- Patients with a job that requires long periods of standing or sitting need to frequently flex and extend their hips, legs, and ankles and change positions.

VENOUS THROMBOSIS

Description

Venous thrombosis involves the formation of a thrombus (blood clot) with vein inflammation. It is the most common disorder of the veins.

Superficial vein thrombosis is the formation of a thrombus in a superficial vein, usually the greater or lesser saphenous vein.

Deep vein thrombosis (DVT) is a disorder involving a thrombus in a deep vein, often the iliac or femoral vein. *Venous thromboembolism* (VTE) is the preferred term to represent the spectrum from DVT to pulmonary embolism (PE). Table 93 compares superficial vein thrombosis and VTE.

Pathophysiology

Three key factors (*Virchow's triad*) that cause venous thrombosis are venous stasis, damage of the endothelium (inner lining of the vein), and hypercoagulability of the blood. The patient at risk for the development of VTE usually has a predisposing condition to these three disorders.

Venous stasis occurs when the venous valves are dysfunctional or the muscles of the extremities are inactive. Venous stasis occurs more often in people who are obese or pregnant, have chronic heart failure or atrial fibrillation, have been on long trips without regular exercise, undergo a prolonged surgical procedure, or are immobile for long periods (e.g., with spinal cord injury or hip fracture).

Damage to the endothelium of the vein may be caused by direct (e.g., surgery, intravascular catheterization, trauma, fracture, burns, prior VTE) or indirect (chemotherapy, vasculitis, sepsis, diabetes) injury. Damaged endothelium stimulates platelet activation and starts the coagulation cascade. This predisposes the patient to thrombus development.

Hypercoagulability of the blood occurs in many disorders, including severe anemias, polycythemia, cancers (e.g., breast, brain, pancreas, GI tract); nephrotic syndrome; high homocysteine levels; and protein C, protein S, and antithrombin deficiency. A patient with sepsis is predisposed to hypercoagulability because

TABLE 93   Comparison of Superficial Vein Thrombosis (SVT) and Venous Thromboembolism (VTE)

	SVT	VTE
Usual location	Typically, superficial leg veins (e.g., varicosities) Sometimes, superficial arm veins	Deep veins of arms (e.g., axillary, subclavian), legs (e.g., femoral), pelvis (e.g., iliac, inferior or superior vena cava), and pulmonary system
Clinical findings	Tenderness, itchiness, redness, warmth, pain, inflammation, and induration along the course of the superficial vein Vein appears as a palpable cord. Edema rarely occurs.	Tenderness to pressure over involved vein, induration of overlying muscle, venous distention Edema of affected extremity May have mild to moderate pain, deep reddish color to area caused by venous congestion *Note:* Some patients may have no obvious physical changes in the affected extremity.
Sequelae	If untreated, clot may extend to deeper veins, and VTE may occur.	Embolization to lungs (pulmonary embolism) may occur and may result in death.[a] Pulmonary hypertension and postthrombotic syndrome with or without venous leg ulceration may develop.

[a]See Pulmonary Embolism.

of endotoxins released from bacteria. Some drugs (e.g., corticosteroids, estrogens) predispose a patient to thrombus formation.

- Women who use tobacco, are of childbearing age, and take estrogen-based oral contraceptives are postmenopausal on oral hormone therapy, are over 35 years old, and have a family history of VTE, are at a very high risk for VTE.

Localized platelet aggregation and fibrin entrap red blood cells (RBCs), white blood cells (WBCs), and more platelets to form a thrombus. A frequent site of thrombus formation is the valve cusp of a vein.

- As the thrombus enlarges, blood cells and fibrin collect behind it, making a larger clot with a "tail" that eventually occludes the vein lumen.
- If a thrombus only partially blocks the vein, endothelial cells cover the thrombus and stop the thrombotic process.
- If the thrombus does not detach, it undergoes lysis or becomes firmly organized and adherent within 5–7 days.
- The organized thrombus may detach and result in an embolus that flows through the venous circulation to the heart and lodges in the pulmonary circulation, resulting in PE.

Superficial Vein Thrombosis
Clinical Manifestations and Diagnosis
The patient may have a palpable, firm, subcutaneous cord-like vein. The surrounding area may be itchy, tender to the touch, reddened, and warm. A mild temperature elevation and leukocytosis may be present. Edema of the extremity may occur.

Duplex ultrasound is used to confirm the diagnosis (5 cm or larger clot) and to rule out clot extension to a deep vein.

Interprofessional and Nursing Management
For patients with a lower leg superficial vein thrombosis, subcutaneous fondaparinux (Arixtra) reduces symptomatic VTE and superficial vein thrombosis extension and recurrence without causing major bleeding problems.

If the superficial vein thrombosis affects a very short vein segment (<5 cm) and is not near the saphenofemoral junction, anticoagulants may not be needed, and oral nonsteroidal antiinflammatory drugs (NSAIDs) can ease symptoms.

- Other interventions to relieve SVT symptoms include telling the patient to wear graduated compression stockings or bandages, elevate the affected limb above level of heart, apply topical NSAIDs, apply warm compresses, and perform mild exercise such as walking.

Venous Thromboembolism
Clinical Manifestations and Diagnosis
The patient with lower extremity VTE may have unilateral leg edema, pain, tenderness with palpation, dilated superficial veins, a sense of fullness in the thigh or the calf, paresthesias, warm skin, redness, or a systemic temperature >100.4°F (38°C).

- If the inferior vena cava is involved, both legs may be edematous and cyanotic.
- About 10% of VTEs involve the upper extremity veins. They may extend into the internal jugular vein or superior vena cava.

If the superior vena cava is involved, similar symptoms may occur in the arms, neck, back, and face.

Diagnosis of an initial VTE is based on clinical assessment combined with D-dimer testing and ultrasound.

Complications

The most serious complications of VTE are PE, chronic thromboembolic pulmonary hypertension, and postthrombotic syndrome (PTS).

- *PTS* can result from chronic venous hypertension caused by valvular destruction (from inflammation and scarring), stiff noncompliant vein walls, and persistent venous obstruction. Symptoms include pain, aching, fatigue, heaviness, sensation of swelling, cramps, pruritus, tingling, paresthesia, bursting pain with exercise, and venous claudication. Manifestations include persistent edema, spider veins (telangiectasia), venous dilation (ectasia), redness, cyanosis, increased pigmentation, eczema, pain during compression, atrophie blanche (white scar tissue), and lipodermatosclerosis

Diagnostic Studies

- Platelet count, hemoglobin (Hgb), hematocrit (Hct), D-dimer testing, and coagulation tests (bleeding time, prothrombin time [PT], and partial thromboplastin time [PTT]) may be altered if underlying blood dyscrasias are present.
- Venous compression ultrasound evaluates deep femoral, popliteal, and posterior tibial veins.
- Duplex ultrasound and color-flow Doppler determine the location and extent of venous thrombi.

Interprofessional Management

In patients at risk for VTE, a variety of interventions are used. Early and aggressive mobilization is the easiest and most cost-effective method to decrease VTE risk.

- Patients on bed rest should change position every 2 hours. Unless contraindicated, teach patients to flex and extend their feet, knees, and hips at least every 2–4 hours while awake.
- Patients who can get out of bed should be in a chair for meals and ambulate at least 4–6 times per day as able. Tell the patient and the caregiver about the importance of these measures.
- Graduated compression stockings (e.g., thromboembolic deterrent [TED] hose) are a part of VTE prevention in hospitalized patients. VTE prevention is enhanced if the stockings are used along with anticoagulation.
- *Intermittent pneumatic compression devices* (IPCs) use inflatable sleeves or boots to compress the calf and thigh and/or foot and ankle to improve venous return. IPCs may be used with

elastic compression stockings. IPCs are not worn when a patient has an active VTE because of the risk of PE.

Anticoagulants are used routinely for VTE prevention and treatment. The goal of anticoagulant therapy for VTE prophylaxis is to prevent clot formation. The goals for treatment of a confirmed VTE are to prevent further clot development and embolization.

- Three major classes of anticoagulants are available: (1) vitamin K antagonists (VKAs), (2) thrombin inhibitors (both indirect and direct), and (3) factor Xa inhibitors. Anticoagulant therapy does not dissolve the clot. Clot lysis begins naturally through the body's intrinsic fibrinolytic system.

- Patients with confirmed VTE should receive initial treatment with either low-molecular-weight heparin (LMWH), unfractionated heparin (UH), or an oral factor Xa drug. Oral VKA therapy may be an option. A therapeutic INR is maintained between 2.0 and 3.0 if VKA therapy is used. Active treatment of VTE should continue for at least 3 months.

- For VTE prevention in the hospitalized medical patient at risk for thrombosis who is not bleeding, low-dose UH, LMWH, or fondaparinux is used. If the patient is at low VTE risk, drug prophylaxis is not needed. Patients with moderate VTE risk (e.g., general, gynecologic, urologic surgery) should receive either UH or LMWH. Patients with high VTE risk (e.g., trauma) should receive UH or LMWH until discharge. Patients having abdominal or pelvic surgery for cancer or major orthopedic surgery (e.g., total knee or hip replacement) should receive VTE prophylaxis.

Another treatment option for patients with a thrombus is catheter-directed administration of a thrombolytic drug (e.g., urokinase, tissue plasminogen activator [tPA]). It dissolves the clot(s), reduces the acute symptoms, improves deep venous flow, reduces valvular reflux, and may help decrease the incidence of PTS. Catheter-directed thrombolysis is an option for select patients who are at a low bleeding risk and present with an acute, extensive, symptomatic, proximal VTE. Systemic anticoagulation is needed before, during, and after catheter-directed thrombolysis.

- Vena cava interruption devices (e.g., Greenfield, Vena Tech, TrapEase filters) can be inserted percutaneously through the right femoral or right internal jugular vein. The filters act as a sieve, permitting filtration of clots without interruption of blood flow.

The interventional radiology procedures for an occluded vein are similar to those used in the treatment of lower extremity peripheral arterial disease (PAD). Such procedures include mechanical thrombectomy, placement of a pharmacomechanical device, and postthrombus extraction, angioplasty, and/or stenting.

Some patients with extensive, acute, proximal VTE who are not candidates for catheter-directed thrombolysis and/or interventional radiology therapies (because of high bleeding risk) may undergo surgery.

Nursing Management

Goals. The patient with VTE will have pain relief, decreased edema, no skin ulceration, no bleeding complications, and no evidence of PE.

Interventions

Focus your nursing care for the patient with VTE on the prevention of thrombi and reduction of inflammation. Review with the patient any drugs, vitamins, minerals, and dietary and herbal supplements that may interfere with anticoagulant therapy.

- Check the results of pertinent tests before initiating, administering, or adjusting anticoagulant therapy. Depending on the anticoagulant ordered, monitor INR, aPTT, ACT, antifactor Xa levels, complete blood count (CBC), creatinine, factor X levels, hemoglobin, hematocrit, platelet levels, and/or liver enzymes. Monitor platelet counts for patients getting UH or LMWH to assess for HIT.
- In case of anticoagulation above target goals, plan to give reversal agents (e.g., protamine, vitamin K) or make dosage adjustments as prescribed
- Monitor for and reduce the risk of bleeding with anticoagulant therapy.
- Early ambulation after VTE results in a more rapid decrease in edema and limb pain. Teach the patient and the caregiver the importance of exercise, and assist the patient in ambulating several times a day.

▼ Patient and Caregiver Teaching

- Focus discharge teaching on modification of VTE risk factors, use of elastic compression stockings, importance of monitoring laboratory values, dietary and medication instructions, and guidelines for follow-up care.
- Once the edema is resolved, measure the patient for custom-fitted elastic compression stockings. Use of such stockings (or sleeves in the case of upper extremity VTE) is recommended for at least 2 years after VTE. For those at high risk for VTE who are planning a long trip, recommend properly fitted, knee-high graduated compression stockings during travel to decrease edema and VTE risk
- Advise the patient to avoid all nicotine products.

- Teach the patient to avoid constrictive clothing.
- When traveling long distances, tell patients to frequently exercise the calf muscles, take short walks, and drink beverages without alcohol or caffeine.
- Tell women with a history of VTE to stop oral contraceptives or hormone therapy.
- Teach the patient and caregiver about signs and symptoms of PE, such as sudden onset of dyspnea, tachypnea, and pleuritic chest pain.
- Instruct the patient and caregiver about drug dosage, actions, and side effects; the need for routine blood tests; and what symptoms need immediate medical attention.
- Teach patients taking low-molecular-weight heparin (LMWH) or fondaparinux and their caregivers how to give the drug subcutaneously.
- Teach patients taking warfarin (Coumadin) to follow a consistent diet of foods containing vitamin K (e.g., dark green leafy vegetables) and to avoid any supplements containing vitamin K. Encourage proper hydration to prevent additional hypercoagulability of the blood, which may occur with dehydration.
- Active patients need to avoid contact sports and high-risk (for trauma) activities (e.g., skiing). Teach older patients about safety precautions to prevent falls (e.g., avoid use of throw rugs).
- Help the patient develop an exercise program with an emphasis on leg strength training and aerobic activity.

WARTS, GENITAL

Description

Genital warts (condylomata acuminata) are caused by the human papillomavirus (HPV). There are around 100 types of HPV. More than 40 types can be sexually transmitted. Most sexually active men and women will be infected with some type of HPV at some point in their lives.

Pathophysiology

"Low-risk" strains of the virus can cause warts on the skin. "High-risk" strains can lead to cancers of the genital tract, anus, or oropharynx in some patients. HPV types 6 and 11 cause about 90% of genital and anal wart cases. HPV is transmitted by skin-to-skin contact, most often during vaginal, anal, or oral sex, but it can be transmitted during nonpenetrative sexual activity. The basal

epithelial cells infected with HPV undergo transformation and proliferation to form a warty growth. The incubation period can range
from weeks to years. Infection with one type of HPV does not prevent infection with another type.

Clinical Manifestations

Most people who have HPV do not know they are infected, because
they have no symptoms. Genital or anal warts are discrete single or
multiple papillary growths. They may grow and coalesce to form
large, cauliflower-like masses, though most patients will have few
lesions. Growths may be pink, pink-flesh colored, or hyperpig-
mented depending on the skin type.

- In men, the warts may occur on the penis, scrotum, in or around
  the anus, or in the urethra.
- In women, the warts may be located on the inner thighs, vulva,
  vagina, cervix, perineum, or internal or external anus.

Diagnostic Studies

- A diagnosis can be made based on the appearance of the lesions.
- Biopsy provides a definitive diagnosis.

Interprofessional and Nursing Management

Genital warts are difficult to treat. The primary goal is the removal
of symptomatic warts.

- In-office treatment consists of chemical or ablative (removal
  with laser or electrocautery) methods. A common treatment is
  trichloroacetic acid (TCA) or bichloroacetic acid (BCA) applied
  directly to the wart surface.
- Options include patient-applied treatments, such as Podofilox
  (Condylox) liquid or gel or Imiquimod cream (Aldara, Zyclara).

Treatment of warts may or may not decrease infectivity as the
HPV causing these may still be present. Anogenital warts are hard
to treat and often need more than one treatment or modality. Therapy should be modified if a patient has not improved or cannot
tolerate the side effects of certain treatments.

- If the warts do not resolve with topical therapies, cryotherapy
  with liquid nitrogen, electrocautery, laser therapy, local α-
  interferon injections, or surgical excision may be needed. Teach
  patients that treatment does not destroy the virus (merely the
  infected tissue), so recurrence and reinfection are possible.
  Long-term follow-up is needed.

HPV vaccines offer protection against strains causing 90% of
genital warts and cervical cancers. They may offer protection from
anal and certain types of throat cancer. Ideally, a person should

receive a vaccine before the start of sexual activity, but even those who are infected with HPV can still get protection against HPV types not already acquired.

See Nursing Management: Sexually Transmitted Infections.

PART TWO

Treatments and Procedures

AMPUTATION

Description

An *amputation* is the removal of a body extremity by trauma or surgery. About 2 million people in the United States live with limb loss. Just over half are due to peripheral vascular disease (PVD) and diabetes. These patients often have peripheral neuropathy that progresses to deep ulcers and gangrene. Trauma is the other major cause. Injuries have affected over 1700 military veterans since 2003. Other reasons for amputation include thermal injuries, tumors, osteomyelitis, and congenital limb disorders.

Interprofessional Management

The goal of surgery is to preserve extremity length and function while removing all infected, pathologic, or ischemic tissue.

The type of amputation depends on the reason for the surgery. A closed amputation creates a weight-bearing residual limb (or stump). An anterior skin flap with dissected soft tissue padding covers the bony part of the residual limb. The skin flap is sutured posteriorly so that the suture line will not be in a weight-bearing area. Disarticulation is an amputation done through a joint. A Syme's amputation is a form of disarticulation at the ankle.

After an open amputation (guillotine amputation), the surface of the residual limb is left uncovered with skin. This type of surgery is generally done to control actual or potential infection. The wound is usually closed later by a second surgery or closed by skin traction surrounding the residual limb.

Nursing Management

Control of illnesses, such as PVD, diabetes, chronic osteomyelitis, and pressure injuries, can prevent or delay the need for amputation.

- Teach patients with these conditions to carefully examine the lower extremities daily for signs of skin infection or breakdown. Teach the patient to report problems to the HCP. These include decreased or absent sensation, tingling, burning pain, cuts, abrasions, and changes in skin color or temperature.

Review safety precautions for people taking part in recreational activities and potentially hazardous work.

Be aware of the tremendous psychologic and social implications of an amputation. The disruption in body image often results in the patient going through the grieving process.

- Use therapeutic communication to assist the patient and caregiver to develop a realistic attitude about the future.

Preoperative Care

Before surgery, reinforce information that the patient and caregiver have received about the reasons for the amputation, proposed prosthesis, and mobility-training program.

- Teach the patient upper extremity exercises, such as push-ups in bed or the wheelchair, to promote arm strength for crutch walking and gait training.
- If a compression bandage will be used after surgery, instruct the patient about its purpose and application. If an immediate prosthesis is planned, discuss general ambulation expectations.

Tell the patient that it may feel as if the amputated limb is still present after surgery. This phenomenon, termed *phantom limb sensation,* occurs for many amputees.

Postoperative Care

Monitor the patient's vital signs and the operative site dressing for hemorrhage. Careful attention to sterile technique during dressing changes reduces the potential for wound infection.

- Proper bandaging ensures the residual limb is shaped and molded for eventual prosthesis fitting. The HCP usually orders a compression bandage to be applied right after surgery to support soft tissues, reduce edema, hasten healing, and minimize pain. Compression also promotes residual limb shrinkage and maturation. This bandage may be an elastic roll applied to the residual limb or a residual limb shrinker, which is an elastic stocking that fits tightly over the residual limb.
- If an immediate postoperative prosthesis has been applied, careful surveillance of the surgical site is needed. Notify the surgeon at once if excess bleeding occurs. Keep a surgical tourniquet available for emergency use.
- Not all patients are candidates for prostheses. The seriously ill or debilitated patient may not have the upper body strength or energy required to use a prosthesis. Mobility with a wheelchair may be the most realistic goal in this situation.

Flexion contractures delay the rehabilitation process. The most common and debilitating contracture is hip flexion. Patients should avoid sitting in a chair for more than 1 hour with hips flexed or with pillows under the surgical extremity. Unless contraindicated, patients should lie on the abdomen for 30 minutes 3–4 times each day and position the hip in extension while prone.

- As recovery and ambulation progress, phantom limb sensation and pain usually subside, although the pain can become chronic. The patient may report shooting, burning, or crushing pain and feelings of coldness, heaviness, and cramping.

A

▼ Patient and Caregiver Teaching
Crutch walking starts as soon as the patient is physically able. Follow orders for weight bearing carefully to avoid injury to the skin flap and delay of tissue healing. Before discharge, teach the patient and caregiver about residual limb care, ambulation, contracture prevention, recognition of complications, exercise, and follow-up care. Table 94 outlines patient and caregiver teaching after an amputation.

TABLE 94   Patient and Caregiver Teaching After an Amputation

After an amputation, include the following instructions when teaching the patient and the caregiver.

- Inspect the residual limb daily for signs of skin irritation, especially redness, excoriation, and odor. Especially evaluate areas prone to pressure.
- Stop using the prosthesis if irritation develops. Have the area checked before resuming use of the prosthesis.
- Wash the residual limb thoroughly each night with warm water and a bacteriostatic soap. Rinse thoroughly and dry gently. Expose the residual limb to air for 20 minutes.
- Do not use lotions, alcohol, powders, or oil on residual limb unless prescribed by the HCP.
- Wear only a residual limb sock in good condition and supplied by the prosthetist.
- Change residual limb sock daily. Launder in a mild soap, squeeze, and lay flat to dry.
- Use prescribed pain management techniques.
- Perform range of motion (ROM) to all joints daily. Perform general strengthening exercises, including the upper extremities, daily.
- Do not elevate the residual limb on a pillow.
- Lie prone with hip in extension for 30 minutes three or four times daily.

ARTIFICIAL AIRWAYS: ENDOTRACHEAL TUBES

Description

The endotracheal (ET) tube is a long, flexible, plastic tube that secures a patient's airway when they need mechanical ventilation. An ET tube consists of a standard adaptor (used to attach the bag-valve-mask [BVM] or ventilator), cuff, pilot balloon, and radiopaque markings along the length of the tube. The markings help

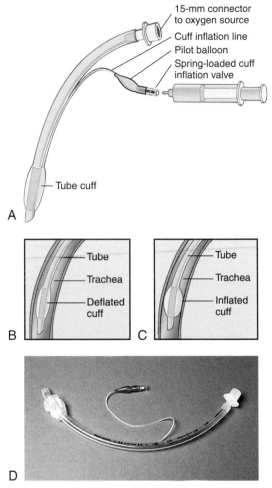

Fig. 32 Endotracheal tube. (A) Parts of an endotracheal tube. (B) Tube in place with cuff deflated. (C) Tube in place with the cuff inflated. (D) Photo of tube before placement.

gauge the distance the tube is inserted. Fig. 32 shows the parts of an ET tube.

- Indications for intubation include acute respiratory distress, apnea, upper airway obstruction (e.g., burns, tumor, bleeding), ineffective clearance of secretions, and high risk for aspiration. ET intubation is done quickly and safely at the bedside by an HCP or respiratory therapist. ET intubation is common in ICU patients requiring mechanical ventilation for short periods of time (e.g., less than 2 weeks).

- In oral intubation, the ET tube is passed into the mouth, through the vocal cords, and into the trachea with the aid of a laryngoscope or a bronchoscope. Oral ET intubation is preferred for intubations because the airway can be secured rapidly.

When oral intubation through the mouth is not possible (e.g., unstable cervical spine injury, dental abscess, epiglottitis), a nasotracheal (NT) tube can help provide an airway. The NT tube is slightly longer than the oral ET tube. It is inserted through the nostril and placed blindly (without seeing the larynx). We attach the patient to the ventilator via the standard adaptor at the end of the NT tube. Nasal intubation is contraindicated in patients with facial fractures or suspected fractures at the base of the skull and postoperatively after cranial surgery.

The most common sizes of ET tubes are 7F and 8F, which refer to the internal diameter of the tube. Often, adult females need a 7F tube and males need an 8F tube. A larger tube reduces the WOB because of less airway resistance. It is also easier to suction and remove secretions, and, if needed, perform bronchoscopy.

Interprofessional and Nursing Management

Managing an artificial airway is often a shared responsibility between you and the respiratory therapist (RT). Agency policy dictates which providers perform which task. Nursing responsibilities include maintaining correct tube placement, maintaining proper cuff inflation, maintaining tube patency, and maintaining alarm systems.

Tell the patient and caregiver the reason for ET intubation and the steps in the procedure. Explain that while intubated, the patient will not be able to speak, but will have other means of communication.

- Have a self-inflating bag-valve-mask (BVM) device (e.g., Ambu bag) available and attached to O_2; have suctioning equipment ready at the bedside; and establish IV access.
- Continuously monitor the patient with an ET tube for placement. Note the exit point from the mouth or nare. Assess the integrity of the tape or securement device. Observe for symmetric chest wall movement. Auscultate to confirm bilateral breath sounds.
- It is an emergency if the ET tube is not positioned properly. If the tube moves or is dislodged, it could easily migrate upward in the

pharynx or enter the right or left mainstem bronchus (thus venti-lating only one lung). This is an airway emergency. Stay with the patient and try to maintain the airway. Support ventilation with a BVM and 100% O_2. Call for the appropriate help to assess or reposition the tube. If a dislodged tube is not repositioned, mini-mal or no O_2 is delivered to the lungs or the entire VT is being delivered to one lung. This places the patient at risk for hypox-emia, pneumothorax, and respiratory and/or cardiac arrest.

The cuff is an inflatable, pliable sleeve encircling the lower, outer wall of the ET tube. The cuff stabilizes and seals the ET tube within the trachea and prevents the escape of ventilating gases.

Excess volume in the ET tube cuff can cause tracheal damage. To avoid this, inflate the cuff with air, then measure and maintain the cuff pressure at 20–25 cm H_2O. Adjust cuff pressure after intuba-tion and on a routine basis (e.g., every 8 hours) using the *minimal occluding volume* (MOV) *technique*.

- To perform the MOV technique in the mechanically ventilated patient, place a stethoscope over the trachea and inflate the cuff to MOV by adding air until you hear no air at peak inspiratory pressure (end of ventilator inspiration). For the spontaneously breathing intubated patient, you inflate until you hear no sound after a deep breath or after inhalation with a BVM. Second, use a manometer to confirm that cuff pressure is between 20 and 30 cm H_2O. Record cuff pressure in the chart.

If adequate cuff pressure cannot be maintained or larger volumes of air are needed to keep the cuff inflated, there could be a leak in the cuff or tracheal dilation at the cuff site. In these situations, notify the HCP.

Closely monitor the patient with an ET tube for adequate oxy-genation and ventilation by assessing clinical findings, arterial blood gases (ABGs), arterial oxygen saturation by pulse oximetry (SpO_2), and other indicators of oxygenation status.

- Do not routinely suction a patient. Regularly assess the patient to determine the need for suctioning. Indications for suction-ing include visible secretions in the ET tube, sudden onset of respiratory distress, suspected aspiration of secretions, increase in respiratory rate or frequent coughing, and sudden decrease in SpO_2. Other signs that may indicate the patient needs suctioning include increased peak airway pressure and adventitious breath sounds over the trachea or bronchi. See Table 95 for closed and open suctioning techniques.

- With an oral ET tube in place, the patient's mouth is always open. Moisten the lips, tongue, and gums with saline or water swabs to prevent mucosal drying. Proper oral care provides

TABLE 95 Suctioning Procedures for Patient on Mechanical Ventilator

General Measures for Closed- and Open-Suction Techniques

1. Gather all equipment.
2. Wash hands and don personal protective equipment and gloves.
3. Explain procedure and patient's role in assisting with secretion removal by coughing.
4. Monitor neurologic and cardiopulmonary status (e.g., LOC, vital signs, ECG, SpO2) before, during, and after suctioning.
5. Check suction source and regulator. Adjust suction pressure to no greater than 125 mmHg pressure with tubing occluded.
6. Press [Silence] on the ventilator (to pause the alarms while suctioning).

Closed-Suction Technique

1. Connect the suction tubing to the end of the in-line suction catheter.
2. Hyperoxygenate the patient by pressing the [100% FIO_2] button on the ventilator. This is the safest way to hyperoxygenate the patient.
   - Another option is to manually increase the FIO_2 to 100%. NOTE: Remember to return FIO_2 to baseline level when done suctioning, if not done automatically after preset time by ventilator.
   - Least preferred method is to disconnect the ventilator tubing and provide manual ventilation with 100% O_2 using a BVM device. Attach a PEEP valve to the BVM for patients on >5 cm H_2O PEEP. Have a second person give 5 or 6 breaths over 30 seconds.
3. Gently but quickly insert the in-line suction catheter into the oral ET tube/tracheostomy, pausing momentarily to pull back on the plastic sleeve containing the catheter. When the patient begins to cough more forcefully, STOP catheter insertion. Note: Do NOT insert the catheter until you meet resistance. This means that the end of the suction catheter is hitting the carina (fragile, vascular tissue that separates right and left mainstem bronchus).

Continued

TABLE 95   Suctioning Procedures for Patient on Mechanical Ventilator—cont'd

4. Apply continuous suction on withdrawal of the catheter over approximately 10 seconds.
5. Observe patient tolerance to procedure.
6. Disconnect the suction tubing from the end of the in-line suction catheter and attach the Yankauer. Gently suction the patient's oral cavity.
7. Ask the patient if they need another suction pass.
8. If the patient does need more suctioning, ensure the ventilator is still providing FIO_2 100%. If not, press the [100% FIO_2] button again.
9. Repeat steps 3 through 7.
10. When the patient does not need more suctioning, ensure the suction tubing is attached to the end of the in-line suction catheter.
11. Rinse the catheter and connecting tubing with the sterile saline solution. Always rinse the tubing away from the patient.
12. Ensure the FIO_2 has returned to its previous setting, or manually return the FIO_2 to the desired value.
13. Reassess the patient for hemodynamic stability and that suctioning was effective. Auscultate to assess changes in lung sounds.
14. Record time, amount, character of secretions and patient's response to suctioning.

Open-Suction Technique

1. Use sterile technique to open catheter package, using the inside of the package as a sterile field.
2. Fill the sterile solution container with sterile normal saline or water.
3. Don sterile gloves. Designate one hand as contaminated for connecting and disconnecting the tubing at the suction catheter and operating the suction control.
4. Pick up the sterile suction catheter with dominant hand. Check function of equipment by suctioning a small volume of sterile saline solution from the container.
5. Have the second person hyperoxygenate the patient with 100% $FIO2$. Disconnect the ventilator tubing from the ET tube/tracheostomy and provide manual ventilation to the patient with 100% O_2 using a BVM device. Attach a PEEP valve to the BVM for patients on >5 cm $H2O$ PEEP. Have the second person give 5 or 6 breaths over 30 seconds.

TABLE 95   Suctioning Procedures for Patient on Mechanical Ventilator—cont'd

A

6. Once hyperoxygenated, have the second person remove the BVM from the end of the oral ET tube or tracheostomy, and gently but quickly insert the in-line suction catheter without suction into the airway. When the patient begins to cough more forcefully, STOP catheter insertion. Do not insert the catheter until you meet resistance. This means that the end of the suction catheter is hitting the carina (fragile, vascular tissue that separates right and left mainstem bronchus).

7. Apply continuous suction on withdrawal of the catheter over approximately 10 seconds.

8. Once the catheter is removed, immediately have the second person reattach the BVM to the oral ET tube/tracheostomy, and hyperoxygenate the patient.

9. Observe patient tolerance of procedure. Immediately stop suctioning the patient and remove the in-line suction catheter from the patient if they become bradycardic or hypotensive. A vagal response may have occurred.

10. Ask the patient if they need another suction pass. Wait at least 30 seconds (ventilator) or 5 to 6 breaths (BVM) in between each suctioning pass.

11. Rinse the sterile suction catheter (with sterile saline solution) between suctioning passes.

12. If the patient needs more suctioning, have the second person remove the BVM from the oral ET tube or tracheostomy, and repeat steps 8 through 12.

13. When the patient does not need more suctioning, the second person will reattach the patient to the ventilator. Discard all used suctioning supplies. Dispose of the catheter by wrapping it around the fingers of gloved hand and pulling glove over catheter.

14. Reassess the patient for hemodynamic stability and that suctioning was effective. Auscultate to assess changes in lung sounds.

15. Record time, amount, character of secretions and patient's response to suctioning.

BVM, Bag-valve-mask; *ECG,* electrocardiogram; *ET,* endotracheal; *FIO₂,* fraction of inspired oxygen; *PEEP,* positive end-expiratory pressure; *SpO₂,* arterial oxygen saturation by pulse oximetry; *SvO₂,* mixed venous oxygen saturation; *ScvO₂,* central venous oxygen saturation; *V_T,* tidal volume.

comfort and prevents injury to the gums and dental plaque formation.

Meticulous care is needed to prevent skin breakdown on the face, lips, tongue, and/or nares because of pressure from the ET tube or from the method used to secure the ET tube to the patient's face. Reposition and resecure or retape the ET tube every 24 hours and as needed.

For the nasally intubated patient, remove the old tape and clean the skin around the ET tube with saline-soaked gauze. For the orally intubated patient, remove the bite block (if present) and the old tape. Provide oral hygiene and then reposition the ET tube to the opposite side of the mouth. Replace the bite block (if appropriate) and reconfirm proper cuff inflation and tube placement. Secure the ET tube again per agency policy.

- Two staff members should always perform the repositioning procedure to prevent accidental ET tube dislodgment. Monitor the patient for respiratory distress throughout the procedure.

BASIC LIFE SUPPORT FOR HEALTHCARE PROVIDERS

Description

Basic life support (BLS) consists of a series of actions and skills performed by the rescuer(s) based on assessment findings. Cardiac arrest is characterized by the absence of a pulse and breathing in an unconscious victim. The current approach for cardiopulmonary resuscitation (CPR) is the chest compressions-airway-breathing (CAB) sequence (See Table 96).

Cardiopulmonary Resuscitation

- The first action the rescuer performs upon finding an adult victim is assessing for responsiveness. This is done by tapping or shaking the victim's shoulder and asking, "Are you all right?" If the victim does not respond, simultaneously scan the victim's chest for signs of absent or abnormal breathing and perform a pulse check by palpating the carotid pulse for at least 5 but no more than 10 seconds. Remember that gasping and/or irregular or agonal respirations are not considered breathing
- To palpate the carotid pulse, maintain a head-tilt position with one hand on the victim's forehead and locate the victim's

trachea using 2 or 3 fingers of your other hand. Slide these fingers into the groove between the trachea and neck muscles where the carotid pulse can be felt. The technique is more easily performed on the side nearest you.

- If a pulse is felt, give one rescue breath every 6 seconds (10–12 breaths/min) and recheck the pulse every 2 minutes. If no pulse is felt, start CAB.

B

TABLE 96 Adult 1- and 2-Rescuer Basic Life Support With Automatic External Defibrillator (AED)

Assess
- Determine unresponsiveness: tap or shake victim's shoulder; shout, "Are you all right?"
- Check for no breathing or abnormal breathing (e.g., gasping) while simultaneously performing a pulse check (5–10 s).

Activate Emergency Response System (ERS)
- Activate ERS (e.g., call 911) and get the AED (if available) (outside of hospital).
- Call a code and ask for the AED or crash cart (in hospital).

Begin High-Quality CPR
- (See Figs. A.1 and A.2 in Appendix A of Harding et al., Lewis' Medical-Surgical Nursing, ed 12).
- If victim has a pulse but is not breathing or not breathing adequately, begin rescue breathing at a rate of 1 breath every 3–5 s, or about 12–20 per minute. Recheck the pulse every 2 minutes.
- If there is no pulse, expose the victim's chest and immediately begin chest compressions
- Deliver compressions at a rate of 100–120 per minute.
- Compress the chest at least 2 inches but not >2.4 inches.
- Allow for complete chest recoil after each compression.
- Deliver a compression-ventilation ratio of 30 compressions to 2 breaths.[a]
- Minimize interruptions in compressions by delivering the 2 breaths in <10 s.

Deliver Effective Breaths
- Open airway adequately.
- Deliver breath to produce a visible chest rise.
- Avoid excessive ventilation.

Continued

TABLE 96   **Adult 1- and 2-Rescuer Basic Life Support With Automatic External Defibrillator (AED)—cont'd**

Integrate Prompt Use of the AED
- Use AED as soon as possible.
- If rhythm is shockable, deliver 1 shock and then resume chest compressions immediately after delivery of shock.
- If the rhythm is not shockable, resume CPR and recheck rhythm every 5 cycles.

Continue CPR
- Continue CPR between rhythm checks and shocks, and until ACLS providers arrive or the victim shows signs of movement.

CPR, Cardiopulmonary resuscitation.
aFor patients with ongoing CPR and an advanced airway in place, a ventilation rate of one breath every 6 seconds (10 breaths per minute) is recommended.
American Heart Association: *Basic Life Support Provider Manual*, Dallas, 2020, The Association.

- If the rescuer is alone, the rescuer shouts for help. If someone responds, the rescuer asks them to activate the emergency response system (ERS) (if outside of the hospital) or call a code (in the hospital) and get an automatic external defibrillator (AED) (if available) or crash cart (in the hospital). If no one responds and the rescuer does not have a mobile phone, the rescuer should leave to activate the ERS, get an AED (if available), and return to the victim before beginning CAB and defibrillation if necessary.

Chest Compressions
- Chest compression technique consists of fast and deep applications of pressure on the lower half of the sternum. The victim must be in the supine position when compressions are performed. The victim must be lying on a flat, hard surface, such as a CPR board (specially designed for use in CPR), a headboard from a unit bed, or, if necessary, the floor. Position yourself close to the side of the victim's chest. More frequently, mechanical chest compression devices are being used to provide chest compressions both prehospital and in the emergency department.
- Chest compressions are combined with rescue breathing for an effective resuscitation effort of the adult victim of cardiac arrest. The compression-to-ventilation ratio for 1- or two-rescuer CPR

is 30 compressions to two breaths. However, if the patient has an advanced airway (e.g., endotracheal tube, laryngeal mask airway), do not pause between compressions for breaths and deliver one breath every 6 seconds (10 breaths/min).

- If a mechanical chest compression device is not used, it is preferable to have two persons performing CPR. One rescuer, positioned at the victim's side, performs chest compressions while the second rescuer, positioned at the victim's head, maintains an open airway and performs ventilations. To maintain the quality and rate of compressions, rescuers should change roles every 2 minutes. Interruptions in CPR should be limited.

Defibrillation

- When the AED or advanced cardiovascular life support (ACLS) team arrives, assess the victim's rhythm. If the victim has a shockable rhythm (e.g., ventricular tachycardia, ventricular fibrillation), deliver one shock and immediately resume CPR for about 2 minutes before checking the rhythm again. If the rhythm is not a shockable rhythm, immediately resume CPR and recheck the rhythm after 2 minutes. CPR should continue between rhythm checks and shocks and until the ACLS team arrives or the victim shows signs of movement (Table 96).

- The American Heart Association includes training in the use of AEDs with BLS instruction of HCPs and laypersons. Survival from cardiac arrest is the highest when immediate CPR is provided and defibrillation occurs within 3–5 minutes. AEDs are found in many out-of-hospital, public settings.

Airway and Breathing

- If a victim has a pulse but is gasping (e.g., agonal breathing) or not breathing, establish an open airway and begin rescue breathing. Open an adult's airway by hyperextending the head. Use the head tilt–chin lift maneuver. This involves tilting the head back with one hand and lifting the chin forward with the fingers of the other hand. Use the jaw-thrust maneuver if you suspect a cervical spine injury. Try to provide ventilation to the victim using a mouth-to-barrier (recommended) device (e.g., face mask or bag-valve-mask) or mouth-to-mouth resuscitation

- For mouth-to-mouth resuscitation, give ventilations with the victim's nostrils pinched. Take a regular (not deep) breath and tightly seal your lips around the victim's mouth. Give one breath and watch for a rise in the victim's chest. Continue rescue breaths at a rate of 10–12 per minute. When the victim has a tracheostomy, give ventilations through the stoma.

- If the victim cannot be ventilated, proceed with CPR. When providing the next rescue breaths, look for any objects in the victim's mouth. If any objects are visible, remove them.
- When providing the next rescue breaths, look for and remove any visible objects from the victim's mouth
- For management of the adult who is choking, see Table 97 and Fig. 33.

TABLE 97   Management of the Adult Choking Victim

Conscious Adult Choking Victim

Assess Victim for Severe Airway Obstruction

Look for any of the following signs:

- Poor or no air exchange
- Clutching the neck with the hands, making the universal choking sign
- Weak, ineffective cough or no cough at all
- High-pitched noise while inhaling or no noise at all
- Increased respiratory difficulty
- Possible cyanosis

Ask the victim if he or she is choking. If the victim nods yes and cannot talk or has any of the symptoms noted earlier, severe airway obstruction is present and you must take immediate action.

Abdominal Thrusts (Heimlich Maneuver) With Standing or Sitting Victim (See Fig. 33)

1. Stand or kneel behind victim and wrap arms around the victim's waist.
2. Make fist with one hand.
3. Place thumb side of fist against victim's abdomen. Position fist midline, slightly above navel and well below breastbone.
4. Grasp fist with other hand and press fist into victim's abdomen with a quick, forceful upward thrust.
5. Give each new thrust with a separate, distinct movement to relieve the obstruction. CAUTION: If victim is pregnant or obese, give chest thrusts instead of abdominal thrusts. Position hands (as described) over lower portion of the breastbone and apply quick backward thrusts.
6. Repeat thrusts until object is expelled or victim becomes unresponsive.

Unconscious Adult Choking Victim

If you see a choking victim collapse and become unresponsive:

TABLE 97   Management of the Adult Choking Victim—cont'd
1. Activate the emergency response system (ERS).
2. Lower the victim to the ground and begin CPR, starting with compressions (do not check for a pulse).
3. Open the victim's mouth wide each time you prepare to give breaths. Look for the object. If you see the object and can easily remove it, do so with your fingers. If you do not see the object, continue with CPR using the chest compression–airway–breathing sequence.
4. If efforts to ventilate are unsuccessful, continue with CPR.

CPR, Cardiopulmonary resuscitation.
American Heart Association: *Basic Life Support Provider Manual,* Dallas, 2020, The Association.

Fig. 33 Abdominal thrusts *(Heimlich maneuver)* administered to a conscious (standing) choking victim.

Hands-Only Cardiopulmonary Resuscitation

Hands-only CPR can be used to help adult victims who suddenly collapse from cardiac arrest outside of a healthcare setting. If you witness this event (as a bystander), you can choose to provide conventional CPR (described previously) or chest compressions only (push fast and deep in the center of the chest). Both methods are effective in the first few minutes of an out-of-hospital cardiac arrest.

CHEMOTHERAPY

Description

Chemotherapy (antineoplastic therapy) is the use of chemicals as a systemic therapy for cancer. It is a mainstay of treatment for most solid tumors and hematologic cancers (e.g., leukemias, lymphomas). The goal of chemotherapy is to eliminate or reduce the number of cancer cells present in the primary and metastatic tumor site(s).

- The two major categories of chemotherapeutic drugs are *cell cycle phase–nonspecific* and *cell cycle phase–specific*. Giving them together maximizes effectiveness by using drugs that function in different ways and throughout the cell cycle.

Classification of Chemotherapeutic Drugs

Chemotherapy drugs are generally classified according to their molecular structure and mechanisms of action (Table 98).

Methods of Administration

The IV route is the most common route for giving chemotherapy. Major concerns associated with IV chemotherapy include venous access problems, device- or catheter-related infection, and *extravasation* (infiltration of drugs into tissues around the infusion site). Many chemotherapy drugs are either irritants or vesicants.

- Irritants damage the intima of the vein, causing phlebitis and sclerosis and limiting future peripheral venous access.
- Vesicants may cause severe local tissue breakdown and necrosis if inadvertently infiltrated into the skin. Monitor for and promptly take action if extravasation of a vesicant occurs.

To minimize discomfort, emotional distress, and risks of infection and infiltration, systemic IV chemotherapy can be given through a central vascular access device placed in a large blood vessel.

Regional chemotherapy delivers the drug directly to the tumor site. Examples include intraarterial, intraperitoneal, intrathecal (intraventricular), and intravesical bladder chemotherapy.

- Only persons specifically trained in chemotherapy handling techniques should be involved with the preparation and administration of cancer drugs. A person preparing, transporting, or giving chemotherapy may absorb the drug through inhalation of particles when reconstituting a powder or through skin contact from exposure to droplets or powder.

TABLE 98 Drug Therapy Chemotherapy

Mechanisms of Action	Examples
Alkylating *Cell Cycle Phase–Nonspecific* Damage DNA by causing breaks in the double-stranded helix. If repair does not occur, cells will die immediately (cytocidal) or when they try to divide (cytostatic).	Bendamustine (Treanda), busulfan (Myleran), chlorambucil (Leukeran), cyclophosphamide, dacarbazine, ifosfamide (Ifex), melphalan, temozolomide (Temodar), thiotepa
Antimetabolites *Cell Cycle Phase–Specific* Mimic naturally occurring substances, thus interfering with enzyme function or DNA synthesis. Primarily act during S phase. Purine and pyrimidine are building blocks of nucleic acids needed for DNA and RNA synthesis.	
• Interfere with purine metabolism	Cladribine, clofarabine (Clolar), fludarabine, mercaptopurine (Purixan), nelarabine (Arranon), pentostatin (Nipent), thioguanine
• Interfere with pyrimidine metabolism	Capecitabine (Xeloda); cytarabine, floxuridine, fluorouracil, gemcitabine (Gemzar)
• Interfere with folic acid metabolism	Methotrexate (Trexall), pemetrexed (Alimta)
• Interfere with DNA synthesis	Hydroxyurea (Hydrea, Droxia)
Antitumor Antibiotics *Cell Cycle Phase–Nonspecific* Bind directly to DNA, thus inhibiting the synthesis of DNA and interfering with transcription of RNA.	Bleomycin, dactinomycin (Cosmegen), daunorubicin, doxorubicin (Doxil), epirubicin (Ellence), idarubicin, mitomycin, mitoxantrone, valrubicin (Valstar)

C

Continued

TABLE 98 Drug Therapy Chemotherapy—cont'd

Mechanisms of Action	Examples
Mitotic Inhibitors	
Cell Cycle Phase–Specific	
Taxanes	
Antimicrotubule agents that interfere with mitosis. Act during the late G$_2$ phase and mitosis to stabilize microtubules, thus inhibiting cell division.	Albumin-bound paclitaxel (Abraxane), docetaxel (Taxotere)
Vinca Alkaloids	
Act in M phase to inhibit mitosis.	Vinblastine, vincristine, vinorelbine
Others	
Microtubular inhibitors.	Estramustine (Emcyt), ixabepilone (Ixempra), eribulin (Halaven)
Nitrosoureas	
Cell Cycle Phase–Nonspecific	
Break DNA helix, interfering with DNA replication. Cross blood-brain barrier.	Carmustine (BiCNU, Gliadel), lomustine (Gleostine), streptozocin (Zanosar)
Platinum Drugs	
Cell Cycle Phase–Nonspecific	
Bind to DNA and RNA, miscoding information and/ or inhibiting DNA replication, and cells die.	Carboplatin, cisplatin, oxaliplatin
Topoisomerase Inhibitors	
Cell Cycle Phase–Specific	
Inhibit topoisomerases (normal enzymes) that function to make reversible breaks and repairs in DNA that allow for flexibility of DNA in replication.	Etoposide, irinotecan (Camptosar), topotecan (Hycamtin)

Note: Many of these drugs are irritants or vesicants that require special attention during administration to avoid extravasation. It is important to know this information about a drug before administering it.

Effects of Chemotherapy

Chemotherapy agents cannot distinguish between normal cells and cancer cells. Side effects are caused by the destruction of rapidly proliferating normal cells including bone marrow, lining of the gastrointestinal tract, and integument (skin, hair, and nails).

The adverse effects of these drugs can be acute, delayed, or chronic.

- *Acute toxicity* includes anaphylactic and hypersensitivity reactions, extravasation or a flare reaction, anticipatory nausea and vomiting, and dysrhythmias.
- *Delayed effects* are numerous and include delayed nausea and vomiting, mucositis, alopecia, skin rashes, bone marrow depression, altered bowel function, and neurotoxicities.
- *Chronic toxicities* involve damage to organs, such as the heart, liver, kidneys, and lungs.

Nursing Management: Chemotherapy and Radiation Therapy

You have an important role in helping patients deal with the side effects of chemotherapy and radiation therapy.

- Myelosuppression is one of the most common effects of chemotherapy. To a lesser extent, it can occur with radiation. Treatment-induced myelosuppression can result in life-threatening and distressing effects. These include infection, hemorrhage, and overwhelming fatigue. Monitor the complete blood count (CBC), particularly the neutrophil, platelet, and red blood cell (RBC) counts.
- Fatigue is a persistent sense of tiredness that interferes with day-to-day functioning. Teach patients energy conservation strategies. Maintaining exercise and activity within tolerable limits is often helpful in managing fatigue.

The intestinal mucosa is sensitive to chemotherapy and radiation therapy, resulting in nausea and vomiting, diarrhea, mucositis, and anorexia. These problems can affect the patient's hydration, nutritional status, and sense of well-being.

- Nausea and vomiting can be managed with antiemetic regimens, dietary modification, and other nondrug interventions. Assess patients for signs and symptoms of dehydration and metabolic alkalosis.
- Both radiation therapy– and chemotherapy-induced diarrhea are best managed with diet adjustments, antidiarrheals, antimotility agents, and antispasmodics (see Table 47.2, Harding et al., *Lewis' Medical-Surgical Nursing*, ed 12).

- Mucositis can be alleviated with systemic and/or topical analgesics and antibiotics (if infection is present). Monitor and get prompt treatment for oral candidiasis. Meticulous oral care during and for a long time after treatment reduces the risk of cavities, which may occur because of decreased saliva. Saliva substitutes or drinking small amounts of water frequently may help patients with xerostomia.
- Monitor the patient who has anorexia to ensure that weight loss does not become excessive. Also observe for dehydration. Small, frequent meals of high-protein, high-calorie bland foods are better tolerated than large meals.

Skin changes with chemotherapy range from mild redness and hyperpigmentation to more distressing effects, such as acral erythema or desquamation. Alopecia caused by chemotherapy is usually reversible. Hair generally begins to grow back 3–4 weeks after the drugs are discontinued.

- With radiation therapy, skin effects occur only in the treatment field. Verify skincare guidelines with your agency's radiation oncology department.

▼ **Patient and Caregiver Teaching**

Teaching is an important part of your role related to chemotherapy.

- Explore the patient's attitude about treatment. You can promote the development of a hopeful attitude about cancer and support the patient and family during the various stages of the process of cancer.
- Provide accurate, essential information about cancer and cancer care to decrease the fear and anxiety often associated with treatment.
- Assess the concerns and emotional responses of patients and their families so that you can connect them with appropriate supportive care resources.

CHEST TUBES AND PLEURAL DRAINAGE

Description

If enough fluid or air accumulates in the pleural space, the normally negative subatmospheric pressure becomes positive and one or both lungs collapse. Inserting a chest tube into the pleural space can reestablish negative pressure, drain the pleural space, and allow for lung expansion. Tubes may also be inserted in the mediastinal space postoperatively to remove air and fluid.

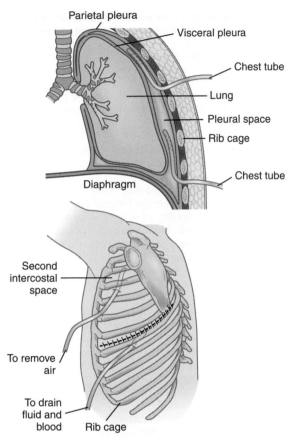

Fig. 34 Placement of chest tubes.

Chest Tube Insertion

Chest tube insertion can be performed in the emergency department (ED), in surgery, or at the bedside. Time permitting, a chest X-ray is used to confirm the affected side.

- The patient is positioned with the arm raised above the head on the affected side to expose the midaxillary area, the standard site for insertion. The area is cleansed with antiseptic solution. The HCP injects a local anesthetic and makes a small incision over a rib. The chest tube is then advanced up and over the top of the rib, to avoid the intercostal nerves and blood vessels (Fig. 34).

- Once inserted, the HCP sutures the tube in place and closes the incision with sutures. The tube is connected to a pleural drainage system.
- The wound is covered with an occlusive dressing. Most HCPs prefer to seal the wound around the chest tube with petroleum (airtight) gauze.
- Inserting a chest tube is painful. Monitor the patient's comfort and use appropriate pain-relieving interventions.

Pleural Drainage

There are two types of pleural drainage systems used to remove air from the pleural space. The first type is a *flutter valve* (Heimlich valve).

- This device consists of a one-way rubber valve within a rigid plastic tube. It is attached to the external end of the chest tube. The inlet nozzle allows the air to pass in the valve through the chest tube attached to it. The outlet nozzle allows the air to pass to the environment or a collecting device during expiration. During inspiration, when pressure in the chest decreases, the valve closes. This prevents air from going back into the patient's chest. During expiration, when intrathoracic pressure increases, the valve opens.
- The flutter valve can be used for a small to moderate-sized pneumothorax. It allows for patient mobility. The patient can hide the smaller drainage bag under clothes when they ambulate. Drainage bags attached to the flutter valve must have a vent to the atmosphere to prevent a tension pneumothorax. This is done by simply cutting a small slit in the top of any drainage bag that does not have a built-in vent. Patients may go home with a flutter valve in place.
- The second type of pleural drainage system is larger and has three basic compartments (Fig. 35). A variety of commercial chest drainage systems are available. The first compartment, or collection chamber, receives fluid and air from the pleural space. The drained fluid stays in this chamber while expelled air vents to the second compartment.
- The second compartment, or *water-seal chamber*, contains 2 cm of water and acts as a one-way valve. Air enters from the collection chamber and bubbles up through the water. The water prevents backflow of air into the patient. Brisk bubbling of air often occurs in this chamber when a pneumothorax is first evacuated. Intermittent bubbling during exhalation, coughing, or sneezing (when intrathoracic pressure is increased) may occur as long as there is air in the pleural space. Eventually, as the air leak

Fig. 35 Chest drainage units. Both units have three chambers: (1) collection chamber, (2) water-seal chamber, and (3) suction control chamber. Suction control chamber requires a connection to a wall suction source that is dialed up higher than the prescribed level. (A) Water suction. This unit uses water in the suction control chamber to control the wall suction pressure. (B) Dry suction. This unit controls wall suction by using a regulator control dial. (Courtesy Atrium Medical Corporation, Hudson, New Hampshire.)

resolves and the lung becomes more fully expanded, bubbling ceases. Normal water fluctuation within the water-seal chamber is called tidaling.

- A third compartment, the suction control chamber, applies suction to the chest drainage unit. Suction pressure is usually $-20\,cm\,H_2O$. For wet suction systems, the suction control chamber uses a column of water to control the amount of suction from the wall regulator. The dry suction chest tube system does not contain water: the amount of suction is determined by turning a dial on the chest tube drainage device to the ordered amount.

Nursing Management: Chest Drainage

Monitor the patient's clinical status.

- Assess vital signs, lung sounds, pain, and need for analgesia.
- Evaluate for subcutaneous emphysema at insertion site.
- Have the patient breathe deeply periodically to promote lung expansion. Encourage ROM exercises to the shoulder on the affected side. Encourage use of incentive spirometry every hour while awake to prevent atelectasis or pneumonia.
- Assess for complications. Auscultate the lungs (decreased or absent breath sounds may indicate air and/or fluid reaccumulating in chest); observe color and characteristics of chest tube drainage (significant bleeding >100 mL/h); observe chest tube insertion site daily (infection may be identified by change in color or amount of drainage, erythema at site, patient fever, increased white blood cell [WBC] count).

Use meticulous sterile technique during dressing changes to reduce the incidence of infection. Change dressing according to policy and HCP preference.

- Remove old dressing carefully. Assess the site for inflammation or infection and culture site as needed. Cleanse the site according to policy, maintaining strict sterile asepsis.
- Redress with occlusive dressing. Some HCPs prefer a petroleum gauze dressing around the tube to prevent air leak. Date the dressing and document dressing change.

Drainage System

- Keep all connections between chest tubes, drainage tubing, and the drainage collector tight. Tape all connections.
- Keep all tubing loosely coiled below chest level. Position so that drainage flows freely. Never raise the drainage system to the level of the patient's chest because fluid can drain back into the lungs.
- Observe for air fluctuations (tidaling) and bubbling in the water-seal chamber.

- Mark the time of measurement and the fluid level on the drainage unit according to policy. Report any change in the quantity or characteristics of drainage (e.g., clear yellow to bloody) to the HCP. Notify HCP if > 100 mL/h drainage.
- Change the unit if the collection chamber is full. Do not try to empty it.
- Never compress, milk, or strip chest tube tubing.
- In the spontaneously breathing patient, if fluid does not rise with inspiration or fall with expiration, the drainage system may be blocked, the lungs have reexpanded, or the system is attached to suction. If the chest tube is connected to suction, disconnect momentarily from wall suction to check for tidaling.
- If bubbling increases, there may be an air leak in the drainage system or a leak from the patient. Suspect a system leak when bubbling is continuous.
- If the drainage system is overturned and the water seal is disrupted, return it to an upright position and encourage the patient to take a few deep breaths.
- If the drainage system breaks, place the distal end of the chest tubing (patient-side) in a container of sterile water as an emergency water seal.

Chest Tube Removal

Chest tubes are removed when the lungs are reexpanded and fluid drainage has ceased or is minimal. Suction is usually discontinued and gravity drainage is used for 24 hours before tube removal. In most settings, the tube is removed by the HCP or an advanced practice nurse.

- Give pain medication about 30–60 minutes before chest tube removal. Gather dressing supplies, including petroleum gauze and dry gauze dressing. Explain the procedure to the patient.
- To remove the tube: (1) cut the suture; (2) have the patient take a deep breath, exhale, and bear down (Valsalva maneuver); and (3) remove the tube.
- The site is immediately covered with the airtight, occlusive dressing to prevent air from entering the pleural space. A dry gauze dressing is placed over top. The wound heals in a few days.
- A chest X-ray is done 30–60 minutes after chest tube removal to check for pneumothorax or fluid accumulation.
- Assess the patient for respiratory distress. This may signify a recurrence of the original problem. If respiratory distress occurs, notify the HCP at once.

DIALYSIS

Dialysis is a technique in which substances move from the blood through a semipermeable membrane and into a dialysis solution (dialysate). It corrects fluid and electrolyte imbalances and removes waste products in renal failure. It also can be used to treat drug overdose.

The two methods of dialysis are *peritoneal dialysis* (PD) and *hemodialysis* (HD) (Table 99).

TABLE 99 Comparison of Peritoneal Dialysis and Hemodialysis

Advantages	Disadvantages
Peritoneal Dialysis (PD)	
• Immediate initiation in almost any hospital	• Bacterial or chemical peritonitis
• Less complicated than hemodialysis	• Protein loss into dialysate
• Portable system with CAPD	• Exit site and tunnel infections
• Fewer diet restrictions	• Self-image problems with catheter placement
• Short training time	• Hyperglycemia
• Useable in patient with vascular access problems	• Surgery for catheter placement
• Less cardiovascular stress	• Contraindicated in patient with multiple abdominal surgeries, trauma, unrepaired hernia
• Home dialysis possible	• Requires completion of education program
• Preferable for patient with diabetes	• Catheter can migrate
	• Best instituted with willing partner
Hemodialysis (HD)	
• Rapid fluid removal	• Vascular access problems
• Rapid removal of urea and creatinine	• Diet and fluid restrictions
• Effective potassium removal	• Heparinization may be necessary
• Less protein loss	• Extensive equipment necessary
• Lowering of serum triglycerides	• Hypotension during dialysis
• Home dialysis possible	• Added blood loss that contributes to anemia
• Can place temporary access at bedside	• Specially trained personnel necessary
	• Surgery for permanent access placement
	• Self-image problems with permanent access

CAPD, Continuous ambulatory peritoneal dialysis.

- In PD, the peritoneal membrane acts as the semipermeable membrane.
- In HD, an artificial membrane (usually made of cellulose-based or synthetic materials) is used as the semipermeable membrane and is in contact with the patient's blood.

Dialysis is begun when the patient's uremia can no longer be adequately treated with conservative medical management. In general, this is when the glomerular filtration rate (GFR) is < 15 mL/min/1.73 m^2. The nephrologist determines when to start dialysis based on the patient's clinical status.

- Uremic complications including encephalopathy, neuropathies, uncontrollable hyperkalemia, pericarditis, and accelerated hypertension indicate the need for immediate dialysis.

Most patients with end-stage renal disease (ESRD) are treated with dialysis because: (1) there is a lack of donated organs, (2) some patients are physically or mentally unsuitable for transplantation, or (3) some patients do not want transplants.

- Age is not a factor in determining candidacy for dialysis. Factors that are important are the patient's ability to cope and the existing support system.

E

ENTERAL NUTRITION

Enteral nutrition (EN, also known as *tube feeding*) is nutrition (e.g., liquefied food or formula) delivered directly into the gastrointestinal (GI) tract through a tube, catheter, or stoma. EN is used for the patient who has a functioning GI tract but is unable to take any or enough oral nourishment, or when it is unsafe to do so. Contraindications for EN include GI obstruction, prolonged ileus, severe diarrhea or vomiting, and enterocutaneous fistula.

EN is easily administered, safer, more physiologically efficient, and typically less expensive than parenteral nutrition. Fig. 36 shows the location of commonly used enteral feeding tubes.

- The type of EN depends on the anticipated length of time enteral feeding will be required, degree of risk for aspiration, patient's clinical status, adequacy of digestion and absorption, and patient's anatomy (e.g., extreme obesity).
- Nasally and orally placed tubes (orogastric, nasogastric [NG], nasoduodenal, or nasojejunal) are most commonly used for short-term feeding (<4 weeks).

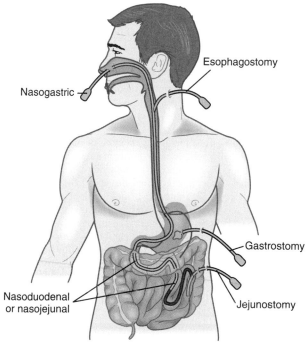

Fig. 36 Common enteral feeding tube placement locations.

- Nasoduodenal and nasojejunal tubes are used when pathophysiologic conditions, such as risk of aspiration, warrant delivering the feeding below the patient's pyloric sphincter. Placement into the small intestine decreases the chance of regurgitating gastric contents into the esophagus and subsequent aspiration. However, the patient can still aspirate gastric secretions if the stomach is not emptying properly.

If the feedings are necessary for an extended time, other tubes are placed in the stomach or small bowel by surgical, endoscopic, or fluoroscopic procedures.

- Common delivery options are continuous infusion or intermittent (bolus) feedings by infusion pump, bolus feedings by gravity, and bolus feedings by syringe. Continuous infusion is most often used for critically ill patients. Bolus feeding may be preferred as the patient improves or at home.

Tube Feedings and Safety

Aspiration and dislodged tubes are important safety concerns. You have a critical role to ensure that tube feedings are safely administered. Obtain X-ray confirmation of newly inserted nasal or orogastric tubes before feeding or administering medications. Maintain proper placement of the tube after feedings are started. To determine if a feeding tube has maintained the proper position, mark the exit site of the feeding tube at the time of the initial X-ray, and observe for a change in the external tube length during feedings. Recheck the tube insertion length at regular intervals.

- Elevate the patient's head of bed to a minimum of 30 degrees, but preferably 45 degrees, to prevent aspiration. Check institution policy for suspending feeding while the patient is supine. If intermittent delivery is used, the head of the bed should remain elevated for 30–60 minutes after feeding.
- Follow your agency policy for checking gastric residual volumes (GRV). Common protocols call for checking GRV every 6–8 hours in noncritically ill patients and before each bolus feeding.
- Flush feeding tubes in adults with 30 mL of warm tap water every 4 hours during continuous feedings or before and after each bolus feeding. Use sterile water in immunocompromised and critically ill patients. Always flush tubes between each medication and after all medications are given.

The types of problems encountered for patients receiving tube feedings and corrective measures are presented in Table 100.

Patient teaching includes skin care, tube care, feeding administration, and potential complications.

TABLE 100 Nursing Management of EN Problems	
Problems and Causes	**Management**
Constipation	
Decreased fluid intake	• Increase fluid intake if not contraindicated. • Give total fluid intake of 30 mL/kg body weight.
Formula	• Change formula to one with more fiber content. • Give as-needed laxative.

Continued

TABLE 100 Nursing Management of EN Problems—cont'd

Problems and Causes	Management
Inactivity	• Encourage ambulation unless contraindicated. • Collaborate with physical therapy to promote activity.
Dehydration	
Diarrhea, vomiting	• Decrease rate or change formula. • Check drugs that patient is receiving, especially antibiotics. • Avoid bacterial contamination of formula and equipment.
Fluid intake	• Increase intake and check amount and number of feedings. • Administer supplemental tube, oral, or IV fluid intake if appropriate.
High-protein formula	• Change formula to one with less protein.
Hyperosmotic diuresis	• Check blood glucose levels often. • Change formula to one with less glucose.
Diarrhea	
Contaminated formula	• Refrigerate unused formula and record date opened. • Discard outdated formula. • Discard formula left standing for longer than manufacturer's guidelines. • 8 hrs for ready-to-feed formulas (cans) • 4 hrs for reconstituted formula • 24 hrs for closed-system enteral formulas • Use a closed system.
Feeding too fast	• Dilute or decrease rate of feeding. • Change to continuous feedings. • Stop excess water boluses.
Formula	• Change to formula that has more fiber or is less hypertonic. • Change to continuous feedings.
Infection	• Obtain stool culture for fecal leukocyte determination, *C. difficile*, and/or toxin assay.

TABLE 100 Nursing Management of EN Problems—cont'd	
Problems and Causes	**Management**
Medications	• Check for drugs that may cause diarrhea (e.g., sorbitol in liquid medications, antibiotics).
Tube moving distally	• Properly secure tube before beginning feeding. • Check placement before each bolus feeding or at least every 4 hrs if continuous feedings.
Vomiting	
Delayed gastric emptying	• Consult with HCP about use of prokinetic drug. • Follow agency policy to manage gastric residual volumes.
Improper tube placement	• Replace tube in proper position. • Check tube position before each bolus feeding and every 4 hrs if continuous feedings.

IMMUNOTHERAPY AND TARGETED THERAPY

Description

Immunotherapy and targeted therapy are cancer treatment modalities that can be effective alone or in combination with surgery, chemotherapy, and radiation therapy.

- *Immunotherapy* uses the immune system, the body's main defense against infection and disease, to fight cancer. Some types of immunotherapy are called *biologic therapy*. Immunotherapy can (1) boost or manipulate the immune system and create an environment that is not conducive for cancer cells to grow or (2) attack cancer cells directly. Types of immunotherapy include cytokines, vaccines, and monoclonal antibodies. Immunotherapy agents alter the biologic response of the host to the tumor cell (Table 101).
- *Targeted therapy* interferes with cancer growth by targeting specific cellular receptors and pathways that are important in tumor growth (see Table 101). Targeted therapy agents are more selective than chemotherapy agents, so they cause less damage to normal cells.

TABLE 101 Select Immunotherapies and Targeted Therapies

Mechanism of Action	Examples
Angiogenesis Inhibitors	
Bind vascular endothelial growth factor (VEGF), thereby inhibiting angiogenesis.	Bevacizumab (Avastin) Pazopanib (Votrient) Ramucirumab (Cyramza)
CD20 Monoclonal Antibodies	
Bind CD20 antigen, causing cytotoxicity and radiation injury.	Ibritumomab tiuxetan/ yttrium-90 (Zevalin)
Bind CD20 antigen, causing cytotoxicity.	Ofatumumab (Arzerra) Rituximab (Rituxan)
CD52 Monoclonal Antibody	
Bind CD52 antigen (found on T and B cells, monocytes, natural killer [NK] cells, neutrophils).	Alemtuzumab (Campath)
Cytokines	
Inhibit DNA and protein synthesis. Suppress cell proliferation. ↑ Cytotoxic effects of NK cells.	α-interferon (Intron A)
Stimulate proliferation of T and B cells. Activate NK cells.	Interleukin-2 (aldesleukin [Proleukin])
Human Epidermal Growth Factor Receptor-2 (HER-2)	
Monoclonal antibody to HER-2 that attaches to the antigen. It is taken into the cells and eventually kills them.	Pertuzumab (Perjeta)Trastuzumab (Herceptin)
Trastuzumab connected to a chemotherapy drug called DM1.	Ado-trastuzumab emtansine (Kadcyla)
Immunomodulatory Drugs (IMiDs)	
Inhibit production of TNF, IL-6, and VEGF, leading to antiangiogenic effects. Stimulate T and NK cells. ↑ γ-interferon and IL-2 production.	Apremilast (Otezla) Lenalidomide (Revlimid) Pomalidomide (Pomalyst) Thalidomide (Thalomid)

TABLE 101 Select Immunotherapies and Targeted Therapies—cont'd

Mechanism of Action	Examples

Kinase Inhibitors

Anaplastic Lymphoma Kinase (ALK) Inhibitors

Mechanism of Action	Examples
Inhibit anaplastic lymphoma kinase (ALK).	Ceritinib (Zykadia) Crizotinib (Xalkori) Entrectinib (Rozlytrek)

BCR-ABL Tyrosine Kinase Inhibitors

Mechanism of Action	Examples
Inhibit BCR-ABL TK. Primarily used in chronic myeloid leukemia.	Bosutinib (Bosulif) Dasatinib (Sprycel) imatinib (Gleevec) Nilotinib (Tasigna)

BRAF and MEK Kinase Inhibitors

Mechanism of Action	Examples
Inhibit BRAF and MEK enzymes.	Dabrafenib (Tafinlar) Trametinib (Mekinist) Vemurafenib (Zelboraf) Cobimetinib (Cotellic)

EGFR Tyrosine Kinase (TK) Inhibitors

Mechanism of Action	Examples
Inhibit epidermal growth factor receptor (EGFR) TK.	Cetuximab (Erbitux) Erlotinib (Tarceva) Gefitinib (Iressa) Panitumumab (Vectibix)
Inhibit EGFR-TK and binds HER-2.	Lapatinib (Tykerb)

Multi-Tyrosine Kinase Inhibitors

Mechanism of Action	Examples
Inhibit multiple TKs.	Axitinib (Inlyta) Cabozantinib (Cometriq) Pazopanib (Votrient) Regorafenib (Stivarga) Sorafenib (Nexavar) Sunitinib (Sutent) Vandetanib (Caprelsa)

mTOR Kinase Inhibitors

Mechanism of Action	Examples
Inhibit a specific protein known as the mechanistic target of rapamycin (mTOR).	Everolimus (Afinitor) Temsirolimus (Torisel)

Continued

TABLE 101 Select Immunotherapies and Targeted Therapies—cont'd

Mechanism of Action	Examples
Programmed Death Receptor (PD)-1 Blockers	
Block PD-1, a protein on T cells that normally helps keep these cells from attacking other cells. This boosts immune response against cancer cells.	Nivolumab (Opdivo) Pembrolizumab (Keytruda)
Proteasome Inhibitors	
Inhibit proteasome activity, which functions to regulate cell growth.	Bortezomib (Velcade) Carfilzomib (Kyprolis)
Vaccines	
Live attenuated strain of *Mycobacterium bovis* induces immune response. Used intravesically to treat bladder cancer.	BCG vaccine
Vaccine against prostate cancer that stimulates the immune system against the cancer.	Sipuleucel-T (Provenge)

BRAF, B-Raf; *HER-2*, human epidermal growth factor receptor 2; *IL*, interleukin; *TNF*, tumor necrosis factor.

Types of targeted therapy agents include tyrosine kinase inhibitors, monoclonal antibodies, angiogenesis inhibitors, and proteasome inhibitors.

- *Tyrosine* kinase *inhibitors* block an important enzyme that activates the signaling pathways that regulate cell proliferation and survival.
- Monoclonal *antibodies* bind to specific target cells. They may also stimulate an immunologic response in the patient.
- Angiogenesis *inhibitors* prevent the vascularization of tumors.
- Proteasome *inhibitors* promote protein accumulation and alter cell function.

Nursing Management

Some problems of immunotherapy and targeted therapy are acute and dose-limited. Capillary leak syndrome and pulmonary edema require critical care nursing. Bone marrow depression with immunotherapy is usually more transient and less severe than that seen with chemotherapy.

- Severe fatigue associated with immunotherapy can be a dose-limiting toxicity. Combining these agents with chemotherapy increases the adverse effects.
- Acetaminophen given before treatment and every 4 hours after treatment can help relieve the flulike syndrome. IV meperidine (Demerol) can help control the severe chills or rigors from agents such as interleukin-2 IL-2.

Other measures include monitoring vital signs, planning for periods of rest for the patient, assisting with activities of daily living (ADLs), and monitoring for adequate oral intake.

M

MECHANICAL VENTILATION

Description

Mechanical ventilation is the process by which a ventilator is used to deliver O_2 to the lungs. It is a means of supporting patients until they recover the ability to breathe independently. It can serve as a bridge to long-term mechanical ventilation or until a decision is made to stop ventilatory support. Mechanical ventilation is not curative.

- Indications for mechanical ventilation include acute respiratory failure (ARF) apnea, inability to breathe or protect the airway, acute respiratory distress, severe hypoxemia and/or hypercarbia, and respiratory muscle fatigue. Other patients who receive mechanically ventilation include those with hemorrhage, trauma, neuromuscular problems, drug overdose, burns, and shock.

Types of Mechanical Ventilation

The two major types of mechanical ventilation are negative pressure ventilation and positive pressure ventilation (PPV).

- *Negative pressure ventilation* involves the use of chambers that encase the chest or body and surround it with intermittent subatmospheric (or negative) pressure. Negative pressure ventilation is noninvasive and does not require an artificial airway. Intermittent negative pressure around the chest pulls the chest wall outward, reducing intrathoracic pressure. Air rushes in the upper airway, which is outside the sealed chamber. Expiration is passive. The machine cycles off, allowing chest retraction.

- A few portable negative pressure ventilators are available for home use for patients with neuromuscular diseases or central nervous system disorders.They are not used routinely for acutely ill patients.
- *Positive pressure ventilation* (PPV) is the main method used with acutely ill patients. It is the main method of mechanical ventilation used with acutely ill patients. During inspiration, the ventilator pushes air into the lungs under positive pressure. Unlike spontaneous ventilation, intrathoracic pressure is increased during lung inflation, not decreased. Expiration is passive, as occurs in normal expiration. Ventilators can deliver positive pressure breaths to the patient by either volume or pressure ventilation. With volume ventilation, a predetermined tidal volume (VT) is delivered with each inspiration. With pressure ventilation, the peak inspiratory pressure is predetermined.

Positive end-expiratory pressure (PEEP) is a ventilator setting in which positive pressure is applied to the airway during exhalation. During exhalation, airway pressure normally drops to near 0. Exhalation occurs passively. With PEEP, exhalation remains passive, but pressure falls to the preset PEEP level, often set between 5 and 10 cm H_2O. PEEP increases functional residual capacity (FRC) and often improves oxygenation by restoring the lung volume that normally remains at the end of passive exhalation.

- PEEP splints open previously collapsed alveoli (increasing the opportunity for O_2 and CO_2 to diffuse across the alveolar capillary membrane) and preventing alveolar collapse throughout the respiratory cycle.

Nursing Management of Mechanical Ventilation

For nursing management of the patient receiving mechanical ventilation, see eNursing Care Plan 28-1, available on the website for Harding et al., *Lewis' Medical-Surgical Nursing,* ed 12.

Noninvasive Ventilation

Noninvasive ventilation (NIV) uses a mask, instead of an ET tube, to help oxygenate and ventilate a patient. The mask can be nasal or full face. NIV is ideal for those who need a higher level of ventilatory support, but their condition is not bad enough to need mechanical ventilation. Good candidates for using NIV are patients with COPD exacerbations and heart failure (HF). The patient with an acute myocardial infarction or gastrointestinal bleed is not a candidate for NIV. Two common modes are continuous positive airway pressure (CPAP) and bilevel positive airway pressure (Bi-PAP).

Continuous positive airway pressure (CPAP) helps restore functional residual capacity (FRC). CPAP is delivered through a tight-fitting face mask, nasal mask, or nasal pillows. It provides one level of pressure delivered continuously, during both inspiration and expiration. CPAP is a common treatment for obstructive sleep apnea.

- CPAP increases work of breathing because the patient must forcibly exhale against the. Therefore, it is used with caution in patients with heart problems. Monitor the patient closely. Report any decline in their condition to the HCP at once.

Bilevel positive airway pressure (Bi-PAP) provides two levels of positive pressure support: inspiratory positive airway pressure (IPAP) and expiratory positive airway pressure (EPAP). IPAP is a higher level of pressure than EPAP. It helps with CO_2 removal. EPAP is a lower level of pressure. It helps keep the alveoli open at end expiration, assisting with oxygenation.

The patient must be awake, alert, able to breathe spontaneously, and tolerate the face piece. Bi-PAP is used for COPD patients with acute conditions (e.g., pneumonia) or exacerbation of chronic conditions (e.g., HF, acute respiratory failure [ARF]). Its use after extubation from mechanical ventilation can help prevent reintubation.

- Patients with shock, altered mental status, or increased airway secretions cannot use Bi-PAP because of the risk for aspiration and the inability to remove the mask.

Nursing Management: Noninvasive Ventilation

Patients with NIV need constant assessment. Assess level of consciousness (LOC), hemodynamic stability, and work of breathing. The patient must be able to remove the mask independently due to the risk of vomiting. Elevate the head of the bed 30–45 degrees to decrease the risk of aspiration.

- Patients who develop a decreased LOC may not be able to maintain a patent airway because they cannot protect their airway or clear secretions. In this situation, they may need intubation and mechanical ventilation. Any degree of hemodynamic instability (e.g., tachycardia, hypotension) warrants immediate reevaluation of NIV.

Provide mouth, nare, and eye care. Provide measures to protect the skin from breakdown and ulceration. Any degree of redness constitutes a Stage I pressure injury (PI). Alleviating pressure from the tight-fitting mask is important. Using masks of different sizes and styles can help. Collaborate with the respiratory therapist (RT).

OSTOMIES

Description

An *ostomy* is a surgically created opening on the abdomen that allows for the discharge of body waste. The outermost portion that is visible is a *stoma*. The stoma is the result of the large or small bowel being brought to the outside of the abdomen and sutured in place. When a stoma is created as a fecal diversion, feces will drain through the stoma instead of the anus.

Ostomies may be temporary or permanent. For example, the person with a draining fistula may need a temporary ostomy to prevent stool from reaching the diseased area. Cancer involving the rectum requires a permanent ostomy if all bowel distal to the ostomy is removed.

Types of Ostomies

Ostomies are named according to location and type (Fig. 37). An ostomy in the ileum is an *ileostomy*. An ostomy in the colon is a *colostomy*. The ostomy is further characterized by its site (sigmoid or transverse). The more distal the ostomy, the more the intestinal contents resemble feces. A comparison of colostomies and ileostomies is shown in Table 102.

The major types of ostomies are end stoma, loop, and double-barrel ostomies.

- An *end stoma* is created by dividing the bowel and bringing the proximal end as a single stoma. The distal portion of the gastrointestinal (GI) tract is surgically removed, or it is oversewn and left in the abdominal cavity. If the distal bowel is removed, then the stoma is permanent.
- A *loop stoma* is constructed by bringing a loop of bowel to the abdominal surface and then opening the anterior part of the bowel to provide fecal diversion. This results in one stoma with a proximal and distal opening and an intact posterior bowel wall that separates the two openings. A loop stoma is usually temporary.
- In a *double-barrel stoma,* the bowel is divided, and both the proximal and distal ends are brought through the abdominal wall as two separate stomas. The proximal one is the functioning stoma; the distal, nonfunctioning stoma is referred to as the *mucus fistula*. The double-barreled stoma is usually temporary.

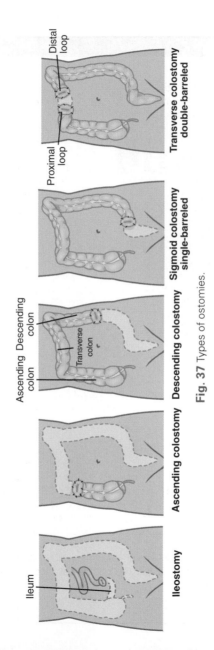

Fig. 37 Types of ostomies.

TABLE 102 Comparison of Ileostomy and Colostomy

Characteristic	Ileostomy	Colostomy		
		Ascending	Transverse	Sigmoid
Stool consistency	Liquid to semiliquid	Semiliquid	Semiliquid to semiformed	Formed
Fluid requirement	↑	↑	Possibly ↑	No change
Bowel regulation	No	No	No	Yes (if there is a history of a regular bowel pattern)
Pouch and skin barriers	Yes	Yes	Yes	Dependent on regulation
Indications for surgery	Ulcerative colitis, Crohn's disease, diseased or injured colon, familial polyposis, trauma, cancer	Perforating diverticulum in lower colon, trauma, rectovaginal fistula, inoperable tumors of colon, rectum, or pelvis	Same as for ascending	Cancer of the rectum or rectosigmoidal area, perforating diverticulum, trauma

Nursing Management

Preoperative Care

Psychologic preparation and emotional support are important as the person begins to cope with the changes in body image and elimination. The patient and caregiver should understand the extent of surgery planned.

- A wound, ostomy, and continence nurse (WOCN) should choose the site where the ostomy will be and mark the abdomen before surgery. The site should be within the rectus muscle, on a flat surface, and in a place that the patient is able to see.

Postoperative Care

Postoperative nursing care includes assessment of the stoma and provision of an appropriate pouching system that protects the skin and contains drainage and odor. The stoma should be dark pink to red. A dusky blue stoma indicates ischemia, and a brown-black stoma indicates necrosis. Assess and document stoma color every 4 hours. Teach the patient that the stoma will be mildly to moderately swollen the first 2–3 weeks after surgery.

Nursing care for the patient with an ostomy is presented in eNursing Care Plan 47-3 on the website.

Colostomy Care

A colostomy in the ascending and transverse colon produces semi-liquid stools. Instruct the patient to use a drainable pouch. A colostomy in the sigmoid or descending colon produces semiformed or formed stools and sometimes can be regulated by the irrigation method. The patient may or may not wear a drainage pouch. A well-balanced diet and adequate fluid intake are important.

Colostomy irrigations may be used to stimulate emptying of the colon. Regularity is possible only when the stoma is in the distal colon or rectum. With bowel control achieved, the patient may need to wear only a pad or cover over the stoma. Irrigation requires manual dexterity and adequate vision. People who irrigate regularly should have ostomy bags available in case they develop diarrhea.

▼ Patient and Caregiver Teaching

Colostomy

- Pouching systems consist of an adhesive skin barrier and a bag or pouch to collect the feces. The skin barrier is a piece of pectin-based or karaya wafer that has a measurable thickness and hydrocolloid adhesive properties. Teach the patient to perform a pouch change, provide appropriate skin care, control odor, care for the stoma, and identify signs and symptoms of complications.
- Instruct the patient about the importance of adequate fluids and a healthy diet and when to seek health care.

- Recommend outpatient follow-up by a WOCN. Give patients written information about the particular ostomy, instructions for pouch changes, supplies and where to purchase them, and outpatient follow-up appointments.
- Emotional support, interventions from skillful WOCNs, and visits from people who have successfully learned to manage their ostomies will help patients learn to cope with and manage the new stoma. Resources such as the United Ostomy Associations of America (www.ostomy.org) may also be helpful.
- For ostomy teaching guidelines, see Table 47.32, Harding et al., *Lewis' Medical-Surgical Nursing,* ed 12.

Ileostomy Care

- Because the stool from an ileostomy is caustic to the skin, a secure pouching system is important. Empty ostomy pouches when they are one-third full to prevent loss of adhesion, as leakage can damage the surrounding tissues. The drainable pouch is usually worn for 4–7 days before being changed unless leakage occurs.
- In the first 24–48 hours after surgery, the amount of drainage from the stoma may be negligible. Once peristalsis returns, the patient may experience a period of high-volume output of 1500–1800 mL/day. Later, the average amount can be 500 mL/day.

▼ Patient and Caregiver Teaching

Ileostomy

- Instruct the patient to drink at least 2–3 L/day when there are excessive fluid losses from heat and sweating. Teach patients signs and symptoms of fluid and electrolyte imbalance so they can take appropriate action.
- A low-fiber diet is ordered initially. Reintroduce fiber-containing foods gradually.
- A stoma bleeds easily because it has a high vascular supply. Tell the patient that minimal oozing of blood is normal.
- Encourage the patient to share concerns and ask questions. Provide accurate information in a clear manner. Recommend support services and assist patients to develop confidence in managing the stoma.
- Help the patient understand if specific aspects of surgery and treatment may affect sexual function or sexual activity. Encourage the patient to discuss concerns.

OXYGEN THERAPY

Description

O_2 therapy is a common treatment for hypoxemia and hypoxia. O_2 is a colorless, odorless, tasteless gas that constitutes 21% of the atmosphere. Giving supplemental O_2 increases the partial pressure of O_2 (PO_2) in inspired air. O_2 therapy requires an HCP order. The dose of O_2 administered to patients is the *fraction of inspired oxygen* (*FIO_2*).

We give O_2 to treat hypoxemia caused by many problems, such as shock, pneumonia, and pulmonary emboli. O_2 therapy is tailored to meet each patient's unique circumstances and physiologic needs.

- For most patients, the goal of O_2 therapy is to keep the SaO_2 greater than 92% during rest, sleep, and activity, or the PaO_2 greater than 60 mm Hg. We may modify these goals depending on the patient's clinical situation. For example, the HCP may accept an SpO_2 and PaO_2 greater than 88% for the patient with longstanding COPD.

Methods of Administration

There are various ways to administer O_2 (Table 103). The device used depends on the patient's underlying condition, the FIO_2 the patient needs, advantages and disadvantages of each device, comfort, cost, and financial resources.

We classify O_2 delivery systems as low-flow or high-flow systems. Low-flow O_2 delivery devices are appropriate for patients who are awake, alert, and spontaneously breathing with a stable, intact respiratory drive. These devices provide O_2 in concentrations that do not meet all of the patient's inspiratory demands. Low-flow devices pull in a proportion of room air, which makes the exact FIO_2 unknown. We do know the range of FIO_2 delivered by each device. Examples include nasal prongs, simple masks, and nonrebreather masks.

High-flow O_2 delivery devices deliver fixed O_2 concentrations (e.g., 28%, 35%) independent of the patient's respiratory rate or pattern. High flow systems provide O_2 in concentrations that meet or exceed the patient's inspiratory demand. These patients are also awake, alert, and spontaneously breathing, but have higher O_2 requirements that low-flow devices cannot meet. High-flow devices help meet achieving specific PaO_2 or SpO_2 targets. Examples include the Venturi mask and high-flow nasal cannula.

TABLE 103 Methods of Oxygen Administration

Description	Nursing Interventions
Low-Flow Delivery Devices *Nasal Cannula* • Most commonly used. • O_2 delivered through plastic tubing (prongs) that fits in the nares. • Used for a patient requiring low O_2 concentrations. • Achieves O_2 concentrations of 24% (at 1 L/min) to 44% (at 6 L/min). • Safe • Easy to set-up and use • Patient can eat, talk, or cough while wearing device. • Allows some freedom of movement.	• Stabilize nasal cannula when caring for a restless patient. • Amount of O_2 inhaled depends on room air and patient's breathing pattern. • Most patients with COPD can tolerate 2–4 L/min through a cannula. • Assess the nares and ears for skin breakdown. May need to pad tubing where it sits on ears. • If flow rates are >5 L/min, nasal membranes may dry and place patient at risk for nose bleeds.

TABLE 103 Methods of Oxygen Administration—cont'd

Description	Nursing Interventions
O_2-Conserving Cannula • Generally indicated for longer-term O_2 therapy at home (e.g., CF, pulmonary hypertension). • Looks like a "moustache" (Oxymizer) or "pendant" type. • Cannula has a built-in reservoir that ↑ O_2 concentration and allows patient to use lower flow, usually 30%–50%, which increases comfort, lowers cost, and can be increased with activities. • Can deliver O_2 flow rates up to 15 L/min.	• More expensive than standard nasal cannula. • Cannula is highly visible. • Assess the nares and ears for skin breakdown. May need to pad tubing where it sits behind ears. • Cannot clean cannula. Change cannula every week. • May need ABGs and oximetry to determine correct flow rate.

Pendant-type O_2-conserving cannula.

Continued

TABLE 103   Methods of Oxygen Administration—cont'd

Description	Nursing Interventions
Partial and Non-Rebreather Masks • Used for short-term therapy for patients with higher O_2 needs • Achieves O_2 concentrations of 60%–90% (with flow rates of 10–15L/min). • O_2 flows into reservoir bag and mask during inhalation. • Bag allows patient to rebreathe about first third of exhaled air (rich in O_2) in conjunction with flowing O_2. • Vents stay open on partial mask. • Some agencies prefer this over nonrebreather as a safety issue.	 • O_2 flow rate must be sufficient to keep bag from deflating during inspiration to avoid CO_2 buildup and rebreathing of CO_2. • If deflation occurs, increase flowrate on flowmeter on wall to keep bag inflated. • Mask should fit snugly. • With nonrebreather masks, make sure valves open during expiration and close during inhalation to prevent decrease in FIO_2 or build-up in CO_2. • Monitor patient closely, since more advanced interventions such as CPAP, Bi-PAP, or intubation with mechanical ventilation may be needed.

TABLE 103 Methods of Oxygen Administration—cont'd

Description	Nursing Interventions
Simple Face Mask	
• Covers the nose and mouth.	• Wash and dry under mask q4h and PRN.
• Achieves O₂ concentrations of 35%–50% with flow rates of 6–12 L/min.	• Mask must fit snugly.
• Mask provides adequate humidification of inspired air.	• Must have flow rates of at least 6 L/min to wash exhaled gases out of mask (if O₂ flow rate not high enough, CO₂ rebreathing is possible)
• Safe	• May change to nasal cannula while patient is eating.
• Easy to set up and use	• Watch for pressure necrosis at top of ears from elastic straps if patient wears for a longer time. Gauze or other padding may alleviate this problem.
• Typically used only for short periods.	

Continued

TABLE 103 Methods of Oxygen Administration—cont'd

Description	Nursing Interventions
High-Flow Delivery Devices	
High-Flow Nasal Cannula	
• Blends O_2 with compressed air to generate high FIO_2	• Nasal cannula must be smaller than 50% of nares to allow flow during exhalation and flush out end-expiratory CO_2.
• Achieves O_2 concentration up to 100% (at flow rate of up to 60 L/min).	• Well tolerated.
• Heated humidifier capable of providing 100% humidity.	• Patients can eat and drink with device in place.
• Soft and flexible nasal prongs.	• Patient may describe feeling of always having to blow nose ("rainout") due to humidification.
• More comfortable than mask.	

TABLE 103 Methods of Oxygen Administration—cont'd

Description	Nursing Interventions
Tracheostomy Collar	
• Collar attaches to neck with elastic strap and can deliver humidity and O_2 through the tracheostomy.	• Secretions collect inside collar and around tracheostomy.
• Some O_2 concentration is lost into atmosphere because collar does not fit tightly.	• Remove collar and clean at least q4hr and PRN to prevent aspiration of fluid and infection.
• Venturi device can be attached to flowmeter and can deliver exact amounts of O_2 through the collar.	• Because condensation occurs in tubing, periodically drain tubing distal to tracheostomy.
Tracheostomy T-Piece	
• Almost identical to tracheostomy collar, but it has a T-connector attached to an O_2 blender.	• Because T-piece connector can disconnect easily, monitor closely.
• Tight fit allows better O_2 and humidity delivery than tracheostomy collar.	• T-piece connector may pull on the tracheostomy tube, causing irritation and potential tissue damage. Monitor closely.
• T-piece allows an inline catheter to be connected for suctioning.	

Continued

TABLE 103 Methods of Oxygen Administration—cont'd

Description	Nursing Interventions
Venturi Mask • Mask can deliver precise, high-flow rates of O_2. • Lightweight plastic, cone-shaped mask Masks are available for delivery of 24%, 28%, 31%, 35%, 40%, and 50% O_2. • Method is especially helpful for giving low, constant O_2 concentrations to patients with COPD. • Adaptors can increase humidification.	• Entrainment device on mask must be changed to deliver higher concentrations of O_2. • Air entrainment ports must not be occluded. • Uncomfortable. • Must be removed for eating. • Patient can talk but voice may be muffled.

Adjustable nose clip

Opening
Exhaled air

Venturi barrel

Room air

BiPAP, Biphasic positive airway pressure; *COPD,* chronic obstructive pulmonary disease; *CPAP,* continuous positive airway pressure; *FIO₂,* fraction of inspired O_2.

O_2 obtained from O_2 cylinders or wall systems is a dry gas. Dry O_2 has an irritating effect on mucous membranes and dries secretions. Humidification involves adding sterile water, attached to the O_2 delivery device, to prevent breathing dry air. A common device used for humidification when the patient has a cannula or mask is a small plastic jar filled with sterile water called a bubble-through humidifier. It is attached to the O_2 source by a flowmeter.

Complications

O_2 supports combustion and increases the rate of burning. Smoking must be prohibited in any patient care area where O_2 is being used.

- Display a "No Smoking" sign on the patient's door and in any area where O_2 is in use. Caution the patient against smoking with an O_2 cannula in place as it can easily ignite and cause significant burns and life-threatening airway issues.

Chemoreceptors control the drive to breathe. They respond to CO_2 and O_2 concentrations in the blood. Normally, an increase in CO_2 in the blood is a major stimulant of the respiratory center. However, some patients (e.g., COPD) develop a tolerance for high CO_2 levels. As a result, the respiratory center loses its sensitivity to high CO_2 levels. For these patients, a major "drive" to breathe is hypoxemia. As a result, there is concern about the dangers of giving O_2 to COPD patients and reducing their drive (stimulus) to breathe. However, the hypoxic drive is complex and involves many other factors. Not all patients with COPD retain CO_2. Therefore, it is good practice to administer O_2 to any patient who will likely benefit from O_2 therapy, whether they actually need it or not. The danger of not giving O_2 to a patient far outweighs the risk of administering O_2 when it is not needed.

- Pulse oximetry and/or arterial blood gases (ABGs) help to determine what FIO_2 level is needed. The goal is a pulse O_2 saturation (SpO_2) of at least 90% or a PaO_2 of at least 60 mmHg. Assess the patient's mental status and vital signs before starting O_2 therapy and frequently thereafter.

O_2 toxicity may result from prolonged exposure to a high level of O_2 (FIO_2). High O_2 concentrations can result in a severe inflammatory response because O_2 free radicals damage the alveolar-capillary membrane. This can cause severe pulmonary edema, shunting of blood, hypoxemia, and pulmonary edema. Preventing O_2 toxicity is essential. The amount of O_2 administered should be enough to maintain the PaO_2 within a normal or acceptable range for that patient.

- Provide FIO_2 at the lowest possible level, while still maintaining acceptable SpO_2 and PaO_2 values for that specific patient. Monitoring ABGs often helps evaluate the effectiveness of therapy and guide the tapering of supplemental O_2.

Infection can be a complication of O_2 administration. Heated nebulizers present the highest risk. Constant use of humidity supports bacterial growth. Whenever possible, use disposable and single patient use equipment. Follow agency policy about the frequency of equipment changes. See Table 98 for nursing interventions specific to different types of oxygen devices.

A home care guide for teaching the patient and family about home O_2 use is given in Table 104.

TABLE 104 Patient and Caregiver Teaching Home Oxygen Use

Home O_2 Use

The company that provides the O_2 and equipment will teach the patient about O_2 delivery and equipment care. The following are some general instructions that you may include when teaching the patient and caregiver about the use of home O_2.

Patient Care
- Set the O_2 flowrate at the rate your HCP told you to set it at. Do not change the rate without first talking to your HCP.
- If you have any shortness of breath, are lightheaded or dizzy, or develop wheezing, call the HCP right away
- Check to make sure you have enough O_2 on hand for weekends and holidays. The company will tell you how to check the O_2 level and when/how you reorder more O_2.

Decreasing Risk for Infection
- Wash hands before and after using your O_2 therapy.
- Wash nasal cannula (prongs) with a liquid soap and thoroughly rinse once or twice a week.
- Brush teeth or use mouthwash several times a day.
- Ask the company providing the equipment how often to change the tubing and filter.
- Replace cannula every 2–4 weeks.
- If you have a cold, replace the cannula after your symptoms pass.

TABLE 104 Patient and Caregiver Teaching Home Oxygen Use—cont'd

Safety Issues

- Keep O_2 tanks at least 5 feet (1.5 meters) away from any source of heat (e.g., gas stoves, fireplaces)
- Post "No Smoking – Oxygen in Use" warning signs on the front and back doors of your home.
- Do not allow smoking in the home, and do not smoke yourself while wearing O_2. Nasal cannulas and masks can catch fire and cause serious burns to face and airways.
- Store O_2 tanks upright.
- Do not use blankets or fabrics that carry a static charge, such as wool or synthetics.
- Do not use flammable liquids such as paint thinners, cleaning fluids, gasoline, kerosene, oil-based paints, or aerosol sprays while using O_2.
- Inform the staff at your electric company if you are using a concentrator. In case of a power failure, they will know the medical urgency of restoring your power.

PACEMAKERS

Description

The artificial cardiac pacemaker is an electronic device used to pace the heart when the normal conduction pathway is damaged. The basic pacing circuit consists of a power source (battery-powered pulse generator), one or more conducting leads (pacing leads), and the myocardium. The electrical signal (stimulus) travels from the pacemaker, through the leads, to the wall of the myocardium. The heart muscle is stimulated to contract.

Demand pacemakers, which are the most common, sense the heart's electrical activity and fire only when the heart rate (HR) drops below a preset rate. Demand pacemakers have two distinct features: (1) a sensing device that inhibits the pacemaker when the HR is adequate, and (2) a pacing device that triggers the pacemaker when no QRS complexes occur within a preset time. In addition to antibradycardia pacing, devices now include antitachycardia and overdrive pacing.

Permanent pacemakers are implanted entirely within the patient's body. The power source is implanted subcutaneously, usually over the pectoral muscle on the patient's nondominant side. It

TABLE 105 Indications for Permanent Pacemakers

- Acquired AV block
- Second-degree AV block
- Third-degree AV block
- Atrial fibrillation with a slow ventricular response
- Bundle branch block
- Cardiomyopathy (dilated or hypertrophic)
- Heart failure
- SA node dysfunction
- Symptomatic bradycardia with unknown cause
- Tachydysrhythmias (e.g., ventricular tachycardia)

AV, Atrioventricular; *SA,* sinoatrial.

is attached to pacer leads threaded transvenously (through a vein) to the right atrium and one or both ventricles. New technology and research are focused on miniaturized, leadless permanent pacemakers. Common reasons for insertion of a permanent pacemaker are listed in Table 105.

Cardiac resynchronization therapy (CRT) is a pacing technique that resynchronizes the heart cycle by pacing both ventricles (biventricular pacing). This is used to improve ventricular function for patients with heart failure. Patients with severe left ventricular dysfunction may have devices that combine CRT with an implantable cardioverter defibrillator (ICD).

A *temporary pacemaker* has a power source outside the body. Temporary pacemakers are used until short-term cardiac conduction problems resolve or more definitive treatment is available. There are three types of temporary pacemakers: transvenous, epicardial, and transcutaneous. Table 106 lists common reasons for temporary pacing.

- A *transvenous pacemaker* consists of a lead or leads that are threaded transvenously to the right atrium and/or right ventricle and attached to the external power source.
- In *epicardial pacing,* atrial and ventricular pacing leads are attached to the epicardium during heart surgery in case pacing is required during the surgical recovery period. The leads are passed through the chest wall and attached to the external power source.
- A *transcutaneous pacemaker* can provide adequate HR and rhythm in an emergency. External electrode pads are connected to the external power source.

TABLE 106 Common Indications for Temporary Pacemakers

- Maintaining HR and rhythm during special circumstances, such as surgery and postoperative recovery, cardiac catheterization or coronary angioplasty, drug therapy that may cause bradycardia, and before implantation of a permanent pacemaker
- Prophylaxis after open heart surgery
- Acute anterior MI with second- or third-degree AV block or bundle branch block
- Acute inferior MI with symptomatic bradycardia and AV block
- Electrophysiologic studies to evaluate patient with bradydysrhythmias and tachydysrhythmias

AV, Atrioventricular; *HR*, heart rate; *MI*, myocardial infarction.

Nursing Management

Patients with temporary or permanent pacemakers are monitored by electrocardiogram (ECG) to evaluate the status of the pacemaker. Pacemaker malfunction primarily involves a failure to sense or a failure to capture.

- *Failure to sense* occurs when the pacemaker fails to recognize spontaneous atrial or ventricular activity and fires inappropriately. Failure to sense is caused by fibrosis around the tip of the pacing lead, battery failure, sensing set too high, or electrode displacement.
- *Failure to capture* occurs when the electrical charge to the myocardium is insufficient to produce atrial or ventricular contraction. This can result in serious bradycardia or asystole. Failure to capture may be caused by pacer lead fracture, battery failure, electrode displacement, electrical charge set too low, or fibrosis at the electrode tip.
- *Failure to pace* occurs if the pacemaker does not initiate an electrical stimulus when it should fire. This can be caused by a wire fracture, lead displacement, oversensing, or electrical interference.

After permanent pacemaker insertion, the patient can be out of bed once stable. Have the patient limit arm and shoulder activity on the operative side to prevent dislodging the newly implanted pacing leads.

- Observe the insertion site for signs of bleeding, and check that the incision is intact. Note any temperature elevation or pain at the insertion site. Stable patients are discharged by the next day.

- After discharge, patients need to check pacemaker function on a regular basis. This can include outpatient visits to a pacemaker clinic or home monitoring using telephone transmitter devices.
- The goals of pacemaker therapy include enhancing physiologic functioning and quality of life. Emphasize these goals to the patient and the caregiver, and provide specific advice on activity restrictions. Table 107 outlines patient and caregiver teaching about pacemakers.

TABLE 107 Patient and Caregiver Teaching Pacemaker

Include the following information in the teaching plan for a patient with a pacemaker and the patient's caregiver.

1. Maintain follow-up care with your healthcare provider (HCP) to begin regular pacemaker function checks. This is often done by interrogating the device using a telephone.
2. Report any signs of infection at incision site (e.g., redness, swelling, drainage) or fever to your HCP immediately.
3. Keep incision dry for 4 days after implantation, or as ordered.
4. Avoid lifting arm on pacemaker side above shoulder until approved by your cardiologist.
5. Avoid direct blows to pacemaker site.
6. Avoid close proximity to high-output electric generators, since these can interfere with the function of the pacemaker.
7. You should not have an MRI scan unless the pacemaker is approved as MRI-safe or there is a protocol in place for patient safety during the procedure.
8. Microwave ovens are safe to use and do not interfere with pacemaker function.
9. Avoid standing near antitheft devices in doorways of department stores and public libraries. Walk through them at a normal pace.
10. Travel is not restricted. Tell security (e.g., airport, train station, public buildings) of the presence of pacemaker because it may set off the metal detector. Handheld screening wands should not be placed directly over the pacemaker. Manufacturer information may vary about the effect of metal detectors on the function of the pacemaker.
11. Monitor pulse and tell your HCP if heart rate drops below predetermined rate.
12. Always carry pacemaker information card and a current list of your medications.
13. Obtain and wear a Medic Alert ID at all times.
14. Consider joining a pacemaker support group (e.g., https://www.pacemakerclub.com).

PARENTERAL NUTRITION

Description

Parenteral nutrition (PN) is a nutrient solution delivered directly into the bloodstream. PN is used when the gastrointestinal (GI) tract cannot be used for the ingestion, digestion, and absorption of essential nutrients (Table 108).

Administration of Parenteral Nutrition

PN may be administered by central or peripheral routes in the patient who is not a candidate for enteral nutrition (EN). The patient receiving PN must be able to tolerate a large volume of fluid.

- *Central PN* is indicated when the patient needs long-term nutritional support or has high protein and caloric requirements. We give central PN through a central venous catheter or a peripherally inserted central catheter (PICC) whose tip lies in the superior vena cava
- *Peripheral PN* (PPN) is administered using a large-bore catheter in a large peripheral vein. PPN is used when nutritional support is needed for a short time, protein and caloric requirements are not high, the risk of a central catheter is too great, or to supplement inadequate oral intake.

Different commercially prepared PN base solutions are available. Some contain dextrose and protein in the form of amino acids. A 3-in-1 or total nutrient admixture containing an IV fat emulsion, dextrose, and amino acids is widely used. Standard electrolytes (sodium, potassium, chloride, calcium, magnesium, phosphate) are available in some premixed solutions or added by pharmacy. The pharmacy also adds prescribed vitamins and trace elements (zinc, copper, chromium, selenium, manganese) to meet the patient's needs..

P

TABLE 108 Common Indications for Parenteral Nutrition

- Chronic severe diarrhea and vomiting
- Complicated surgery or trauma
- GI obstruction
- GI tract anomalies and fistulas
- Intractable diarrhea
- Severe anorexia nervosa
- Severe malabsorption
- Short bowel syndrome

GI, Gastrointestinal.

TABLE 109 Complications of Parenteral Nutrition

Catheter-Related Problems
- Air embolus
- Catheter-related sepsis
- Dislodgment
- Hemorrhage
- Occlusion
- Phlebitis
- Pneumothorax, hemothorax, and hydrothorax
- Thrombosis of vein

Metabolic Problems
- Altered renal function
- Essential fatty acid deficiency
- Hyperglycemia, hypoglycemia
- Hyperlipidemia
- Liver dysfunction
- Refeeding syndrome

Refeeding syndrome is the body's response to the switch from starvation to a fed state in patients who are severely malnourished. Serious outcomes include dysrhythmias and respiratory arrest.

- Hypophosphatemia is the hallmark of refeeding syndrome. Other manifestations include hyperglycemia, fluid retention, hypokalemia, and hypomagnesemia.
- Conditions that predispose patients to refeeding syndrome include long-standing malnutrition states, such as chronic alcohol use, vomiting and diarrhea, chemotherapy, and major surgery.

Other complications of PN are listed in Table 109.

Home Nutritional Support

Home PN nutrition is an accepted mode of therapy for the person who needs continued nutritional support. Nutritional therapies are expensive. Specific criteria must be met for expenses to be reimbursed. Involve the discharge planning team early on to help address such issues.

- Teach the patient and caregiver about catheter or tube care, proper technique in handling the solutions and tubing, and side effects and complications.
- Tell the family about support groups such as the Oley Foundation (www.oley.org) that provide peer support and advocacy.

RADIATION THERAPY

Description

Radiation therapy is one of the oldest methods of cancer treatment. High-energy beams, when absorbed into tissue, produce ions in the cells. The energy in ionizing radiation breaks the chemical bonds in DNA and causes cell death.

- Radiation doses are expressed in units called a *gray* (Gy) or centigray (cGy). A *centigray* is equal to 1 rad; 100 cGy equals 1 Gy.
- The total radiation dose is divided into daily fractions. Daily doses between 180 and 200 cGy/day are considered standard fractionation. They are typically delivered once a day Monday through Friday for a period of 2–8 weeks, depending on the desired total dose.
- Radiation only affects tissues in the treatment field, so it is not the main treatment for systemic disease. However, radiation therapy may be used alone or in combination with chemotherapy or surgery to treat primary tumors or for palliation of metastatic lesions.
- Radiation can be delivered externally (*external beam radiation therapy*) or internally (*brachytherapy*). *Gamma knife technology* is used to deliver highly accurate stereotactic treatment to a localized treatment volume.

Rapidly dividing cells in the gastrointestinal (GI) tract, oral mucosa, and bone marrow show early acute responses to radiation. Tissues with slowly proliferating cells, such as cartilage, bone, and kidneys, show later responses to radiation. Some cancers are more susceptible to radiation than others (Table 110).

TABLE 110 Tumor Radiosensitivity

High Radiosensitivity	Mild Radiosensitivity
• Hodgkin's lymphoma	• Colon adenocarcinoma
• Neuroblastoma	• Gastric adenocarcinoma
• Non-Hodgkin's lymphoma	• Renal adenocarcinoma
• Ovarian dysgerminoma	• Soft tissue sarcomas
• Testicular seminoma	(e.g., chondrosarcoma)
• Wilms' tumor	
	Poor Radiosensitivity
Moderate Radiosensitivity	• Malignant glioma
• Bladder carcinoma	• Malignant melanoma
• Breast adenocarcinoma	• Osteosarcoma
• Esophageal carcinoma	• Testicular nonseminoma
• Oropharyngeal carcinoma	
• Prostate carcinoma	
• Uterine and cervical carcinoma	

R

Nursing Management: Radiation Therapy and Patient and Caregiver Teaching

See Nursing Management of Chemotherapy and Radiation Therapy.

TRACHEOSTOMY

Description

A *tracheostomy* is a surgically created stoma (opening) in the anterior trachea. It is used to: (1) establish a patent airway, (2) bypass an upper airway obstruction, (3) simplify removal of secretions, (4) permit long-term mechanical ventilation, and (5) facilitate weaning from mechanical ventilation.

Most surgical tracheostomy procedures are done electively in the operating room using general anesthesia. When swelling, trauma, or upper airway obstruction prevents endotracheal intubation, an *emergent cricothyroidotomy* (also known as a "cricothyrotomy") involves making an incision through the skin and cricothyroid membrane on the anterior neck.

A *percutaneous tracheostomy* can be performed using local anesthesia and sedation and analgesia. A needle is placed into the trachea, followed by a guide wire. The opening is progressively dilated until it is large enough for insertion of a tracheostomy tube.

- A tracheostomy tube provides a more secure airway and allows more freedom of movement than an endotracheal tube. The tracheostomy tube is shorter in length and slightly wider in diameter than an ET tube. This makes it easier to keep the tube clean and promotes better oral and bronchial hygiene. A tracheostomy (compared to an ET tube) may increase patient comfort because no tube is present in the mouth. There is also less risk of long-term damage to vocal cords.

A variety of tracheostomy tubes are available to meet patient needs (see Fig. 38).

- *Cuffed* and *uncuffed* tracheostomy tubes are available. A tracheostomy tube with an inflated cuff is used the most, especially if the patient needs mechanical ventilation. Cuffs ensure the patient receives the volume of air delivered by the ventilator and decrease the risk of aspiration. Cuffless tubes are often used for patients with longer-term tracheostomies, when mechanical ventilation is not needed, and the risk of aspiration has decreased. With some tracheostomies, talking and eating are possible.

Fig. 38 Tracheostomy tube. (A) Tracheostomy tube inserted in airway with inflated cuff. (B) Parts of a tracheostomy tube.

- The outer and/or inner cannula may be *fenestrated* or *non-fenestrated*. A fenestrated tube has an opening (a hole) on the dorsal surface of the tube. This helps promote spontaneous breathing. With a cuffed, fenestrated tracheostomy tube, when the cuff is deflated and the inner cannula removed, air can pass from the lungs up through the opening in the tracheostomy tube and through the vocal cords (including larynx) and into the upper airway (including the mouth and nose). This allows the patient to breathe spontaneously and speak with the tracheostomy tube in place. When the cuff is reinflated and the inner cannula reinserted, air cannot pass from the lungs through the vocal cords.

Nursing Management

Before the tracheostomy, explain the purpose of the procedure and inform the patient and family that the patient will not be able to speak if an inflated cuff is used. Do not dislodge the tracheostomy tube during the first 5–7 days, when the stoma is not healed.

- Because tube replacement is difficult, several precautions are required: (1) keep a replacement tube of equal or smaller size at the bedside, readily available for emergency reinsertion; (2) do not change tracheostomy tapes for at least 24 hours after the insertion procedure; and (3) let a healthcare provider (HCP) perform the first tube change, usually no sooner than 7 days after the tracheostomy.
- If the tube is accidently dislodged, immediately attempt to replace it. Insert the obturator in the replacement tube, lubricate with saline, and insert the tube into the stoma. Once the tube is inserted, remove the obturator at once so that air can flow through the tube.
- If the tube cannot be replaced because of tract immaturity (less than 1 week old) or other circumstances, immediately place the patient in semi-Fowler's position to decrease dyspnea. Cover the stoma with a sterile dressing and ventilate the patient with the BVM over the nose and mouth.
- If a patient has had a total laryngectomy, there will be complete separation between the upper airway and trachea. Ventilate this patient through the tracheostomy stoma.

Care of the patient with a tracheostomy involves suctioning the airway to remove secretions, cleaning around the stoma, changing tracheostomy ties, and inner cannula care if a nondisposable inner cannula is used. See Table 111 for a detailed description of tracheostomy care.

TABLE 111   Tracheostomy Care

The following are general guidelines for basic tracheostomy care. Become familiar with the specific policies and/or procedures in your institution.

1. Explain procedure to patient.
2. Use tracheostomy care kit or collect sterile equipment (e.g., suction catheter, one pair of sterile gloves, one pair of nonsterile gloves, water basin, tracheostomy ties, tube brush or pipe cleaners, 4 × 4-inch gauze pads, sterile water or normal saline, tracheostomy dressing [optional]).
   • Note: Clean technique is used for the patient with a tracheostomy at home.
3. Position patient in semi-Fowler's position.
4. Assemble supplies on bedside table.
5. Wash hands. Put on PPE.
6. Open sterile equipment. Pour sterile H_2O or normal saline into two compartments of sterile container or two basins, then apply sterile gloves.
7. If present, unlock and remove inner cannula. Many tracheostomy tubes do not have inner cannulas. Care for these tubes includes all steps listed below, except for inner cannula care.
8. Inner cannula care
   • Disposable: If using a disposable inner cannula, replace with new cannula.
   • Non-Disposable:
     • Immerse inner cannula in sterile solution and clean inside and outside of cannula using tube brush or pipe cleaners.
     • Rinse cannula in sterile solution. Remove from solution and shake to dry. Insert inner cannula into outer cannula with the curved part downward, and lock in place.
9. Stoma care: Remove dried secretions from stoma using 4 × 4-inch gauze pad soaked in sterile water or saline. Gently pat area around the stoma dry. Be sure to clean under the tracheostomy flange (faceplate), using cotton swabs to reach this area.

After the tracheostomy tube from a temporary tracheostomy is removed, apply a sterile occlusive dressing and monitor the site for bleeding. Instruct the patient to splint the stoma with the fingers when coughing, swallowing, or speaking. The opening closes in a few days.

▼ **Patient and Caregiver Teaching**

■ Assess ability of the patient and caregiver to provide care at home.

T

- Include instructions for tracheostomy tube care, stoma care, suctioning, airway care, and responding to emergencies.
- Make a referral to a home healthcare nurse to provide ongoing assistance and support.
- Teach patient and caregiver the signs and symptoms to report to healthcare professionals, such as changes in secretions (color and consistency) and elevated temperature.

URINARY CATHETERIZATION

Indications for short-term urinary catheterization are listed in Table 112. The risk of infection is too high to perform catheterization for routine acquisition of a urine specimen for laboratory analysis or the convenience of the healthcare team or caregivers. Catheterization for sterile urine specimens may be needed if the patient has a history of complicated urinary tract infection (UTI). A catheter should be the last resort to provide the patient with a dry environment to prevent skin breakdown and protect dressings or skin lesions.

- Complications seen with long-term use (more than 28 days) of indwelling catheters include catheter-associated urinary tract infection (CAUTI), bladder spasms, periurethral abscess, chronic pyelonephritis, urosepsis, urethral trauma or erosion, fistula or stricture formation, and stones. CAUTIs are the most common HAI.

Aseptic technique is mandatory when inserting a urinary catheter. See Table 113 for urinary catheter management. Address patient concerns, which may include embarrassment, an altered body image, and fear that the catheter will result in increased dependency.

- Catheters vary in materials, tip shape, and lumen size. Catheters coated with antimicrobial agents may prevent CAUTIs.
- Catheters are sized according to the French scale. Each French unit (F) equals 0.33 mm of diameter. The diameter listed is the internal diameter of the catheter. The size used varies with the patient's size and the purpose of catheterization. In women, urethral catheter sizes 10F–12F are the most common. In men, sizes 14F–16F are used. Balloon sizes are 5 or 30 mL.

The most common route of catheterization is *urethral catheterization*, insertion of the catheter through the external meatus into the urethra, past the internal sphincter, and into the bladder.

Suprapubic catheterization requires surgical placement through an open approach with a small incision made in the abdominal wall

TABLE 112 Indications for Urinary Catheterization

U

Indwelling Catheter

- Relieve urinary retention caused by lower urinary tract obstruction, paralysis, or inability to void
- Bladder decompression preoperatively and operatively for lower abdominal or pelvic surgery
- Facilitate surgical repair of urethra and surrounding structures
- Splinting of ureters or urethra to facilitate healing after surgery or other trauma in area
- Accurate measurement of urine output
- Contamination of stage III or IV pressure ulcers with urine that has impeded healing, despite appropriate personal care for the incontinence
- Terminal illness or severe impairment, which makes positioning or clothing changes uncomfortable, or which is associated with intractable pain

Intermittent (Straight, in-and-out) Catheter

- Relieve urinary retention caused by lower urinary tract obstruction, paralysis, or inability to void
- Study of anatomic structures of urinary system
- Urodynamic testing
- Collect sterile urine sample in certain situations
- Instill medications into bladder
- Measure residual urine after voiding (postvoid residual [PVR]) if portable ultrasound not available

or through a percutaneous approach. The catheter is placed while the patient is under general anesthesia for another procedure or at the bedside with a local anesthetic. The catheter may be sutured in place.

- The care of the suprapubic catheter is similar to that of the urethral catheter. Tape the catheter to prevent dislodgement. A pectin-based skin barrier (e.g., Stomahesive) is effective in protecting the skin around the insertion site from breakdown.
- A suprapubic catheter is prone to poor drainage because of mechanical obstruction of the catheter tip by the bladder wall, sediment, and clots. To ensure patency of the tube: (1) prevent tube kinking by coiling the excess tubing and maintaining gravity drainage, (2) have the patient turn from side to side, and (3) milk the tube. If these measures are not effective, obtain a

TABLE 113 Care of the Patient With a Urethral Catheter

The following measures can be used to manage the patient with a urethral catheter and prevent catheter-associated urinary tract infection (CAUTI).

- Determine need for catheterization, but HCP must order.
- Choose appropriate type and size of catheter.
- Insert catheter using sterile technique.
- Develop plan of care to decrease risk for CAUTI.
- Teach catheter care to the patient, especially one who is ambulatory.
- Maintain a sterile, closed drainage system.
- Do not disconnect the distal urinary catheter and proximal drainage tube except for catheter irrigation (if ordered).
- Use sterile technique whenever the collecting system is open. If frequent irrigations are needed in short-term catheterization to maintain catheter patency, a triple-lumen catheter may be preferable, permitting continuous irrigations within a closed system.
- A routine catheter change is not needed if the patient is catheterized for less than 2 weeks. For long-term use of an indwelling catheter, replace the catheter based on patient assessment and not on a routine changing schedule.
- If ordered, aspirate small volumes of urine for culture from the catheter sampling port using a sterile syringe and needle. Prepare the puncture site with an antiseptic solution.
- With long-term use of a catheter, a leg bag may be used. If the collection bag is reused, wash it in soap and water and rinse thoroughly. When it is not reused immediately, fill it with ½ cup of vinegar and drain. Vinegar is effective against *Pseudomonas* and other organisms and eliminates odors.
- Remove the catheter as early as possible. Intermittent catheterization and external catheters are alternatives that have less risk of CAUTI.
- Ensure that APs:
  - Maintain unobstructed downhill flow of urine.
  - Empty the collecting bag regularly and accurately record the urine output.
  - Provide perineal care (once or twice a day and when needed), cleaning the meatus-catheter junction with soap and water.
  - Do not use lotion or powder near the catheter.
  - Anchor catheter using a securement device. Anchor catheter to upper thigh in women and lower abdomen in men to prevent catheter movement and urethral tension.

healthcare provider's (HCP's) order to irrigate the catheter with sterile technique.

■ Bladder spasms may cause urinary leakage. Oxybutynin or solifenacin can decrease bladder spasms.

A *ureteral catheter* is often called a *ureteral stent*. It is placed through the ureters into the renal pelvis. The catheter is inserted either by being threaded up the urethra and bladder to the ureters under cystoscopic observation or by surgical insertion through the abdominal wall into the ureters. The ureteral catheter is used either during surgery with removal immediately afterward or after surgery to splint the ureters and prevent them from being obstructed by edema. Care of these catheters is similar to that of urethral catheters. Avoid situations that could cause dislodgement or displacement of the catheter.

■ If the output from a ureteral catheter is decreased, notify the HCP immediately.

An alternative approach to a long-term indwelling catheter is *intermittent catheterization* of the urethra, also referred to as "straight" or "in-and-out" catheterization. The main goal of intermittent catheterization is to prevent urinary retention, stasis, and compromised blood supply to the bladder caused by prolonged pressure. It is used in conditions such as neurogenic bladder.

■ A urethral catheter is inserted into the bladder every 3–5 hours. Some patients perform intermittent catheterization only once or twice each day to measure residual urine and ensure an empty bladder.

■ Instruct patients to wash and rinse the catheter and their hands with soap and water before and after catheterization. Using a lubricant makes catheterization more comfortable and minimizes trauma.

■ The patient, caregiver, or HCP may insert the catheter.

■ In the hospital or long-term care facility, sterile technique is used for catheterizations. For home care, a clean technique that includes good hand washing with soap and water is used.

■ Teach the patient to observe for signs of UTI so that treatment can be instituted early.

PART THREE

Reference Appendix

ABBREVIATIONS

A

ABG	arterial blood gas
ACE	angiotensin-converting enzyme
ACLS	advanced cardiac life support
ACS	acute coronary syndrome
ACTH	adrenocorticotropic hormone
ADH	antidiuretic hormone
AED	automated external defibrillator
AIDS	acquired immunodeficiency syndrome
AKA	above-knee amputation
AKI	acute kidney injury
ALL	acute lymphocytic leukemia
ALS	amyotrophic lateral sclerosis
AMI	acute myocardial infarction
ANA	antinuclear antibody
ANS	autonomic nervous system
AORN	Association of periOperative Registered Nurses
APD	automated peritoneal dialysis
aPTT	activated partial thromboplastin time
ARDS	acute respiratory distress syndrome
ATN	acute tubular necrosis
BCLS	basic cardiac life support
BKA	below-knee amputation
BMI	body mass index
BMR	basal metabolic rate
BMT	bone marrow transplantation
BPH	benign prostatic hyperplasia
BSE	breast self-examination
BUN	blood urea nitrogen
CABG	coronary artery bypass graft
CAD	coronary artery disease; circulatory assist device
CAPD	continuous ambulatory peritoneal dialysis
CAVH	continuous arteriovenous hemofiltration
CBC	complete blood count
CCU	coronary care unit; critical care unit
CDC	Centers for Disease Control and Prevention
CIS	carcinoma in situ
CKD	chronic kidney disease
CLL	chronic lymphocytic leukemia
CML	chronic myelocytic leukemia

Continued

ABBREVIATIONS—cont'd

CMP	cardiomyopathy
CN	cranial nerve
CNS	central nervous system
CO	cardiac output
COPD	chronic obstructive pulmonary disease
CPAP	continuous positive airway pressure
CPR	cardiopulmonary resuscitation
CRRT	continuous renal replacement therapy
CRNA	certified registered nurse anesthetist
CSF	cerebrospinal fluid
CT	computed tomography
CVA	cerebrovascular accident; costovertebral angle
CVAD	central venous access device
CVI	chronic venous insufficiency
CVP	central venous pressure
D&C	dilation and curettage
DDD	degenerative disc disease
DI	diabetes insipidus
DIC	disseminated intravascular coagulation
DJD	degenerative joint disease
DKA	diabetic ketoacidosis
DM	diabetes mellitus; diastolic murmur
DRE	digital rectal examination
DVT	deep vein thrombosis
ECF	extracellular fluid
ECG	electrocardiogram
ED	emergency department; erectile dysfunction
EEG	electroencephalogram
EMG	electromyogram
ENT	ear, nose, and throat
ERCP	endoscopic retrograde cholangiopancreatography
ERS	emergency response system
ESR	erythrocyte sedimentation rate
ESRD	end-stage renal disease
ET	endotracheal
FEV	forced expiratory volume
FRC	functional residual capacity
FUO	fever of unknown origin
GCS	Glasgow Coma Scale

ABBREVIATIONS—cont'd

GERD	gastroesophageal reflux disease
GFR	glomerular filtration rate
GH	growth hormone
GTT	glucose tolerance test
GU	genitourinary
GYN, Gyn	gynecologic
H&P	history and physical examination
HAV	hepatitis A virus
HBV	hepatitis B virus
HCP	health care provider
Hct	hematocrit
HCV	hepatitis C virus
HD	hemodialysis; Huntington's disease
HDL	high-density lipoprotein
HF	heart failure
Hgb	hemoglobin
HIV	human immunodeficiency virus
HPV	human papillomavirus
HSCT	hematopoietic stem cell transplantation
I&D	incision and drainage
IABP	intraaortic balloon pump
IBS	irritable bowel syndrome
ICP	intracranial pressure
IE	infective endocarditis
IFG	impaired fasting glucose
IGT	impaired glucose tolerance
INR	international normalized ratio
IOP	intraocular pressure
IPPB	intermittent positive pressure breathing
ITP	idiopathic thrombocytopenic purpura
IUD	intrauterine device
IV	intravenous
IVP	intravenous push
JVD	jugular venous distention
KUB	kidney, ureters, and bladder (x-ray)
KS	Kaposi sarcoma
KVO	keep vein open
LAD	left anterior descending
LDL	low-density lipoprotein

Continued

ABBREVIATIONS—cont'd

LLQ	left lower quadrant
LMN	lower motor neuron
LMP	last menstrual period
LOC	level of consciousness
LP	lumbar puncture
LUQ	left upper quadrant
LVH	left ventricular hypertrophy
MAP	mean arterial pressure
MD	muscular dystrophy
MDS	myelodysplastic syndrome
MG	myasthenia gravis
MI	myocardial infarction
MICU	medical intensive care unit
MODS	multiple organ dysfunction syndrome
MRB	manual resuscitation bag
MS	multiple sclerosis
MVP	mitral valve prolapse
NAFLD	nonalcoholic fatty liver disease
NASH	nonalcoholic steatohepatitis
NG	nasogastric
NHL	non-Hodgkin's lymphoma
NPO	nothing by mouth
NS	normal saline
NSR	normal sinus rhythm
OA	osteoarthritis
OD	right eye; optical density; overdose
OOB	out of bed
OR	operating room
ORIF	open reduction and internal fixation
OS	left eye
OSA	obstructive sleep apnea
OTC	over-the-counter
PA	posteroanterior; physician's assistant
PAC	premature atrial contraction
$PaCO_2$	partial pressure of carbon dioxide in arterial blood
PaO_2	partial pressure of oxygen in arterial blood
PACU	postanesthesia care unit
PAD	peripheral artery disease
PAP	pulmonary artery pressure

ABBREVIATIONS—cont'd

A

PAWP	pulmonary artery wedge pressure
PCA	patient-controlled analgesia
PCI	percutaneous coronary intervention
PCO_2	partial pressure of carbon dioxide
PCWP	pulmonary capillary wedge pressure
PD	Parkinson's disease; peritoneal dialysis
PE	pulmonary embolism; physical examination
PEEP	positive end-expiratory pressure
PEFR	peak expiratory flow rate
PERRLA	pupils equal, round, and reactive to light and accommodation
PET	positron emission tomography
PICC	peripherally inserted central catheter
PID	pelvic inflammatory disease
PKD	polycystic kidney disease
PMH	past medical history
PMI	point of maximal impulse
PMS	premenstrual syndrome
PN	parenteral nutrition
PND	paroxysmal nocturnal dyspnea
PNS	peripheral nervous system
PO, po	orally
PO_2	partial pressure of oxygen
POC	point-of-care
PPD	purified protein derivative
PSA	prostate-specific antigen
PT	prothrombin time
PTT	partial thromboplastin time
PVC	premature ventricular contraction
PUD	peptic ulcer disease
R/O	rule out
RA	rheumatoid arthritis
REM	rapid eye movement
RF	rheumatic fever
RHD	rheumatic heart disease
RLQ	right lower quadrant
RLS	restless legs syndrome
ROM	range of motion
ROS	review of systems

Continued

ABBREVIATIONS—cont'd

RUQ	right upper quadrant
SA	sinoatrial
SCD	sickle cell disease; sudden cardiac death
SCI	spinal cord injury
SDB	sleep-disordered breathing
SICU	surgical intensive care unit
SIRS	systemic inflammatory response syndrome
SLE	systemic lupus erythematosus
SNS	sympathetic nervous system
SOB	shortness of breath
STI	sexually transmitted infection
SVR	systemic vascular resistance
SVT	superficial vein thrombosis
TAH	total abdominal hysterectomy
TB	tuberculosis
TBSA	total body surface area
TCDB	turn, cough, and deep breathe
TENS	transcutaneous electrical nerve stimulation
THR	total hip replacement
TIA	transient ischemic attack
TJC	The Joint Commission
TKO	to keep open
TNM	tumor, node, metastasis
TPR	temperature, pulse, and respirations
TURP	transurethral resection of the prostate
UA	unstable angina
UAP	unlicensed assistive personnel
UGI	upper gastrointestinal
UI	urinary incontinence
UMN	upper motor neuron
URI	upper respiratory infection
UTI	urinary tract infection
VAD	venous access device; ventricular assist device
VDH	valvular disease of the heart
VF	ventricular fibrillation
VS	vital signs
VT	ventricular tachycardia
VTE	venous thromboembolism
WHR	waist-to-hip ratio
WNL	within normal limits

THE JOINT COMMISSION OFFICIAL "DO NOT USE" LIST

Do Not Use[a]	Potential Problem	Use Instead
U, u (unit)	Mistaken for "0" (zero), the number "4" (four) or "cc"	Write "unit"
IU (International Unit)	Mistaken for IV (intravenous) or the number 10 (ten)	Write "International Unit"
Q.D., QD, q.d., qd (daily)	Mistaken for each other	Write "daily"
Q.O.D., QOD, q.o.d., qod (every other day)	Period after the Q mistaken for "I" and the "O" mistaken for "I"	Write "every other day"
Trailing zero (X.0 mg)[b]	Decimal point is missed	Write X mg
Lack of leading zero (.X mg)		Write 0.X mg
MS	Can mean morphine sulfate or magnesium sulfate	Write "morphine sulfate"
MSO_4 and $MgSO_4$	Confused for one another	Write "magnesium sulfate"

[a]Applies to all orders and all medication-related documentation that is handwritten (including free-text computer entry) or on preprinted forms.
[b]Exception: a "trailing zero" may be used only where required to demonstrate the level of precision of the value being reported, such as for laboratory results, imaging studies that report size of lesions, or catheter/tube sizes. It may not be used in medication orders or other medication-related documentation.

Additional Abbreviations, Acronyms, and Symbols

Do Not Use	Potential Problem	Use Instead
> (greater than) < (less than)	Misinterpreted as the number "7" (seven) or the letter "L" confused for one another	Write "greater than" Write "less than"
Abbreviations for drug names	Misinterpreted because of similar abbreviations for multiple drugs	Write drug names in full
Apothecary units	Unfamiliar to many practitioners. Confused with metric units	Use metric units
@	Mistaken for the number "2" (two)	Write "at"
cc	Mistaken for U (units) when poorly written	Write "mL" or "ml" or "milliliters" ("mL" is preferred)
Mg	Mistaken for mg (milligrams), resulting in 1000-fold overdose	Write "mcg" or "micrograms"

BLOOD GASES

NORMAL VALUES

	Arterial (Sea Level)
pH	7.35–7.45
PaO_2[a]	80–100 mm Hg (10.6–13.33 kPa)
$PaCO_2$	35–45 mm Hg (4.66–5.98 kPa)
HCO_3	21–28 mEq/L (21–28 mmol/L)
O_2 saturation	>95%

[a]In a patient >60 years of age, normal PaO_2 is equal to 80 mm Hg minus 1 mm Hg for every year over 60. When supplemental oxygen is provided, expected PaO_2 = $FIO_2 \times 5$.

Interpreting Arterial Blood Gases (ABGs)

1. Check pH
   ↑ = Alkalosis; ↓ = acidosis
2. Check $PaCO_2$
   ↑ = CO_2 retention (hypoventilation); respiratory acidosis or compensating for metabolic alkalosis
   ↓ = CO_2 blown off (hyperventilation); respiratory alkalosis or compensating for metabolic acidosis
3. Check HCO_3
   ↑ = Nonvolatile acid is lost; HCO_3 is gained (metabolic alkalosis or compensating for respiratory acidosis)
   ↓ = Nonvolatile acid is added; HCO_3 is lost (metabolic acidosis or compensating for respiratory alkalosis)
4. Determine imbalance
5. Determine if compensation exists

DETERMINING THE IMBALANCE IN ABGS

If pH ↑ and $PaCO_2$ ↓ or pH ↓ and $PaCO_2$ ↑	then respiratory disorder
If pH ↑ and HCO_3 ↑ or pH ↓ and HCO_3 ↓	then metabolic disorder
If $paCO_2$ ↑ and HCO_3 ↑ or $paCO_2$ ↓ and HCO_3 ↓	then compensation is occurring
If $paCO_2$ ↑ and HCO_3 ↓ or $paCO_2$ ↓ and HCO_3 ↓	then mixed imbalance

BLOOD PRODUCTS

Description	Special considerations	Indications for use
Albumin		
Prepared from plasma. Can be stored for 5 year. Available in 5% or 25% solution. Heat treated. Does not transmit viruses.	Albumin 25% expands the blood volume by about 3.5 times. Hyperosmolar solution acts by moving water from extravascular to intravascular space.	Hypovolemic shock, hypoalbuminemia, after large-volume paracentesis, replacement in plasmapheresis.
Cryoprecipitates and commercial concentrates		
Prepared from fresh frozen plasma. 10–15 mL/bag. Can be stored for 1 year. Once thawed, must be used within 4–6 h.		Replacement for fibrinogen deficiency, usually due to DIC, severe liver disease, or massive transfusion. Has other clotting factors, especially factor VIII, factor XIII, and von Willebrand factor.
Fresh frozen plasma		
Liquid part of whole blood is separated from cells and frozen. 1 unit is about 250 mL. Rich in clotting factors but has no platelets. Can be stored for up to 1 year, depending on storage. Must be used within 24 h after thawing.	Use in treating hemorrhagic shock is being replaced by pure preparations, such as albumin and plasma expanders.	Bleeding caused by deficiency in clotting factors (e.g., DIC, bleeding, massive transfusion, liver disease, vitamin K deficiency, excess warfarin).

Description	Special considerations	Indications for use
Frozen RBCs		
Prepared from RBCs using glycerol for protection and frozen. Can be stored for up to 10 year.	Successive washings with saline solution remove most WBCs and plasma proteins.	Autotransfusion. Stockpiling or rare donors for patients with alloantibodies.
Packed RBCs		
Prepared from whole blood by sedimentation or centrifugation. 1 unit is 250–350 mL. Can be stored up to 42 days depending on processing (anticoagulants and preservatives).	Use of RBCs for treatment allows remaining components of blood (e.g., platelets, albumin, plasma) to be used for other purposes. Less risk of fluid overload. Preferred RBC source because they are more component specific. Leukocyte depletion (leukoreduction) by filtration, washing is frequently used, Decreases non-hemolytic febrile or mild allergic reactions in patients who receive frequent transfusions. Reduces transmission of viruses. Irradiation prevents graft versus host disease in immunocompromised patients.	Severe or symptomatic anemia, acute blood loss. 1 unit of RBCs can be expected to ↑ Hgb by 1 g/dL or Hct by 3% in a typical adult. 1 unit can replace a blood loss of 500 mL.

Continued

B

BLOOD PRODUCTS—cont'd

Description	Special considerations	Indications for use
Platelets Prepared from fresh whole blood. An apheresed single donation is usually 200–400 mL in volume. May be pooled from multiple donors.	Can obtain multiple units from 1 donor by plateletpheresis. Can be kept at room temperature in the blood bank under gentle agitation for 1–5 days depending on type of collection and storage. For patients who receive frequent transfusions and become refractory, may give leukocyte reduced, HLA, or type specific to prevent alloimmunization to HLA antigens.	Bleeding caused by thrombocytopenia. May be contraindicated in TTP and HITT except in life-threatening hemorrhage. Average corrected count increment is 10×10^9/L. Failure to have an increase may be due to fever, sepsis, splenomegaly, or DIC or development of antibodies (*refractory*).

DIC, Disseminated intravascular coagulation; *Hct,* hematocrit; *Hgb,* hemoglobin; *HITT,* heparin-induced thrombocytopenia and thrombotic syndrome; *HLA,* human leukocyte antigen; *RBC,* red blood cell; *WBC,* white blood cell.

BREATH SOUNDS

Auscultation finding	Description	Common etiology and significance
Absent breath sounds	No sound heard over entire lung or area of lung	Pneumothorax, pleural effusion, mainstem bronchi obstruction, large atelectasis, pneumonectomy, lobectomy
Bronchophony, whispered pectoriloquy	Spoken or whispered syllable more distinct than normal on auscultation	Pneumonia
Coarse crackles	Louder, discontinuous, low-pitched sounds caused by air passing through airway intermittently occluded by mucus, unstable bronchial wall. May be heard on inspiration, expiration, or both. Similar sound to blowing through straw under water	Excess fluid within the lungs, heart failure, pulmonary edema, pneumonia with severe congestion, COPD
Egophony	Spoken "E" similar to "A" on auscultation because of altered transmission of voice sounds	Pneumonia, pleural effusion
Fine crackles	Short, discontinuous, high-pitched sounds heard just before the end of inspiration. Result of rapid equalization of gas pressure when collapsed alveoli or terminal bronchioles suddenly snap open. Similar sound to that made by rolling hair between fingers	Interstitial edema (early pulmonary edema), alveolar filling (pneumonia), loss of lung volume (atelectasis), early phase of heart failure, idiopathic pulmonary fibrosis

Continued

B

BREATH SOUNDS—cont'd

Auscultation finding	Description	Common etiology and significance
Pleural friction rub	Creaking or grating sound from roughened, inflamed pleural surfaces rubbing together. Evident during inspiration, expiration, or both. No change with coughing. Often uncomfortable, especially on deep inspiration	Pleurisy, pneumonia, pulmonary infarct
Stridor	Continuous musical or crowing sound of constant pitch. Result of partial obstruction of larynx or trachea	Croup, epiglottitis, vocal cord edema after extubation, foreign body
Wheezes	Continuous high-pitched squeaking or musical sound caused by rapid vibration of bronchial walls. First evident on expiration but possibly evident on inspiration as obstruction of airway increases. May be audible without stethoscope	Bronchospasm (caused by asthma), airway obstruction (caused by foreign body, tumor), COPD

COPD, Chronic obstructive pulmonary disease.

COMMONLY USED FORMULAS

Parameter	Formula	Normal range
Anion gap	$Na - \left(HCO_3^+ + Cl\right)$	8–16 mEq/L
Body mass index (BMI)	$\dfrac{\text{Weight in pounds}}{\text{Height inches}^2} \times 703$	18.5–24.9 kg/m^2
Cardiac index (CI)	$\dfrac{CO}{\text{Body surface area (BSA)}}$	2.2–4.0 L/min/m^2
Cardiac output (CO)	$HR \times SV$	4–8 L/min
Cerebral perfusion pressure (CPP)	$MAP - ICP$	80–100 mm Hg
Ejection fraction (EF)	$\dfrac{SV}{\text{End} - \text{diastolic volume}} \times 100$	55% or greater
Mean arterial pressure (MAP)	$\dfrac{2(DBP) + SBP}{3}$	70–105 mm Hg
Stroke volume (SV)	$\dfrac{CO}{HR}$	60–150 mL/beat

DBP, Diastolic blood pressure; *HR,* heart rate; *ICP,* intracranial pressure; *SBP,* systolic blood pressure.

C

CHARACTERISTICS OF COMMON DYSRHYTHMIAS

Normal rhythm/ Dysrhythmia	Rate and rhythm	PATTERN		
		P wave	PR interval	QRS complex
Normal sinus rhythm (NSR)	60–100 beats/min and regular	Normal	Normal	Normal
Sinus bradycardia	<60 beats/min and regular	Normal	Normal	Normal
Sinus tachycardia	101–200 beats/min and regular	Normal	Normal	Normal
Premature atrial contraction (PAC)	Usually 60–100 beats/ min and irregular	Abnormal shape	Normal	Normal (usually)
Paroxysmal supraventricular tachycardia (PSVT)	150–220 beats/min and regular	Abnormal shape, may be hidden in the preceding T wave	Normal or shortened	Normal (usually)
Atrial flutter	Atrial: 200–350 beats/min and regular Ventricular: > or < 100 beats/min and may be regular or irregular	Flutter (F) waves (sawtoothed pattern); more flutter waves than with QRS complexes. May occur in a 2:1, 3:1, 4:1 (etc.) pattern	Not measurable	Normal (usually)

Atrial fibrillation	*Atrial:* 350–600 beats/min and irregular *Ventricular:* > or < 100 beats/min and irregular	Fibrillatory (f) waves	Not measurable	Normal (usually)
Junctional dysrhythmias	40–180 beats/min and regular	Inverted; may be hidden in QRS complex	Shortened, if present	Normal (usually)
First-degree AV block	Normal and regular	Normal	>0.20 s	Normal
Second-degree AV block				
• Type I (Mobitz I, Wenckebach heart block)	*Atrial:* Normal and regular *Ventricular:* Slower and irregular	Normal	Progressive lengthening	Normal QRS width, with pattern of 1 nonconducted (blocked) QRS complex
• Type II (Mobitz II heart block)	*Atrial:* Usually normal and regular *Ventricular:* Slower and regular or irregular	More P waves than QRS complexes (e.g., 2:1, 3:1)	Normal or prolonged but consistent for every QRS	Widened QRS, preceded by ≥ 2 P waves, with nonconducted (blocked) QRS complex

C

CHARACTERISTICS OF COMMON DYSRHYTHMIAS—cont'd

Normal rhythm/ Dysrhythmia	Rate and rhythm	PATTERN		
		P wave	PR interval	QRS complex
Third-degree AV block (complete heart block)	*Atrial:* Regular but may appear irregular because of P waves hidden in QRS complexes *Ventricular:* 20–60 beats/min and regular	Normal, but no connection with QRS complex	Inconsistent	Normal or widened, no relationship with P waves
Premature ventricular contraction (PVC)	PVCs occur at variable rates underlying rhythm can be regular or irregular	Not usually visible, hidden in the PVC	Not measurable	Wide and distorted
Ventricular tachycardia (VT)	150–250 beats/min and regular or irregular	Not usually visible	Not measurable	Wide and distorted
Accelerated idioventricular rhythm	40–100 beats/min and regular	Not usually visible	Not measurable	Wide and distorted
Ventricular fibrillation (VF)	Not measurable and irregular	Absent	Not measurable	Not measurable

AV, Atrioventricular.

ELECTROCARDIOGRAM (ECG) MONITORING

ECG Waveforms and Normal Sinus Rhythm

ECG WAVEFORMS AND INTERVALS AND SOURCES OF POTENTIAL VARIATIONS[a]

Description	Normal duration (sec)	Source of possible variation
P wave		
Represents time for the passage of the electrical impulse through the atrium causing atrial depolarization (contraction). Should be upright.	0.06–0.12	Disturbance in conduction within atria
PR interval		
Measured from beginning of P wave to beginning of QRS complex. Represents time taken for impulse to spread through the atria, AV node and bundle of His, bundle branches, and Purkinje fibers, to a point immediately before ventricular contraction.	0.12–0.20	Disturbance in conduction usually in AV node, bundle of His, or bundle branches but can be in atria as well
QRS complex		
Q wave: first negative (downward) deflection after the P wave, short and narrow, not present in several leads.	<0.03	MI may result in development of a pathologic Q wave that is wide (≥0.03 s) and deep (≥25% of the height of the R wave)
R wave: first positive (upward) deflection in the QRS complex.	Not usually measured	
S wave: First negative (downward) deflection after the R wave.	Not usually measured	

Description	Normal duration (sec)	Source of possible variation
QRS interval Measured from beginning to end of QRS complex. Represents time taken for depolarization (contraction) of both ventricles (systole).	<0.12	Disturbance in conduction in bundle branches or in ventricles
ST segment Measured from the S wave of the QRS complex to the beginning of the T wave. Represents the time between ventricular depolarization and repolarization (diastole). Should be isoelectric (flat).	0.12	Disturbances (e.g., elevation, depression) usually caused by ischemia, injury, or infarction
T wave Represents time for ventricular repolarization. Should be upright.	0.16	Disturbances (e.g., tall, peaked; inverted) usually caused by electrolyte imbalances, ischemia, or infarction
QT interval[b] Measured from beginning of QRS complex to end of T wave. Represents time taken for entire electrical depolarization and repolarization of the ventricles. Normal adult women have slightly longer QT intervals than men.	0.34–0.43	Disturbances usually affecting repolarization more than depolarization and caused by drugs, electrolyte imbalances, and changes in heart rate

AV, Atrioventricular; *MI,* myocardial infarction.

[a]Heart rate influences the duration of these intervals, especially the PR and QT intervals (e.g., QT interval shortens in duration as heart rate increases).

[b]A corrected QT interval (QTc) is calculated to account for the influence of heart rate.

E

GLASGOW COMA SCALE

Appropriate stimulus	Response	Score
Eyes open		
Approach to bedside	Spontaneous response	4
Verbal command	Opening of eyes to name or command	3
Pain	Lack of opening of eyes to previous stimuli but opening to pain	2
	Lack of opening of eyes to any stimulus	1
	Untestable[a]	U
Best verbal response		
Verbal questioning with maximum arousal	Appropriate orientation, conversant—correct identification of self, place, year, and month	5
	Confusion—conversant, but disorientation in 1 or more spheres	4
	Inappropriate or disorganized use of words (e.g., cursing), lack of sustained conversation	3
	Incomprehensible words, sounds (e.g., moaning)	2
	Lack of sound, even with painful stimuli	1
	Untestable[a]	U

GLASGOW COMA SCALE—cont'd

Appropriate stimulus	Response	Score
Best motor response		
Verbal command (e.g., "raise your arm," "hold up 2 fingers")	Obedience of command	6
Pain (pressure on proximal nail bed)	Localization of pain, lack of obedience but presence of attempts to remove offending stimulus	5
	Flexion withdrawal,[a] flexion of arm in response to pain without abnormal flexion posture	4
	Abnormal flexion, flexing of arm at elbow and pronation, making a fist	3
	Abnormal extension, extension of arm at elbow usually with adduction and internal rotation of arm at shoulder	2
	Lack of response	1
	Untestable[a]	U

[a]Added to the original scale by some centers.

HEART SOUNDS

Angle of Louis
2nd rib
Aortic area (base)
2nd ICS
MSL   MCL   AAL
Pulmonic area
Erb's point
Tricuspid area
Left ventricle
Epigastric area
Mitral area (apex) and PMI

H

HEART SOUNDS—cont'd

Sound	Auscultation site	Clinical occurrence
S_1 (M_1 T_1)	Apex	Closing of mitral and tricuspid valves; signals the beginning of systole
S_2 (A_2 P_2)	A_2 at second ICS, RSB; P_2 at second ICS, LSB	Closing of aortic and pulmonic valves; signals the beginning of diastole
S_2 physiologic split	Second ICS, LSB (pulmonic area)	A split sound. Due to a normal delay of pulmonic valve during inspiration; abnormal if heard during expiration or constantly during the respiratory cycle. Louder during exercise or in individuals with thin chest walls; more common in children/young adults
S_3 (ventricular gallop)	Apex	Extra heart sound heard in early diastole closely after S_2, similar to sound of a gallop. Low-intensity vibration of the ventricular wall associated with decreased compliance of the ventricles during filling. Common in children/young adults and during late pregnancy. Also in hypertension; left ventricular failure; volume overload; and mitral, aortic, or tricuspid regurgitation.
S_4 (atrial gallop)	Apex	Low-frequency vibration caused by atrial filling and contraction against increased resistance precedes S_1 of next cycle. May be normal in infants, children, and athletes. Pathologic in patients with left ventricular hypertrophy, aortic stenosis, hypertension, coronary artery disease.

HEART SOUNDS—cont'd

Sound	Auscultation site	Clinical occurrence
Murmurs	Apex Second ICS, LSB, or RSB	Turbulent blood flow across diseased heart valves. Graded on a 6-point Roman numeral scale of loudness and recorded as a ratio. The numerator is the intensity of the murmur, and the denominator is always VI, which indicates that the 6-point scale is being used. Grade I/VI indicates a murmur that is barely audible, heard only in a quiet room and then not easily; grade VI/VI indicates a murmur that can be heard with stethoscope lifted off chest wall.
Pericardial friction rubs	Usually heard best at the apex, with patient upright and leaning forward, and after expiration	High-pitched, scratchy sounds that may be transient or intermittent and may last several hours to days. Heard when inflamed surfaces of pericardium (pericarditis) move against each other.

ICS, Intercostal space; *LSB,* left sternal border; *RSB,* right sternal border.

H

INTRACRANIAL PRESSURE MONITORING

Intraventricular monitoring can be used to continuously measure intracranial pressure (ICP). The ICP tracing shows normal, elevated, and plateau waves. At high ICP, the P2 peak is higher than the P1 peak, and the peaks become less distinct and plateau.

LABORATORY VALUES

Test	Conventional units	SI units[a]
Complete blood count		
Red blood cells (RBCs)	*Male:* $4.7–6.1 \times 10^6/\mu L$ *Female:* $4.2–5.4 \times 10^6/\mu L$	*Male:* $4.7–6.1 \times 10^{12}/L$ *Female:* $4.2–5.4 \times 10^{12}/L$
White blood cells (WBCs)	$5000–10,000/mm^3$	$5.0–10.0 \times 10^9/L$
Hemoglobin (Hgb)	*Male:* 14–18 g/dL *Female:* 12–16 g/dL	*Male:* 140–180 g/L *Female:* 120–160 g/L
Hematocrit (Hct)	*Male:* 42%–52% *Female:* 37%–47%	*Male:* 0.42–0.52 *Female:* 0.37–0.47
Chemistry		
Alanine aminotransferase (ALT)	4–36 U/L	
Albumin	3.5–5 g/dL	35–50 g/L
Aspartate aminotransferase (AST)	0–35 U/L	0–0.58 µkat/L
Ammonia	10–80 mcg/dL	6–47 µmol/L
Amylase	60–120 Somogyi U/dL	30–220 U/L
Bicarbonate	21–28 mEq/L	21–28 mmol/L
Bilirubin		
• Total	0.3–1.0 mg/dL	5.1–17 µmol/L
• Direct	0.2–0.8 mg/dL	3.4–12.0 µmol/L
• Indirect	0.1–0.3 mg/dL	1.7–5.1 µmol/L
b-Type natriuretic peptide (BNP)	<100 pg/mL	<100 pmol/L
Calcium (total)	9.0–10.5 mg/dL	2.25–2.62 mmol/L
Calcium (ionized)	4.5–5.6 mg/dL	1.05–1.3 mmol/L
Cholesterol	<200 mg/dL	<5.2 mmol/L
• High-density lipoprotein (HDL)	*Male:* > 45 mg/dL *Female:* > 55 mg/dL	*Male:* > 0.75 mmol/L *Female:* > 0.91 mmol/L
• Low-density lipoprotein (LDL)	*Recommended:* < 130 mg/dL	

Continued

LABORATORY VALUES—cont'd

Test	Conventional units	SI units[a]
• Very low-density lipoproteins (VLDLs)	7–32 mg/dL	
Chloride	98–106 mEq/L	98–106 mmol/L
Creatinine	*Male*: 0.6–1.2 mg/dL *Female*: 0.5–1.1 mg/dL	*Male*: 53–106 µmol/L *Female*: 44–97 µmol
Glucose (fasting)	74–106 mg/dL	4.1–5.9 mmol/L
Hemoglobin, glycosylated (A1C)	4.0%–5.9%	4.0%–5.9%
Iron, total	*Male*: 80–180 mcg/dL *Female*: 60–160 mcg/dL	*Male*: 14–32 µmol/L *Female*: 11–29 µmol/L
Lactic dehydrogenase (LDH)	100–190 U/L	100–190 U/L
Lipase	0–160 U/L	
Magnesium	1.3–2.1 mEq/L	0.65–1.05 mmol/L
Osmolality	285–295 mOsm/kg	285–295 mmol/kg
Phosphorus (phosphate)	3.0–4.5 mg/dL	0.97–1.45 mmol/L
Phosphatase, alkaline	30–120 U/L	0.5–2.0 µkat/L
Potassium	3.5–5.0 mEq/L	3.5–5.0 mmol/L
Protein (total)	6.4–8.3 g/dL	64–83 g/L
Sodium	136–145 mEq/L	136–145 mmol/L
Triglyceride	*Male*: 40–160 mg/dL *Female*: 35–135 mg/dL	*Male*: 0.45–1.81 g/L *Female*: 0.40–1.52 g/L
Urea nitrogen (BUN)	10–20 mg/dL	3.6–7.1 mmol/L
Coagulation		
Activated partial thromboplastin time (aPTT)	30–40 s	30–40 s
Fibrin split (degradation) products, FSP	<10 mcg/mL	<10 mg/L
Platelets (thrombocytes)	150–400 × 10^3/µL	150–400 × 10^9/L
Prothrombin time (Protime, PT)	11–12.5 s	11–12.5 s

[a]*SI*, Système International (i.e., International System of Units).

LUNG VOLUMES AND CAPACITIES

Parameter	Definitions	Normal Value[a]
Volumes		
Expiratory reserve volume (ERV)	Additional air that can be forcefully exhaled after normal exhalation is complete	1.0 L
Inspiratory reserve volume (IRV)	Maximum volume of air that can be inhaled forcefully after normal inhalation	3.0 L
Residual volume (RV)	Amount of air remaining in the lungs after forced expiration. Air available in lungs for gas exchange between breaths	1.5 L
Tidal volume (V_T)	Volume of air inhaled and exhaled with each breath. Only a small proportion of total capacity of the lungs	0.5 L
Capacities		
Functional residual capacity (FRC)	Volume of air remaining in lungs at end of normal exhalation (FRC = ERV + RV). Increase or decrease possible with lung disease	2.5 L
Inspiratory capacity (IC)	Maximum volume of air that can be inhaled after normal expiration (IC = V_T + IRV)	3.5 L
Total lung capacity (TLC)	Maximum volume of air that lungs can contain (TLC = IRV + V_T + ERV + RV)	6.0 L
Vital capacity (VC)	Maximum volume of air that can be exhaled after maximum inspiration (VC = IRV + V_T + ERV). Higher VC for men (generally)	4.5 L

[a]Normal values vary with patient's height, weight, age, race, and gender.

MEDICATION ADMINISTRATIONS

Equivalent Weights and Measures.

Metric	Apothecary	Household
Weight		
1 kg	2.2 pounds	
1000 mg = 1 g	gr xv	
60 or 65 mg	gr i	
30 mg	gr ss (one-half)	
0.4 mg	1/150 gr	
1 mcg = 0.0001 mg		
Volume		
1000 mL = 1 L	Approx. 1 quart	Approx. 1 quart
1 L distilled water weighs	1 kg	
500 mL	Approx. 1 pint	16 ounces
240 or 250 mL	viii (8 ounces)	1 cup
30 mL	i (1 fluid ounce)	2 tablespoons
15 mL	iv (4 fluid drams)	1 tablespoon
4–5 mL	i (1 fluid dram)	1 teaspoon
1 mL	Minims xv or xvi	

Drug Calculations

Ratio and Proportion

1. To set up a ratio and proportion, put on the right-hand side what you already have, or what you already know (e.g., 1000 mg: 1 mL).
2. On the left-hand side put X, or what you want to know (e.g., 750 mg: X).
3. The equation should look like this:

$$750 \text{ mg} : X = 1000 \text{ mg} : 1 \text{ mL}$$

4. Multiply the two inside numbers. Multiply the two outside numbers.

$$1000 \text{ X} = 750$$

5. Solve for X:

$$X = \frac{750}{1000} = 0.75 \text{ mL}$$

IV Drip Rate

$$\frac{\text{Total number of milliliters to be infused}}{\text{Total number of minutes infusion}} \times \text{Drop factor} = \text{Rate (Drops per minute)}$$

Techniques of Administration
Angles of Injection

Injection Sites
Subcutaneous

Intramuscular: Ventrogluteal Muscle

Intramuscular: Dorsogluteal Muscle

Intramuscular: Deltoid Muscle

Intramuscular: Vastus Lateralis Muscle

Z-Track Technique

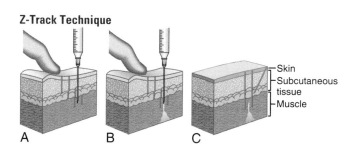

IV Site Complications.

	Infiltration	Phlebitis
Assessment		
Color	Pale	Red
Temperature	Cool to cold	Warm to hot
Swelling	Rounded	Cordlike vein path
Pain	Yes, usually	Yes
Flow	Slowed or stopped	No change or may be slowed
Nursing actions		
	Discontinue IV infusion	Discontinue IV infusion; usually call IV team
	Call IV team	
	Get order for warm compresses and elevate part	Note irritating solution. Warm compresses; elevate and immobilize part

M

TEMPERATURE EQUIVALENTS

°C	°F	°C	°F	°C	°F
34.0	93.2	37.2	99.0	40.2	104.4
34.2	93.6	37.4	99.3	40.4	104.7
34.4	93.9	37.6	99.7	40.6	105.2
34.6	94.3	37.8	100.0	40.8	105.4
34.8	94.6	38.0	100.4	41.0	105.9
35.0	95.0	38.2	100.8	41.2	106.1
35.2	95.4	38.4	101.1	41.4	106.5
35.4	95.7	38.6	101.5	41.6	106.8
35.6	96.1	38.8	101.8	41.8	107.2
35.8	96.4	39.0	102.2	42.0	107.6
36.0	96.8	39.2	102.6	42.2	108.0
36.2	97.2	39.4	102.9	42.4	108.3
36.4	97.5	39.6	103.3	42.6	108.7
36.6	97.9	39.8	103.6	42.8	109.0
36.8	98.2	40.0	104.0	43.0	109.4
37.0	98.6	—	—	—	—

°C, Celsius (centigrade) degrees; °F, Fahrenheit degrees.

Conversion Factors

To convert from °C to °F:

$$\left(°C \times \frac{9}{5} \right) + 32 = °F$$

To convert from °F to °C:

$$(°F - 32) \times \frac{5}{9} = °C$$

TNM CLASSIFICATION SYSTEM

Primary tumor (T)

T_0	No evidence of primary tumor
T_{is}	Carcinoma in situ
T_{1-4}	Ascending degrees of increase in tumor size and involvement
T_x	Tumor cannot be measured or found

Regional lymph nodes (N)

N_0	No evidence of disease in lymph nodes
N_{1-4}	Ascending degrees of nodal involvement
N_x	Regional lymph nodes unable to be assessed clinically

Distant metastases (M)

M_0	No evidence of distant metastases
M_{1-4}	Ascending degrees of metastatic involvement, including distant nodes
M_x	Cannot be determined

ENGLISH/SPANISH COMMON MEDICAL TERMS

Hints for Pronunciation of Spanish Words

- *h* is silent.
- *j* is pronounced as *h*.
- *ll* is pronounced as a *y* sound.
- *r* is pronounced with a trilled sound, and *rr* is trilled even more.
- *v* is pronounced with a *b* sound.
- A *y* by itself is pronounced with a long *e* sound.
- Accent marks over the vowel indicate the syllable that is to be stressed.

T

Common Words/Phrases for Clinical Situations

Introductory

I am _____.	Soy _____.
What is your name?	¿Cómo se llama usted?
I would like to examine you now.	Quisiera examinarlo(a) ahora.

General

How do you feel?	¿Cómo se siente?
Good	Bien
Bad	Mal
Do you feel better today?	¿Se siente mejor hoy?
Where do you work?	¿Dónde trabaja? (Cuál es su profesión o trabajo?) (¿Qué hace usted?)
Are you allergic to anything?	¿Es usted alérgico(a) a algo?
Medications, foods, insect bites?	¿Medicinas, alimentos, picaduras de insectos?
Do you take any medications?	¿Toma usted algunas medicinas?
Do you have any drug allergies?	¿Es usted alérgico(a) a algún médicamento?
Do you have a history of:	¿Ha sufrido antes:
Heart disease?	Del corazón?
Diabetes?	De diabetes?
Epilepsy?	De epilepsia?
Bronchitis?	De bronquitis?
Emphysema?	De enfisema?
Asthma?	De asma?

Pain

Have you any pain?	¿Tiene dolor?
Where is the pain?	¿Dónde le duele?
Do you have any pain here?	¿Le duele aquí?
How severe is the pain?	¿Qué tan fuerte es el dolor?
Mild, moderate, sharp, or severe?	¿Ligero, moderado, agudo, severo?
What were you doing when the pain started?	¿Qué estaba haciendo cuando comenzó el dolor?
Have you ever had this pain before?	¿Ha tenido este dolor antes?
Do you have a pain in your side?	¿Tiene usted dolor en el costado?
Is it worse now?	¿Es peor ahora?
Does it still pain you?	¿Le duele todavía?

Common Words/Phrases for Clinical Situations—cont'd

Did you feel much pain at the time?	¿Sintió mucho dolor entonces?
Show me where.	Muéstreme dónde.
Does it hurt when I press here?	¿Le duele cuando aprieto aquí?

Head

Head	La cabeza
Face	La cara
Eye	El ojo

Ears/Nose/Throat

Ears	Los oídos
Eardrum	El tímpano
Laryngitis	La laringitis
Lip	El labio
Mouth	La boca
Nose	La naríz
Tongue	La lengua

Cardiovascular

Heart	El corazón
Heart attack	El ataque del corazón
Heart disease	La enfermedad del corazón
Heart murmur	El soplo del corazón
High blood pressure	Presión alta

Respiratory

Chest	El pecho
Lungs	Los pulmones

Gastrointestinal

Abdomen	El abdomen
Intestines/bowels	Los intestinos
Liver	El hígado
Nausea	Náusea
Gastric ulcer	La úlcera gástrica
Stomach	El estómago, la panza, la barriga
Stomachache	El dolor de estómago

Continued

T

Common Words/Phrases for Clinical Situations—cont'd

Genitourinary

Genitals	Los genitales
Kidney	El riñón
Penis	El pene, el miembro
Urine	La orina

Musculoskeletal

Ankle	El tobillo
Arm	El brazo
Back	La espalda
Bones	Los huesos
Elbow	El codo
Finger	El dedo
Foot	El pie
Fracture	La fractura
Hand	La mano
Hip	La cadera
Knee	La rodilla
Leg	La pierna
Muscles	Los músculos
Rib	La costilla
Shoulder	El hombro
Thigh	El muslo

Neurologic

Brain	El cerebro
Dizziness	El vértigo, el mareo
Epilepsy	La epilepsia
Fainting spell	El desmayo
Unconsciousness	Pérdida del conocimiento (inconsciente, sin sentido)

Reproductive

Uterus	El útero, la matríz
Vagina	La vagina

URINALYSIS

Test	Normal	Abnormal finding	Possible etiology and significance
Color	Amber yellow	Dark, smoky color	Hematuria
		Yellow-brown to olive green	Excessive bilirubin
		Orange-red or orange-brown	Normal side effect of phenazopyridine
		Cloudiness of freshly voided urine	Urinary tract infection (UTI)
		Colorless urine	Excessive fluid intake, kidney disease, or diabetes insipidus
Odor	Aromatic	Ammonia-like odor	Urine allowed to stand
		Unpleasant odor	UTI
Protein	Random protein (dipstick): 0–Trace 0–8 mg/dL	Persistent proteinuria	Acute and chronic kidney disease, heart failure
	24-hr protein (quantitative): 50–80 mg/day		Heart failure, inflammatory process of urinary tract, nephritis, nephrosis, strenuous exercise
Glucose	None	Glycosuria	Diabetes mellitus, pituitary disorders

Continued

URINALYSIS—cont'd

Test	Normal	Abnormal finding	Possible etiology and significance
Ketones	None	Present	Diabetes mellitus, starvation, dehydration
Bilirubin	None	Present	Liver disorders
Specific gravity	1.005–1.030	Low	Diabetes insipidus
	Maximum concentrating ability of kidney in morning urine (1.025–1.030)	High	Dehydration, albuminuria, glycosuria
		Fixed at about 1.010	Renal inability to concentrate urine; end-stage kidney disease
Osmolality	50–1200 mOsm/kg (50–1200 mmol/kg)	<50 mOsm/kg (<50 mmol/kg)	Aldosteronism, diabetes insipidus, hypokalemia, pyelonephritis.
		>1200 mOsm/kg (>1200 mmol/kg)	Heart failure, liver disease, shock, SIADH.
pH	4.6–8.0	4.6–8.0	UTI, urine allowed to stand at room temperature. Respiratory or metabolic acidosis

hpf, High-power field; *SIADH,* syndrome of inappropriate antidiuretic hormone secretion.

INDEX

Note: Page numbers followed by *f* indicate figures and *t* indicate tables.